Synopsis of surgery

Synopsis of surgery

RICHARD D. LIECHTY, M.D.

Professor of Surgery, University
of Colorado Medical Center,
Denver, Colorado

ROBERT T. SOPER, M.D.

Professor of Surgery, Director,
Pediatric Surgical Services, University
of Iowa College of Medicine,
Iowa City, Iowa

with a Foreword by
Thomas E. Starzl, M.D.

Third edition
with 741 illustrations

The C. V. Mosby Company

Saint Louis   1976

Third edition

Copyright © 1976 by The C. V. Mosby Company

Previous editions copyrighted 1968, 1972

Printed in the United States of America

Distributed in Great Britain by Henry Kimpton, London

Library of Congress Cataloging in Publication Data

Liechty, Richard D
  Synopsis of surgery.

  Bibliography: p.
  Includes index.
  1. Surgery—Handbooks, Manuals, etc. I. Soper, Robert T., joint author. II. Title. [DNLM: 1. Surgery, Operative. W0500 L718s]
RD31.5.L5   1976   617   75-30917
ISBN 0-8016-3015-0

CB/CB/CB 9 8 7 6 5 4 3 2 1

Contributors

WILLIAM H. BAKER

Associate Professor of Surgery, University of Iowa
College of Medicine, Iowa City, Iowa

WILLIAM C. BOYD, M.D.

Assistant Professor of Surgery, University of Iowa
College of Medicine, Iowa City, Iowa

HERBERT J. BUCHSBAUM, M.D.

Professor of Obstetrics and Gynecology, Director, Oncology
Service, University of Iowa College of Medicine,
Iowa City, Iowa

CHARLES A. BUERK, M.D.

Assistant Professor of Surgery, University of Colorado
Medical Center, Denver, Colorado

F. K. CHAPLER, M.D.

Associate Professor of Obstetrics and Gynecology, University
of Iowa College of Medicine, Iowa City, Iowa

REGINALD R. COOPER, M.D.

Professor and Chairman, Department of Orthopaedics,
University of Iowa College of Medicine, Iowa City, Iowa

ROBERT J. CORRY, M.D.

Associate Professor of Surgery, Director, Transplantation
Service, University of Iowa College of Medicine, Iowa City, Iowa

LAWRENCE DEN BESTEN, M.D.

Professor and Vice Chairman, Department of Surgery,
University of Iowa College of Medicine; Chief,
Surgical Service, Iowa City Veterans Administration
Hospital, Iowa City, Iowa

DONALD B. DOTY, M.D.

Associate Professor of Division of Thoracic and
Cardiovascular Surgery, University of Iowa
College of Medicine, Iowa City, Iowa

ADRIAN E. FLATT, M.D., M.Chir., F.R.C.S.

Professor of Orthopaedic Surgery, Director, Division of
Hand Surgery, Department of Orthopaedic Surgery, University
of Iowa College of Medicine, Iowa City, Iowa

†RUBIN H. FLOCKS, M.D.

Professor of Urology, University of Iowa College
of Medicine, Iowa City, Iowa

JOEL B. FREEMAN, M.D., F.R.C.S.(C)

Assistant Professor of Surgery, University of Iowa
College of Medicine, Iowa City, Iowa

DAVID W. FURNAS, M.D., M.S., F.A.C.S., F.R.C.S.(C)

Professor and Chairman, Division of Plastic Surgery,
University of California, Irvine, Irvine, California

DARYL K. GRANNER, M.D.

Professor of Medicine and Biochemistry, Director, Division of
Endocrinology and Metabolism, University of
Iowa College of Medicine, Iowa City, Iowa

WILLIAM K. HAMILTON, M.D.

Professor and Chairman, Department of Anesthesia, University
of California, San Francisco, San Francisco, California

---

†Deceased.

CHARLES E. HARTFORD, M.D.

Associate Professor of Surgery, Director, Burn Unit,
University of Iowa College of Medicine,
University Hospitals, Iowa City, Iowa

A. CURTIS HASS, M.D.

Hall Radiation Center, Cedar Rapids, Iowa

JOHN C. HOAK, M.D.

Professor of Medicine, Director, Division of
Hematology-Oncology, University of Iowa College of Medicine,
Iowa City, Iowa

CHARLES J. KRAUSE, M.D., F.A.C.S.

Associate Professor of Otolaryngology
and Maxillofacial Surgery, University of Iowa
College of Medicine, Iowa City, Iowa

RICHARD L. LAWTON, M.D.

Professor of Surgery, University of Iowa
College of Medicine, Iowa City, Iowa

RICHARD D. LIECHTY, M.D.

Professor of Surgery, University of Colorado
Medical Center, Denver, Colorado

EDWARD E. MASON, M.D., Ph.D.

Professor of Surgery, University of Iowa
College of Medicine, Iowa City, Iowa

BRIAN F. McCABE, M.D.

Professor and Head, Department of Otolaryngology
and Maxillofacial Surgery, University of Iowa
College of Medicine, Iowa City, Iowa

ROBERT Y. McMURTRY, M.D., F.R.C.S.(C)

Consultant of Orthopaedic Surgery, Sunnybrook Medical
Center; Lecturer of Orthopaedics, University of Toronto,
Toronto, Ontario, Canada

HIRO NISHIOKA, M.D.
Assistant Clinical Professor of Neurosurgery, Medical
College of Wisconsin, Milwaukee, Wisconsin

**ISRAEL PENN, M.D., F.R.C.S. (England and Canada),
F.A.C.S.**
Associate Professor of Surgery, University of Colorado
Medical Center; Chief of Surgery, Veterans Administration
Hospital, Denver, Colorado

SAMUEL D. PORTER, M.D., F.A.C.S.
Clinical Assistant Professor of Surgery, University of Iowa
College of Medicine, Iowa City, Iowa

KENNETH J. PRINTEN, M.D., F.A.C.S.
Associate Professor of Surgery, University of Iowa
College of Medicine, Iowa City, Iowa

NICHOLAS P. ROSSI, M.D.
Professor of Division of Thoracic and Cardiovascular
Surgery, University of Iowa College of Medicine,
Iowa City, Iowa

JOSEPH D. SCHMIDT, M.D., F.A.C.S.
Professor of Urology, University of Iowa
College of Medicine, Iowa City, Iowa

SIROOS S. SHIRAZI, M.D., F.A.C.S.
Assistant Professor of Surgery, University of Iowa
College of Medicine, Iowa City, Iowa

ROBERT T. SOPER, M.D.
Professor of Surgery, Director, Pediatric Surgical Services,
University of Iowa College of Medicine, Iowa City, Iowa

SIDNEY E. ZIFFREN, M.D.
Professor and Head, Department of Surgery, University of
Iowa College of Medicine, Iowa City, Iowa

This book is dedicated to

Valerie and Hélène

Foreword

It is paradoxical that a field such as surgery, which has undergone an explosion of developments in the last three decades, should generate a textbook that has decreased in size. The need for such an abbreviated book was recognized by Liechty and Soper from the beginning, and the correctness of their views has been vindicated by the popularity among students of their *Synopsis of Surgery*, which is entering the third edition.

The main justification for any textbook is that it conveys the essence of a subject matter in an efficient and readable manner. *Synopsis of Surgery* meets this objective for the surgical tyro. The information given can be a base upon which the student may rest his or her case. Or it may provide a platform upon which is built specialized knowledge from more detailed texts or from journals.

This is a materialistic justification for another book. It is interesting that Liechty and Soper also see a more spiritual rationalization. They obviously hope that their work will aid professional development, but with some time left over for humanitarian pursuits, and that the union of interests will make for a more complete and compassionate physician. With this sensitivity to the needs of students, it is not surprising that both Liechty and Soper have been singled out to receive a number of student awards. Most recently, Dale Liechty was selected the Outstanding Faculty Member in the Clinical Departments of the University of Colorado during 1973-1974.

At its beginning in 1968, *Synopsis of Surgery* was almost completely the product of staff members of the University of Iowa. Although the

Iowa faculty still dominates the book, the effort has become more bi-institutional with Liechty's move to Colorado in 1972. Despite this change, a great advantage of the book has been retained, namely a short time lag of less than nine months between the submission of the material and publication. In larger texts with geographically separated and multiple co-authors, this period may extend to two or three years and assure obsolescence on the day of birth.

Thomas E. Starzl, M.D.

Professor and Chairman, Department of Surgery, University of Colorado Medical Center, Denver, Colorado

Preface

Some years ago an esteemed older colleague, with tongue in cheek, compared medical students to the ancient "covered vessels." His extended metaphor went somewhat as follows: As teachers, we receive them as freshmen, bright and eager, but nearly empty. We proceed over the next four years to stuff these vessels with innumerable facts, tamping down the contents in the final year, hoping that somehow the lids will fit back on. At the end of four years, if they can retrieve enough data from within to answer our questions, we award them degrees and our congratulations. But along the way, we discover an almost insurmountable problem: our stores of information could fill the interiors many times over, leaving virtually no room for other knowledge—from philosophy, literature, religion, or art—to filter in and enliven the drabness.

Recently at one of our universities, some medical students agonized over this same issue. Shocked by the suicide of a classmate, the class met to unload their feelings. The upshot of their discussion was this: although they were being trained to become healers of mankind, not one of them sensed their fellow student's despair. Their lament, echoing from all sides of the room, came straight on: medical schools dehumanize students. They meant, of course, that the overwhelming amount of information they were expected to master usurped their time, their energy, and, finally, even their sensitivities. Their plaints seemed to reflect a kind of arithmetic of futility: to a person, all stated their longing to enlarge their humanity, but none felt that he was allowed the time.

We, again, quote the editorial that appeared in our first two editions.

> In all probability, the present type of medical textbook will eventually disappear, to be succeeded by two quite different types. There will be the textbook carefully designed for a particular audience (the student, whether still in school or 15 years out of school). . . . Quite distinct will be the reference books which discuss specific topics in substantial detail. . . . Whoever tries to mix these two types is, at the present complex level of medicine, performing only a disservice. (JAMA 197:133, July 25, 1966)

The writer admonishes us, as teachers, to select carefully our material for a "particular audience." Although we have grudgingly watched this book expand, we nevertheless continue to write for a special audience, for the beginning student, whether a junior ward clerk (perhaps headed for a career in psychiatry) or a seasoned physician who needs only a brief updating in some surgical field unfamiliar to him.

From researcher to family practitioner, we all share the students' dilemma, enforced on us by the information explosion. As the time for teaching—and learning—traditional courses has shortened, the mass of scientific information has expanded even more. As teachers, we have no other choice, then, but to compress this knowledge into digestible portions.

Any author who attempts to select this core information runs the dual risk of omitting essentials or including trivia, but we accept these risks as our only option. Encouraged by many kind comments concerning our past editions, we believe that we have arrived at a reasonable balance, perhaps one that will allow the student some occasional extra moments—with a Kierkegaard, Dostoevsky, or Bach—to leaven his data-filled existence.

We welcome our new authors and thank all of our contributors for sharing their rich teaching experiences in *Synopsis of Surgery*. Especially, we appreciate their enthusiastic endorsement of our common philosophy: any successful curriculum depends upon a core of basic medical knowledge, designed for the beginning student.

Richard D. Liechty, M.D.

Robert T. Soper, M.D.

Contents

Synopsis of surgery

CHAPTER 1

Origin of surgical disease

RICHARD D. LIECHTY
ROBERT T. SOPER

Each day of the year our medical school libraries add the equivalent of three new *volumes* of medical literature to their already extensive collections. As in other scientific fields, the medical profession, and especially the medical student, face an "information crisis." The volume and scope of medical literature dramatically emphasize the diversity of specialization. But common bonds do exist across the specialty fields. Obstruction is still obstruction whether in the lacrimal duct, ureter, or spinal canal. We would like to begin by emphasizing some of these common concepts that link one specialty to another.

All somatic diseases, regardless of the specialty fields treating them, have their origins in the following six basic pathological processes:

1. Congenital defects
2. Inflammations
3. Neoplasms
4. Trauma
5. Metabolic defects and degeneration
6. Collagen defects

Four phenomena that result from these fundamental pathological processes are responsible for almost all surgical diseases and for many nonsurgical diseases as well. These phenomena are (1) obstruction, (2) perforation, (3) erosion, and (4) tumors (or masses).

OBSTRUCTION

Cerebrovascular disease (strokes) and coronary heart disease (coronaries) are two of the leading causes of death in the United States. Both result from obstruction of vital arteries carrying blood to the brain or to the heart muscle. Glaucoma, one of the two leading causes

Table 1-1. Diseases resulting from obstruction

System	Disease	Nature of obstruction
C.N.S.	Hydrocephalus	Congenital obstruction of C.S.F.
E.N.T.	Middle ear infection	Eustachian tube obstruction
Eye	Glaucoma	Obstruction of aqueous humor
Lung	Atelectasis	Mucous plug in bronchus
Biliary tract	Cholecystitis	Cystic duct stone
G.I.	Appendicitis	Fecalith, appendix
G.U.	Prostatism	Prostatic hypertrophy
Extremity	Intermittent claudication	Arteriosclerosis

Table 1-2. Examples of perforation

System	Disease	Nature of perforation
C.N.S.	Cerebral hemorrhage	Rupture of central nervous system artery
E.N.T.	Perforation of tympanic membrane	Infection with pressure
Lung	Spontaneous pneumothorax	Rupture of bleb
Biliary tract	Rupture of gallbladder	Obstruction, distension, necrosis
G.I.	Duodenal ulcer	Perforation of ulcer
G.U.	Ruptured bladder	Obstruction and distension
Vascular	Aortic aneurysm	Rupture of aneurysm

of blindness in our country, also results from obstruction, in this case obstruction to the outflow of fluid from the anterior chamber of the eye.

Free flow of blood, urine, cerebrospinal fluid, lymph, and other fluids, as well as air, is essential for health. Note in Table 1-1 the wide variety of diseases that result from obstruction.

PERFORATION

Perforation, similarly, is the direct cause of many surgical diseases. Perforation is often such an intensely dramatic event that few medical students will forget the "boardlike" abdomen of the patient with a ruptured peptic ulcer or the shock that overwhelms the patient with a ruptured aortic aneurysm. Examples are given in Table 1-2.

Table 1-3. Examples of erosion

System	Disease	Nature of erosion
C.N.S.	Meningitis	Erosion of abscess wall; mastoiditis
E.N.T.	Pharyngeal carcinoma	Bleeding; erosion into blood vessels
Lung	Tuberculosis	Bleeding; granulomatous erosion into blood vessels
G.I.	Duodenal ulcer	Bleeding; ulcer erosion into blood vessels
G.U.	Bladder stone	Bleeding; erosion of bladder wall
Extremity	Raynaud's phenomenon	Digital ulceration; ischemic erosion of skin

EROSION

Erosion is a "partial perforation," a slower process of ulceration (i.e., a break in the continuity of a tissue surface). Examples of erosion are given in Table 1-3.

TUMORS

The most subtle of these four phenomena is a tumor or a mass. This explains, in large measure, why cancer is so often detected only after it induces one of the previous three processes; e.g., we occasionally see tumors of the breast that have grown to astonishingly large size. Because no vital flow is obstructed and perforation or erosion of the skin occurs very late, symptoms and consequently diagnosis are delayed, often tragically.

These four phenomena, *obstruction, perforation, erosion,* and *tumors,* are the underlying direct causes of most surgical diseases. Like the theme of a symphonic work, they recur in many different forms. Sometimes they appear unmistakably loud and clear; at other times soft, muted, and elusive. The able physician will learn to recognize them. The core and the concern of this book are to aid the student in his recognition and understanding of these processes.

CHAPTER 2

Wounds, wound healing, and drains

DAVID W. FURNAS
RICHARD D. LIECHTY

Although the healing of wounds is a vital part of surgery, it also plays an important role in other medical fields. For example, the fibrous healing of myocardial infarcts often leads to life-threatening arrhythmias or ventricular aneurysms, and fibrous vegetations threaten embolization from rheumatic valvular disease. In posthepatitic patients, scar tissue infiltrates the liver and in some cases fatally encases the regenerating liver cells or produces portal venous hypertension. In these examples, fibrous tissue healing in its exuberant, sometimes misdirected, growth may eventually prove fatal. Wound healing, the surgeon's constant concern, is of more than casual interest to other physicians as well.

Healing by regeneration in man is limited to simple tissues, such as epithelium, and one compound organ, the liver. All other organs (skin, bowel, heart, brain) heal by merely sealing or patching of the wound. Paraplegia, for example, results from transection of the upper spinal cord. Scar tissue joins the severed cord ends, but blocks all nerve impulses; the distal neurons, separated from their cell nuclei, degenerate and die. Unfortunately man has, in his evolutionary past, virtually lost the ability to regenerate compound tissues. There remains, however, this remarkable process of sealing or patching that man depends on to survive his hostile environment.

Tissues heal by three main processes: *epithelization, fibrous tissue synthesis,* and the powerful force of *contraction.* Many surgical decisions depend on a clear knowledge of these extraordinary phenomena. When to remove sutures, where to make incisions, when to release a postoperative patient for normal activities, when to splint a wound, when to primarily close a wound, and when to leave it open are practical applications that the student should keep in mind as he studies the fundamental aspects of wound healing.

We first discuss the healing of *incised wounds, avulsed wounds,* and *contaminated wounds.* Pathological wound healing, wound complications, placement of incisions, suture materials, and wound drainage complete this chapter.

INCISED WOUNDS AND SUPERFICIAL WOUNDS

A simple *clean incised wound* heals by *primary intention* after accurate surgical closure *(primary closure).* Within the first few hours of injury the cut edges of the wound are coapted by a fibrinous coagulum, which serves as a scaffold for granulation tissue to form. During the first day leukocytes, mast cells, and macrophages enter the area to dispose of local debris and bacteria. The *epithelial cells* of the neighboring epidermis dedifferentiate, flatten out, multiply, migrate into and across the wound, and redifferentiate. Within 24 hours the epidermal surface is intact in an incised and sutured wound. This same sequence of fibrin deposition, granulation tissue, and epithelization serves to replace and heal the surface of broader wounds, such as second-degree burns or light abrasions, within a few days or weeks.

During the first few days that an incision is healing, the *inflammatory phase,* almost no tensile strength is gained. Meanwhile, *capillary buds* begin to sprout from the wound edges and differentiate into functioning networks, and *fibroblasts* migrate into the wound area, probably from nearby loose connective tissue. These fibroblasts form *collagen,* the material that knits the wounded dermis and deeper structures and gives strength to the wound. First the fibroblasts secrete *tropocollagen,* which aggregates into large *procollagen* fibers. These herald the *collagen phase,* the earliest evidence of tensile strength. Procollagen, through polymerization and cross linkages, becomes collagen, and from the fifth through the fifteenth days there is a rapid gain in tensile strength.

The young collagen fibers mature, link with one another, and orient along lines of stress. The wound reaches almost its full strength within 6 weeks. Although a slight gain continues over a number of months, the scar seldom, if ever, becomes stronger than the surrounding skin and fascia.

The *rate of healing* is accelerated by a rich blood supply and perhaps by warmth of the wounded part. Thus the face heals rapidly and sutures may be removed in a few days. In contrast, sutures must be left for 10 to 14 days in wounds of the lower leg because of its poorer blood supply.

As *wound maturity* progresses, the fibroblasts and capillaries greatly diminish in number, and the resultant scar is composed chiefly of collagen connective tissue, capped with epithelium. This progress is observed clinically as an initial red, raised, hard *immature scar* that molds into a flat, soft, and pale *mature scar* over a period of 3 to 12 months or more, as collagen molecules and cross links rearrange.

An *excised wound* or defect closes slower but in identical fashion, except that *contraction* of the wound edges plays the principal role. The edges of the defect advance into the defect probably from the action of contractile *myofibroblasts,* recently described cells now being investigated. *Wound contraction* is a consistent, powerful force that all experienced surgeons respect (Figs. 2-3 and 2-4).

"EXCISED" OR AVULSIVE WOUNDS

If a wound cannot be primarily closed, it must heal by *secondary intention* by means of the mechanisms of contraction and epithelization. Examples are wounds that are excessively contaminated, wounds

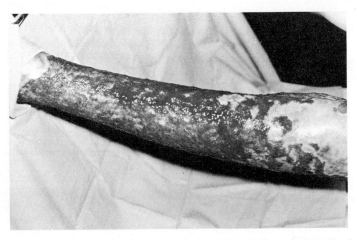

Fig. 2-1. Granulation tissue. Red, moist bed of fibroblasts and capillaries covering the surface of a leg that sustained full thickness burns 6 weeks before.

in which treatment has been delayed, or burns and wounds that involve necrosis of large skin surfaces. In a few days, the raw, exposed area becomes filled with *granulation tissue* ("proud flesh") (Fig. 2-1) composed of sprouting capillaries and fibroblasts. The wound edges creep toward each other by *contraction* and *epithelial migration*. If a mantle of necrotic skin clings to the surface of the defect, it is called an *eschar*. Formed of coagulated collagen and debris, it is much thicker and tougher than the scab of a superficial wound (Fig. 2-2). Tightly attached at first, it eventually separates from the underlying granulation tissue and falls away.

Healing is speeded by removing dead tissue, debris, and secretions by surgical excision (debridement) and by applying intermittent dressings moistened with antibacterial solutions to the wound. The capillarity of the dressings drains away bacterial exudate. Dead tissue adherent to the dressings is removed when the dressings are changed. There soon emerges a clean granulating surface that resists reinfection. Wound closure can be hastened by *secondary closure* (if the wound edges can be apposed) undertaken a few days after injury. Sutures are used to appose the wound edges, usually after first excising

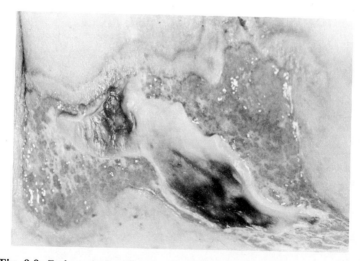

Fig. 2-2. Eschar. A deep burn coagulated the full thickness of the skin several weeks before. The eschar is in the process of separating from the underlying bed of granulation tissue. The copious exudate from local bacterial activity speeds the process.

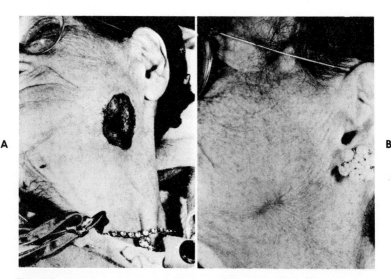

A

B

Fig. 2-3. Useful wound contraction. **A,** Wide removal of carcinoma of skin with electrocoagulation leaving an open 3 × 4 cm. defect. **B,** Defect several months later after spontaneous closure by contraction and epithelialization. (Courtesy Department of Dermatology, University of Iowa Hospitals.)

granulation tissue. Larger wounds are closed with split skin grafts. If the defect is *too* large, an unstable scar may result.

In many instances healing by *secondary intention* is convenient and desirable (Fig. 2-3). However, when the wound is located on the face or over a joint (where mobility of the part favors excessive displacement), contracture is likely and it results in diminished motion and sometimes grotesque deformity (Fig. 2-4). This is prevented by early closure of the wound with skin grafts or pedicles before contraction occurs. In addition, splints and physical therapy may help prevent skin grafts from contracting.

CONTAMINATED WOUNDS

Wounds received outside of the operating room are contaminated wounds. They may be *grossly clean* or *dirty, neat,* or *ragged* and contused.

A "golden period" of approximately *6 hours* was cited several

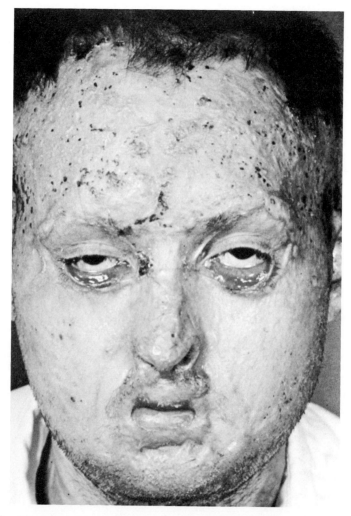

Fig. 2-4. Inimical wound contraction. Ectropion of eyelids and stenosis of mouth resulted from spontaneous closure of burn wounds of the face by contraction and epithelialization.

decades ago as the optimum time to close a contaminated wound, after which the wound should be left open to prevent infection. This concept should not be entirely ignored; but more important is the answer to the question: Can this *contaminated wound* be converted into a surgically *clean wound,* or is this a *contaminated wound* in which bacterial activity is already so advanced that it *cannot* be converted?

We now have antibiotics and more refined surgical techniques so that, with an *excellent blood supply, we can take liberties with the golden period.* A 2-day-old wound of the foot that shows no sign of infection can be closed with appropriate preparation (not simply "putting in stitches") with small risk of infection. A grossly clean, neat wrist laceration, 12 hours old, can be repaired safely. However, a 3-hour-old wound of the lower leg received from a dirty barnyard source should probably be left open.

A contaminated wound is always converted to a *surgically clean wound* prior to early closure, by the following steps:
1. Take culture; start antibiotics if wound large; tetanus prophylaxis
2. *Cleaning* of all foreign material and loose debris by use of syringes, scrub brushes, and curettes; avoid traumatic tattoos
3. *Hemostasis*
4. *Irrigation* with several liters of sterile solutions (saline, hydrogen peroxide, benzalkonium chloride) to dilute the number of bacteria remaining in the wound and to carry away microscopic debris
5. *Matching* the landmarks of the wound so that a tentative plan for debridement, shifting of tissues, and closure can be made
6. *Debridement,* i.e., scalpel excision of ragged wound edge, all dead or questionably viable tissue, and tissues that contain embedded foreign material
7. *Closure* with sutures, grafts, or pedicle, *or* if heavy contamination or missing tissue:
8. Dress frequently with moist antibiotic dressings and carry out delayed closure several days later *or* dress and await secondary healing

PATHOLOGICAL WOUND HEALING

At times an excessively hard, raised, red, itching, unsightly *hypertrophied scar* (Fig. 2-5) may result from excessive tension on the wound, unfavorable site, inaccurate wound closure, or unknown factors. Exuberant hypertrophied scars sometimes result from partial thickness burns in children (Fig. 2-6). Improvement usually occurs with time; surgical excision and revision of the scar may be necessary.

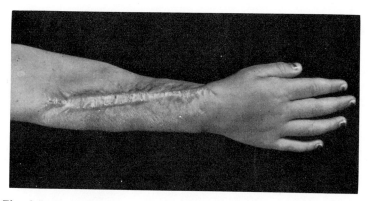

Fig. 2-5. Hypertrophied scar resulting from closure of forearm defect under tension.

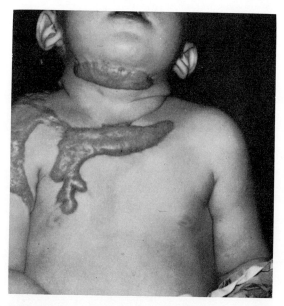

Fig. 2-6. Exuberant hypertrophied scar resulting from scalds (deep partial thickness burn).

The patient must understand that *scar "removal" can never eradicate scarring but can only minimize it.*

Occasionally a massive overgrowth of scar tissue invades the normal surrounding skin and creates unsightly, gnarled protuberances called *keloids* (Fig. 2-7). Keloids occur only in susceptible individuals, most often in pigmented races. They have great propensity for *recurrence* when excised.

If a granulating wound defect is too large, closure by the process of contraction will be unsuccessful and will leave an open expanse of granulation tissue. In time the capillaries and fibroblasts diminish, and the granulation tissue is gradually transformed into avascular scar tissue. Epithelial migration yields only a thin, fragile mantle over the scar. The result is an *unstable scar* that is prone to reinjury

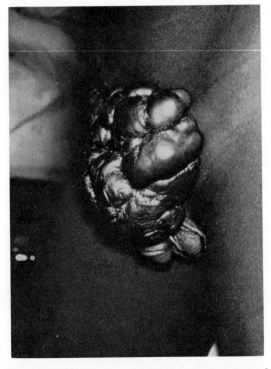

Fig. 2-7. Keloid in right inguinal hernioplasty wound.

and chronic ulceration. If recurring ulceration proceeds for several decades, metaplasia and finally squamous carcinoma *(Marjolin's ulcer)* may occur at the site of the injury. To prevent an unstable wound, the surgeon converts exposed granulation tissue into a closed wound by application of a split skin graft or pedicle.

WOUND COMPLICATIONS

Healing of wounds is retarded by the *protein deficiency* seen in severely depleted patients (particularly deficiency of the amino acid methionine), but healing is not greatly affected in patients who have moderate deficiencies. *Ascorbic acid deficiency* interferes with formation of collagen from collagen precursors, and the wounds develop little tensile strength. Because all collagen, and especially wound collagen, is continually being built up and destroyed, lack of vitamin C can cause a disruption in wounds that are years old. This explains the mystifying wound disruptions in scorbutic sailors, so well described in seafaring tales. Excessive *adrenocortical hormones* suppress fibroblastic activity. *Diabetes mellitus* sometimes engenders poor healing. *Infection, excessive motion, hematomas, seromas, edema, venous stasis, foreign material,* and *heavily traumatized tissue* in the wound area all impede satisfactory healing. *Reduced vascular supply* from any cause retards or prevents wound healing, e.g., *excessive tension* on the wound edges, *radiation changes, heavy scarring,* or *arteriosclerosis.*

Meticulous attention to nutrition, antisepsis, operative technique, hemostasis, and postoperative care will favor satisfactory wound healing.

PLACEMENT OF INCISIONS

Minimum scar formation and maximum camouflage are most likely to result when incisions are placed in the *wrinkle lines* of Kraissl and Conway (Fig. 2-8). These lines fall at right angles to the direction of pull of the underlying muscles. On the face they are most easily identified by having the patient grimace and perform exaggerated expressions. Elsewhere they are found by close inspection of the skin. Sometimes incisions may be hidden at or above the hairline, in the eyebrows, behind the ears, in the mouth, or along the areolar border of the nipple (Fig. 2-8, *A* and *B*). If an incision must cross the flexor surface of a joint, it is important that it curve or zigzag, nearly paralleling the transverse joint crease for part of its distance. Access to the flexor surface of the finger is made through the midlateral line or *neutral border* of the finger (Fig. 2-8, *C*). Straight longitudinal incisions across flexor surfaces of joints are notorious for the contractures they cause. On the abdomen, transverse (wrinkle line) incisions generally offer superior healing, although the need for

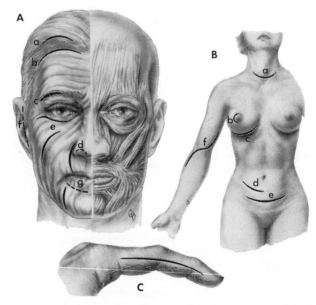

Fig. 2-8. A, Incisions camouflaged, *a,* in scalp, *b,* at scalp line, *c,* in eyebrow, *d,* in nostril, *e,* in wrinkle lines, *f,* in retroauricular area, and, *g,* inside mouth. **B,** Incisions camouflaged in, *a,* neck creases, *b,* areolar border, *c,* submammary fold, *d,* skin creases of abdomen, *e,* wrinkle line and pubic hair of abdomen, and, *f,* design of incision across the flexor surface of a joint to avoid contracture. **C,** Incision along neutral border of finger (where flexor skin creases meet extensor creases) to avoid contracture.

extensive exposure sometimes dictates vertical incisions. Because the main muscular pull is transverse, transverse incisions paralleling these tensions have less tendency to disrupt. Transverse incisions are preferable on the chest also. Vertical incisions on the sternal region are noted for their tendency to hypertrophy.

SUTURE MATERIALS

Catgut and *chromic catgut* are made from intestinal submucosa of sheep. They are *absorbed* by the tissues, an advantage in contaminated wounds. They cause more inflammatory reaction, i.e., they are more *reactive* than other suture materials, and they are not as easy to manipulate as sutures of natural fiber. *Polyglycollic acid sutures* and some other new polymers are also absorbed.

Natural-fiber sutures, silk, cotton, and linen, are *not absorbed,* are *much less reactive,* and have more tensile strength. They are the *easiest of all sutures to handle.* If buried in a contaminated wound, they act as a nidus for bacteria and tend to cause small draining sinuses that persist for many months until the sutures are finally expelled or removed.

Synthetic-fiber sutures, nylon, Dacron, polyester, polypropylene, etc., are *not absorbed.* They are *stronger* and *less reactive* than silk, with much less tendency to cause draining sinuses after closure of contaminated wounds, particularly if they are *mono*strand rather than *poly*strand. The monostrand sutures are *more difficult to handle* than natural-fiber sutures, but they have an advantage of minimum capillary action.

Wire sutures, stainless steel, silver, or tantalum, are *not absorbed,* have minimum capillarity and minimum reactivity, and are the *strongest* of sutures. They are *more difficult to handle* than the other materials and tend to cut through tissues.

WOUND DRAINAGE

Drains are placed in wounds only when *abnormal fluid collections* are present or expected. The purpose of drainage is to provide an exit for these fluids. Collections of body fluids can be harmful in the following ways:

1. Provide culture media for bacterial growth
2. Cause tissue irritation or necrosis, e.g., bile, pancreatic juice, pus, urine
3. Cause elevation of skin flaps with loss of vascularity and sloughing
4. Cause pressure on adjacent organs

In clean wounds, when no abnormal collection of fluids is expected, drainage is *unnecessary,* i.e., after a thyroidectomy or hernia repair. Bleeding should seldom, if ever, be used as an alibi for draining. Hemostasis should be attained at the time of operation. Blood clots may obstruct drains and entice the surgeon into a sense of security while bleeding proceeds in the wound.

Surgeons vary somewhat in their indications for drainage. Table 2-1 lists surgical procedures in which drains are commonly used.

Soft rubber or plastic drains are commonly used for wound drainage; when large amounts of drainage material are expected or when a "dry wound" is important, suction applied to hollow tube drains is effective.

Drains act as foreign bodies. Granulation tissue forms about them

Table 2-1. Surgical procedures commonly followed by drainage

Procedure	*Material to be drained*
Cholecystectomy	Bile from accessory bile ducts—from liver to gallbladder
Pancreatic resection	Pancreatic juice, from many tiny pancreatic ducts
Parotidectomy	Secretions from transected parotid gland
Thoracotomy	Air or serous fluid drained from intrapleural space; important to keep lung expanded
Splenectomy	Tail of pancreas is often very close to splenic hilum; drainage of pancreatic juice
Nephrectomy	Drainage of perinephric fat that is susceptible to infection
Incision and drainage of furuncles	Drain pus, allow wound to heal from bottom
Large flaps	Serum blood prevented from collecting with suction catheters

and walls them off rapidly. Thus the area in which drains are effective is soon limited by this "isolating effect" of healing tissue. Drains are usually removed slowly as the amount of drainage decreases over a period of days or rarely weeks.

T TUBES AND OTHER "FISTULA"-FORMING TUBES

Hollow drainage tubes are often used to form *fistulas* (hollow connections) from internal organs, either to drain a body fluid (bile) to the outside or to instill materials into body organs (feeding jejunostomy).

The short member of the T tube is placed in the common bile duct while the longer member leads outside the body, thus providing a bypass for the bile to the outside. It is also used to inject radiopaque dye for roentgen-ray studies of the bile ducts. Granulation tissue soon forms a fibrous wall about the T tube, walling it off from the remainder of the peritoneal cavity—the rubber tube is a foreign body. After 7 to 10 days a T tube can be removed with no fear of internal bile leak. However, if a T tube is pulled out within 48 hours of its insertion, a bile leak invariably occurs into the peritoneal cavity with consequent bile peritonitis. This same walling-off process occurs around *gastrostomy, jejunostomy, cecostomy, cystostomy,* and other tubes.

If these tubes become dislocated before the fibrous tract forms, extravasation will almost always result, often with serious or fatal consequences. Because of their important function, these tubes are stitched securely to the skin and should seldom be removed before 7 days after insertion.

Urinary catheters, nasogastric tubes, and rectal tubes pass through natural orifices that are lined by epithelium, and therefore can be removed at any time with no heed to this important principle of fibrous sealing-off of the tube. *Thoracotomy tubes* are discussed in Chapter 30.

CHAPTER 3

Fluids and electrolytes

EDWARD E. MASON

The subject of fluids and electrolytes is sometimes neglected because of both its simplicity and its potential complexity. Probably 95% of surgical patients require only short-term, routine replacement of fluids. When patients resume oral intake, they regulate themselves. Furthermore, with short-term intravenous therapy, patients can withstand gross insults. Normal kidneys, by excreting excess fluids, readily compensate for most fluid overloads, and when fluid replacement is inadequate, the kidneys conserve fluids.

This chapter is dedicated to the presentation of a simple scheme for rational analysis of the daily fluid requirements for all patients whether the problem is simple or complex, but especially to the recognition, understanding, and logical analysis of requirements for the occasional difficult patient whose kidneys are not functioning well and whose life may depend on this portion of the treatment.

Three major questions must be answered in order to provide optimum parenteral fluids:

1. What metabolic fluids (urine and insensible loss) are needed?
2. What abnormal body fluids (vomiting, diarrhea) currently being lost must be replaced?
3. What fluids are needed to correct accumulated fluid and electrolyte imbalances?

The first two questions are commonplace. Serious, neglected illnesses and injudicious fluid therapy underlie the last question.

A clear comprehension of this chapter is best attained by an initial rapid reading, followed by methodical study with concentration on those areas each student finds most difficult.

COLLECTION OF INFORMATION

What information is required to answer these questions about a particular patient, and how is it obtained? Four major sources are used: (1) history (including accurately maintained records of intake and output), (2) physical examination, (3) laboratory analyses, and (4) diagnosis ex juvantibus (the response to treatment).

History

If the patient is seen by a physician for the first time, only an estimate may be available for the amounts of *fluid loss* such as vomitus, liquid stools, and urine. Similar rough estimates should be made for *fluid intake* in terms of containers familiar to the patient and relatives.

For the hospitalized patient with intake and output recorded, a table should be made of all the solutions that have been given to the patient, starting from the time the patient was last thought to be in balance. The total amounts of the following should be determined: (1) electrolyte solutions given, (2) urine excreted, and (3) the electrolyte-containing fluids lost from the body by gastric suction or other routes. An estimate must also be made of the insensible loss by evaporation from skin and lungs. In the average adult at normal temperatures and humidity, this loss will total about 800 ml. per day.

Physical examination

During the physical examination an estimate should be made of the amount of subcutaneous extracellular fluid present. This requires an awareness of the effect of varying amounts of subcutaneous fat and elastic tissue upon skin turgor. Skin turgor can be evaluated by pinching the skin into a fold and observing the rate of return to normal. In the very obese patient, severe dehydration may be masked by fatty turgor of the skin. In the elderly and often poorly nourished patient with little fat and elastic tissue, poor skin turgor often suggests dehydration even though the extracellular fluid volume is normal. In a young, lean, acutely ill adult, severe deficiency of extracellular fluid is marked by skin that can be pinched up into a fold and remains in that position for several seconds.

Overexpansion of extracellular fluid is sometimes difficult to determine until the patient develops dependent edema along the back or buttocks or, if the patient has been in a standing or sitting position, pitting edema of the ankles. Sometimes, even though definite edema cannot be found, the jellylike movement of the tissues upon percussion will suggest that the subcutaneous tissues are waterlogged. *Changes* in the findings are often much more helpful than the static findings at any single examination. These changes in *extracellular fluid* (skin turgor, edema, and ascites) are easier to detect than changes in total body water. *Rapid* changes in total body water, either overhydration or dehydration, do lead to mental confusion, coma, and convulsions (which may mimic the signs and symptoms of a poorly localized cerebrovascular accident). However, total body water abnormalities, in contrast to extracellular fluid changes, produce no detectable changes in skin turgor.

Physical examination not only reveals signs of gross abnormalities of total body water and extracellular fluid volumes but also may provide clues to abnormal *chemical composition* of body fluids. A patient with suspected potassium deficiency will often have weakness of his muscles and distension of the bowel with poor bowel sounds. A high serum potassium may cause rhythm disturbances of the heart as the potassium approaches a lethal level of 8 to 10 mEq./L. High serum calcium levels cause mental confusion, nausea and vomiting, and profound weakness. Low calcium levels are accompanied by muscle spasm and neuromuscular irritability, so that tapping over the facial nerve causes contraction of the facial muscles (Chvostek's sign).

Central nervous system disease, such as encephalitis and cirrhosis, often results in comatose states. The consequent rapid ventilation causes "blowing off" of carbon dioxide, which results in *respiratory alkalosis*. This causes a decrease in ionized calcium and may be accompanied by the signs of calcium deficiency. Patients with metabolic acidosis breathe rapidly and deeply in an effort to blow off sufficient carbon dioxide to lower carbonic acid levels and, by virtue of this respiratory alkalosis, to compensate for the *metabolic acidosis*. The physician who is familiar with the patient's basic underlying disease is in an excellent position to recognize various physical signs of abnormal fluid and electrolyte balance. Reexamination of the patient is important. Changes in physical findings not initially evident are often recognized during repeated examinations. Changes in body weight, skin turgor, alertness, and breathing rate *during treatment* also contribute to the evaluation.

ANALYSIS OF DATA
Estimation of body fluid volumes in health

The average healthy adult male who is well nourished, but with a minimum of fat (fat contains almost no free water), has about 60% of his body weight made up of fluid components. Women have more fat than men. By finding out what an obese patient weighed before becoming obese (or, if necessary, by simply estimating what the patient should weigh after a satisfactory regimen of weight reduction), one can arrive at a rough idea of the patient's expected normal lean (nonfat) body mass. From *lean body mass,* estimates of the volume of fluids in the body compartments can be calculated easily.

The lean body weight is converted from pounds into kilograms by using the factor 2.2 pounds per kilogram. The patient's extracellular fluid volume is estimated by multiplying the lean body mass by 20%. This leaves, therefore, 40% of the lean body mass as intracellular fluid; 15% of the lean body mass is fluid between the cells, or interstitial fluid, and 5% is fluid in the circulating blood volume exclusive of the blood cells. A 70 kg. lean man should therefore possess about 3.5 liters (L.) of plasma; 7% to 8% of the lean body mass is the usual estimate of normal blood volume (plasma + cells).

VOLUME, TONICITY, AND BODY SOLUTES

Every solution has a characteristic solute curve, illustrated by Fig. 3-1, where the horizontal axis is the *volume,* the vertical axis is *con-*

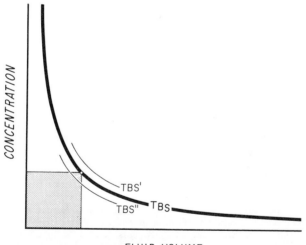

FLUID VOLUME

Fig. 3-1. Concentration-volume relationship. Concentration of electrolytes on vertical axis against fluid volume on horizontal axis. Because total body solutes (**TBS**) is a fixed amount of solutes, any point on the curving line equals any other point. Since concentration × volume = TBS, then if volume increases, concentration must decrease; if volume decreases, concentration must increase. **TBS'**, Increase in solutes (electrolyte overinfusion). **TBS''**, Decrease in solutes (from vomiting and diarrhea).

centration, and the curving line represents a given amount of *solute.* Since the amount of solute is fixed, any volume increase causes a reciprocal decrease in concentration. Similarly, with decreasing volume the concentration rises.

The equation *Volume × Concentration = Total body solute* depicts this relationship mathematically. The body solutions share this same relationship, but obviously life depends on these three variables remaining within a limited, physiological range.

Body solutions differ from simple, in vitro solutions because the body has two distinct fluid compartments (cellular and extracellular). Cells separate the body solutes by pumping sodium out and allowing potassium to replace the displaced sodium. But the concentration of solute in the cellular compartment *always equals* the concentration of

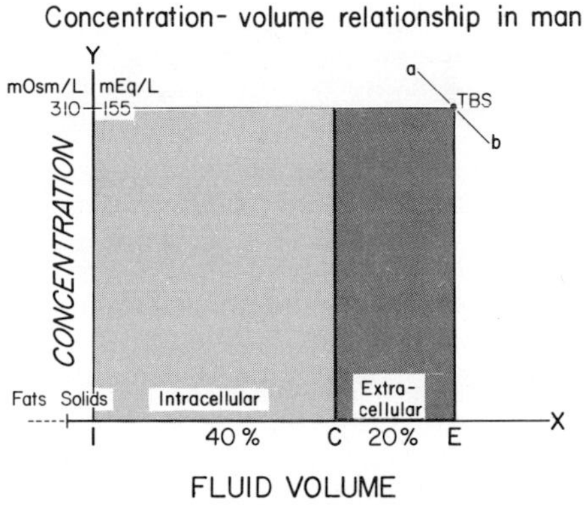

Concentration- volume relationship in man

Fig. 3-2. Concentration of electrolytes on vertical axis against fluid volume on horizontal axis. Distribution of body fluids into, **I,** intracellular (40%) and, **E,** extracellular compartments (20%). Remaining 40% of body weight is composed of solids and normally distributed fat. Total body solutes, **TBS,** are depicted by a curving line, **a-b,** which is a *mathematical constant.* (Concentration × volume = total solutes in *any* solution.) This line naturally falls at the intersection of volume and concentration. This diagram depicts the mathematical relationship of these three important variables (concentration × volume = total solutes) in body fluids. When one changes, another *must* also change. A clear understanding of these diagrams in health and in the disease states that follow is as fundamental to understanding fluid and electrolyte problems as are the multiplication tables to understanding mathematics.

solute in the extracellular compartment. This is the *law of osmotic equilibrium*. The concentration of intracellular cations (chiefly potassium) always equals the concentration of extracellular cations (chiefly sodium). Water diffusing freely between the two body compartments maintains this osmotic equality. Fig. 3-2 shows the concentration–volume–total solute relationship as it applies to man.

Although we depend on extracellular fluid (serum) samples for concentration measurements, we know they reflect intracellular concentrations as well. Despite the dual fluid compartments and the physiological segregation of cations in the body, the *Concentration* × *Volume* = *Total body solute* relationship is equally valid in living organisms as in the test tube.

Sodium concentration, the dominant extracellular cation, holds the key to body tonicity and volume. Since sodium represents 92% of all extracellular cations, we can use it as if it were the only cation. The body zealously guards sodium concentration between 136 and 145 mEq./L. in a healthy man. Despite wide individual variations in the intake of salt and water, control of thirst and antiduretic hormone stabilizes sodium concentration within this narrow range.

Sodium concentration is a measure of *tonicity* of body fluids: sodium concentrations below 136 mEq./L. denote *hypotonicity;* concentrations above 145 mEq./L. indicate *hypertonicity*.

We can estimate acute body volume changes by determining weight changes, skin turgor, pulse rate, dryness of tongue, hematocrit, hemoglobin* etc. We can also accurately determine body tonicity (sodium concentration) in the laboratory. With the aid of these two measurements and clear understanding of the volume–concentration–total solute relationship, we can diagnose and treat most body fluid abnormalities. The six chief abnormalities are total body water loss,

---

*Red blood cells and concentration defects: Another concentration measurement helpful in the diagnosis of extracellular fluid deficit is the concentration of the red blood cells. Plasma is part of the extracellular fluid. Plasma volume contracts along with the interstitial fluid volume. The result is an increase in the hemoglobin concentration and hematocrit. Often a hemoglobin or hematocrit has not been determined before the patient loses extracellular fluid. An estimate can still be helpful, however, if the patient has not had signs or symptoms of anemia or polycythemia. Under such circumstances a hematocrit of 60 or above or a hemoglobin of 19 Gm.% allows a strong presumption that contraction of the extracellular fluid volume has occurred. The single measurement is interpreted as *a change in concentration due to a change in compartment volume*.

total body water gain, extracellular fluid loss, extracellular fluid gain, pure salt deficit, and malnutrition. We will discuss and illustrate these abnormalities in terms of the volume–concentration–total body solute diagrams.

BODY FLUID ABNORMALITIES
Total body water loss

An estimate is made of the total body water deficit incurred, by lack of oral intake and the duration of desiccation from loss of urine and continued evaporation from skin and lungs. This number of liters of water is subtracted in the diagram by moving the line *E* appropriately closer to *I;* e.g., if a 70 kg. man has been unable to drink for 2½ days and during this time has continued to evaporate water, he has an estimated loss of 2 L. Also, if during this time he has excreted 1 L. of urine, his total body water deficit would amount to 3 L. (approximately 7% of his lean body weight). This is depicted by a 7% decrease in the distance between *I* and *E*. (See Fig. 3-3.)

The cells also participate in this loss depicted by a 7% decrease in the distance between *I* and *C.* Any change in total body water is a change both in the *cellular volume* and in the *extracellular fluid volume.* Water moves freely across the cell membranes, equalizing

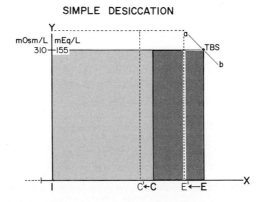

Fig. 3-3. In simple desiccation, volume decreases, concentration increases, and total body solutes (the product of volume × concentration) remain the same. Remember, the curving line, **a-b,** is a constant. (Any point on this line equals any other point.) Both extracellular and intracellular compartments share in water loss.

the osmotic pressure *outside* the cell and *inside* the cell. Since no solutes are lost, the concentration rises.

Total body water gain

If the patient has a retention of water without any change in total body salt, concentration of salt decreases; e.g., if the retention is 4 L. in a 70 kg. man (total body water is about 42 L.), this is a 10% increase in total body water, and the concentration of solutes (as depicted by sodium) can be expected to decrease by 10% (Fig. 3-4). This means that the sodium should now be 129 mEq./L. instead of 143.

Extracellular fluid loss

The extracellular fluid volume is altered when the patient loses electrolyte-containing fluids as in vomiting and diarrhea or after a severe burn. In major trauma (as after prolonged and extensive operations and after major hemorrhage), a decrease in extracellular fluid occurs. An effort should be made to estimate the actual number of liters of electrolyte-containing fluid lost—this is depicted by moving the line *E* to the left, but with no change in the intracellular fluid volume *IC* (Fig. 3-5). Sometimes the diagnosis of extracellular fluid

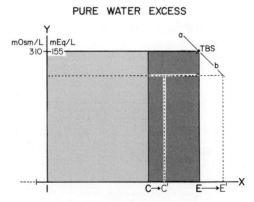

Fig. 3-4. In pure water excess (usually renal failure), fluid volume increases and concentration decreases. Total body solutes remain the same. Note that this excess water is distributed throughout the total body water.

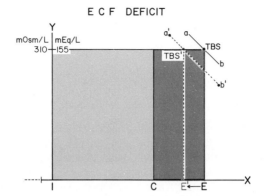

Fig. 3-5. Extracellular fluid deficit. Because body solutes are *lost* from the body (vomiting, diarrhea, burns), **TBS** changes to **TBS'** (the new constant is an identical curving line **a'-b'**). Note that concentration stays the same but volume of extracellular fluid decreases.

deficit can be made, but the historical data necessary for quantitation are deficient. The degree of ECF contraction must be estimated from physical findings plus response to treatment. A loss of one-fourth to one-third of the extracellular fluid volume is sufficient to cause signs of circulatory disturbance such as a lowered blood pressure, especially with the patient in a sitting position. Urinary output is low. A patient who has vomiting and diarrhea and who has very poor skin turgor may therefore need as much as 3 to 4 L. expansion of extracellular fluid before he begins to look well, to resume normal renal function, and to have a normal blood pressure and normal peripheral circulation.

Extracellular fluid gain

Patients with heart failure or with cirrhosis and increased aldosterone, or patients with decreased renal function who are given too much sodium-containing fluid, may develop edema, ascites, or pleural fluid. This retention can be estimated by knowing the increase in *total body weight*, and it should be depicted in the diagram as an increase in extracellular fluid volume *EC*. Congestive heart failure and overtransfusion of blood and salt solutions are two common examples.

Pure salt deficit

The patient who loses extracellular fluid (containing electrolytes) and receives nonelectrolyte fluid may have a normal body weight and

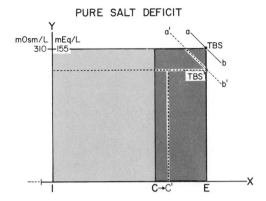

Fig. 3-6. Vomiting or diarrhea followed by drinking water is a common cause of pure salt deficit. Volume stays the same; concentration decreases. Again, since body solutes have been lost, the position of **TBS** changes to **TBS″**. The excess water distributes evenly between the intracellular and the extracellular compartments. The overall effect is a shrinking of the extracellular compartment. The hematocrit reflects this shrinkage by rising. Intracellular fluid volume is increased.

a normal total body water volume, but a *decrease* in total body solute. This is depicted in Fig. 3-6 by TBS″. With simple loss of extracellular fluid (Fig. 3-5), the position of the cell membrane, C, does not change. However, in pure salt deficiency (with vomiting of electrolyte solution and replacement with water), an internal shift to C' (water goes into cells) occurs. Even though the patient's body weight is normal, the concentration of sodium is low and the hematocrit and hemoglobin are elevated. This paradoxical decrease in sodium concentration and rise in hematocrit and hemoglobin concentration strongly suggest a pure salt deficit. The white blood count is usually markedly elevated. This may suggest infection, but the body temperature is usually below normal and when the salt is replaced, the white count falls toward normal along with the hematocrit.

Total body water excess versus pure salt deficiency

Sometimes the information from history and physical findings is insufficient to make a complete diagnosis in a patient with a *low* concentration of serum sodium, and the differential diagnosis must be made between total body water excess and pure salt deficiency. Examination of Figs. 3-4 and 3-6 reveals how this diagnosis can be settled. The lowered concentration of serum sodium indicates that if

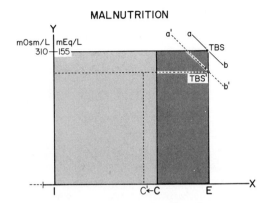

Fig. 3-7. The chronically malnourished patient has a low concentration of serum sodium but the total body sodium is increased. The deficit in body solute is in exchangeable potassium. There is movement of sodium into cells as well as expansion of extracellular fluid and total body water. Plasma volume is actually above normal and hematocrit is reduced. The history and physical findings should distinguish this condition from pure water excess. The low hematocrit distinguishes malnutrition from pure salt deficiency.

total body solute is normal (a simple total body water excess), extracellular fluid volume is increased (*E'* would now be opposite *b*). With the increase in extracellular fluid volume, intracellular fluid volume (including red blood cells) would be equally increased. The hematocrit would be normal. In contrast to this, if the problem is one of loss of electrolyte solution and replacement with nonelectrolyte solution (a pure salt deficiency), total body water and body weight are unchanged. There is, however, an internal shift of fluids into the cells depicted by an increase in *IC* and a decrease in *EC*, with *C'* the position of the cell membranes. Since the extracellular fluid volume is contracted, the hematocrit will be high. The rise in hematocrit with pure salt deficit distinguishes it from total body water excess in which the hematocrit is unchanged.

There is still another possibility for explaining a low concentration of serum sodium—protein malnutrition. Under such circumstances serum albumin is decreased and plasma volume tends therefore to be inadequate. Retention of sodium occurs and water retention also occurs to the extent that an effective plasma volume is established by increase in extracellular fluid and total body water. A simplified sum-

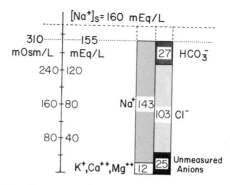

Fig. 3-8. Total anions must always equal total cations. Dilution or concentration of the body electrolytes will affect both sides of the Gamble diagram so that the change in anion concentration is proportional to the change in cation (sodium) concentration.

mary of these changes is shown in Fig. 3-7. Because of the decrease in cellular tissue and potassium, total body solate is decreased.

Assessing laboratory data

Two concepts must be mastered regarding the interpretation of serum sodium concentration. These are the rules of (1) *osmotic equilibrium,* which we have already discussed, and (2) *electrical neutrality.* The second rule states that *total anions must equal total cations* in an electrolyte solution. It implies that any change in concentration of sodium must be accompanied by an equal change in anions.

Once the use of sodium concentration as an index of tonicity of body fluids and the rule of electrical neutrality are accepted, the clinician may evaluate the accuracy of a set of laboratory data (Fig. 3-8). The internal consistency of a set of laboratory data should be carefully scrutinized. If the concentration of chloride plus CO_2 (as bicarbonate) approaches or exceeds the value given for sodium, obviously a laboratory error involves at least one of these ions. All three of the determinations must be repeated.

If the concentration of sodium is excessively high in comparison to the concentration of CO_2 plus chloride, this may be a laboratory error, but it may also indicate an abnormal accumulation of unmeasured anions as occurs in uremia, ketosis, severe infection, and circulatory insufficiency. If the patient has no disease or condition that would

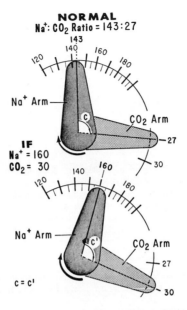

Fig. 3-9. Arms of the circular slide rule are set as the normal ratio of CO_2 to sodium. The arms with this fixed ratio are then moved to the observed sodium, and the expected CO_2 is read. The expected chloride for any observed sodium is determined in the same fashion.

cause an elevation of unmeasured anions, laboratory error should be suspected. In good laboratories 10% of the sets of data may contain internal inconsistencies that demand a repeat analysis.

Bedside proportions and a circular pocket slide rule

A small circular slide rule is helpful (Fig. 3-9) for these proportions and for other calculations at the bedside. The ratio of normal concentration of chloride to sodium can be established (143 to 103), and then with this ratio maintained as a fixed angle, the sodium arm can be moved to the observed, abnormal value of, shall we say, 160. For such a patient, with a relative deficiency in total body water (Figs. 3-3 and 3-9), the expected chloride should be 115. Changes in concentration of major anions should be proportional to changes in concentration of sodium unless an associated disturbance of electrolyte *composition* of the extracellular fluid exists.

The normal ratio of CO_2 content to sodium concentration is 27 to 143. This ratio (or fixed angle) is established on the arms of the slide rule (Fig. 3-9). As the sodium arm is moved over to 160, it is observed that the normal CO_2 content for the patient becomes 30. In this way, the rule of electrical neutrality allows determination of the internal consistency of a set of data as well as determination of whether an observed chloride or CO_2 concentration is simply altered by virtue of the change in *total body water* or whether it is altered by a true change in the *composition* of the electrolytes in extracellular fluid.

A reciprocal relationship is also seen between CO_2 content (HCO_3 in Fig. 3-8) and chloride. A compositional change in which the concentration of one of the anions increases markedly cannot exist without a decrease in another of the anions, e.g., when a patient with a peptic ulcer vomits acid gastric juice containing high concentrations of chloride, the remaining fluid in the body has a deficit of chloride (hypochloremia). This is a deficit of chloride in the entire extracellular fluid. The bicarbonate anion will be above normal. When the CO_2 content (bicarbonate) is normal or decreased and the chloride is markedly decreased, some cause for elevation of the *unmeasured anions*, such as phosphate, ketone bodies, or organic acids, must be sought. One of the more common causes of this is renal insufficiency; the blood urea nitrogen and creatinine will be elevated.

The other ions exist in such low concentrations that they do not participate in the reciprocity with total body water, nor are they influenced in a significant way by considerations of electrical neutrality. One trace cation is normally present in a concentration of 40 nM/L. This is the hydrogen ion, and in so-called *metabolic* disturbances of acid-base balance (diabetic acidosis, uremia) the serum CO_2 content in mEq./L. may permit a very good estimate of the severity of hydrogen ion increase (acidosis) or decrease (alkalosis). If the patient has been vomiting, the resultant hypochloremia and an increase in the bicarbonate (or CO_2) content indicate a *hypochloremic alkalosis*. In situations in which chloride and/or other anions are increased in concentration and bicarbonate is decreased, a diagnosis of *metabolic acidosis* is made. Whether this is a primary metabolic acidosis or is compensatory to respiratory alkalosis is a question that is discussed in the section on acid-base balance (p. 36).

WRITING THE PRESCRIPTION

The physician at the bedside who understands the concentration volume relationships *and* the clinical status of his patient is well prepared to order replacement fluids. In order that nothing be left out of this order, he should consider THREE ITEMS: *metabolic fluid losses, current abnormal fluid losses, and accumulated imbalances.*

Replacing urine and insensible fluid loss

First the patient needs metabolic fluids for urine and insensible loss. This fluid is relatively low in electrolyte concentration and can be supplied by the use of 5% glucose. The average patient will produce about 1,000 ml. of urine in 24 hours and will require some 800 ml. of the same fluid for replacement of insensible loss from skin and lungs. This does *not* include sweat, which should be considered as an abnormal fluid and would require some replacement with salt. This may approach 2,000 or 3,000 ml. in hot weather or with fever. Accurate body weights are essential when losses occur that cannot be measured. They are indicated in all patients receiving intravenous fluids.

Replacing abnormal fluid losses

The second type of fluid required depends on abnormal losses. Usually the orders are written on morning rounds. At this time about 8 hours of the day have passed, and it is a simple calculation to determine the amount of juice in the gastric suction or drainage from other parts of the gastrointestinal tract and simply to multiply the amount of fluid by 3 to estimate total 24-hour requirements. If the patient has no abnormal fluid losses, this item can be ignored. If the fluid being lost is acid gastric juice, as determined by a quick bedside determination with pH-sensitive paper, replacement should be with 0.9% saline. If the intestinal juices are quite alkaline, as is the case with a fresh ileostomy or leakage from a duodenal fistula, replacement should be with saline and one-sixth molar sodium lactate in the ratio of 2 parts and 1 part. If the patient is losing extracellular-like fluid with a normal body fluid pH, e.g., the removal of a large volume of pleural or peritoneal fluid, this should be replaced with a fluid that has the composition of normal extracellular fluid. This can be approximated by using isotonic saline and one-sixth molar sodium lactate in the proportions of 4:1, which is the ratio of the major anions in extracellular fluid—chloride and bicarbonate, 103 and 27.

Restoring normal balance

The third and most complex item to be considered is the portion of the prescription that will return the patient to normal fluid and electrolyte balance if he is out of balance. The concentration volume diagram is of great help in situations of imbalance. A few examples of the various abnormalities just discussed are given in the following paragraphs:

1. If the patient is deficient in *total body water* as is evidenced by a 10% increase in sodium concentration (and weight loss of 8 pounds), he will require a 10% increase in total body water, which can be supplied as 5% glucose. This means that to change a sodium concentration from 158 to 143 in a lean 70 kg. man, it would be necessary to provide 4 L. of 5% glucose. Remember, this is *in addition to* the fluids required for metabolic purposes (urine and insensible loss) and replacement of current abnormal losses.

2. If the patient has a *deficit* of *extracellular fluid* estimated to be approximately one-fourth of his normal expected extracellular volume, this can be replaced with lactated Ringer's solution or with a mixture of saline and M/6 sodium lactate in the proportions of 4 and 1. For the hypothetic 70 kg. lean man, this would require 20% of 70, which is 14 L. times a one-fourth deficit, or 3.5 L. of extracellular fluid replacement.

3. For the patient who has a *pure salt deficiency* and a normal total body water (Fig. 3-6), corrective salt replacement is calculated as follows:

Given a serum sodium concentration of 121 mEq./L., the deficiency is 143 mEq./L. – 121 mEq./L. = 22 mEq./L. Since, in this situation, the "excess" water has shifted into cells (remember, water moves freely across cell membranes), the deficit in sodium (22 mEq./L.) must be multiplied by the *total body water* (42 L.) to give 924 mEq. This is the total deficit, which is the amount of salt contained in 6 L. of extracellular fluid. An alternate method of calculating this deficit may be used. Twenty-two mEq. is roughly 15% of the normal sodium concentration (143 mEq./L.). This 15% deficit is multiplied by the total body water (42 L.) to give 6 L. of extracellular fluid.

This much salt should never be given as a single order. Initially a hypertonic salt solution can be used, but not more than 9 to 10 Gm. of salt should be given without reevaluating the patient. This is the amount of salt present in 200 ml. of 5% sodium chloride or 300 ml. of 3% sodium chloride. In such a severe extracellular fluid salt deficiency, this order may be repeated twice, but then the remainder of the deficit should be made up of isotonic electrolyte solution. Additional salt can thus be administered in the fluids needed for metabolic requirements for urine and insensible loss. Usually these are non-electrolyte solutions, but in the patient with a salt deficit the entire intravenous fluid therapy can consist of electrolyte solution over a period of several days until the deficiency is corrected.

4. If the patient has a *hypochloremia,* the replacement solutions should be composed of 0.9% saline. *Saline is an acidifying solution* and will correct a metabolic alkalosis because saline has 155 mEq. of chloride per liter in comparison with normal extracellular fluid, which has only 103 mEq./L. This means that in every liter of 0.9% saline approximately 50 mEq./L. of extra chloride is provided to increase the chloride concentration. The *extracellular fluid total chloride deficit* and the number of liters of 0.9% saline required to supply this amount of excess chloride can be calculated.

5. If the patient has a *metabolic acidosis* with a bicarbonate of 17 mEq./L. and one desires to increase this to 27, the deficit of 10 mEq. is multiplied by the estimated liters of *extracellular fluid,* which in the 70 kg. person should be 14 L., for a total of 140 mEq. A molar solution of sodium lactate contains 1,000 mEq./L. of lactate. The lactate is metabolized, and the result is bicarbonate. One-sixth molar sodium lactate solution contains one-sixth as much bicarbonate as molar lactate, or 166 mEq., in a liter. This means that some 850 ml. of one-sixth molar sodium lactate would supply the required 140 mEq. of bicarbonate. Additional requirements for some of the other ions can be added to the total order.

Selecting and administering fluids

As the various requirements of fluid and electrolytes are added up, some of the electrolytes may be placed in metabolic fluids if necessary to avoid using hypertonic electrolyte solutions. In a patient who has large current losses and an extensive past deficit (in addition to his metabolic needs), the administration of 8 to 9 L. of fluid in 24 hours may be required. If this is the case, the order should be written so that the nurse will run the fluids at a rate to approximate 9 L. in 24 hours. The size of drops varies, but the average is about 16 drops per ml.; 9 L. of fluid contain 144,000 drops. There are 60 minutes in the hour, and in 24 hours there are 1,440 minutes. A simple division reveals that the intravenous fluid should run at the rate of 100 drops per minute. Always specify the rate at which intravenous fluids should be infused.

Recording intake and output

The various bottles of fluid ordered should be numbered. The nurse should write the numbers on the bottles when they are prepared for the patient, so that they correspond with the physician's orders. When each bottle is empty, it should be kept in a box under the patient's bed—at any time the numbered bottles can be reviewed to determine what fluids have been given and what fluids are yet to be given. At least once every 24 hours, usually at midnight, all of the bottles are gathered together and the total 24-hour urine volume is measured as well as the volume of gastrointestinal juices. This information must then be recorded accurately in the chart.

Bedside tests

Much of the information is now available for writing a new set of fluid orders for the next 24 hours. Either the nurse or the physician can obtain additional useful information at the bedside by measuring the specific gravity of the urine. With color-coded test tape, pH should be measured for the urine and all other fluids removed from the patient. A patient who is losing acid gastric juice will develop an alkalosis, and his urine will tend to become more alkaline. A patient who is losing alkaline juices in excess of what is replaced will gradually develop a metabolic acidosis, and his urine will become more acid. A patient who is not receiving enough water will develop a high specific gravity of the urine. A patient who is receiving gavage feedings with a high-protein, high-calorie feeding and an inadequate amount of water may have 1 L. of urine but the specific gravity may be 1.035, indicating that the water intake is inadequate for this solute load.

Bedside tests are available for estimation of the *urine chloride* (the Fantus test) or the *urine sodium* (the zinc uranyl acetate precipitation test). These tests show whether the urinary salt excretion is normal or high or low; e.g., if a patient with a low or normal serum sodium concentration has 8 to 9 Gm. of salt in the urine continuously in spite of the fact that a seemingly adequate amount of salt is being given intravenously each day, either adrenal insufficiency or a salt-losing disease of the kidney should be suspected. Such a patient can be given 8 to 10 mg. of desoxycorticosterone acetate (DOCA). If this causes an immediate reduction in the salt excretion, the patient has adrenal insufficiency and will need treatment with corticosteroids. If steroids are ineffective, a renal abnormality exists and the salt loss will have to replaced as an abnormal loss in the same way that loss of electrolyte in gastrointestinal secretions is replaced.

Clinical reevaluation

When the fluids have been ordered, the physician should examine the patient again periodically to make sure that the diagnosis is correct and that the patient is responding to the fluid therapy as anticipated. A patient with a severe metabolic acidosis who is receiving one-sixth molar sodium lactate should have a progressive decrease in the rate and depth of respiration. A patient with a severe extracellular fluid volume deficit who is receiving 3 to 4 L. of extracellular fluid should have an improvement in his skin turgor, pulse, blood pressure, and rate of urinary output. A patient with a total body water deficit should have improvement in his sensorium, an increase in output, and a decrease in specific gravity of the urine. If such a patient has an excessive amount of urine and seems to be losing urine as fast as 5% glucose is given, diabetes insipidus should be suspected and tested for by giving vasopressin (Pitressin). These examples are of *diagnosis ex juvantibus.* If the response to treatment is not as expected, the entire collection and analysis of information must be reviewed since the basis for the fluid orders may have been erroneous.

SPECIAL PROBLEMS

The healthy, young, thin patient with a surgical problem such as inguinal hernia or appendicitis receives parenteral fluids for a very short time and will tolerate gross errors of fluid therapy ranging from receiving no fluids to receiving only glucose solution or saline. Since the majority of patients do not require careful analysis, real danger exists that a physician will become careless and fail to think through the logical analysis, which may be lifesaving in the critically ill patient. The general analysis has been presented, and after some experience in its use it actually requires only a few minutes to complete in the majority of patients. In addition to the preceding outline, the experienced physician will apply additional reasoning when he recognizes certain specific problems such as complicated acid-base imbalance, disturbances in potassium metabolism, acute trauma, and other problems, some of which will be discussed briefly.

ACID-BASE BALANCE

The hydrogen ion concentration in body fluids plays a critical role in enzyme systems and other physiological processes (conservation of base by the kidneys and the binding of oxygen by hemoglobin, for example). Remarkable *buffer systems* dampen or moderate any rapid changes in hydrogen ion concentration. The main buffer system, the bicarbonate ion–carbonic acid buffer, is aided first by pulmonary regulation or excretion of volatile acids as CO_2 and second by renal excretion of nonvolatile acids such as those of phosphate and ammonium. The ratio of bicarbonate ion to carbonic acid in body fluids is normally 20:1. The Henderson-Hasselbalch equation expresses this important relationship of body pH, bicarbonate ion (nonvolatile), and carbonic acid (volatile) in mathematical terms:

$$pH = pK + \log \frac{BHCO_3}{H_2CO_3}$$

In clinical concepts, this may be expressed as:

$$\text{Acid-base balance} = \text{Constant} + \frac{\text{Kidney function}}{\text{Ventilation}}$$

Primary diseases in the kidneys, which cause ineffective excretion of nonvolatile acids, are compensated for by increased excretion of volatile (carbonic) acid by the lung. The converse is also true. In assessing acid-base disturbances, CO_2 content, which measures volatile *and* nonvolatile acids, is of limited value in patients with complicated metabolic, renal, and pulmonary problems.

Two pieces of data and a diagram (Fig. 3-10) are necessary to analyze acid-base disturbances more completely. These are pH and P_{CO_2}. They are obtained rapidly and accurately from arterial blood samples.

Concept of pH

pH is the negative log of the hydrogen ion concentration and is a convenient way of stating a very small number. The normal arterial pH is 7.4. With increasing hydrogen ion concentration, the pH de-

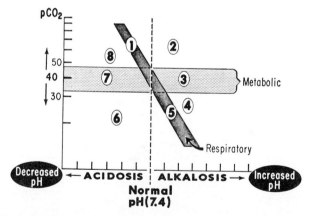

Fig. 3-10. This illustration shows all possible acid-base abnormalities in terms of P_{CO_2} and pH. (Modified from Siggaard-Andersen, O.: The acid-base status of the blood, Baltimore, 1964, The Williams & Wilkins Co.)

1. Respiratory acidosis
2. Mixed respiratory acidosis and metabolic alkalosis
3. Metabolic alkalosis
4. Mixed metabolic and respiratory alkalosis
5. Respiratory alkalosis
6. Mixed metabolic acidosis and respiratory alkalosis
7. Metabolic acidosis
8. Mixed metabolic and respiratory acidosis

creases, and this is referred to as a state of *acidosis*. Hydrogen ion concentration decrease is associated with an increased pH and is called *alkalosis*.

Two types of pH disturbance are classified according to whether they are caused by a change in the body carbonic acid, *respiratory disturbances,* or whether they are caused by a change in concentration of nonvolatile, nonrespiratory substances, *metabolic disturbances.* Whenever fluids that are excreted, secreted, or lost from the body differ in their hydrogen ion concentration from normal body fluids, an opposite change occurs in the hydrogen ion concentration of the fluids remaining in the body; e.g., if a patient loses acid gastric juice, the body changes toward an alkalosis. If the patient excretes very alkaline urine, the body fluids change toward a state of acidosis. Acidosis and alkalosis (or basosis) are, for the clinician, terms signifying a deviation around a normal body pH of 7.4.

Concept of P_{CO_2}

The second important datum is the partial pressure of carbon dioxide (P_{CO_2}) in the body fluids and in the alveolar air, which is in equilibrium with these fluids.* A normal P_{CO_2} is usually about 40 mm. Hg. The rate of excretion of carbon dioxide by ventilation regulates the carbonic acid in the body. A P_{CO_2} above normal (hypercarbia) indicates *respiratory acidosis*. If the ventilation is above normal so that the patient is blowing off excessive amounts of CO_2 (hypocarbia), the P_{CO_2} will be below normal, *respiratory alkalosis*.

Types of acid-base imbalances

Acid-base deviations from normal can be classified as *primary, compensatory,* or *mixed;* e.g., a patient with a *primary metabolic acidosis* from retention of lactic acid (attributed to poor circulation or shock) will usually respond to the increased concentration of hydrogen ions by breathing more rapidly and increasing the rate of excretion of carbonic acid. This is *compensatory respiratory alkalosis. Primary respiratory alkalosis* may occur in a patient with portal hypertension and cirrhosis. Portacaval shunt causes increased amounts of ammonia in the blood and, as a result of this, stimulation of the respiratory center. Increased ventilation results in "blowing off" carbonic acid, which eventuates in primary respiratory alkalosis. Some-

---

*Usually the alveolar CO_2 concentration is about 5.6%. Partial pressures, measured in mm. Hg, vary with barometric pressure and vapor pressure.

times a patient develops two primary conditions, one of which is respiratory and the other metabolic, and yet neither of these is compensating. Both are the result of some disease process or its complication, and these are referred to as *mixed forms of acid-base imbalance;* e.g., a patient with emphysema may be unable to excrete carbon dioxide normally and develops an elevated P_{CO_2}, or a *primary respiratory acidosis,* from the retained carbonic acid. At the same time such a patient may have one of several different conditions that might also cause a *primary metabolic alkalosis,* such as an obstructing duodenal ulcer causing vomiting of acid gastric juice.

Graphic summary of acid-base abnormalities

The pH, P_{CO_2} diagram (Fig. 3-10) makes it possible to summarize all of the possibilities of primary, compensatory, and mixed acid-base abnormalities. Pure abnormalities of nonrespiratory, or metabolic, origin are depicted in areas 7 and 3, and pure deviations from normal (caused by decreased or increased excretion of carbonic acid or respiratory abnormalities) are shown in areas 1 and 5. Areas 2, 4, 6, and 8 are all mixed areas. Area 6 is a common location for patients who have a primary metabolic acidosis and a compensatory respiratory alkalosis. Area 2 includes patients with mixed primary problems but also *respiratory compensation for a metabolic alkalosis.* If a patient with a primary metabolic alkalosis moves into area 2, it may signify that he also has a primary abnormality in his pulmonary function, and one should look for airway obstruction, pneumonia, pulmonary embolism, or other cause of impaired gas exchange.

Importance of clinical correlation

The preceding examples illustrate that *understanding of the particular patient's acid-base problem requires more than just laboratory data.* The clinician must know what primary acid-base abnormalities might be present according to the disease process; e.g., increased ventilation may result because the lungs and the central nervous system function in a normal manner to compensate for a metabolic acidosis. If a patient has a high blood urea nitrogen and diseased kidneys fail to excrete excess organic acids, the retention of these acids will cause a metabolic acidosis. If the patient has severe ketosis, secondary to uncontrolled diabetes, and the lungs are clinically normal, then the excessive ventilation is compensatory, and the clinician knows, before he enlists the help of the laboratory, that the patient's P_{CO_2} and pH will converge somewhere in area 6.

With accurate clinical knowledge of the patient, measurement of P_{CO_2} and pH is usually unnecessary. The CO_2 content of blood will provide a sufficiently accurate estimation of the abnormality in base excess. Normally the CO_2 content is 27 mEq./L. in such samples, and in the patient described, the CO_2 content might be 17 or even 7. The difference from normal in CO_2 content is -10 or -20 and is the deficit in base; e.g., if the CO_2 content is only 7, this means a 20 mEq. deficit. A 70 kg. lean patient with 14 L. of extracellular fluid would need 20 times 14 or 280 mEq. of bicarbonate or lactate to bring the CO_2 content back to 27. This would require about 1,700 ml. of M/6 sodium lactate since 166 mEq. are present in 1 L.

When pH and P_{CO_2} measurements are necessary

Situations arise in the seriously ill patient (often found in post-operative and intensive care areas) in which the patient probably has both metabolic and respiratory abnormalities. In these complex situations, measurements of P_{CO_2} and pH are invaluable guides to determine whether the primary abnormality is metabolic, respiratory, or both.

From the examples given, simple calculations will determine the amount of one-sixth molar sodium lactate required for treatment of a metabolic acidosis or the amount of 0.9% saline, with its 50 mEq. chloride excess per liter, required to treat a metabolic alkalosis (provided that it is not secondary to potassium deficiency). Primary respiratory abnormalities, of course, are best treated by measures to restore normal ventilation rather than by administration of any particular type of intravenous fluid. Alkaline solutions (one-sixth molar sodium lactate) may be necessary to correct a compensatory metabolic acidosis before sedation is given to correct the primary respiratory alkalosis (inappropriate overactivity of respiratory center).

POTASSIUM

Special thought must be given to potassium balance because potassium is the chief cation within cells (94% of total body potassium is in the cells). Young adult women have 2,000 to 3,000 mEq., and men have up to 5,000 mEq. total potassium. The correlation in humans between total exchangeable potassium and energy consumption (in calories per day with moderate activity) is around 0.90. The total exchangeable body potassium can be measured by dilution with radioactive potassium, but this is not a practical clinical test. The clinician must rely on analyses of serum potassium. There are only about 70 mEq. of potassium in the extracellular fluid. The normal serum potassium ranges between 3.5 and 5 mEq./L. If as much as 70 mEq. of potassium moves out of its location in cells into extracellular fluid or if this much potassium is retained in extracellular fluid during intravenous potassium administration, the patient will probably die of cardiac arrest.

Recognition of potassium abnormalities

Recognition of body potassium deficiency is, like the recognition of sodium deficiency, dependent to a great extent on the suspicion of the clinician. His suspicion is raised by knowledge of circumstances that cause potassium loss. Potassium is continually excreted in the urine. In contrast to sodium, despite cessation of potassium intake, the kidneys continue to excrete potassium (minimum rate, 10 to 20 mEq. per day). It is also lost in gastrointestinal juices. If a patient has been losing large amounts of such fluids and the replacement solutions have contained no potassium, total body potassium deficiency will eventually occur, usually accompanied by a lowering of serum potassium concentration. The degree of lowering of serum potassium concentration, however, tells little about the magnitude of total body potassium deficiency.

Patients unable to take food by mouth or subjected to trauma, burns, and major operative procedures, or treated previously with steroids or diuretics are likely to have a potassium deficiency. The physical signs are nonspecific. Such patients have weakness (occasionally almost to paralysis), decreased deep reflexes, and commonly ileus, abdominal distension, and a picture easily confused with chronic bowel obstruction. The deep tendon reflexes are decreased. The electrocardiogram shows a flattening or even inversion of the T-wave. These patients are quite sensitive to digitalis and may, if treated with digitalis, show signs of intoxication with nausea and abnormal rhythm.

Patients with high serum potassiums also may have muscular paralysis and complain of paresthesias. The electrocardiogram shows elevated and peaked T-waves and, with near lethal potassium levels, the electrocardiogram loses all of its normal components.

Potassium problems are divided into (1) those patients in whom the extracellular fluid potassium concentration is abnormal, but without any intracellular deficit, and (2) those patients who have a total body potassium deficiency. The extracellular fluid potassium is affected by the rate of potassium absorption or absence of intake, the rate of loss from the body in various fluids, and the maintenance of a normal cellular metabolism. Sodium is continuously pumped out of cells, allowing a high concentration (or gradient) of potassium within the cells compared with the concentration of potassium in extra-cellular fluid. If the patient becomes severely ill so that metabolism is impaired and the sodium pump begins to fail, then sodium tends to remain in cells and potassium tends to leak out; the extracellular fluid potassium will rapidly reach a level incompatible with life.

Potassium excess

If a heavy object crushes large masses of muscle, potassium leaks out into the extracellular fluid along with myoglobin. The kidneys may become damaged from the pigment and from impaired circulation, and such a patient will die of potassium poisoning within 18 to 24 hours after the crushing injury. Severe burns and major operative procedures are also followed by elevation of serum potassium, because of tissue damage and impaired renal function.

In most instances all that is required relative to potassium balance is to restrict potassium during the first 24 hours after a major operation or during the first few days after a burn. The patient with crush syndrome has to have vigorous treatment with peritoneal dialysis or use of the artificial kidney, and the dialyses may have to be carried on almost continuously during the first few days while the large amounts of potassium are being lost from the crushed muscle. The patient in negative nitrogen balance who is burning his own cellular protein also loses potassium, and the amounts of potassium entering extracellular fluid can be reduced by supplying 400 to 800 calories a day by the administration of glucose in the intravenous fluids so as to minimize protein catabolism.

Potassium and hydrogen ion concentration

The concentration of potassium in extracellular fluid is influenced by the hydrogen ion concentration. Increasing concentrations of hydrogen ion in the extracellular fluid (acidosis) cause hydrogen to move into cells and potassium to move out of cells so that the serum potassium will rise. If the acidosis is treated with sodium bicarbonate or sodium lactate, the serum potassium concentration will fall as the patient becomes less acidotic. If a patient has an alkalosis, this will cause the serum potassium to fall. The patient with severe diabetic acidosis may, upon initial examination, have a serum potassium that is high and then in the course of treatment (and in a matter of hours if the acidosis is rapidly corrected) the potassium may fall to a very subnormal level partly as a result of the change in acid-base balance and also because of the fact that the patient may have a severe total body deficit of potassium.

Potassium deficit

Total body potassium deficit may arise in a variety of situations, but one of the classic examples is the patient who develops pyloric obstruction from a duodenal ulcer; vomiting produces a *hypochloremic alkalosis*. The physician prescribes an amount of saline that he feels should correct the hypochloremic alkalosis and, after treatment with this, finds that the patient still has a low chloride concentration and a high CO_2 content in blood. He may also observe that the patient has an acid urine, which seems inconsistent in a patient with alkalosis. In the days before the flame photometer, this was sufficient to justify a diagnosis of potassium deficiency, but with potassium analysis it is possible to document this by finding a low serum potassium.

For every 3 mEq. of potassium lost from the cells, 2 mEq. of sodium and 1 mEq. of hydrogen ion enter the cells. The hydrogen, of course, is bound to protein and other buffers, but as a result of this exchange the cells become more acid. The cells lining the renal tubules participate in potassium deficiency and cellular acidosis so that the

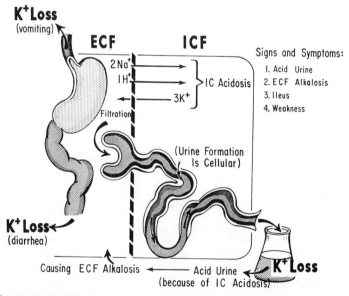

Fig. 3-11. Hypokalemic alkalosis is a common clinical problem seen after vomiting because of obstructing duodenal ulcer or pyloric stenosis with replacement of NaCl but *not* K⁺. K⁺ leaves cells. H⁺ and Na⁺ enter cells. Intracellular *acidosis* results from this exchange. Kidney cells are also acidotic and therefore secrete acid urine; ECF alkalosis is exaggerated. This situation is reversed only by replacing K⁺ deficit.

urine formed is acid (Fig. 3-11). Excretion of acid urine produces hypochloremic alkalosis in extracellular fluid. In the patient who has been vomiting acid gastric juice and also losing potassium, there are therefore two reasons for developing hypochloremic alkalosis. Both potassium and chloride are required to correct the potassium deficiency and the extracellular alkalosis.

Notice that two different problems related to potassium and hydrogen ion have been discussed. In the first situation, a primary *extracellular acidosis* occurs and hydrogen ion moves into the cell forcing potassium out, causing an increase in concentration of serum potassium. In the other situation, the primary abnormality is an *intracellular potassium deficiency* and an increase in cellular hydrogen-ion concentration along with movement of sodium into the cell, followed by the production of an extracellular alkalosis. In the first situation the acidosis begins in extracellular fluid and also involves intracellular fluid. In the second situation, an intracellular acidosis initiates and sustains extracellular alkalosis. As you might expect, some patients who develop an extracellular acidosis, as in diabetic ketosis or with diarrhea, also develop a depletion of cellular potassium.

Treating potassium imbalances

The best treatment is prevention; potassium imbalance, like other fluid and electrolyte problems, can be prevented by replacing abnormal fluid losses as they occur and providing adequate calories and metabolic fluids together with 40 mEq. of urinary loss potassium per day. The potassium requirements may be slightly higher if the patient is receiving steroids or diuretics. The requirements are nil if the patient is oliguric, is acidotic, or has recently undergone a major operation.

Gastrointestinal juice losses should be replaced in the same quantity and at the same rate as they are being lost. For each liter of intravenous electrolyte solution required, 40 mEq. of potassium chloride should be added. Potassium should almost always be diluted in intravenous fluids so that 40 mEq. is distributed in at least a liter of fluid. If, however, the serum potassium is below 3 mEq./L., as much as 80 mEq. can be placed in each liter of intravenous fluid. In some instances, several hundred mEq.'s will need to be given in a day, and perhaps for a number of days, until the total body potassium deficit is repaired. This must be monitored with serum potassium analyses, and the treatment is tapered to maintenance levels as soon as the serum potassium reaches a normal range.

High potassium levels in patients who are markedly acidotic and who have adequate renal function will return to normal as the patient's acidosis is corrected. In oliguria or acute renal failure, a serum potassium of 7 mEq./L. or above should be treated with emergency measures such as the administration of one-sixth molar sodium lactate to correct the acidosis, calcium to counteract the effect of potassium on myocardial irritability, and the administration of glucose and insulin to cause deposition of potassium along with phosphate and glycogen in the liver. If the patient can take sodium polystyrene sulfonate (an exchange resin) with sorbitol by mouth, this will remove potassium but should not be relied upon in the emergency situation. The exchange resin can also be given as a retention enema. Peritoneal dialysis or hemodialysis is often required to restore the potassium to normal in the patient with renal failure; delay is deadly.

CALCIUM AND PHOSPHATE
Hypocalcemia

The administration of parenteral calcium or phosphate is infrequently required, but the circumstances in which it is required may be very dramatic. Tetany usually occurs within 2 days after parathyroidectomy or injury of the blood supply of the parathyroids during radical thyroidectomy. Recognition may be delayed for several weeks if the deficiency is mild. Hypocalcemia also occurs after removal of parathyroid adenomas or hyperplastic parathyroids and is to be expected if the patient has osteitis fibrosa cystica or other evidence of bone demineralization such as an elevated alkaline phosphatase.

Hypocalcemia is common in chronic acidosis and becomes manifest when the acidosis is treated. Acidosis tends to sustain a relatively high concentration of *ionized* calcium. When the acidois is treated and the body fluids become more alkaline, rapid reduction in ionized calcium causes onset of symptoms. This is seen in patients with chronic renal insufficiency and occasionally in patients treated for acidosis from other causes such as diabetic ketosis or acidosis secondary to chronic diarrhea. Patients with malabsorption and steatorrhea, such as that occurring after the removal of small bowel or sidetracking of small bowel for purposes of treating obesity, may develop a chronic hypocalcemia.

The symptoms of low serum calcium are tingling of the fingers and feet and paresthesias about the face and especially around the lips and tongue. Some patients have severe spasm of various muscles, more commonly the back muscles and the muscles of the hands and feet, so that the patient develops a characteristic flexion of the wrist and the metacarpophalangeal joint with extension of the distal phalangeal joints, referred to as carpopedal spasm. The muscular irritability can be demonstrated by tapping over the facial nerve and noting the contraction of the facial muscles, especially the orbicularis oris (Chvostek's sign). Production of carpopedal spasm by application of a tourniquet (Trousseau's sign) is less often demonstrable but is equally pathognomonic of hypocalcemia.

The muscle spasm and paresthesias cause anxiety, which commonly causes the patient to hyperventilate. The subsequent reduction in carbonic acid and respiratory alkalosis leads to a further decrease in the ionized calcium, which increases the symptoms and frightens the patient, causing further hyperventilation. This is similar to the hyperventilation syndrome with tetany occasionally seen in a patient who has a normal serum calcium, but it is much more likely to occur in a patient with hypoparathyroidism.

The suspected diagnosis is confirmed by a serum calcium below 8 mg.% and, probably of even more importance, a serum phosphorus that is above 4.5 mg.%. If both calcium and phosphorus are below normal, it suggests a problem of inadequate nutrition rather than hypoparathyroidism. Patients with uremia have retention of phosphate and a lowering of serum calcium so that the laboratory values may imitate primary hypoparathyroidism, and in the chronic forms of uremia, a compensatory hyperplasia of the parathyroid glands may result.

Treating hypocalcemia

Parathyroid tetany is safely and dramatically treated by the administration of 10 ml. of 10% calcium gluconate intravenously. This should be given slowly, and if the patient is not completely relieved of his symptoms, a second 10 ml. can be administered. This may have to be repeated several times in the first few days, and for the patient who has had hyperparathyroidism and depletion of his bone minerals, it may be necessary to add up to 80 ml. of 10% calcium gluconate to each liter of intravenous fluids and to run the intravenous infusion of 5% glucose continuously at a rate sufficient to keep the patient from having tetany.

Vitamin D_2 (calciferol) is given in oral doses of 50,000 units per day along with oral calcium gluconate. This calcium salt is rather insoluble and must be given in a saturated solution or in a suspension. Vitamin D has a slow action requiring at least a week for its full effect. If a patient still has hypocalcemia after several weeks, the dosage can be increased to 100,000 units. Occasional patients require as much as 200,000 units per day of vitamin D_2 to maintain a normal serum calcium. The patients are taught how to test their own urine with Sulkowitch reagent, and they are advised to report immediately if the urinary calcium precipitation is too dense to see newsprint through. The hypoparathyroidism that occurs after thyroidectomy may be temporary, and it is important to avoid vitamin D poisoning. These are toxic doses of vitamin D for a patient whose parathyroid function returns to normal. The urinary calcium test is not very accurate, and serum calcium determinations are also required until the patient is well regulated. Even then the serum calcium should be measured several times a year. The use of calcium in the intravenous fluids can be discontinued as soon as the patient is able to get along without the medication for several days without any signs or symptoms of tetany. Mild tetany is not dangerous. Prolonged hypocalcemia should not be tolerated, however, because such patients develop cataracts.

Hypercalcemia

Hypercalcemia causes many nonspecific symptoms that are related to the gastrointestinal tract, the kidneys, and the neuromuscular and skeletal tissues. These patients complain of anorexia, nausea, vomiting, constipation, diarrhea, abdominal pain, nocturia, polyuria, thirst, headache, backache, bone pain, aching thigh muscles, weakness, lethargy, loss of interest, exhaustion with mild physical effort, dizziness, fainting, and confusion, as well as symptoms of acute peptic ulcer, pancreatitis, renal stones, and kidney infection. Hyperparathyroidism has been referred to as "a disease of stones, bones, abdominal groans, and psychic moans with fatigue overtones." In spite of all these symptoms the diagnosis was often not made for months or years, and many patients developed parathyroid crisis with serum calcium levels of 17 mg.% or above and serum phosphorus levels below 3 and often in the range of 1.5 mg.%. We now almost routinely measure serum calcium and phosphorus levels in surgical patients. This practice detects hypoparathyroidism before severe complaints or serum chemical alterations have had time to develop.

There are no typical physical signs. The patients are irritable, seclusive, distracted, and dull. They often have laxity of their joints, which makes them able to put their feet behind their head and also causes them to have a peculiar and unsteady gait. The diagnosis is made from the typical serum calcium elevation and extremely low serum phosphorus. Once these chemical abnormalities are found, a differential diagnosis arises that involves hyperparathyroidism, multiglandular adenomas, cancer of the breast and other cancers with bone metastases (or cancerous production of parathormone), sarcoidosis, and milk-alkali syndrome. The last condition is infrequent but results when a patient with peptic ulcer drinks several quarts of milk a day and ingests large amounts of alkaline powders in the treatment of his ulcer.

Treating hypercalcemia

Albright suggested in 1932 that sodium phosphate might be used in the treatment of hyperparathyroidism, since excessive excretion of phosphates by the kidney and a consistently low serum phosphorus were found in those patients who had not yet developed uremia. The retention of phosphorus is greatly in excess of the observed rise in serum phosphorus during the recovery of patients who have had hyperparathyroidism, and this has suggested that these patients probably have a great deficit of phosphate in extraskeletal tissues. Recently hypercalcemia has been treated successfully by isotonic disodium phosphate and monopotassium phosphate (Goldsmith and Ingbar). This causes a prompt reduction in serum calcium levels from the dangerous areas above 17 mg.% to normal levels and is effective whether the hypercalcemia is caused by hyperparathyroidism or cancer. Improvement in stupor, nausea, renal function, and other symptoms and signs of hypercalcemia is immediate.

This treatment should not take the place of appropriate diagnostic measures and surgical treatment of the underlying cause of the hypercalcemia, but it does solve the emergency problem and allows the surgeon to perform a necessary operation under more optimum conditions. High serum calcium also causes renal damage. In animals even 24 hours of hypercalcemia will cause calcification in the kidney, with resultant decrease in glomerular filtration rate and elevation of blood urea nitrogen. Myocardial and brain damage may also occur during the phosphate depletion and hypercalcemia of parathyroid intoxication.

MAGNESIUM
Magnesium deficiency

Magnesium deficiency is likely to be present in patients with delirium tremens, in patients with cirrhosis in whom fluid and salt retention require the use of diuretics, and in patients with ulcerative colitis and chronic diarrhea. The signs and symptoms of magnesium deficiency in such patients may be mimicked by other deficiencies likely to be present at the same time. Prolonged parenteral fluid therapy without magnesium supplement is a common precedent now to magnesium deficiency, just as in similar patients a few years ago prolonged parenteral fluid therapy without addition of potassium was a common antecedent to hypokalemia. Another similarity between potassium and magnesium deficiencies is their occurrence in those patients with chronic renal disease who have a high urine output, but without uremia. Magnesium deficiency may appear in the patient who has been operated upon for severe hyperparathyroidism.

The serum magnesium concentration tends to fall parallel to the decrease in calcium concentration during the early hypocalcemic phase of recovery from hyperparathyroidism. This is undoubtedly related to the repletion of magnesium in the bones. Magnesium is also localized in cells, particularly in the mitochondria. The intracellular fluid magnesium is around 28 mEq./L., whereas the serum levels normally range between 1.5 and 2.5 mEq./L.

Deficiency of magnesium causes central nervous system and neuromuscular hyperirritability with hallucinations, jerking, plucking at the bedclothes, and movements of the hand that simulate the so-called hepatic flap of liver failure. Convulsions may occur. The reflexes are usually hyperreactive, and the patient may develop nystagmus or a positive Babinski and other signs suggesting central nervous system disease. This picture is easily confused with water intoxication, which can also cause convulsions and coma. Treatment is usually given intramuscularly with 50% magnesium sulfate in doses of 2 Gm. at a time repeated every 6 hours until the serum magnesium is again normal. One gram a day of magnesium sulfate is sufficient for maintenance, but in the majority of patients parenteral fluids are not required over a long enough period of time so that a significant magnesium depletion would occur.

Magnesium excess

Magnesium intoxication is difficult to separate from hyperkalemia and other associated abnormalities that occur in uremia. A patient with acute renal failure who is treated frequently with peritoneal or extracorporeal dialysis should not develop magnesium intoxication.

EXTRACELLULAR FLUID LOSS

Internal sequestration of sodium-containing fluids is a common circumstance in the surgeon's practice and is difficult to recognize or to treat quantitatively because the fluid is hidden. Extracellular fluid loss occurs in patients with burns, intestinal obstruction, peritonitis, serum sickness, and multiple soft tissue injuries. This also occurs in connection with hemorrhage if the blood is not immediately replaced. Since bleeding is a part of major operations and extensive fractures, such patients require a mixed type of replacement with both blood and extracellular-like fluid. Physicochemical changes occur in the collagen in burned skin and cause it to swell by taking up extracellular fluid. Anyone who has seen an obstructed bowel with its severe edema or exudate of peritonitis involving large surface areas, including both visceral and parietal peritoneum, can readily understand the mechanism of sodium fluid sequestration.

Trauma and hemorrhage

If blood is lost by simple hemorrhage and is immediately replaced and if no tissue damage occurs either from the injury or from a period of shock, then no electrolyte solution is required. If a few hours transpire during or after the hemorrhage before treatment, then sodium-containing fluids become sequestered within the body. The resultant reduction in effective extracellular fluid volume requires both replacement of the blood and restoration of the effective extracellular fluid volume. In the average adult, one should give as much as 2 L. of extracellular-like fluid while waiting for the blood to be cross matched. If more than 1,000 ml. of blood are required, some additional electrolyte solution may also be given.

During major prolonged operations, a reduction in effective extracellular fluid volume of 15 to 20% is often seen. Administration of this fluid during the operation will reduce the amount of blood required to maintain normal vital signs. This does not obviate the replacement of blood loss. The electrolyte fluid should be given in addition to blood.

In all of these patients with burns, trauma, hemorrhage, and operative procedures (lasting longer than $2\frac{1}{2}$ hours), the extracellular-like fluid can be made up of 0.9% saline and one-sixth molar sodium lactate in the proportions of 4:1. In most hospitals lactated Ringer's solution is available and has the composition of extracellular fluid.

When extracellular fluid is sequestered as a result of a burn, trauma, or shock-induced tissue injury, and the patient receives appropriate electrolyte solutions to replace this fluid, there must follow a mobilization and excretion of such fluid. If the kidneys do not function well and the fluid is retained, pulmonary edema may occur. After resuscitation, electrolyte-containing solutions should be withheld and, if necessary, diuretics used until the fluid overload is corrected.

Patients should be prepared for major operative procedures by having blood volume and hemoglobin levels restored to normal before the operation. Severe depletion of body proteins should also be corrected by the administration of either plasma or human serum albumin. The normal patient has approximately 60% of his blood volume in veins, including the large veins leading into the right side of the heart; he may lose 1 to 1.5 L. of blood before he becomes hypotensive simply because of the constriction of these veins, thereby maintaining venous return.

The normal patient also has about 60% of his albumin in extravascular areas and can lose this much of his total body albumin before he begins to show the signs and symptoms of reduced plasma volume. If a patient with reduced blood volume and reduced body albumin is subjected to a major operation and does not have more than his operative blood loss replaced, he may in the postoperative period demonstrate a failing renal function, poor peripheral circulation (even with the appearance of arterial thromboses in major vessels), and an extremely high hematocrit. If the problem is not recognized and treated vigorously with electrolyte solution, plasma, and blood, such a patient will succumb. Deficiencies of albumin and whole blood should be repaired *before* the operation. Lactated Ringer's solution is given as needed *during* the operation.

REPLACEMENT OF GASTROINTESTINAL FLUID LOSS

Much of the imbalance in fluid and electrolytes could be avoided if gastrointestinal fluids were properly replaced at the time of their loss. This implies, of course, accurate records of the type and volume of fluid lost. In the adult, this is a loss of isotonic fluid and it is simply replaced with isotonic fluid, such as 0.9% saline or saline plus one-sixth molar sodium lactate. Since all of the fluids lost and the two replacement solutions have the same concentration of electrolytes, the chief difference relates to the anion *composition and therefore the pH* (Table 3-1). The pH of the fluid being lost can be determined at the bedside with pH paper. If acid juice is lost from the stomach (and not all juice aspirated from the stomach is acid gastric juice), the fluids remaining in the body are more alkaline. Fluid lost from the upper small bowel (through a long intestinal tube or a duodenal fistula) is alkaline, resulting in an acidosis. If the loss is a balanced loss of gastric and intestinal juices having a pH of approximately 7.4, then the acid-base balance of the patient is unchanged.

If the juice being lost is acid with an excess of chloride, then the replacement solution should be isotonic saline, which has an excess of 50 mEq. of chloride per liter as compared with the chloride con-

Table 3-1. Treatment of acid-base disturbances

Type of fluid loss	*Resultant acid-base disturbances*	*Treatment I. V. fluid ratio (0.9% NaCl:M/6 NaHCO₃)*		
		Neutral (4:1)	*Acidifying (1:0)*	*Alkalinizing (2:1)*
Balanced loss	None	Balance	Acidosis	Alkalosis
Acid juice loss	Alkalosis	Alkalosis	Balance	Severe alkalosis
Alkaline juice loss	Acidosis	Acidosis	Severe acidosis	Balance

centration in normal extracellular fluid. If the fluid being lost is alkaline, the replacement solution should be made up of only two parts of saline and one part of one-sixth molar sodium lactate. If the solution lost is approximately that of extracellular fluid, then the proportions of isotonic saline and one-sixth molar sodium lactate should be 4:1, which is the proportion of bicarbonate to chloride in extracellular fluid.

A few physicians stubbornly maintain that the kidney will take care of any imbalance, that any electrolyte loss may be treated by the administration of 0.9% saline. If a patient is losing alkaline intestinal juices, therefore having a metabolic acidosis, and is then treated with saline, which causes its own hyperchloremic acidosis, the result will be a severe metabolic acidosis that even a normal kidney could not correct. The kidneys in a patient with severe acidosis do not function normally.

The patient with ulcerative colitis who has a total colectomy and ileostomy illustrates the need for continuous monitoring of the type of intestinal fluids lost. During the early postoperative period the loss is primarily one of acid gastric juice from the stomach that tends to produce an alkalosis and requires treatment with saline. As the intestine begins to function several days after the operation and acid gastric suction fluid loss ceases and alkaline ileostomy fluid loss begins, a large loss of alkaline intestinal juices results in acidosis. At this time the treatment must suddenly be changed from the administration of the acidifying saline solution to an alkalinizing replacement solution containing 2 parts saline and 1 part one-sixth molar sodium lactate. In the replacement of all intestinal fluid loss, 20 to 40 mEq. of potassium should be added for each liter of fluid lost. Gastric juice potassium concentration is usually around 8 to 10 mEq./L. Intestinal juices may contain as high as 50 or 60 mEq. potassium per liter.

ACUTE RENAL FAILURE

Kidney shutdown is usually the result of a combination of several factors such as hypotension, intravenous hemolysis (infusion of mismatched blood or distilled water), dehydration, extensive trauma, crushing of muscle, and release of myoglobin. *Ischemia* is the common denominator of most causes of acute renal failure.

All degrees of injury from mild tubular injury to complete renal cortical infarction are seen. In most patients there is a lysis of tubular cells with varying numbers of breaks in basement membranes. The latter results in permanent tubulovenous fistulas or obstructed nephrons. Tubulolysis is a reversible lesion, analogous to a burn, with remaining islands of viable cells from which regeneration occurs. Recovery of function requires a few days to as long as 3 weeks. During the period of regeneration the patient remains oliguric. As the nephrons begin to retain the glomerular filtrate, polyuria develops. As the living cells mature and begin to show subcellular organelles such as mitochondria, normal concentrating function is restored and the diuretic phase of recovery is replaced by normal renal function.

Prevention of acute renal failure requires adequate and early replacement of blood and extracellular fluid, as discussed on pp. 26 and 50. A traumatized patient requiring four units of blood replacement may, in addition, need 3 or 4 L. of lactated Ringer's solution before the urine output is adequate.

Mannitol or furosemide may restore urine flow even though there is a persistent inadequacy of blood and extracellular fluid volume, but it will not correct, and may obscure, the circulatory insufficiency at fault.

Progressive decrease in urine volume to less than 500 ml. per day or a rising blood urea nitrogen and creatinine with a greater volume of urine indicates probable acute renal failure. Persistent circulatory insufficiency must be ruled out, and a trial of blood or lactated Ringer's solution may be given to see if normal urine volume can be restored. Simple retention must be ruled out by catheterization or irrigation of an indwelling catheter. The urine is examined for blood cells and casts; tests for urea, creatinine, and electrolytes in the urine are not usually necessary. With renal failure, the urine approaches the chemical composition of the blood.

Acute renal failure causes a retention of any fluids that are administered to the patient; the dilution of total body solute depends on the magnitude of accumulated water, as illustrated in Fig. 3-4. The percent decrease in serum sodium concentration will be equal to the percent increase in lean body mass calculated from change in body weight. If acute renal failure is recognized early and if fluid is restricted adequately, serum sodium concentration remains normal.

Potassium and organic acids accumulate with a resultant progressive fall in CO_2 content. If the patient vomits or has loss of acid gastric juice by nasal gastric suction, then the CO_2 may remain normal, with decrease in the serum chloride. This is ideal, since retained *organic acids* do not cause acidosis. A low serum chloride never requires treatment if the CO_2 content is normal. As phosphate is retained the serum calcium falls. Death occurs after about 10 to 12 days from high potassium, from retained fluids and pulmonary edema, or from pneumonia. Death may occur in 24 hours with crushing injuries, as mentioned on p. 42. No patient should die from renal failure.

Emergency treatment of a high serum potassium requires (1)

glucose and insulin to force potassium into glycogen stores, (2) *correction of the acidosis* to force potassium into cells, (3) *elevation of serum calcium* to counteract the effect of potassium on myocardial irritability, and (4) dialysis as soon as possible.

Patients without recent abdominal operations can be subjected to peritoneal dialysis within a very short time. Peritoneal dialysis or hemodialysis is required at intervals of every few days to maintain body chemistries reasonably normal while the kidneys are recovering. Peritoneal dialysis is less efficient than hemodialysis with an artificial kidney, and it must be used more frequently and for longer periods of time—but peritoneal dialysis can be used when an artificial kidney is not available.

In addition to the treatment of hyperkalemia, management of acute renal failure should include (1) replacement of only insensible and renal water losses, (2) weighing the patient daily—about 1 pound is the anticipated daily loss, (3) calories given in the form of sugar-sweetened butterballs for protein-sparing effect, and (4) oral ion-exchange resins that bind potassium and increase its excretion in the stool.

SUMMARY

The surgeon is a physician who operates. He is responsible for the complete day-to-day care of his patients and should make a habit on rounds of asking himself what each patient needs for (1) metabolic fluids, (2) replacement of abnormal loss, and (3) restoration of any imbalance that exists. The latter should be defined on the basis of the data available from history, physical findings, intake and output records, and any laboratory analyses of abnormalities of (a) volume, (b) tonicity and chemical composition, and (c) acid-base balance. The diagrams: (1) volume versus concentration, (2) bar graph of ECF cations and anions, and (3) pCO_2, pH should be drawn in the patient's chart, progress notes together with appropriate modifications from normal. Inconsistencies in the analyses should be adjudicated by collecting additional data, repeating examinations of patient and laboratory tests, and reviewing the logic of the diagnostic analysis. Finally the needs for fluids, electrolytes, and nutrients should be totaled for the day and incorporated into a simple prescription that the nurse can supply, with prepared intravenous solutions.

CHAPTER 4

Hemostatic defects and bleeding: diagnosis and treatment

JOHN C. HOAK

Abnormalities of hemostasis, whether congenital or acquired, may lead to significant complications at operation or during the postoperative period. If forewarned about the likelihood of hemostatic problems, the surgeon can often forestall disastrous, unexpected bleeding by selective preoperative studies and treatment. The dangers of massive blood loss from such defects are obvious, but it is seldom appreciated that minor episodes of bleeding may favor subsequent complications of poor wound healing and local or systemic infections. The purpose of this chapter is to consider the more common conditions that impede normal hemostasis and to help avert these immediate and delayed complications.

HEMOSTATIC MECHANISMS

Normal hemostasis involves the interaction of several components, which are (1) structure and vasoconstrictive properties of the vessel wall, (2) normal platelets (both number and function), (3) coagulation factors, and (4) normal fibrinolytic parameters.

Surgical bleeding begins with injury to blood vessels that damages the endothelium. This usually exposes the blood to subendothelial tissue components that cause platelets to adhere to collagen or microfibrillar structures. Additional platelets aggregate in response to the release of adenosine diphosphate from platelets to form a hemostatic plug. Under the influence of thrombin, platelets undergo irreversible changes, which, together with newly formed fibrin, reinforce the hemostatic plug. Disorders caused by platelet deficiencies (numbers or function) and to a lesser extent coagulation factor deficiencies may disrupt this early phase of hemostasis.

The current concept of the blood coagulation mechanism is shown in Fig. 4-1. The present concept of the mechanisms involved in fibrinolysis is shown in Fig. 4-2.

The physician can usually suspect a hemorrhagic disorder from a careful history. He should never rely on a "few screening laboratory tests" to substitute for the vitally important history. The following sequence may be helpful in the diagnosis of a hemorrhagic disease:

1. History of bleeding
   a. Familial
   b. In spontaneous episodes
   c. During or after operative procedures and trauma

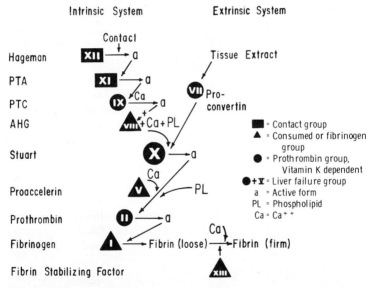

Fig. 4-1. Blood coagulation mechanism. The partial thromboplastin time reflects changes in clotting factors shown under the intrinsic system (XII, XI, IX, VIII, X, V, II, I). The one-stage prothrombin time reflects changes in clotting factors involved with the extrinsic system (VII, X, V, II, I).

2. Physical examination
   a. Skin and mucous membranes (ecchymoses, petechiae, hematomas)
   b. Retina (hemorrhages)
   c. Joints (hemarthroses)
   d. Teeth (bleeding after extraction)
3. Concurrent disease known to cause secondary bleeding (e.g., leukemia, liver disease, carcinoma of the prostate)
4. History of drug ingestion (e.g., anticoagulants, aspirin)
5. Diet (e.g., deficiency of vitamin K or vitamin C)
6. Initial laboratory studies (urine, stool, and blood count)

Clinical examination usually provides a satisfactory appraisal of hemostatic activity. Blood clotting tests are then useful to elucidate the nature and severity of a clotting defect. They, of course, may not reflect other defects in the hemostatic mechanism, e.g., vascular defects. Also there are a few patients with mild forms of clotting disorders (e.g., hemophilia) who are asymptomatic until they bleed excessively after minor trauma or an operation. Laboratory tests may reveal the abnormality in these instances. But the student should remember that about 50% of patients with classical hemophilia have normal whole blood clotting times.

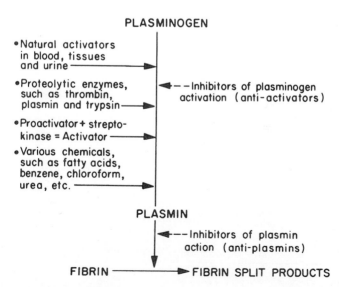

Fig. 4-2. Fibrinolysis mechanism. (After Harker, L. A.: Hemostasis manual, Seattle, 1970, University of Washington Press.)

At the University of Iowa Hospitals, we recommend certain coagulation tests to evaluate possible hemorrhagic disorders. The initial set of tests includes the following:

1. Bleeding time
2. Prothrombin time
3. Partial thromboplastin time
4. Platelet count

If any of these tests is abnormal or if clinical judgment suggests abnormal hemostasis, additional coagulation studies are performed in association with hematological consultation.

Bleeding profile
   Bleeding time
   Clot retraction
   1-Stage prothrombin
   Fibrinogen
   Plasma clot lysis
   Euglobulin clot lysis
   Thrombin time
   Partial thromboplastin time
   Prothrombin utilization
   Urea solubility for factor XIII
   Specific factor assays
   Test for circulating anticoagulant

Consumption-fibrinolysis profile
   Platelet count
   Thrombin time
   1-Stage prothrombin
   Partial thromboplastin time
   Fibrinogen
   Euglobulin clot lysis
   Fi test on serum
   Test for fibrin monomer
   Assay of fibrin split products
   Reptilase time

Platelet profile (to be considered when platelet dysfunction, rather than deficiency, is suspected)
   Platelet count
   Bleeding time
   Clot retraction
   Platelet adhesiveness
   Platelet aggregation (ADP, collagen, epinephrine, Ristocetin)
   Prothrombin utilization
   Platelet morphology
   Adenine nucleotide content of platelets

MANAGEMENT OF THE PATIENT WITH DEFECTIVE HEMOSTASIS

Hemophilioid disorders

Classical hemophilia is characterized by a deficiency of factor VIII and is considerably more common than Christmas disease (congenital deficiency of factor IX). Both disorders are transmitted by female carriers and occur in males. They have similar clinical features and cannot be differentiated except by special coagulation studies. Von Willebrand's disease, a hemophilioid disorder, occurs with equal incidence in both men and women. Patients with this disorder have a deficiency of factor VIII, but unlike classical hemophiliacs, usually have a prolonged bleeding time, decreased platelet adhesiveness, and platelets that do not aggregate with Ristocetin. Transfusion of normal or hemophilic plasma to patients with von Willebrand's disease causes a delayed rise in factor VIII activity that is thought to result from increased VIII synthesis. Similar results are not found when von Willebrand's plasma is given to a classical hemophiliac.

It is now possible to perform surgery on classical hemophiliacs if they are given concentrates of factor VIII before and after operation. In general, cryoprecipitate or other types of VIII concentrates are preferable to plasma or blood to minimize the volume transfused. An amount of factor VIII to raise the factor VIII activity to 80% of normal is given just before operation. Half that amount is then given every 12 hours after surgery for 10 to 14 days. The half-life of factor VIII is approximately 12 hours.

Formula for calculating amount of factor VIII required

$$\frac{\text{Units}}{\text{required}} = \text{Body weight (kg.)} \times 0.4 \times \text{Desired VIII increase in } \%$$

1 unit = factor VIII activity of 1 ml. normal pooled plasma. About 100 units of factor VIII are contained in one sack of cryoprecipitate.

Cryoprecipitate is also useful for treating patients with von Willebrand's disease but is ineffective for patients with Christmas disease.

Concentrates of factors IX, X, VII, and II are commercially available and are satisfactory for the management of patients with Christmas disease at surgery. A factor IX activity of at least 60% is desirable before operation. Half of that amount of concentrate required to increase the IX activity to 60% is then given every 24 hours for 10 to 14 days after operation. The half-life of factor IX is approximately 24 hours.

Formula for calculating amount of factor IX required

$$\frac{\text{Units}}{\text{required}} = \text{Body weight (kg.)} \times 0.5 \times \text{Desired IX increase in }\%$$

1 unit = factor IX activity of 1 ml. normal pooled plasma.

Concentrates of these clotting factors should be used with care since they are expensive and carry a potential risk of hepatitis. Some factor IX concentrates have produced thrombosis. If an emergency operation is required in a patient with a hemophilioid disorder when no concentrates are available, we have found a technique that can be of considerable benefit. We have infused large volumes of normal plasma (2 L. in 1½ to 2 hours) coincident with the intravenous injection of the diuretic furosemide. In this manner, satisfactory factor IX activity was achieved in a patient with Christmas disease who had to undergo an emergency operation.

Platelet disorders

Infusions of fresh whole blood, platelet-rich plasma, or platelet concentrates may promote hemostasis temporarily in patients with thrombocytopenia or impaired platelet function. The cause of thrombocytopenia should be determined and corrected when possible. The physician must always consider drug effects as a cause of platelet deficiency or dysfunction.

Vitamin K disorders

As shown in Fig. 4-1, vitamin K is necessary for the synthesis of prothrombin (II) and factors VII, IX, and X by the liver. Deficiencies of these factors occur in patients with impaired utilization of vitamin K (liver disease), in those being treated with coumarin type of anticoagulants, or in those who have impaired absorption of vitamin K related in extrahepatic biliary obstruction or sprue. Vitamin K is available as vitamin K_1, which is used to prepare patients preoperatively with suspected vitamin K deficiency. Rapid reversal (4 to 24 hours) of the anticoagulant effect of coumarin is achieved by parenteral injection of vitamin K_1. Large doses of vitamin K_1 may cause resistance to further coumarin therapy.

Patients with extrahepatic biliary obstruction producing an increased prothrombin time may be given vitamin K_1 parenterally or orally. If the prothrombin time remains prolonged after 2 days of vitamin K therapy, it signifies sufficient liver disease to interfere with the utilization of vitamin K and the synthesis of the aforementioned coagulation factors. This is a sign of severe hepatic disease.

Disseminated intravascular coagulation (consumption coagulopathy)

Disseminated intravascular coagulation as a clinical problem should be suspected when a patient develops bleeding in association with hypofibrinogenemia, thrombocytopenia, a prolonged thrombin time, and positive tests for fibrin monomer and fibrin split products. Treatment should be aimed at correcting the precipitating problem (sepsis, malignancy, abruptio placentae, etc.). Heparin may help to prevent further intravascular clotting. Fresh whole blood transfusions help treat the anemia, thrombocytopenia, and hypofibrinogenemia. Fibrinogen without heparin may potentiate clotting and also entails the risk of hepatitis.

Fibrinolytic states

Excessive fibrinolysis may produce local or systemic bleeding. Fibrinolysis most often occurs secondary to intravascular clotting, but occasionally the fibrinolysis appears to be the primary cause of the impaired hemostasis, and bleeding ceases with administration of epsilon aminocaproic acid (EACA) to block fibrinolysis. Usually 2 Gm. of EACA is given intravenously, followed by an infusion of EACA in saline or glucose solution (10 to 20 Gm. every 24 hours). The drug may also be given orally. Great caution should be used when EACA is given to patients with impaired renal function.

Bleeding after heparin

Bleeding after heparin should be suspected in patients who received heparin before surgery or as part of an extracorporeal procedure during operation. It results from an excessive dose of heparin, or inadequate neutralization of the heparin effect with protamine. Excessive amounts of protamine may also impair hemostasis.

Unexplained bleeding

When bleeding cannot be ascribed to surgical sources or any specific coagulation defect, consideration should be given to a combined defect. In particular, attention should be directed to platelets and fibrinolysis. Administration of calcium has not proved helpful. Similarly, hemostatic tonics have no place in the management of such problems.

TRANSFUSION THERAPY

With the development of improved blood banking techniques, transfusion of blood components has largely replaced transfusion of whole blood. A single unit of fresh whole blood can provide a unit of packed RBCs, a unit of platelets, a unit of cryoprecipitate for treating classical hemophilia, and plasma proteins for preparing albumin and gamma globulin.

Packed RBCs are given to increase the red cell volume in the treatment of symptomatic anemia unresponsive to other measures. Albumin solution is used to restore the plasma volume in patients with hypovolemia caused by the loss of plasma into the tissues as seen with some inflammatory conditions. Platelet concentrates are used to control thrombocytopenic bleeding in patients with bone marrow failure or leukemia, occasionally for those who have thrombocytopenia secondary to multiple transfusions of stored blood, and if necessary in the preparation of patients with idiopathic thrombocytopenic purpura for splenectomy. The survival of transfused platelets varies with the mechanism of the thrombocytopenia. The half-life of transfused platelets is usually $2\frac{1}{2}$ to 4 days but varies with collection and storage techniques.

Determination of the patient's blood volume and serial measurements of central venous pressure may be useful aids in assessing adequacy of blood replacement in surgical patients.

Consideration of the potassium content of stored blood may be important in some patients with existing hyperkalemia or with certain types of impaired renal function. The RBCs in older banked blood have a very low 2,3-DPG level. It takes several hours after a transfusion for the cells to replenish their supply of 2,3-DPG and function effectively in oxygen delivery. Consequently, older banked blood should be avoided in the replacement of the RBC volume in the critically ill patient with severe tissue hypoxia.

Complications of blood transfusions
Intravascular hemolysis

Intravascular hemolysis is the most common and the most serious complication of blood transfusion. The hemolysis may be transient and mild, or it may be serious, or even fatal. Hemolysis produces hemoglobinemia and hemoglobinuria. The serum bilirubin reflects the severity of the hemolysis.

It is the responsibility of the physician who administers blood to understand the causes, signs, symptoms, and proper management of transfusion reactions. Blood transfusion reactions are heralded by chills, fever, and restlessness, followed by dyspnea, cyanosis, peripheral vascular collapse, hemoglobinemia, and hemoglobinuria. Shortly thereafter the patient may experience pain in the flanks and develop urticaria. Oliguria followed by anuria, jaundice, and anemia may appear within 24 to 48 hours. The signs and symptoms are proportionate to the severity of the hemolytic reaction. Thus, oliguria, anuria, jaundice, and anemia signify a severe hemolytic reaction.

The key to managing a patient with a transfusion reaction rests in its early recognition and the immediate termination of the transfusion. The blood and a sample of the patient's blood are sent immediately to the blood bank for immunological tests and culture. Another sample of the patient's blood is tested for hemolysis and the urine for hemoglobin. These tests usually establish the diagnosis. An intravenous infusion of 100 ml. of 20% mannitol solution can be tried over 5 minutes to initiate diuresis. The patient should be catheterized and the urinary output monitored. Treatment is tailored to the severity of the transfusion reaction.

Pyrogenic reactions

Pyrogenic reactions are caused by chemical contaminants in the equipment used for the transfusion. The use of disposable equipment has virtually eliminated them.

Leukocyte immune reactions

Transfusion of blood containing leukocytes into sensitized individuals may cause a reaction characterized by fever, chills, and signs of pulmonary edema. The recipient may appear to have fluid overload, pneumonitis, or pulmonary emboli. Steroid therapy may be helpful. The reaction can be prevented by transfusing RBCs free of WBCs (washed RBCs or RBCs prepared from frozen blood).

Bacterial reactions

Blood, contaminated by bacteria, triggers a reaction in the recipient ranging from transient fever to shock and death. Massive contamination with gram-negative organisms is usually fatal. The only truly effective therapy is prevention by meticulous aseptic handling of blood.

Allergic reactions

Occasionally a transfusion will be followed by angioneurotic edema, hives, and asthma. The cause of allergic reactions is often obscure. Foods or drugs ingested by the donor are responsible in some cases. Usually these allergic reactions are mild and require no treatment. Antihistamines will control most reactions.

Anti-IgA in IgA-deficient recipient

Patients with this reaction may develop either anaphylactic shock or a more mild reaction with erythema and urticaria. Fever is usually absent but profound hypotension may occur. Such patients lack immunoglobulin A (IgA) and have developed an IgG-type anti-IgA from previous transfusions. It is uncommon. The diagnosis requires demonstrating the absence of IgA in the recipient and the presence of anti-IGA in the circulation. The reaction can be prevented by using washed RBCs.

Overtransfusion

When blood is given to a patient with limited cardiac reserve (the elderly, frail, or debilitated patient), circulatory overload is a threat. Circulatory overload is suggested by signs and symptoms of pulmonary congestion and edema. The blood transfusion is stopped, and venesection, alternating tourniquets, and digitalization may be required.

Transmission of hepatitis and other infectious diseases

Both infectious hepatitis (incubation period 30 to 38 days) and serum hepatitis (incubation period 41 to 108 days) can be transmitted by whole blood and all blood components except albumin and gamma globulin. The incidence of icteric and anicteric hepatitis varies but may be as high as 10%, depending on the donor population. About 20 to 40% of donors whose blood will transmit viral hepatitis can be shown to have the hepatitis-associated antigen (HAA) in their serum. There is a 3- to 5-fold increase in the incidence of hepatitis in recipients who receive HAA-positive blood as compared to those who receive only HAA-negative blood.

Cytomegalovirus infection, syphilis, malaria, brucellosis, and Chaga's disease can also be transmitted by blood transfusion.

Whole blood substitutes

Plasma has a limited place as a substitute for whole blood. In general, when whole blood is not immediately available for a patient with blood loss shock, dextran or electrolyte solutions should be used rather than pooled plasma. Specific indications for giving plasma include (1) the treatment of burns and other varieties of shock not associated with the loss of red blood cells and (2) the correction of hypoproteinemia and protein depletion. The principal complication of plasma is serum hepatitis, which occurs approximately once in every four pooled plasma infusions. Type-specific plasma is much less risky than pooled plasma.

Another whole blood and plasma substitute is dextran, which is available in low or high molecular weight. Infusion of more than 500 ml. of dextran solution may produce red cell aggregation and agglutination. Dextran in large volumes may interfere with the hemostatic mechanism and produce bleeding. Dextran also may induce blood typing difficulties.

CHAPTER 5

Shock

ROBERT T. SOPER
ROBERT J. CORRY

Shock may be defined as a condition of inadequate vascular perfusion to satisfy the minimal metabolic demands of cells or the inability of tissues to utilize oxygen and other nutrients. The clinical situation triggering shock produces a defect, or a combination of defects, somewhere along the critical pathways of body fluid flow to upset cellular utilization of high energy substrates.

Shock is the terminal event in all deaths. Trauma with attendant shock is said to be the most common primary factor causing death during the first four decades of life in the United States. Recent studies have provided new and intriguing concepts to the understanding of shock. We now recognize that shock, although usually associated with systemic hypotension, may occur with normal arterial pressures such as in patients with gram-negative septicemia. Conversely, low arterial pressures do not necessarily signify shock.

Shock may result from many different causes, but all have the common effect of reducing vascular perfusion of body cells leading to tissue hypoxia, metabolic acidosis, and cellular death, if uncorrected. The absence of a single simple test to measure effective blood flow to tissues accounts for much of the confusion about the diagnostic criteria of shock and for the widely divergent approaches to its classification and treatment. Lacking such a test, the physician must base his diagnosis of shock on signs, symptoms, and measurements that suggest, but do not absolutely prove, the presence of shock.

NORMAL CELLULAR PERFUSION

Normal perfusion of body tissues begins with the heart, which pumps oxygenated blood and nutrients into the major arteries of the

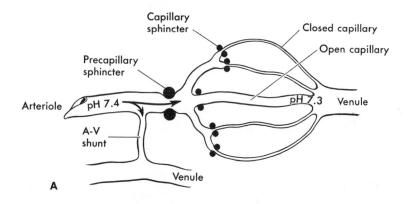

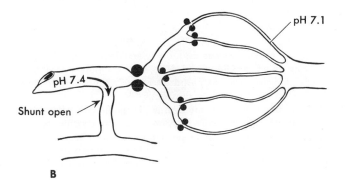

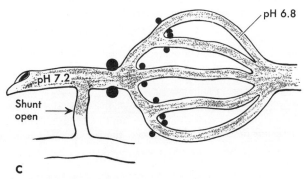

Fig. 5-1. For legend see opposite page.

body in a pulsatile manner. Regulators of organ blood flow are concentrated in the precapillary sphincters of the metarterioles of the body. These regulators produce resistance to arterial flow to maintain blood pressure and convert the pulsatile circulating stream to an even flow (Fig. 5-1, *A*). A single precapillary sphincter regulates flow to several capillaries. Normally, only about 20% of the capillaries of the body are perfused at any one time (the other 80% are closed). If all the capillaries were open simultaneously, the circulating blood volume would have to be increased many times to fill all vascular channels of the body. The capillaries carrying blood at a given time are rotated, so that all cells are periodically perfused with oxygen and nutrients. This orderly rotation of perfused capillaries is probably assured by the following mechanism: as the cells of inactive capillaries become anoxic, some vasoactive substance is released (histamine? lactic acid?) that dilates the capillary sphincters to allow perfusion through these channels, diverting flow from capillaries nourishing freshly oxygenated tissue.

The blood flow through the few capillaries open at a given time is rapid, and the decrease in pH of the blood is small. End products of cellular metabolism are picked up on the venous end of the capillaries, and the blood is returned in the venous channels to the heart pump. Arterial blood not needed by its capillary branches at that moment is diverted directly back to the veins via arteriovenous shunts by contraction of metarteriole sphincters. Maintenance of flow discourages clumping of cells and increased blood viscosity to prevent intravascular clotting.

A derangement of one or more of these components of normal circulation may impair cellular perfusion and produce shock. The physi-

---

Fig. 5-1. A, Diagram of normal microcirculation. The precapillary sphincter is partially constricted, diverting some of the arterial blood directly to the veins via the arteriovenous shunt. The blood entering the capillary system is perfusing only about 20% (1 out of 5 capillaries in the diagram) of the cells nourished by this system at any given time. The intermittent opening and closing of the capillary sphincters assure periodic perfusion of all tissue. Blood flow is rapid through the perfused capillary, and the decrease in the blood pH is small. **B,** Vasoconstriction phase of shock. The majority of the blood in the arteriole is diverted across the arteriovenous shunt to the venous side by constriction of the precapillary sphincter. Capillary perfusion is reduced and blood flow slowed to produce a greater drop in capillary blood pH. **C,** Vasodilatation phase of shock. Capillaries and venules dilate, blood volume is inadequate to fill the large vascular bed, blood flow stagnates, pH drops, and thrombosis may occur.

cian must pinpoint and correct these derangements to treat shock adequately.

INADEQUATE CELLULAR PERFUSION: THE BASIS OF SHOCK

The inadequate perfusion of tissue that occurs during shock deprives the affected cells of oxygen and substrates essential to normal cell function. A series of complex chemical transformations are necessary for the synthesis of adenosine triphosphate (ATP), the ultimate source of energy for life processes. In the absence of oxygen, ATP is inefficiently produced via anaerobic metabolism, or fermentation. Lactic and pyruvic acid accumulate in the tissues, helping to produce the metabolic acidosis of shock. Stored high-energy phosphate compounds decrease, the cellular enzyme systems become disorganized, and the cell ultimately dies.

Most shock states are associated with hypovolemia and hypotension, nonspecific stimuli that provoke the release of catecholamines and result in marked compensatory vasoconstriction (Fig. 5-1, *B*). Constricted metarteriole sphincters divert more of the arteriolar blood across the arteriovenous shunts to increase venous return to the heart, reducing blood flow in the capillary systems controlled by the metarteriole. The scanty blood that does enter the capillaries flows slowly and has more oxygen extracted and a lower pH than normal. The stagnant, viscid capillary blood tends to sludge and clot.

As cellular anoxia increases, vasoactive substances are released, causing capillary channels to dilate and expand the vascular bed (Fig. 5-1, *C*). This increases the vascular bed volume to well above that which could be filled by even a "normal" circulating blood volume. This phenomenon materially worsens the relative hypovolemia that already exists.

To recap, hypovolemia induces slow passage of blood through the capillaries, produces tissue anoxia, favors anaerobic metabolism, increases the production of lactic and pyruvic acids, and results in a smaller amount of more viscid and acidified blood reaching the venous side of the circulation. Venous return to the heart is diminished, central venous pressure decreases, and cardiac output falls because of reduced filling of the heart. Metabolic acidosis stimulates hyperpnea, and excess carbon dioxide is "blown off" in the lungs. The factors of *stagnation* of capillary flow, *acidemia,* and *capillary thrombosis* are a vicious cycle that, if not corrected, leads to cellular death, organ failure, and death of the organism.

The following definite priorities are assigned to the organ systems relative to the order in which they are deprived of adequate blood flow in hypovolemic shock: (1) skin and subcutaneous fat first, (2) intestine and skeletal muscle next, (3) then major viscera such as the kidney and liver, and, finally, in the terminal stages of shock, (4) the coronary and cerebral blood flow begin to fail.

Clinical criteria and bedside tests roughly parallel the selective perfusion of tissues just noted. *Pale, cold,* and *clammy skin and mucous membranes* reflect the skin and subcutaneous vasoconstriction, *weakness* and *ileus,* the reduction of blood to muscle and intestine, *oliguria,* the renal vasoconstriction, and the state of *consciousness* roughly reflects the cerebral blood flow. *Arterial blood pressure* measures the adequacy of compensatory vasoconstriction in tailoring the size of the vascular tree to the circulating blood volume, *central venous pressure* is a rough estimate of the adequacy of venous return to the heart, and the *cardiac rhythm, rate,* and *output* reflect the response of the pump to shock.

COMPENSATORY MECHANISMS

Many compensatory mechanisms cushion the magnitude and deleterious effect of the shock state. As we have seen, hypovolemia increases the serum catecholamines to produce vasoconstriction, which reduces the size of the vascular bed, elevates arterial pressure, shunts blood away from the capillaries and back to the veins, increases the venous return to the heart, and improves the pumping action of the heart. The circulating blood volume is replenished by two mechanisms: (1) a major shift of extracellular fluid into the vascular bed and (2) a retention of water and sodium by the kidney caused by a rise in antidiuretic hormone and aldosterone secretion. Hyperpnea rids the body of excess CO_2, and tachycardia circulates available blood more rapidly.

CLASSIFICATION

Shock may be classified in several ways. One of the simplest is on the basis of cause of the shock and is outlined as follows:

1. *Hypovolemic shock:* Hemorrhage, burns, trauma, intestinal obstruction, diarrhea, fractures, dehydration
2. *Septic shock:* Septicemia, endotoxemia, exotoxemia
3. *Cardiogenic shock:* Myocardial infarct, cardiac tamponade, cardiac arrhythmias
4. *Vasogenic shock:* Spinal anesthesia or trauma, anaphylaxis, arsenic poisoning, overdose of vasodilating agents
5. *Neurogenic shock:* Simple fainting

Hypovolemic shock occurs when there is a significant loss of circulating blood volume, extravascular fluid, or both. This is the most common type of shock seen in surgical practice and is characterized clinically by cold skin, tachycardia, lowered blood pressure, decreased central venous pressure, decreased urine flow, increased arterial blood lactate level, and decreased cardiac index. Whole blood loss may occur either externally by surface injury or internally into tissue planes such as occurs from crush injuries, pancreatitis, and peritonitis. Bleeding into the lumen of the gastrointestinal tract is another major cause of hypovolemic shock in the surgical patient. External blood loss is easy to recognize, quantitate, and treat, while internal bleeding or third space sequestration of fluid is frequently more difficult to quantitate and manage.

When the arterial blood pressure falls from any cause, the compensatory response is mediated primarily through the sympathetic nervous system by increasing peripheral resistance (arteriolar constriction) and increasing the cardiac output. In addition, venomotor tone is increased to deliver more blood from venous reservoirs into the circulation. The vessels of the heart and brain are not involved in arteriolar constriction and thus remain protected.

Additional endocrine responses occur such as the release of the antidiuretic hormone (ADH) and aldosterone, both of which act to retain salt and water. Renin is released from the juxtaglomerular apparatus in response to decreased pressure. This proteolytic enzyme forms angiotensin from plasma precursers, and after conversion to angiotensin 2, leads to increased production and release of aldosterone from the adrenal gland. When plasma-like fluid is the primary constituent of the blood that is sequestered in tissues injured by burn cellulitis or trauma, hemoconcentration occurs with a consequent increase in viscosity. Under these circumstances blood sludging occurs in the microcirculation with the added risk of intravascular coagulation. When whole blood is lost, the additional deleterious effect on the tissue of sludging does not occur because of subsequent hemodilution.

Septic shock

Septic shock has at least two distinctly different mechanisms for producing shock: (1) extensive cellulitis or diffuse infections of body cavities (peritonitis) sequester large amounts of plasma-like fluid into the injured tissue to produce hypovolemia (the so-called third-space loss) and (2) toxins produced by the infecting organisms exert profound effects upon circulation.

Septic shock may be produced by either gram-negative or gram-positive organisms. The most common cause is gram-negative organisms and is found most often in gynecological or urological patients. In contrast to hypovolemic shock, the patient with septic shock is usually warm, has pink extremities, and is in a moderate state of alkalosis. Cardiac output is increased and peripheral resistance is decreased. Circulating blood volume is usually normal or above normal, but oxygen utilization is maintained at a lower than normal level. This seems to indicate inability of the cell to utilize oxygen in septic shock. Many mechanisms have been studied with respect to this peculiar cellular paralysis and, of the systems studied, 2,3-DPG (diphosphoglycerate) is the most promising to explain the inefficient oxygen utilization by the cells.

Sepsis may produce profound shock, with a high mortality. Shock produced by gram-positive organisms tends to be less severe than that occasioned by gram-negative organisms. Often, septic and hypovolemic shock occur simultaneously to compound each other. However, it is clear that septic shock can occur alone, such as the shock occasionally provoked by instrumentation of the lower urinary tract with release of endotoxin from a small prostatic abscess or urinary tract infection. Endotoxin will occasionally produce an abnormal acceleration of the clotting process known as disseminated intravascular coagulation (DIC). When massive DIC causes consumption of platelets and fibrin, diffuse hemorrhage occurs. Under these circumstances, the patient may die of hypovolemic shock.

Cardiogenic shock

Cardiogenic shock occurs when there is inadequate cardiac output despite a normal blood volume. Many conditions may produce a fall in cardiac output. For example, the heart may not fill adequately because of pericardial tamponade, tension pneumothorax, or venocaval obstruction. The heart may not pump the circulating volume efficiently because of poor emptying of the chambers (atrial and ventricular arrythmias), sudden changes in myocardial conduction or contraction (myocardial infarction), or total cessation of heartbeat (cardiac arrest). Obviously, cardiac arrest always occurs as a terminal event in all forms of shock but only with a severe myocardial infarction is it the *primary cause of shock*. Pulmonary embolus may produce profound shock and presents classically with hemoptysis, dyspnea, cyanosis, and splinting of the chest. Only about one-third of these patients have demonstrable phlebitis.

Vasogenic shock

Vasogenic shock occurs when the vascular bed is suddenly expanded by generalized vasodilatation, thereby rendering a "normal" blood volume totally inadequate to fill the expanded vascular space. This type of shock is seen under a variety of clinical conditions, but as a result of two basic mechanisms: (1) interference with sympathetic autonomic activity (spinal cord injury caused by trauma or operation, spinal or epidural anesthesia, overdosage with antihypertensive and alpha receptor blocking drugs) and (2) rapid release of histamine into the blood (major antigen-antibody reaction, severe cellular anoxia occurring in the terminal stages of hypovolemic shock).

Neurogenic shock

Neurogenic shock is associated with simple syncope, and results from a sudden diminution of sympathetic autonomic activity by means of a reflex phenomenon that involves the central nervous system. The resulting vasodilatation enlarges the vascular bed to produce shock similar to the mechanism outlined under vasogenic shock. Simple syncope is triggered by unpleasant experiences, pain, and fright. Compensation is generally rapid, and the sequelae are not serious.

FUNCTIONAL DISTURBANCES OF SHOCK

No single classification of shock is universally satisfactory. The preceding classification is based on the cause or etiology of the shock state and is used because it is simple and based on clinical phenomena with which most of us are familiar. Recognition of the primary cause of shock allows the clinician to take effective action to halt the progress of shock and rapidly begin effective treatment.

In some cases, however, the cause of the shock is not readily apparent, and one must then recognize and treat the functional disturbances that occur as a result of the shock. Furthermore, many different causes of shock may act simultaneously, and again the functional derangements in circulation must be corrected.

As an example, the renal ischemia that occurs in many types of shock results in oliguria and ultimately in anuria if not reversed; renal circulation must be improved (volume replacement, vasodilators) to allow formation of urine. Acidosis associated with severe shock must be treated by buffers and alkaline fluids, regardless of the cause of shock. Shock caused by endotoxemia responds poorly to fluid and blood administration and requires appropriate antibiotic treatment and perhaps vasodilators. A heart that begins to fail because of the increased work load and tachycardia imposed by shock must be supported by inotropic drugs or digitalis. Vasoconstrictor drugs are dangerous when used to treat the hypotension of ordinary shock when maximum compensatory vasoconstriction already exists. Vasodilating drugs are then indicated, but only after correction of the body fluid deficit.

TREATMENT OF SHOCK
General principles

The goal of the treatment of shock is to restore normal cellular perfusion. Shock must first be recognized and a quick clinical assessment made of its degree of severity. The patient is placed at rest in bed in the Trendelenburg position, airway and adequate respiratory exchange are assured, and base line monitors of the vital signs are taken: temperature, pulse rate and volume, arterial blood pressure. A urethral catheter is inserted, and the hourly urine output is recorded. If the cause of the shock is readily apparent, one must then prevent its progression, if possible: control of bleeding, splinting of fractures, nasogastric suction, etc. Life-threatening aspects of shock must be controlled before any strenuous manipulations are carried out to determine the more exact and complex cause of shock.

If the cause is not apparent, the functional derangements imposed by the shock are assessed, and steps are taken to treat them appropriately: the efficiency of the heart pump is restored if necessary, the volume of circulating blood and extracellular fluid is replenished, peripheral vasomotor activity is evaluated, and the pH and viscosity of blood are restored to normal. The patient is observed frequently and carefully by the same person to note the response to treatment, to direct changes in therapy, and to detect complications of treatment. The goal of treatment is a patient who is alert and no longer complaining of thirst or air hunger, who has warm, pink, and dry skin with prompt capillary refill upon compression of the nail beds, and who is excreting satisfactory amounts of urine.

Specific measures

The physician must first be certain that the patient's heart is beating. Cardiac arrest is the inevitable end result of severe shock and must be treated by (1) establishing an adequate airway, (2) assisting respirations, and (3) beginning external cardiac massage. An emergency electrocardiogram distinguishes between ventricular fibrillation and asystole as cause of the arrest, the former being treated by electrical shock to defibrillate. Sodium bicarbonate buffer is given to correct acidosis, and finally cardiac stimulants are introduced intravenously or directly into the heart, if the preceding measures are unsatisfactory.

If the heartbeat is present but the pumping action is inefficient and sluggish, digitalis or inotropic agents are indicated. Distant heart tones with a large heart suggest pericardial tamponade, which is treated by needle aspiration of the blood or fluids sequestered within the pericardial sac.

Hypovolemia is next corrected by volume replacement, preferably of the volume and type of body fluids that have been lost. Large-bore needles or catheters are placed into two veins. Ideally, a catheter is advanced into either the superior or inferior vena cava to allow monitoring of central venous pressure. A specimen of the patient's blood is removed for immediate type and cross match. Until blood becomes available, fluid is infused in the form of saline, bicarbonate, Ringer's solution, plasma, or dextran, depending on the needs of the patient and the fluids available. The immediate effect of electrolyte solution in increasing blood volume is as good as that of coloid, although colloid (plasma or dextran) does remain in the vascular tree longer than electrolyte solution does. Low molecular weight dextran pulls in additional extracellular fluid into the vascular space and also decreases blood viscosity to improve sluggish capillary flow and discourage intravascular clotting. When blood becomes available, it is given to the point of restoring the red blood cell count to normal. Fluids in excess of this are often needed, but they are better supplied by electrolyte or dextran rather than additional blood.

If blood has been lost, a crude estimation of the amount of hemorrhage is helpful in estimating the replacement need. Mild blood loss of 10 to 15% of blood volume does not produce clinical signs of shock unless it has been lost rapidly, and replacement is often optional. However, shock will be produced by a 10% blood loss in the elderly or otherwise debilitated patient, and replacement is wise. With moderate blood loss of 20 to 30% of blood volume, clinical signs of shock appear, and a corresponding amount is replaced. After replacement of lost blood, additional amounts of electrolyte solution should be given to replenish the extracellular fluid that earlier had been drawn into the vascular space to compensate for lost blood. Fluids in addition to these estimated losses are necessary if the vascular space has been abnormally enlarged in response to poor tissue perfusion. Even a "normal" blood volume is inadequate to fill this enormous vascular space, and additional electrolyte solution is necessary to maintain adequate central venous pressure and venous return to the heart. During the recovery phase of shock, fluid in excess of the "normal" blood volume is excreted by diuresis.

The vasomotor status of the circulatory system must then be evaluated. Generally, compensatory vasoconstriction is found, which is known to decrease capillary flow and tissue perfusion. Therefore, after adequate volume replacement, vasodilating agents (phentolamine, phenoxybenzamine hydrochloride) may be used judiciously in an attempt to relax the precapillary sphincters and improve capillary perfusion. If vasodilators are given when the circulating blood volume is deficient and when maintenance of arterial blood pressure is dependent on vasoconstriction, a disastrous fall in arterial blood pressure will occur. However, if the vascular space is full and venous return to the pump is adequate, vasodilatation improves tissue perfusion and increases the efficiency of organ function. Vasoconstrictor drugs are indicated only when vasodilatation exists with a normal blood volume (absence of sympathetic autonomic function).

Intravascular coagulation occurs in severe stages of shock because of stagnation of excessively viscid and acid blood within capillaries, to which is frequently added hypercoagulability associated with trauma, red cell hemolysis, and bacterial toxins. This tendency is reduced by expanding blood volume, increasing flow rates through capillaries and veins, and reducing blood viscosity with drugs such as low molecular weight dextran. Acidosis is corrected by administration of bicarbonate, tromethamine (THAM), or lactated Ringer's solution.

Septic shock is treated with replacement of body fluids that have been sequestered in areas of cellulitis or peritonitis, if present. There is no drug to counteract the bacterial toxins, other than bactericidal antibiotics to remove the source of the toxins. Blood cultures are obtained, and broad-spectrum antibiotics are administered. These may need to be changed when the bacterial sensitivity studies become available. Obviously, surgical drainage or removal of the septic source is of paramount concern, if feasible. Vasodilators are useful in modifying the potent vasopressor effects of gram-negative endotoxemia, and severe acidosis also needs to be corrected. Body temperature should be monitored carefully in septic shock, cooling blankets often being necessary to reduce dangerous hyperthermia. The role of corticosteroids in septic shock is still debated but probably should be considered after all the preceding derangements have been corrected. Vasopressor drugs are contraindicated, except when fluid deficits have been replenished in patients known to have gram-positive sepsis.

Monitors and guideposts to adequate treatment

The *general appearance* of the patient is important in judging how appropriate and adequate the shock treatment has been. The mental status of the patient offers a crude indication of cerebral perfusion, the goal being an alert and communicative patient. The skin and mucous membranes should be pink and warm, and the skin should be dry and of a normal temperature. Capillary refill should be prompt, as evaluated by the speed with which the color returns to the nail beds after compression.

The *vital signs* (pulse, arterial blood pressure, and respiratory rate) are monitored frequently and preferably by the same techniques. A return toward normal of all these parameters indicates a favorable response to treatment.

Urinary output is one of the most valuable monitors of all during shock treatment. Hourly measurements of the urinary output are especially valuable in determining the rate of fluid replacement. This monitor is important enough to justify passing a urethral catheter into each patient who is seriously shocked. Hourly urine output should be as follows:

> 10 to 20 ml./hr. in an infant or child
> 30 to 50 ml./hr. in a normal adult
> 20 to 30 ml./hr. in the elderly

The urine specific gravity and pH are measured on each of the hourly specimens.

Venous pressure determinations are a useful guide to the rate of fluid volume replacement in shock. A crude estimation of venous pressure is made by observing the filling of the neck and extremity veins at various elevations from the heart. Far more accurate than this is the central venous pressure, which is measured with a catheter in the superior or inferior vena cava, where no valve dampens the pressure between the end of the catheter and the heart. Normal central venous pressure varies from 5 to 15 cm. of water. It is elevated by positive pressure respiration and the Valsalva maneuver. Most patients in shock initially have a low central venous pressure, which rises to normal with adequate replacement of fluid volumes. High central venous pressure indicates right heart failure, pulmonary venous obstruction (massive pulmonary embolus), left heart failure, pericardial tamponade, or excess fluid and blood administration. The correct cause must be determined, and appropriate efforts must be made to bring the venous pressure back to normal. The central venous pressure is not infallible, and foolish reliance cannot be placed on it. If the catheter slips, becomes misplaced, or the end comes to lie against the vein wall, the recorded pressure is misleading. This is especially likely when massive amounts of blood have been given through the catheter, requiring checks of position and placement periodically.

Left atrial pressure measurements with the Swan-Ganz catheter are a useful tool to guide volume replacement, since pressure in the left atrium is a more reliable index of blood volume than right atrial pressure.

Arterial blood gas studies are helpful in determining the degree of acidosis and the efficiency of respiration. A low blood pH in a severely shocked patient justifies treatment with a buffer solution such as sodium bicarbonate. High P_{CO_2} or low P_{O_2} indicate that respiratory assistance is needed.

Serum electrolyte determinations are often helpful, especially when the shock results from major body fluid losses, to aid in the choice of repair solutions (Chapter 3).

Serial hematocrit determinations are useful if the shock results from blood or body fluid loss. The hematocrit is normal immediately after blood loss and gradually decreases as extracellular fluid is drawn into the vascular space to replenish circulatory volume. The hematocrit of the bank blood is 35 to 37%, and in massive blood replacement the patient's hematocrit is limited to this level, Conversely, the hematocrit rises with plasma loss and falls back toward normal when extracellular fluid is drawn into the vascular tree, or is administered in therapy.

All of the preceding parameters are useful in judging the degree of shock and the response to treatment. None of them is used alone, and *total patient evaluation* is the most important single criterion in evaluating the response to therapy. Restoration of adequate tissue perfusion assures successful therapy.

CHAPTER 6

Surgical infections

WILLIAM C. BOYD

The importance of infection in the field of surgery is underscored by reports on nosocomial infections from the Communicable Disease Center. Nationwide surveys have shown the infection rate of hospitalized patients to be highest (7.5%) among university surgical services. A nosocomial rate of 7.5% represents 2 million infections per year at an estimated annual cost of $10 billion. The infection rate is lower in obstetrics-gynecology departments, and medical services usually boast the lowest infection rate. Studies have reported a gram-negative sepsis incidence of 1:1,000 hospital admissions with a mortality rate of 25%, resulting in approximately 79,000 deaths per year in the United States; by comparison, there are 40,000 deaths per year in the United States attributed to carcinoma of the colon. The problem is further emphasized if one realizes that each surgical wound infection costs approximately $7,000, based upon lengthened hospitalization, physician fees, medications, increased insurance rates, and time lost from employment. It is self-evident that understanding the causes and proper treatment of surgical infections is a worthwhile goal for every medical student. Lack of these basic cornerstones severely limits the surgeon's ability to render service and protect the patient's well-being.

"SURGICAL" VERSUS "MEDICAL" INFECTION

The term "surgical infection" generally implies certain basic differences from a "medical infection." Medical infections are characteristically monomicrobic infections that are diffuse and associated with little tissue reaction but a marked systemic response by the host. In contrast, surgical infections are usually polymicrobic and invasive, with rapid growth and spread of bacteria into surrounding tissues or systems. The host response is more likely local, is unlikely to resolve spontaneously, and if untreated results in suppuration, necrosis, gangrene, prolonged morbidity, and death. The treatment of surgical infections is based on excision or incision and drainage. Antimicrobial agents play an important but secondary role in treating surgical infections as compared to their use for medical infections.

PATHOPHYSIOLOGY OF INFECTION
General factors

Many factors influence the incidence of surgical infection. Microorganisms are ubiquitous and the host is technically always infected. Clinical infection is manifested by invasion of microorganisms. The balance between the host defense mechanisms and the microorganisms determines the degree of health. The most important host defense against infection is a properly functioning natural immune mechanism. Maintenance of intact skin, mucous membranes, and normal bacterial flora also defends against invasive infection. Passive immunity provides temporary host protection from certain infections.

Once microorganisms have penetrated the intact skin or mucous membrane, the major battle against infection is waged by the immune response and normal functioning leukocytes. Systemic diseases that weaken the normal host defense mechanisms include: leukemia, lymphomas and other malignancies, diabetes mellitus, Cushing's syndrome, dysgammaglobulinemia, and agammaglobulinemia. If the host has another major illness at the time of bacterial invasion (thermal burn, uremia, cardiovascular failure, malnutrition, major trauma) or is immunosuppressed, he is less able to withstand invasion. Remote infection at the time of operation favors development of a wound infection. These clinical settings reduce the effectiveness of the natural immune response. Stasis or obstruction to flow of material such as bile, urine, intestinal contents, and mucus all enhance the likelihood of infection.

Local factors

Local wound factors such as crushing or necrosis of tissue, hemorrhage, dead space, and foreign bodies affect the balance in favor of the microorganism. The size of the bacterial inoculum and the length of time the bacteria are in the wound relate directly to the incidence of wound infection. By definition, a wound is clinically infected if it contains more than 10^5 organisms per gram of tissue. The so-called golden period in which one may clean a wound to reduce its bacterial count and lessen the chance of infection is approximately 6 hours. The host defense mechanisms are maximally mobilized in 4 to 5 hours;

since invasion of the host has not yet started, careful cleansing of the wound reduces the size of the inoculum and forestalls infection. Foreign material in the wound (dirt, wood, cloth, and metal) also favors infection. Experimentally, clinical infection requires 7.6×10^6 staphylococcal organisms in the dermis of a normal host; however, addition of a foreign body such as silk suture reduces this number of organisms to less than 100. Reducing the size of the bacterial population and removing foreign material help avoid wound infection.

CLASSIFICATION OF INFECTION

There are several terms that describe different types of surgical infection. These will be discussed in a natural progression from the earliest entry by microorganisms to the subsequent severe invasive stages, which may lead to death if untreated.

Cellulitis, the earliest host response to invasion by microorganisms, is characterized by polymorphonuclear leukocyte infiltration, capillary dilatation, rapidly multiplying bacteria, increased capillary permeability, and edema. Clinical manifestations are pain intensified by motion, redness (erythema), heat, and edema. Many bacteria produce collagenases, hyaluronidases, proteinases, and leucocidins, which augment their ability to spread and multiply.

Suppuration is tissue liquefaction and results in abscess formation. An *abscess* is a collection of liquified tissue cells, bacteria, lymphocytes, polymorphonuclear leukocytes, and bacterial toxins. Furuncles, carbuncles, paronychias, and felons are special types of abscesses because of anatomical features and not pathophysiology. Bacteria often enter a lag growth phase when they are sequestered in an abscess cavity; this factor, coupled with poor access of circulating blood to the abscess, accounts for the inability of systemic antibiotics to eradicate abscesses. Proper treatment therefore must include surgical drainage.

Lymphangitis is produced by bacterial invasion of the lymphatic channels draining the local site of infection. It is characterized by tenderness and streaking erythema of the skin overlying the lymphatic channels leading from the site of infection to the regional lymph nodes. The reaction in the draining lymph nodes causes tenderness and swelling, referred to as *lymphadenitis.* This mechanism of bacterial spread is common to most infections. *Suppurative lymphadenitis* is an abscess in a lymph node.

Bacteremia represents the transient appearance of bacteria in the bloodstream. This is clinically characterized by chills, rigors, and fever but may occur without clinical signs or symptoms. Blood cultures are required to diagnose the offending organism and should be obtained at the time of the chill, which corresponds to the bacteremia, rather than the fever spike, which follows their appearance.

Septicemia is a clinical syndrome caused by the continual presence of bacteria and/or their toxins in the bloodstream rather than the transient appearance of bacteria. Clinically, it is commonly associated with hypotension, tachycardia, low urinary output, fluid retention, and deterioration of respiratory function.

Pyemia is pus in the bloodstream and is usually fatal.

Each of these processes may be caused by a variety of organisms. Diagnosis is incomplete without identifying the offending organism. Gram-negative organisms have caused the majority of the severe surgical infections during the last decade, but optimal treatment demands *precise* identification of the organism.

In addition to these common mechanisms of surgical infections, there are specific infections that demand special mention.

INFECTIONS OF SPECIAL INTEREST

Chronic progressive cutaneous gangrene (Fig. 6-1, *A* and *B*), Meleny's ulcer, results from the combined growth of microaerophilic nonhemolytic *Streptococcus* and *Staphylococcus* organisms. This infection is characterized by an advancing border of erythema with a purplish rolled edge surrounding a zone of central necrosis and ulceration. Treatment of choice is excision of the ulcer and surrounding necrotic border plus administration of systemic penicillinase-resistant penicillin or vancomycin. An antibiotic for gram-negative organisms is often included, since *Proteus* organisms are frequently cultured from the ulcer.

Tetanus is caused by the obligatory anaerobic organism *Clostridium tetani*. The disease is 100% preventable if the host has been properly immunized with tetanus toxoid. In spite of this fact, over 100 people in the United States die each year because they lack proper immunization.

Clostridium tetani organisms are present in the soil and the feces of both wild and domesticated animals. Only rarely is it found in the feces of man. Its hardy spores frequently gain access to contaminated traumatic or surgical wounds, where they may germinate and produce the potent neurotoxin that causes tetanus. The incubation period in the human is usually between 6 and 10 days; there is an inverse relationship between the severity of the disease and the length of incubation. The organism requires a strict anaerobic environment to grow and produce its neurotoxin. There is no specific diagnostic test for the disease; diagnosis is made on clinical grounds with occasional recovery of large gram-positive rods on Gram stain from the wound.

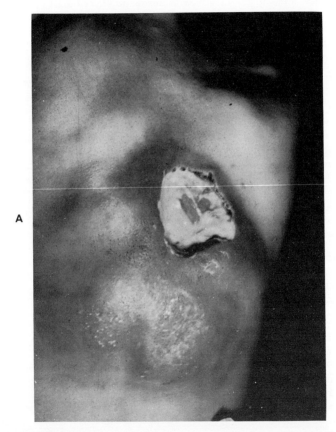

A

Fig. 6-1. Chronic progressive subcutaneous gangrene in area of right scapula. **A,** Note obvious swelling with discoloration and central necrosis at 5 days after onset. **B,** Much more extensive gangrene extending deeply into soft tissues 14 days after onset.

The onset of trismus (spasm of the masseter muscles) is the usual presenting sign, followed by spasm of other skeletal muscles. Generalized convulsions herald a grave prognosis.

Although tetanus is usually associated with major trauma, tissue necrosis, and devitalized tissue, a simple wound may allow entry of the organism. If by secondary infection and local conditions the proper anaerobic conditions are met, the organism will proliferate and produce its neurotoxin.

A patient previously immunized with tetanus toxoid requires a booster dose only every 10 years to maintain immunity; however, if he receives open, penetrating trauma the booster should always be given at that time. Patients with a tetanus-prone wound who have not been previously immunized should receive human hyperimmune globulin to induce temporary passive immunity. Presently, the recommended dose is 500 units, but the exact amount required is under review. The patient should also receive 0.5 cc. of tetanus toxoid given via a dif-

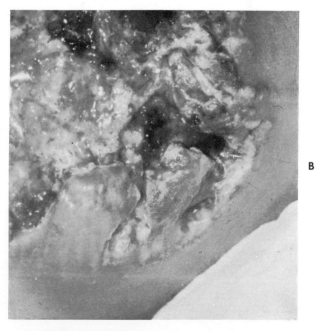

B

Fig. 6-1, cont'd. For legend see opposite page.

ferent syringe into a different intramuscular site, and be instructed to complete the series of three toxoid injections required for proper active immunization. Horse tetanus antiserum is of historical interest only and is no longer used.

Patients with tetanus should have the site of infection excised or widely drained to eliminate the anaerobic conditions. High doses of penicillin are given as the drug of choice against any residual *Clostridia* organisms. Good supportive care is vital in managing these patients. Poor respiratory toilet with atelectasis, aspiration, and pneumonia is a common cause of death. Prevention of respiratory complications is best achieved by tracheostomy and good pulmonary toilet. Muscle spasms and convulsions are controlled with pharmacological agents, primarily intravenous valium. Patients who are severely ill may require curare, respirator support, and sedation with barbiturates.

Although reduction of external stimuli is desirable, sequestering tetanus patients in a dark room is not required. Successful care can be provided in well-staffed intensive care units. Death from tetanus is usually secondary to pulmonary complications of pneumonia or suffocation. Mortality from tetanus remains 50% despite intensive supportive care. Patients who recover from the clinical disease but were not previously immunized should also undergo immunization, since having the disease does not confer immunity.

Gas gangrene is more properly known as "anaerobic myonecrosis." It is an anaerobic infection of muscle characterized by marked local edema, massive death of tissue, profound toxemia, and a variable amount of gas production.

The causative agent is of the genus *Clostridium: Clostridium perfringens* (most common), *C. novyi, C. septicum, C. bifermentans, C. histolyticum,* and *C. fallax.* Clostridia are gram-positive, spore-forming rods that have very fastidious growth requirements. They are primarily saprophytic organisms with very low invasiveness. Although often cultured from an open wound, they will not germinate and produce toxins unless there are strict anaerobic conditions. These organisms are ubiquitous and common in soil and the gastrointestinal tract of man and animals.

The Clostridia species responsible for gas gangrene produce twelve different toxins which are used in their identification. The more important toxins are lecithinase, collagenase, hyaluronidase, and fibrinolysin.

The disease is diagnosed on clinical grounds rather than by laboratory tests. The classical clinical picture is characterized by acute onset (after incubation of 6 hours to 3 days) of severe local wound pain, tachycardia, tachypnea, and hypotension. Some fever is usual, but not in proportion to the other findings.

The histopathological picture is one of invasion and destruction of viable muscle. Destruction of white blood cells by leucocidins accounts for notable absence of polymorphonuclear cells microscopically in gas gangrene. The wound exudes a sweet mousy-smelling serosanguineous to clear fluid, and the overlying skin is tense and white to bronze colored.

Wounds that are predisposed to gas gangrene are those contaminated with foreign material (soil, clothing, metal) or that have devitalized tissue from arterial injuries or tight casts or dressings. Thorough wound debridement is the cornerstone in preventing and treating the disease. Antibiotics (penicillin and chloromycetin) play a minor role in controlling other bacteria and will kill *Clostridia*, but are not curative. In contrast to *Clostridium tetani*, there is no effective antitoxin or antiserum available for treating gas gangrene.

The introduction of hyperbaric oxygen therapy for gas gangrene by Borema has increased survival of these patients. The patient is placed in a hyperbaric chamber and the oxygen is delivered at 3 atmospheres pressure for one to eight treatments of 30 minutes each. Wound debridement is then performed on a nontoxic patient.

Surgical treatment relies upon removal of all involved muscle and tissue, converting the wound to aerobic conditions free of necrotic tissue. Gas gangrene treated under optimum conditions still carries a 22% mortality.

Ecthyma gangrenosum is caused by emboli of *Pseudomonas aeruginosa*. This disease is most commonly seen in severely debilitated patients. The lesion is characterized by a black necrotic area appearing in normal skin or wounds. Treatment consists of high doses of carbenicillin and/or gentamycin and in some cases excision of the lesions. Even with vigorous therapy survival is uncommon (Fig. 6-2).

Bites, both human and animal, pose special problems. Human bites are notoriously dirty, contaminated wounds containing a multitude of organisms. Anaerobic nonhemolytic *Streptococcus, Bacteroides,* as well as spirochetes and *Staphylococcus* lead the list in frequency. Thorough cleaning and delayed closure of the wound plus antibiotics constitute proper treatment.

By comparison, animal bites are relatively clean wounds, the major contaminant being *Pasteurella multocida,* which is sensitive to penicillin. Animal bites should also be carefully cleaned and debrided and wound closure delayed. Tetanus prophylaxis should be instituted in all wounds of trauma, particularly bites.

Rabies is of special concern following animal bites. If possible, the offending animal should be quarantined by a veterinarian. If the risk of rabies is low, then a course of vaccine is begun after local care of the wound, and continued until the fate of the animal is known. Both

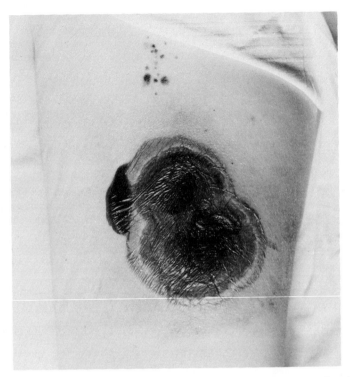

Fig. 6-2. Ecthyma gangrenosum diagnostic of *Pseudomonas* septicemia.

the rabies vaccine and antirabies serum should be given in high-risk cases or if the bite occurred from an unmolested wild animal. Dogs, skunks, and bats are numerically the most common sources of rabies in North America (Table 6-1).

FUNGAL INFECTIONS

Fungal infections recently have entered the sphere of surgical infections. The large numbers of immunosuppressed patients, longer survival among thermal burn patients, and increased use of powerful broad-spectrum antibiotics have all contributed to an increased incidence of fungal infections. The more commonly encountered fungi are *Actinomyces bovis, Candida albicans, Nocardia asteroides,* blastomycosis, aspergillosis, and sporotrichosis.

Table 6-1. Guide for postexposure antirabies prophylaxis*

Biting animal		Treatment		
		Exposure		
Species	Status at time of attack	No lesion	Mild†	Severe‡
Dog or cat	Healthy	None	None[1]	S[1]
	Signs suggestive of rabies	None	V[2]	S + V[2]
	Escaped or unknown	None	V	S + V
	Rabid	None	S + V	S + V
Skunk, fox, raccoon, coyote, bat	Regard as rabid in unprovoked attack	None	S + V	S + V

Code: V = Rabies vaccine (duck embryo).
  S = Antirabies serum.§
  1 = Begin vaccine at first sign of rabies in biting dog or cat during holding period (preferably 7 to 10 days).
  2 = Discontinue vaccine if biting dog or cat is healthy 5 days after exposure, or if acceptable laboratory negativity has been demonstrated in animal killed at time of attack; if observed animal dies after 5 days and brain is positive, resume treatment.

*The recommendations in this table are intended only as a guide; they may be modified according to knowledge of the species of biting animal and circumstances surrounding the biting incident.

†Scratches, lacerations, or single bites on areas of the body other than the head, face, neck, hands, or fingers; open wounds, such as abrasions, that are suspected of being contaminated with saliva also belong in this category.

‡Multiple or deep puncture wounds, and any bites on the head, face, neck, hands, or fingers.

§If antirabies serum is indicated, a portion of the total dose should be infiltrated thoroughly around the wound; as in all instances in which horse serum is used, a careful history should be taken and tests for hypersensitivity performed.

From Public Health Service Advisory Committee, Morbidity and mortality weekly report, May 13, 1967, pp. 152-155.

There are three major clinical types of *actinomycosis:* cervicofacial, thoracic, and abdominal. The infection is characterized by nodular or granulomatous areas that break down and suppurate, discharging pus through sinus tracts. Diagnosis may tentatively be made by a Gram stain showing "sulfur granules," which are masses of mycelia. Treatment of actinomycosis is long-term, high-dose penicillin and, when appropriate, surgical excision and drainage (Fig. 6-3).

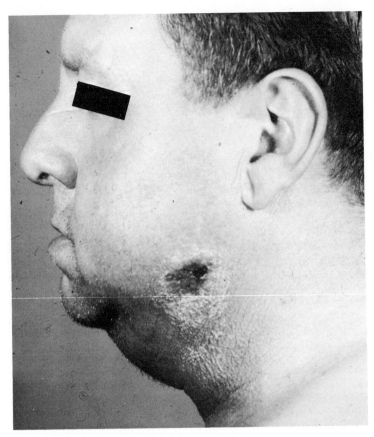

Fig. 6-3. Actinomycosis of the jaw.

Candidiasis is an opportunistic yeast infection caused by *Candida albicans. Candida* organisms are commonly found in the vagina, alimentary tract, and urine of debilitated patients, and have become an increasingly frequent problem in burn patients. Oral candidiasis (thrush) and superinfection of the gastrointestinal tract with *Candida* is frequent after long-term, broad-spectrum antibiotic therapy. Drugs used in treating candidiasis are nystatin, 5-fluorocytosine, and amphotericin B (Fig. 6-4).

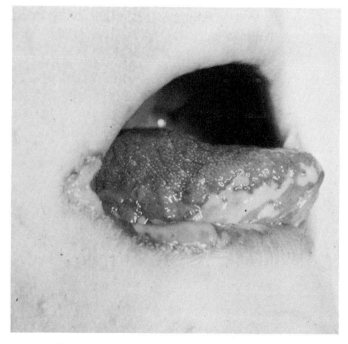

Fig. 6-4. Superinfection with *Candida albicans.*

Nocardia asteroides is an aerobic, gram-positive, partially acid-fast fungus that affects the respiratory and central nervous systems. It is frequently seen in transplant patients on immunosuppression, causing cavitary lesions of the lung. Treatment consists of administration of sulfonamides plus surgical drainage, when feasible.

Blastomycosis is a chronic granulomatous, suppurative disease that originates as a respiratory infection and disseminates with pulmonary, osseus, and cutaneous involvement. The possibility of direct cutaneous implantation of the organisms has not been resolved. The causitive agent is usually *Blastomycosis dermatitidis.* The cutaneous lesion is characterized by an ulcerated or verrucose granuloma with a serpiginous advancing border elevated 1 to 3 mm. This lesion may be confused with basal cell carcinoma. Diagnosis is made by culture and demonstration of budding yeast in a KOH slide mount. Treatment includes administration of stilbamidine, 2-hydroxystilbamidine, or amphotericin B.

Aspergillosis is a granulomatous, necrotizing, cavitary disease of the lungs, often with hematogenous spread to other organisms. The lung lesion is referred to as a "fungus ball" and may be associated with massive bleeding. As with most fungus infections, treatment of aspergillosis is difficult, but the best results are obtained with surgery and 5-fluorocytosine or amphotericin B.

Sporotrichosis, caused by *Sporotrichum schenckii,* is a chronic subcutaneous lymphatic mycosis that may remain localized for months, only to become generalized involving bones, joints, lungs, and the central nervous system. It is commonly contracted by puncture wounds with thorns or splinters and is not uncommon among rose gardeners. The typical lesion is characterized by an ulcer at the tip of a finger with an associated chain of swollen lymph nodes extending up the arm. Treatment with oral saturated solution of potassium iodine is usually very successful. Amphotericin B is used in resistant cases or in patients who do not tolerate iodides.

FEVER OF UNKNOWN ORIGIN

Fever of unknown origin may be defined as one which persists for more than 3 weeks and is undiagnosed after extensive medical evaluation. The surgeon's dilemma revolves around how to deal with this situation. There are certain steps that should be taken in evaluating a fever of unknown origin.

The first and most important step is a complete, thorough physical examination with special attention given to the ears, nose, throat, lungs, and abdomen; such examination often reveals the source of fever. Masses in the abdomen must be evaluated regarding possible abscesses.

Laboratory studies such as CBC with differential, erythrocyte sedimentation rate, urinalysis, sputum culture, and chest x-rays are often helpful. A Gram stain of fluids collected may be of great help in diagnosis before culture reports are available.

Drugs as a cause of the fever must always be evaluated. Antibiotics themselves have been incriminated, including penicillins, sulfonamides, streptomycin, gentamycin, tetracycline, vancomycin, and nitrofurantoin. Tuberculosis is evaluated by history of contact and skin testing with intermediate strength PPD. One should also maintain a high index of suspicion that occult malignancy may be responsible for the fever.

The final question that requires consideration when other causes are excluded is whether the fever is real or factitious. Factitious fevers require very tactful investigation on the part of the surgeon and the nursing personnel.

If after careful and complete evaluation the cause of the fever is still unknown, exploratory laparotomy should be considered. Complete exploration of the abdominal cavity with biopsy of the liver, lymph nodes, and removal of the spleen and occasionally the gallbladder provide material help in diagnosing 70% of cases. Removal of the spleen remains a controversial subject but if there is any suggestion of enlargement or abnormality, it should be removed for pathological and bacteriological study. The same principles apply to the gallbladder.

Once an infectious cause for the fever is verified, the next question relates to its proper treatment. Gram stain of the specimens may guide early antibiotic treatment while awaiting culture and sensitivity reports. Proper gathering, labelling, and rapid transport of the specimens to the laboratory for culture are very important. The specimen should not be allowed to dry out. The original culture, unclouded by antibiotic therapy, provides the most reliable information. Anaerobic organisms may cause very serious infections, but if not cultured properly will not be detected by the laboratory.

TREATMENT OF SURGICAL INFECTIONS

Surgical infections, by definition, usually require some form of excision or drainage. Drainage must be adequate and dependent so that pus drains freely. Administration of antibiotics restores the well-being of the patient more quickly, after proper surgical care. Antibiotics do not rid the patient of all bacteria but only control the growth of selected organisms. Furthermore, antibiotics will not control an infection that has been improperly treated surgically.

In all types of illness, but particularly infection, maintaining the patient in a good nutritional status in positive nitrogen balance enhances recovery. This task is often of herculean proportions in seriously ill patients such as thermal burn patients. A patient with 50% total BSA burn may require 5,000 calories/day in order to maintain positive nitrogen balance.

Choice of antibiotics

There are two major clinical groups of antibiotics, those which are bacteriocidal and cause death of the organism, and those which are bacteriostatic and only inhibit further microbial growth. A bacteriostatic agent would not suffice in a patient lacking normal white blood cells and macrophages.

Because of the vast numbers of commercially available antibiotic preparations, it is best to classify them by their mode of action: (1) those which interfere with cell wall synthesis—penicillins including penicillinase-resistant penicillins, cephalosporins, bacitracin, vancomycin; (2) those which interfere with protein synthesis—tetracyclines, chloramphenicol, erythromycin, lincomycin, clindamycin, kanamycin, gentamycin, streptomycin, neomycin; and (3) those which interfere with the cell membrane—polymyxin B, colistin, amphotericin B, and nystatin.

From this list of antimicrobial agents the following guidelines help in choosing the best agent. (1) The best antibiotic is one with the narrowest spectrum and least toxicity to the host. This requires accurate

Table 6-2. Antibiotics for serious infections requiring intravenous therapy*

	Total daily dose	Interval between doses (hrs.)	S. viridans	S. pyogenes (group A or B)	Enterococci	Pneumococci	S. aureus penicillinase (−)	S. aureus penicillinase (+)	N. meningitidis
Penicillin G	10-20x10⁶ mU	4	1	1		1	1		1
Ampicillin	12 gm.	4			1				
Oxacillin	8-10 gm.	6						1	
Carbinicillin	24-40 gm.	4							
Cephalothin	8-12 gm.	4	2	2	3	2	2	2	3
Erythromycin	2-4 gm.	6	3	3		3	3	3	3
Lincomycin	4-8 gm.	6	3	3		3	3	3	
Clindamycin	2-5 gm.	6-8							
Tetracycline	2 gm.	6							3
Chloramphenicol	50 mg./kg.	6							2
Kanamycin	15 mg./kg.	8-12							
Gentamicin	3-6 mg./kg.	8							
Polymyxin B+	2.5-3 mg./kg.	12							
Amphotericin	40-70 mg.	24-48							
Vancomycin	2 gm.	6			2			3	

*1 = first choice; 2 = second choice; 3 = third choice. Dosage based on function is abnormal. In several instances either of two agents is equally
†Colistimethate may be used at dose 5 mg./kg.
‡Both agents should be used.

culture and sensitivity testing. (2) For maximum benefit, the antibiotic should be present in the tissue before the bacteria arrive. This means that administration of antibiotics should be begun 3 to 4 hours prior to contamination, when possible. (3) The antibiotic agent should be given long enough and in high enough doses to allow the natural host defense mechanisms to return the host to a healthy state. (4) Antibiotics will not cure improperly treated surgical infections. (5) After treatment is well under way, repeat cultures help ascertain if the bac-

E. coli—domiciliary	E. coli—hospital acquired	Klebsiella	Klebsiella—hospital acquired	Enterobacter	Serratia	P. mirabilis	Indole-positive Proteus	Pseudomonas	Bacteroides	Haemophilus	Salmonella	Mima-Herellea	Clostridium	Candida
													1	1
1						1				1	1			
				1	2									
1	1	1	2			2	1	1†		3			2	
													2	
									2					
									2				3	
									1	2	2			
2	2		2	2	2	3	3						1	
2	2		1	1	1	3	2	1‡					1	
			3	3				2					2	
														1

normal renal function. Table should be consulted to adjust dose if renal effective and offers equal toxic hazards.

teria present are still susceptible to the antibiotic being used. (6) Finally, an appropriate route of administration of the antibiotic must be chosen.

The best route of administration is the intravenous one; in most cases to deviate from this should be the exception rather than the rule. The patient in shock will not absorb intramuscular antibiotics and intravenous administration is mandatory. A patient with ileus or other malfunction of the gastrointestinal tract will not utilize oral antibiotics. Thermal burn patients are an exception to the aforementioned rule, topical antibiotics seeming to be the best route of administration for the burn wound. If the oral route is chosen, the rate of absorption from the gastrointestinal tract and the effect of gastric acid on the agent must be considered (Table 6-2).

Avoiding infection in the surgical patient remains the best policy and reduces the need to utilize the preceding information. The surgeon should be alert to certain high-risk situations that lead to infection. Plastic intravenous catheters are associated with an increased incidence of thrombophlebitis; intravenous sites should be changed every 48 hours and rarely should catheters be left in place longer than 72 hours. Foley catheters should be placed aseptically and connected to a closed drainage system to minimize cystitis and urinary tract infections. Tracheostomies must be cared for with sterile technique and tracheal suctioning performed with sterile catheters.

Preparation of the colon prior to elective surgery is commonly performed to lower the risk of postoperative infection. Many different methods have been used, the efficacy of each method being debatable. Reduction in the amount of stool and hence the number of bacteria present is common to all methods. One popular regimen has the patient eat a low residue diet for 3 days, shifting to clear liquids 24 to 48 hours prior to surgery. In addition, the patient is given a daily cathartic of either neoloid or castor oil. Many combinations of oral nonabsorbable antibiotics are used, one of the better being erythromycin and neomycin for 24 hours before operation.

Preoperative systemic antibiotics have reduced postoperative infection in high-risk patients. They should be started at least 6 hours prior to surgery in order to achieve good tissue levels, such as intravenously at 6 P.M., midnight, and 6 A.M. prior to operation. In trauma cases with suspected contamination from a perforated viscus, intravenous antibiotics begun preoperatively result in a lower incidence of infection than when they are begun intraoperatively or postoperatively.

Wound infections are minimized when tissues are cut rather than crushed, are handled gently, and good hemostasis is obtained. A minimum of foreign substances in the wound also reduces infection.

Infection continues to be one of the major causes of hospital morbidity and mortality in surgical patients in spite of many new and powerful antibiotic agents. Understanding the basic pathogenesis of infection is essential to the practice of surgery. Careful attention to surgical technique, avoiding undue contamination, and attention to indwelling catheters help minimize this problem.

CHAPTER 7

Total parenteral feeding

ROBERT T. SOPER
JOEL B. FREEMAN

Total intravenous feeding (parenteral hyperalimentation) is a technique of prolonged intravenous administration of all required proteins, calories, and essential minerals. A sterile hypertonic solution of the appropriate nutrients is delivered at a steady rate through catheters into a large vascular channel where blood flow is rapid. The solution is quickly diluted to isotonic concentration and disseminated throughout the body.

Total parenteral feeding is reserved for those occasions when the gastrointestinal tract should not or cannot be used for nutritional purposes. In general terms, then, this nutritional technique is employed in the already malnourished patient who cannot eat and in patients facing lengthy periods of starvation because of some medical or surgical problem that precludes gastrointestinal feedings.

Total parenteral feedings are different from the conventional parenteral fluids, which are discussed in Chapter 3. The latter provide body requirements for fluids, electrolytes, pH adjustments, and vitamins. They capably sustain most patients for short-term periods of starvation until they can eat again. However, conventional fluids lack proteins and are deficient in calories so that if the starvation period is lengthy enough, serious malnutrition ensues. It is for this small group of patients that parenteral hyperalimentation has become an important and occasionally life-saving therapeutic modality.

INADEQUACIES OF CONVENTIONAL PARENTERAL FEEDING

Conventional parenteral fluids contain no protein; since the daily requirements for protein average about 2.5 Gm./kg. in young children and 1 Gm./kg. in adults, a negative balance of this magnitude accrues each day. Parenteral fluids contain inadequate calories. With intestinal alimentation, calories are ingested as carbohydrate and fat. When there are inadequate calories, body protein breakdown is further accelerated. Let us examine how the calorie-poor conventional parenteral fluids produce severe caloric deficiencies.

Fig. 7-1 graphically presents a method for estimating maintenance body fluid and caloric requirements based on body weight. For each of the first 10 kg. of body weight, maintenance fluid and caloric requirements per day are roughly 100 ml. and 100 calories (kilocalories, or large calories) per kilogram, respectively. For the second 10 kg. of body weight, or from 10 to 20 kg., the daily requirements drop to about 50 ml. and 50 calories/kg. For body weight in excess of 20 kg., the maintenance requirements are roughly 20 ml. and 20 calories/kg./day.

Thus, a baby weighing 5 kg. needs 500 ml. of fluid and 500 calories per day for maintenance purposes. Likewise, a youngster weighing 15 kg. requires 1,250 ml. and 1,250 calories each day (1,000 ml. and calories for the first 10 kg., and 50 × 5 = 250 ml. and calories for the next 5 kg. of body weight). The 70 kg. prototype adult requires 2,500 ml. and 2,500 calories each day for maintenance purposes (1,000 ml. and calories for the first 10 kg. of weight, 500 ml. and calories for the second 10 kg. of weight, and 20 × 50 = 1,000 ml. and calories for the next 50 kg. of body weight).

Remember, the formula listed in Fig. 7-1 estimates only *maintenance* fluid and calorie requirements. Medical or surgical disease in-

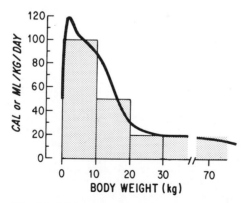

Fig. 7-1. Maintenance needs, caloric or fluid.

Table 7-1. Conventional parenteral feeding

Size (kg.)	Normal (cal./day)	Calorie (5% glucose)	Calorie deficit/day	Diseased (cal./day)	Calorie deficit/day
3	300	60	240	450	390
10	1,000	200	800	1,500	1,300
20	1,500	300	1,200	2,250	1,950
40	1,900	380	1,520	2,850	2,470
70	2,500	500	2,000	3,750	3,250

creases calorie requirements significantly above maintenance levels. However, fluid needs are unaltered unless the disease itself produces excessive fluid loss from diuresis, perspiration, hyperthermia, gastro-intestinal losses, etc. The exact increment of calorie requirements that disease imposes above maintenance varies with the type and severity of illness. A useful estimate is 50%.

Table 7-1 uses this estimate to calculate the daily caloric deficiencies accruing in sick patients of five different weights (and ages) from the 3 kg. newborn up to the 70 kg. prototype adult. This table reminds us how quickly serious caloric deficits occur in a sick patient nourished only by fluids containing 5% glucose (200 Kcal./L.) and no protein.

Thus, the 3 kg. prototype newborn requires 300 ml. of maintenance fluid each day (100 ml. × 3 kg. = 300 ml.). If 5% glucose is used, only 60 calories are delivered to the patient each day. Since normal daily requirements of this 3 kg. newborn are 300 calories, he is deficient 240 calories daily (300 − 60 = 240). However, if the calorie requirements are increased by 50% because of disease, the net daily calorie needs approach 450 calories. The fluid requirements are unchanged, so that still only 60 calories are delivered, the net caloric deficit rising to 390 calories per day (450 − 60 = 390 calories). Since the newborn has little subcutaneous fat or other nutritional reserve, he quickly becomes malnourished with a calorie deficit of this magnitude.

Referring again to Table 7-1, we see that the 10 kg. 18-month-old ill baby maintained on 5% dextrose suffers a daily calorie deficit of 1,300 calories. The 20 kg. 4-year-old has a net calorie deficit approaching 2,000 calories per day, and the 40 kg. school child accrues nearly a 2,500 calorie deficit each day. The 70 kg. adult is given only 500 calories per day when the 2,500 ml. fluid requirement is provided by 5% glucose. If the calorie requirements are increased to 3,750 calories per day because of disease, the individual suffers a daily deficit of 3,250 calories.

The maleffects of caloric deficits of this magnitude are proportionate to a number of variables: duration, current nutritional status, magnitude of the medical or surgical illness, etc. The tolerance is roughly inversely proportionate to age and size, the otherwise healthy adult tolerating a daily deficit of 3,250 calories better than the term newborn tolerates a 390 calorie deficit.

INDICATIONS FOR TOTAL PARENTERAL FEEDING

Parenteral hyperalimentation is indicated whenever it can be documented that a patient has consumed less than 50% of his caloric requirements for several days without any prospect for improvement or use of the intestinal tract. Parenteral hyperalimentation is not used in place of conventional parenteral fluids for the patient who is starved for only a short period of time, nor when the gastrointestinal tract can be satisfactorily utilized.

In the newborn, parenteral hyperalimentation is begun when the predicted starvation period is as short as 7 days, particularly if the patient is recovering from a major operative procedure or is premature. There are certain medical diseases in which lengthy periods of gastrointestinal rest are useful, such as prolonged diarrhea, disaccharidase deficiencies, protein-losing enteropathies, severe gastrointestinal allergies, or inflammatory bowel disease. However, the majority of diseases for which parenteral hyperalimentation is indicated fall within the realm of surgery and include patients who have had massive bowel resection, prolonged and multiple intestinal obstruction, gastroenteric fistulas, prolonged paralytic ileus, massive burns, wound dehiscence, etc.

The deleterious effects of a prolonged catabolic state briefly include decreased resistance to infection, poor healing of wounds (favoring dehiscence or hernia), tardy healing of intestinal anastomoses (leading to leaks and fistulas), weight loss, anemia, muscle wasting, retarded growth and development, generalized edema, and even central nervous system affects such as apathy and depression. Parenteral hyperalimentation prevents these sequelae of prolonged starvation.

The formula

A normal diet in man consists of protein, which is used for synthesis of new body tissues, and carbohydrate and fat, which are used for energy purposes. When calories are inadequately provided, body protein is broken down and the constituent amino acids are converted to glucose (gluconeogenesis). During this process, nitrogen is released and excreted in the urine. Therefore, measuring the amount of nitrogen administered and the nitrogen excreted in urine (and feces) gives

Table 7-2. Parenteral feeding mixtures

	Concentration	Calorie/kg./day	
Dextrose	25%	120	} 129
Fibrin hydrolysate	2%	9	
Dextrose	20%	96	
Fibrin hydrolysate	2%	9	} 118
Alcohol	2%	13	
Dextrose	17.5%	84	
Fibrin hydrolysate	2.5%	12	} 123
Lipid	2.5%	27	

one a reasonable estimate of the anabolic or catabolic status of the body physiology (nitrogen balance).

Although energy requirements may be met by either proteins or carbohydrates, body tissue may be repleted only by protein. There is no enzymatic pathway for conversion of glucose into tissue protein. Conversely, if protein solutions are administered intravenously but energy requirements are not met, the body will selectively use the administered protein for energy requirements rather than buildup of new tissues. Hence all intravenous nutrition formulas are constituted so that each gram of nitrogen (16% of protein) is accompanied by at least 150 non-protein calories as dextrose, alcohol, or fat. These calories permit the amino acids to be used for tissue synthesis rather than gluconeogenesis.

Table 7-2 lists the calorie-producing ingredients of three total parenteral feeding mixtures. They all contain hypertonic glucose and protein and about the same number of calories per unit of volume. The best calorie provider of all the nutrients is fat, containing 9 calories/ Gm. Regrettably, there is no intravenous fat preparation that has Food and Drug Administration clearance in the United States and so lipid cannot be incorporated into our formulas.* In England, Canada, and Europe, however, the product Intralipid has been safely used for at least 15 years and may ultimately pass FDA clearance in the United States. Intralipid derives its fat from soybean oil and is tolerated very well for lengthy periods of time even when administered by peripheral vein. When Intralipid is used, the concentration of glucose may be reduced and therefore urinary losses are less problematic. Alcohol also contains more calories than glucose (7 calories/Gm.) and is used in certain parenteral hyperalimentation formulas. Its primary disadvantage lies in its potential hepatotoxicity.

*Intralipid was approved for use in the United States by the Food and Drug Administration in November, 1975.

Table 7-3. Parenteral feeding formula

Protein hydrolysate or pure amino acids 5%			200 ml.
Dextrose 50%			160 ml.
Distilled water			40 ml.
Contents			0.9 calories and 25 mg. amino acids/ml.
Calorie: nitrogen ratio			225:1
Electrolytes			
NaCl	30 mEq./L.	Ca	500 mg./L.
KHPO₄	20 mEq./L.	Mg	50 mg./L.
Heparin			1,000 units/L.
Multiple vitamin infusion			3-5 ml. (daily)
Vitamin K₁			10 mg. (weekly)
Folic acid			15 mg. (weekly)
Vitamin B₁₂			100 μg. (weekly)
Iron (by deep intramuscular injection)			When indicated by low serum iron

Table 7-3 contains the formula for the parenteral feeding solution used at The University of Iowa Hospitals. Hypertonic glucose and amino acids provide the calories. The five electrolytes are routinely added with a certain amount of day-to-day variation to meet individual patient needs. At least eight additional trace elements are given when lengthy periods of parenteral hyperalimentation are required. A dilute heparin concentration discourages clotting around the catheter. A broad spectrum of fat- and water-soluble vitamins completes the list.

Note that the formula delivers to the patient 1 calorie/ml. and about 25 mg. of amino acids/ml., which are satisfactory amounts for normal growth and development. It is believed that essential fatty acid and trace metal deficiencies are prevented by administering small plasma transfusions once or twice weekly. The formula is made up daily by the hospital pharmacy in a laminar airflow hood under the strictest aseptic conditions. An aliquot of each mixture is cultured to prove its sterility before being released to the ward. The shelf life of this mixture is short, so that each day's supply is manufactured shortly before it is used. Commercial preparations of parenteral hyperalimentation formulas are now on the market but these must still be mixed shortly before use because of the short shelf life.

The delivery system

Because all parenteral hyperalimentation formulas are hypertonic compared to serum, they must be delivered into a high-flow part of the vascular system for rapid dilution and to prevent endothelial damage and thrombosis. The superior vena cava is admirably suited for this purpose. The inferior vena cava has been used, but problems of sterility and immobilization of the catheter in the groin make it much less desirable.

In the school child and older patient, the catheter is introduced into the subclavian vein percutaneously from just below the clavicle and the catheter is threaded easily into the superior vena cava. However, in the infant and younger child, it is safer to insert the catheter by a surgical cutdown into either the external jugular vein or a branch of the internal jugular vein (Fig. 7-2). Accurate placement of the tip of the catheter into the superior vena cava must be confirmed either by cinefluoroscopy or roentgen-ray examination, since malplacement is common (and dangerous).

For sterility purposes, one should widely separate the point where the catheter penetrates the skin from where it enters the vein. In the infant and young child we tunnel the catheter subcutaneously to exit from the skin over the flat portion of the mastoid bone behind the ear. The head and neck must be shaved and prepared as though for an operation, and the entire procedure is generally carried out in the operating room.

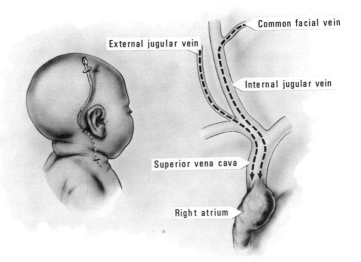

Fig. 7-2. Insertion of delivery-system catheter into external or internal jugular vein in infant.

We prefer an intravenous catheter constructed of Silastic impregnated with silver, so that the catheter is radiopaque. Silastic is much softer than the conventional plastic catheters. It is nonirritating and nonreactive, and can lie in the venous system for years without provoking phlebitis. The catheter is anchored by a suture (preferably nylon) both at the point where it penetrates the vein and at skin level so as to discourage inadvertent removal.

The entire system, including the intravenous tubing from the formula bottle to the Silastic catheter, is changed daily and must be maintained as a completely closed system. Under no condition should the intravenous line be broken for drawing blood, administering other intravenous fluids, or determining central venous pressure. A small sterile dressing covers the Silastic catheter where it exits from the skin. This dressing is changed three times weekly by specially trained nurses; the skin is defatted with acetone and cleaned with an appropriate antiseptic, and Betadine ointment is placed over the entire area.

It is of paramount importance that the formula be administered at a constant hourly rate over each 24-hour period. A gravity drip will suffice if monitored closely by skilled personnel. When the volume is critical, as in pediatric patients, constant flow rates are more readily achieved by incorporating a small variable speed infusion pump into the system. We use Millipore filters (with a diameter of 0.22 μ) only when infusion pumps are used and specifically to prevent air embolism.

SPECIAL CONSIDERATIONS OF PARENTERAL HYPERALIMENTATION

During the first few days of hyperosmolar intravenous feeding, amino acids and sugar are commonly lost in the urine, hence posing the threat of osmotic diuresis and dehydration. This is combatted by using a half-strength solution the first day, a three-fourths solution the second day, and then the full-strength parenteral hyperalimentation formula the third day. Frequent examinations of the urine for sugar provide guidelines for administering exogenous insulin on a sliding scale so as to prevent serious hyperglycemia and glycosuria. After several days of parenteral hyperalimentation, endogenous insulin production increases so that blood and urine sugars are maintained within normal limits. Hence it is dangerous to administer insulin routinely without regard for the urinary and blood sugar values. By the same token, the hyperalimentation infusion must never be abruptly discontinued or hypoglycemia will ensue.

When parenteral hyperalimentation is first started, the body weight, fluid balance, serum electrolytes, and blood and urine sugar and osmolality are monitored daily. After the patient is stabilized on parenteral hyperalimentation, only weekly checks are generally necessary for proper monitoring although urine sugars must be monitored four times daily until therapy is discontinued. During parenteral nutrition the body is in an anabolic state and potassium requirements are often increased above maintenance. Potassium, like nitrogen, is incorporated intracellularly and is usually given in direct ratio to the amount of administered nitrogen (10 to 15 mEq./Gm. nitrogen).

As the patient recovers, oral feedings are begun and gradually increased as tolerated. Parenteral hyperalimentation is proportionately reduced in a stepwise manner. Once the patient resumes normal oral feedings equivalent to 50% of his caloric requirements, parenteral hyperalimentation is terminated.

Special problems

Thrombosis around the catheter has not occurred since we switched from plastic to Silastic catheters and added dilute heparin to the formula. Malplacement is avoided by roentgen-ray or fluoroscopic check. As long as the catheter is radiopaque, no dye need be injected to ascertain its position.

Septicemia is unquestionably the most serious complication of parenteral hyperalimentation. It occurs when any foreign body (catheter) dwells in the vascular system for lengthy periods of time, especially in debilitated patients who frequently have other sites of infection concomitant with their surgical problem. However, the rate of infection appears to be directly proportional to the care that is exercised during the initial placement and the subsequent day-to-day management of the catheter. Meticulous attention to detail and close daily scrutiny by trained personnel will keep the rate of infection to a minimum. Absoute sterility is also required during mixing of the formula.

With careful attention to these points, infection should not be a problem for the first 3 weeks and we have frequently been able to avoid infection with a single catheter in place for a period of 3 months. Ultimately, however, infection will occur with lengthy superior vena cava catheterization. Sepsis which occurs under these circumstances is often caused by bizarre organisms such as fungi and yeast or by skin bacteria which are not usually considered to be pathogenic.

At the first sign of infection (unexplained temperature, leukocytosis, hyperglycemia, or simply an unexpected deterioration of the patient's general condition) the parenteral feeding catheter is withdrawn and its tip cultured. Serial blood cultures direct appropriate antibiotic treatment. The patient's general condition is carefully assessed for possible infection elsewhere. After treatment of septicemia is begun, the catheter can be replaced in another vein within 48 to 72 hours.

CONCLUSION

Parenteral hyperalimentation is a very useful and sometimes life-saving technique to prevent or treat serious malnutrition in patients whose medical or surgical illness precludes enteral feeding. There is objective evidence of nutritional improvement in the form of weight gain, wound healing, closure of intestinal fistulas, reversal of severe inflammatory gastrointestinal disorders, improvement in serum albumin concentration, etc. Gastrointestinal secretions virtually cease as the intestine is "put to rest." Many patients enjoy a general feeling of well-being. Blood-borne infection, the most dreaded complication of parenteral hyperalimentation, is minimized by strict attention to asepsis in the manufacture and delivery of the formula. It is no longer necessary for a patient to starve simply because he temporarily is unable to eat.

CHAPTER 8

Preoperative care

RICHARD D. LIECHTY

Judging precisely which patients will survive, or succumb to, any specific operations for a disease, or diseases, is impossible. The many obvious variables such as age, seriousness of the primary disease, and coexisting diseases, account for the intangible nature of risk in any operation. Healthy, good-risk patients have died after simple operations, and aged, poor-risk patients have eased through procedures of astonishing magnitude. Therefore, estimation of surgical risk is at best an educated guess based on past experiences. When asked to guarantee an operation (and this happens not infrequently), the experienced surgeon refuses to guarantee anything but his professional concern and competence. Sound surgical judgment, nevertheless, requires an estimation of surgical risk, especially in difficult cases when surgical risk must be cautiously weighed against any expected benefit from the operation. Important factors in surgical risk can be summed up as the kind of patient, the disease, and the treatment. This risk is in the form of the following equation:

$$\textit{The patient} + \textit{The disease} + \textit{The treatment} = \textit{Surgical risk}$$

THE PATIENT
Age

Prematurity and extreme old age are associated with increased operative risk. Little difference is seen, however, in operative mortality in the third decade as compared to the eighth decade with *brief procedures* that disturb physiological functions minimally, such as thyroidectomy or hernia repair; with operations of greater magnitude, involving increased physiological stress, the mortality is substantially greater in older patients. The mortality of combined abdomino-perineal resection, for example, rises strikingly with age. (For further discussion, see Chapter 29.)

Cardiopulmonary status

The following factors increase the operative risk in ascending order.

1. No cardiac disease
2. Hypertension
3. Angina infrequent with normal EKG
4. Angina frequent
5. Angina infrequent with abnormal EKG
6. Previous myocardial infarction, 2 years; asymptomatic
7. Previous myocardial infarction, 2 years; symptomatic
8. Recent myocardial infarction, 3 to 6 months
9. Associated pulmonary disease
10. Other heart disease—FC III and IV
11. Recent myocardial infarction, 3 months

Emergent or vitally necessary (cancer) operations in patients at severe risk demand extra caution. The surgeon and the anesthesiologist should enlist the cardiologist in caring for these patients. Cardiac drugs, pacemakers, continuous monitoring, careful blood replacement and oxygen therapy can save many lives.

Hypovolemia and anemia increase operative risk, especially in the aged. The old dictum "One should never give a single unit of blood" is fallacious, particularly in the aged patient with marginal perfusion of coronary and cerebral vessels.

Renal factors

Advanced renal insufficiency increases operative risk. Meticulous attention to fluid and electrolyte administration during the operative and postoperative periods in these patients can lessen the problem. (See Chapter 3.) The surgeon should correct all remedial renal diseases prior to elective operations. Renal dialysis can clear azotemia in advanced renal disease.

Hepatic factors

Jaundice and ascites may indicate severe liver disease. Unremitting, progressive jaundice signals a need for urgent remedial operation for the jaundice, if the jaundice is "surgical." The following factors increase surgical risk: albumin below 2.5 gm.%, bromsulphalein retention above 10%, and ascites unresponsive to medical treatment. (See Chapter 17.)

Endocrine system

Endocrine factors are discussed in the relevant chapters (7, 13, 14, and 15). *Diabetes* is a frequent complicating factor with many surgical problems. Uncontrolled diabetes is a distinct hazard that must be treated vigorously prior to induction of anesthesia.

Dehydration states

Varying states of simple desiccation, extracellular fluid loss, hemorrhage, or loss of specific electrolytes can appreciably affect operative risk. They are discussed at length in Chapter 3.

Nutritional status

As learned from experiences in prisoner-of-war camps, starvation in itself should not be a deterrent to necessary operations. Although severe protein depletion can impede wound healing, operations to correct protein deficiencies (total colectomy for ulcerative colitis) should proceed in the face of the disease, if the aim of the operation is to correct the source of the deficiency. Delay may be lethal. Vitamin K to correct prothrombin deficiencies and vitamin C to aid in wound healing in the depleted patients have, without question, been beneficial. Parenteral hyperalimentation has aided the preoperative preparation of these patients immensely (see Chapter 7).

Obesity increases operative risk in almost direct proportion to its severity. This increased hazard is most obvious in abdominal and pelvic operations. Operative time, septic complications, and cardiovascular and pulmonary complications are all increased with obesity.

THE DISEASE

The variability of the physical status of patients parallels the wide range of diseases that may afflict them. The nature of the disease (malignant or benign, infected or sterile), the physiological disturbances it causes, the site, and the length of time it has been present are all important factors affecting surgical risk.

With critical disorders (cancers or disease causing exsanguinating hemorrhage), consideration of surgical risk becomes a clear, hard question of life or death. When the alternative to operative treatment is so obvious, most surgeons (and patients) would choose an operation with even the slight probability of saving life as the hoped-for reward.

Malignant versus benign disease

Operations upon specific organs are, by and large, more hazardous for malignant than for benign diseases. A gastric operation for cancer, for example, carries a higher mortality than one for benign gastric ulcer. Operations for thyrotoxicosis are less hazardous than cancer operations on the thyroid gland.

Septic versus sterile disease

Septic diseases are more complicated, with a higher mortality, than are sterile or relatively sterile diseases. Perforated appendicitis has a higher mortality than early acute appendicitis. Septic cholecystitis is more often fatal than aseptic, uncomplicated cholecystitis.

Site of the disease

The site of the disease is an important determinant of surgical risk. Operative risk decreases in descending order in the following sites: heart, thoracic esophagus, brain, rectum, colon, stomach, and lung. The nature and extent of the disease is, of course, an important factor in each specific site.

The time factor

The greater the length of time the patient has had the disease, the poorer the operative risk. The increase in mortality with perforations from any source within the abdominal cavity is well known. Debilitating effects from cancer that has lurked undetected for long periods also increase surgical risk.

THE TREATMENT

Treatment strongly influences both the *patient* and the *disease*. This is the only one of the three factors of surgical risk over which the surgeon has much control. Discrimination based on wide knowledge of the patient's overall status and the disease that afflicts him keynotes successful management. After assessing the patient and the disease as completely as possible, the surgeon plans the operative treatment.

Magnitude of the operation

After restoration of the ill patient to as near normal as possible, the extent of the operation must be considered. One thought should be clearly in mind: *surgical risk increases with the magnitude of the procedure.* Blood loss, trauma to the patient, and operating time are all cofactors. Replacement of an intracardiac valve is obviously more hazardous than the comparatively simply mitral valvulotomy. Cholecystostomy is a shorter, simpler, and safer procedure than cholecystectomy for acute cholecystitis. A wide variety of other such examples illustrate the importance of surgical judgment. In choosing among whatever therapeutic options are possible, the surgeon must weigh this critical factor of surgical magnitude carefully. In most instances, decisions are relatively easy; in a few they are immensely difficult.

An additional important, but largely unassessable factor, is the skill of the surgeon and his team. What can be performed expeditiously with a well-trained team in a modern hospital may, unfortunately, become catastrophic under less favorable conditions.

Postoperative care

The quality of postoperative care is another important, yet variable, factor in operative risk. Experienced nursing personnel in intensive care units have reduced postoperative mortality more than any other factor. Their efficiency, skill, and dedication are more important than electronic monitors, suction and inhalation equipment, or any of the other mechanical devices that aid in the care of the postoperative patient. Their continued training is the responsibility of the surgeons who work with them.

• • •

Operative risk is an intangible yet invaluable and practical concept. The spectrum of variables inherent in the *patient,* the *disease,* and the *treatment* defy precise analysis. Eventually computers may help in assessing operative risk; at the present time valid statistical analyses of the many variables (to program a computer) exist only as research projects. Estimation of surgical risk must, as always, be based on experience, intuition, and a generous measure of common sense.

CHAPTER 9

Anesthesia

WILLIAM K. HAMILTON

This chapter is written with the idea that it is more important to present to the medical student concepts and principles than to clutter his mind with details and small bits of information. Inherent in such generalization are incompleteness and broad statements that suffer from lack of complete accuracy. This choice seems a preferable alternative to providing great detail that, although more complete, would probably be more inaccurate in a very short time.

The application of operative therapy to patients almost always provides a need for anesthesia of some type. The purpose of anesthesia is primarily amelioration of pain, but it has as associated important functions the relief of fear and anxiety. The simple relief of pain and the provision of comfort during an operation could easily be supplied by many means. Perhaps the easiest would be to accomplish unconsciousness with a blow on the head or administration of some very potent long-lasting potion. This obviously is not a satisfactory method. We must provide this anesthetic state by some means that is completely reversible and that involves a minimum of physiological or pharmacological trespass.

The provision of the anesthetic state, then, is easy; *regulation* and *control* are moderately complex and determine the success of the procedures.

Anesthesia at the time of surgery is obviously desirable; like many things that are desirable, it extracts a cost from the user. It must be considered as a comatose state produced by severe drug poisoning during which the patient is subjected to trauma, hemorrhage, starvation, and other abnormal conditions.

Anesthetic agents affect many functions of the body. Though we are unable to observe many of these, we do see some, and the most

111

important are considered as costs of anesthesia and the causes of anesthesia mortality and morbidity.

The most common and perhaps most severe cost of anesthesia is that of *respiratory inadequacy,* which occurs from one or any combination of three basic factors. The first is *airway obstruction.* The airway, which should be considered as the air passages extending from the lips and nares to the alveolar surfaces, is easily obstructed in unconscious patients. Many of the activities that we undertake in the awake state, such as movement, coughing, deep breathing, yawning, and sighing, serve to maintain clear airways. Glands in respiratory mucosa keep secretions from drying out and ciliary action keeps secretions moving within the respiratory tract. The function of these involuntary protecting mechanisms is likewise depressed by anesthetic agents. An awake person maintains a degree of muscular tone that keeps the anterior and posterior pharyngeal walls separated. The asleep person often allows the anterior pharyngeal wall to fall against the posterior pharyngeal wall, and the result is obstruction of the air passages on attempted inspiration. The common snore is an example of this. As compared to normal sleep, a patient depressed by drugs may obstruct more completely and not be arousable to overcome this obstructive pattern.

The second cause of respiratory inadequacy occurs as a result of *central nervous system depression.* The central nervous system has a complex system of receptors, integrators, and effectors that maintain some degree of respiratory homeostasis. Nearly all depressant drugs cause this system to function improperly, especially when drugs are given in concentrations sufficient to provide surgical anesthesia. As a result of this, the response may not be appropriate when carbon dioxide accumulates or when hypoxia is allowed to develop.

The third cause of respiratory inadequacy is *disruption* of the integrity of the *peripheral neuromuscular system.* The classic example in this area is the muscle-relaxant drugs that prohibit transmission of impulses from nerves to muscles; the same type of abnormality can occur with regional anesthesia when conduction along nerve pathways is interrupted and muscle paralysis results. Any one of these three abnormalities or any combination of the three might exist to produce varying degrees of respiratory abnormality up to and including death.

The adequacy of circulation is also challenged by an anesthetic state. Like respiration, one may categorize the causes for this circulatory inadequacy as follows: (1) diminished venous return, (2) depression of heart muscle, and (3) maldistribution of circulation.

Diminished venous return occurs as a result of the effect of anesthetic agents on autonomic regulation of veins or vein walls, to allow venous dilatation to occur. As a result, pooling of blood exists within the veins, even at low venous pressure, and blood does not return to the heart. The veins contain much more of the circulating blood volume than do the arteries. Therefore, an increase in the diameter of this system provides a large reservoir for pooling of blood. Anything that then mechanically obstructs the return of blood will be more effective if the veins are looser or more compliant. Intermittent positive pressure breathing and abnormal positioning of patients on the operating table may therefore be much more serious impediments to venous return than in the awake state.

All depressant drugs used for anesthesia probably *depress* contractility of *cardiac muscle*. Whether there is a significant difference in this effect of various anesthetic agents is subject to some argument, but if a difference exists, it is not of great magnitude. Apparently ether and cyclopropane either allow or stimulate reflex release of catecholamines, which then counteract to some extent the agent-induced myocardial depression. Evidence is not available, however, to prove that these agents provide more adequate perfusion of the entire organism or selected organs than those agents that do not have this compensatory mechanism or that patients anesthetized with these agents fare any better than others.

Of great importance is the fact that some of the controlling mechanisms for regulating distribution of cardiac output are lost when the anesthetic state is produced. Because of this, blood may be allowed to flow to tissues that need it very little at the expense of tissues that need it a great deal; e.g., while sleeping and lying still, one needs to perfuse muscles very little; a small proportion of the cardiac output would suffice to perfuse and nourish muscle adequately. However, organs such as the liver, kidney, and heart may need the same amount of blood flow as they would if more physical activity were being undertaken. Presumably, the autonomic nervous system serves in the awake but inactive patient to divert blood flow from muscle to more needy tissues. Anesthetic agents may depress the autonomic nervous system sufficiently to disrupt this regulatory mechanism and therefore provide a *maldistribution of cardiac output*. Thus it is possible for cardiac output to be numerically unchanged but for vital tissues to be underperfused and undernourished.

Another problem for the anesthetized patient is a loss of the protection that the ability to perceive pain and discomfort provides. Patients who are anesthetized cannot complain, and considerable harm to the body has occurred as a result. Examples are nerve paralyses, burns from cautery or heating blankets, trauma from restraining straps and bands, and the aspiration of inhaled gastric contents.

There is probably some disruption of function of all organ systems during this state of acute drug poisoning. The effects are now known in great detail, and it appears that generally they are reversible and without great significance to patients' welfare. Examples are loss of gastrointestinal motility, a depression of renal function, and alterations in endocrine secretion.

(4) A minor cost of the anesthetic state is the specific toxicity of some agents. The classic form of this toxicity has been liver damage caused by chloroform anesthesia. Instances of this type of abnormality and their definite proof are difficult to establish.

It is inherent in production of the anesthetic state by many agents that danger of fire and explosion exists. The current tendency is to use fewer anesthetic agents that are combustible or explosive, and this danger will be further minimized in the future. However, the use of explosive agents is still widespread, and one needs to be aware of this fact and to follow simple rules of common sense in the operating room.

MEANS OF PRODUCING ANESTHESIA

Anesthesia may be roughly categorized into regional and general. Regional anesthesia is the production of anesthesia in just one region of the body, whereas general anesthesia implies the production of a total state of unconsciousness or anesthesia of the entire organism. The categorization is obviously not an absolute one since the anesthetization of large regional areas produces generalized effects, and there are such wide variations in the degrees of general anesthesia produced that it can hardly be considered one class or category.

Regional anesthesia

Regional anesthesia can be produced by the deposition of the proper drug on the nerve or nerve pathway anywhere between the site of the painful stimulus and the receptors of the painful stimuli in the central nervous system (Fig. 9-1). As general rules, one may state that the more central the application of this drug, the more anesthesia is produced per milligram of drug, and that if specific nerves or groups of nerves can be so treated, more satisfactory and comfortable anesthesia would result than with the diffuse use of drugs. If the drug is deposited upon the surface of the area to be anesthetized, it produces *topical anesthesia.* If it is infiltrated in skin or subcutaneous tissues by use of a needle and syringe, the method is considered to be *local infiltration.* If specific areas of the body are blocked by the infiltration of a surrounding perimeter with a local infiltration technique, it is referred to as a *field block.* If individual nerves or

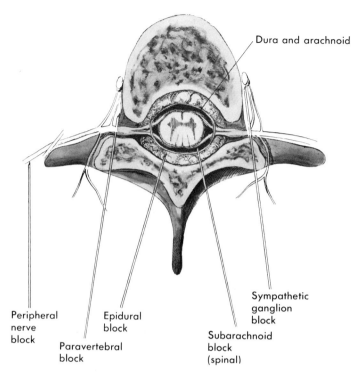

Dura and arachnoid

Sympathetic
ganglion
block

Peripheral
nerve
block

Epidural
block

Subarachnoid
block
(spinal)

Paravertebral
block

Fig. 9-1. Types of nerve blocks.

plexuses of nerves are blocked, it is referred to as a *nerve block*. Drugs may also be deposited in the epidural space or in the subarachnoid space in the production of spinal anesthesia (Fig. 9-1).

Advantages of regional anesthesia are somewhat debatable. The patient is awake—this may be good or bad, but advantages that result from preservation of the awake state are airway control and spontaneous respiration. For many operations this is a definite advantage and avoids serious respiratory complications that were discussed earlier. Good regional anesthesia provides excellent operating conditions in that the muscular relaxation approaches cadaveric degrees, and for abdominal surgery the bowel is constricted, providing extra room. Spinal anesthesia provides a pharmacological bargain unequaled in other forms of anesthesia; for instance, a very small amount of drug deposited in the subarachnoid space will provide excellent anesthesia for a large portion of the body. Therefore, there is minimum detoxifying to do, and there is minimum actual cellular depression by the anesthetic agent itself.

Disadvantages of regional anesthesia are also relative. A false security often exists. The widespread belief that local or regional techniques are "safer" is often far from true. There can be much circulatory and respiratory abnormality with regional anesthesia, and frequently a trained anesthetist is not present to tend to the needs of the patient during operations performed with regional anesthesia. An especially bad concept is that of using heavy sedation and "local" with no attendants. This method combines many of the bad effects of regional and general anesthesia and deprives the patient of the good effects of either. The fact that patients are awake can be a disadvantage at times; the sights, sounds, and smells of the operating room are quite undesirable for some, and therefore regional anesthesia may not provide patient comfort.

Regional anesthesia is not readily adaptable to all situations. Although any operation can probably be performed with some type of regional anesthesia, it cannot always be accomplished with comfort and facility. This would be especially true in young children or in uncooperative patients of any age. The techniques for good nerve blocking require considerable finesse and practice and frequently are not comfortable for patients. Blocks are frequently incomplete either because of faulty technique or overlapping nerve supply. The fact that many operations take hours to complete makes regional anesthesia quite unsatisfactory, as patients do not tolerate the necessary immobility.

There is some disadvantage as a result of systemic depression of the body from the drugs used. These reactions should be considered as toxic and not allergic. Systemic allergy from regional anesthetic agents is extremely rare if it occurs at all.

The most important disadvantages of regional anesthesia are the lack of flexibility in either time or extent of the procedure. One must therefore provide anesthesia for time durations and anatomic extent greater than anticipated for surgery; and if for some reason these dimensions are exceeded by the operative procedure, supplementation with some form of general anesthesia is required.

General anesthesia

General anesthesia, as stated before, is associated with complete loss of consciousness. There are many agents capable of producing satisfactory and desirable general anesthesia, and it is not within the intended scope of this chapter to discuss these agents individually or to compare them in any fashion. Drugs may be administered intravenously, by rectum, by mouth, or, as is most commonly done, by inhalation. It is of basic importance to consider that whatever the route of administration, the effects are essentially the same, and patients require the same care and attention. It is a tempting concept that anesthesia or drug depression produced by heavy premedication or by intravenous sedation does not carry with it the same risk and need for observation and care that inhalation anesthesia does. Probably the opposite is more nearly true, in that inhalation drugs are excreted rapidly, and the recoverability or reversibility of their effects is infinitely greater than that of nonvolatile drugs administered by other routes.

Anesthesia may be produced by one or a combination of several drugs. Arguments for the superiority of one approach over the other are still unsettled, and it is not known whether production of the anesthetic state by one or by a combination of drugs is superior as far as effect on patient welfare is concerned.

The advantages and disadvantages of general anesthesia are in a sense covered by the same discussion concerning regional anesthesia if one looks at the opposite side of the coin. The flexibility of general anesthesia is highly desirable and perhaps is its greatest advantage; it can be adapted for any operation for any age and for any anatomic problem. Operations can be completely comfortable for a few moments or for many hours. Patients are oblivious of nonoperating stimuli and are comfortable during long periods of time on the operating table. Production of the unconscious state allows the anesthetist to control respiration and demands a skilled and trained attendant to care for the patient's needs throughout the entire operative procedure.

The disadvantage of general anesthesia is largely significant depression of vital functions of circulation and respiration. Most, if not all, anesthetic deaths from general anesthesia are caused by this depression. These agents are potent drugs and are applied in near lethal concentrations.

The choice between general or regional anesthesia is one for which no hard and fast rules may be applied. These will vary with the needs of the surgeon, the skill of anesthesia personnel, and the desires and personality of the patient. The combination of regional and general anesthesia is often appealing; though it adds some dangers of both, it also adds some benefit of both types of techniques.

CONDUCT OF ANESTHESIA
Preoperative evaluation and management

Anesthesia is better and safer if it is prepared and planned for. For this reason, persons administering the anesthetic have an obligation to become acquainted with patients and their medical problems.

Preoperative and preanesthetic evaluation should provide enough knowledge of the patient's physical state to base a judgment as to whether the patient is in optimal condition or not. In the past, considerable emphasis was placed upon specific indications and contraindications for various types and techniques of anesthesia and whether anesthesia should or should not be administered. Currently, few such contraindications or indications are taught. The change in attitude results from increased knowledge about effects of anesthetic agents and procedures. Most indications and contraindications were empirically based. Sober thought and investigation does not provide much evidence supporting choice of particular anesthetic agents for particular patients. Additionally, many illnesses at one time considered contraindications for anesthesia and surgery are now indications for major surgical intervention. The classical example of this situation is that of heart disease. Patients were once denied the benefits of surgery because of cardiac failure or congenital heart disease; these are now indications for surgery of the greatest magnitude.

Prior to administering anesthesia the anesthesiologist must have a knowledge of the surgical requirements for the operation at hand. This would include, for example, the *position* in which the patient is to be placed, the approximate *duration* of the operation, the *degree of relaxation* necessary, anticipated *blood loss,* and the presence or absence of *explosive hazards.* He must then incorporate these facts into his plans for the operation. Of equal importance, he must establish some degree of rapport with the patient. A preoperative visit and an explanation of subsequent events will often develop a high degree of confidence and is a safer and more desirable way of providing relief from anxiety and fear than is the use of depressant drugs.

Premedicant drugs, however, are used almost routinely. Their primary purposes are to sedate the patient and to prevent excess secretions from accumulating in the respiratory tract because of the absence of cough and swallowing actions. A great variety of drugs have been used. In general, they fall into three categories: (1) the *sedatives,* such as barbiturates and tranquilizers, (2) the *drying agents,* such as atropine and scopolamine, and (3) *analgesics,* such as morphine and meperidine. There is obviously some overlap in functions of these agents, and again superiority of one approach over another is difficult to prove. Drugs must be given on an individual basis rather than by routines and generalizations. These drugs are depressant drugs and will extract some toll from the patient; as with all depressant drugs, they should be used only when needed.

It is important to ascertain that patients are in an optimum condition for surgery. There is, and probably always will be, some morbidity and mortality from the administration of anesthesia and application of surgical therapy. It is reasonable to assume that morbidity and mortality will be greater if surgery and anesthesia are added to preexisting abnormalities, such as myocardial failure or respiratory tract infections. If these abnormalities are present, they should not be considered as reasons to deny surgery to patients, but if time allows, they should be controlled to the best degree they can by treatment during the preoperative period. Obviously, emergent situations occur in which preoperative preparation is minimal, and the need for preoperative therapy must be balanced against the urgency of the surgical intervention.

The purpose of this chapter does not include discussion of technical details of the management of patients during anesthesia; however, certain concepts are worthy of mention.

Operating room management

Upon arrival in the operating room, the anesthesiologist must accept the responsibility of protecting the patient from harm. He must ascertain proper identity and that fever or other complication has not arisen in the immediate preoperative period. A patient must be positioned on the operating table in such fashion as to avoid injury and provide comfort. One must establish that foreign bodies such as gastric contents, removable dental appliances, chewing gum, etc. are not available for aspiration. Provision must be made to evaluate the patient's condition adequately during the anticipated surgery by applying blood pressure–monitoring equipment, stethoscopes, and perhaps more sophisticated monitors.

Induction of anesthesia is an extremely critical time because of the rapidity of change that occurs. It is at this time that severe overdoses and acute respiratory and circulatory problems are most likely to occur.

During anesthesia constant and undivided attention must be given to the maintenance of adequate respiration and circulation with the knowledge that one cannot easily determine the adequacy of either.

The airway must be maintained, either by appropriate manipulation and positioning of the head and neck or by the insertion of artificial airway support. The latter includes oropharyngeal airways, endotracheal airways, and occasionally even tracheotomy. *No patient should be anesthetized unless and until the person administering anesthesia can guarantee maintenance of an adequate airway.* This may on occasion involve preoperative tracheotomy or the insertion of an endotracheal catheter with the patient awake. A patient who has a full stomach is quite likely to vomit during induction of anesthesia.

Vomitus filling the mouth, pharynx, and perhaps the trachea is quite an uncontrollable situation and is the cause of much anesthetic morbidity, especially in the area of obstetric anesthesia. Therefore, patients who have a full stomach must be guaranteed that their airway will not become occluded during the time when they are unable to handle vomited materials by themselves. This has been attempted by many means.

The safest method for preventing occlusion of the airway is to insert an endotracheal catheter while the patient is awake. The catheter is equipped with an inflatable cuff, assuring an airtight seal in the trachea. This obviously has the disadvantages of discomfort to the patient and may be technically very difficult to do to patients who are uncooperative for any reason. Therefore, many compromises have been suggested. Practice and persistence will allow intubation when the patients are awake without tremendous discomfort to them in a high majority of cases, and other approaches to this problem must be attempted, with the realization that they are substitutes and probably less satisfactory methods.

Because all of our agents are capable of compromising respiration and circulation, we must prepare to monitor and assist or control breathing. The latter is accomplished by intermittent application of positive pressure to the proximal airway. Pressure may be generated by compressing the anesthesia reservoir bag manually or by a mechanical respirator. Such intermittent positive pressure breathing is a common practice and a very useful one; it has some hazards or disadvantages. Among the latter are decreased venous return because of the decreased venous pressure gradients from periphery to the chest. This, of course, leads to decreased cardiac output. Overdistension of the lung can occur, especially in patients with obstructive lung disease. In these and perhaps in others, lung rupture can occur. Spontaneous respiration acts as a guide to the depth of anesthesia. Controlled respiration, therefore, deprives one of this valuable guide and offers a dangerous opportunity for overdosage of potent drugs. Overventilation and respiratory alkalosis are common accompaniments of controlled respiration but seem to be of minimal consequence.

The monitoring of circulation is an equally important function of the person administering anesthesia. Efforts have to be directed toward maintaining adequate perfusion of tissues. Unfortunately, however, there are few, if any, methods to evaluate this accurately. At least we should think of perfusion rather than of pressure alone. Far too much effort has been directed at maintaining arterial blood pressure at some predetermined level rather than abolishing the cause of hypotension or evaluating tissue perfusion that is resulting. We can roughly assess perfusion in the operating room by observing the color and temperature of the skin, pupillary reaction, urine flow, and changes in depth of anesthesia when the inspired concentrations are altered.

Special anesthesia techniques

For various reasons, special complicated techniques may be undertaken to provide anesthesia. They include *purposeful hypotension* for times when the performance of surgery is aided by a "bloodless" field and the *reduction of body temperature* to varying degrees when circulation must be so compromised that decreased metabolism of tissues needs to be provided. Purposeful hypotension may be provided either by drugs that paralyze the autonomic nervous system or by deep levels of general anesthesia. Hypothermia may be produced either by surface cooling in ice water or by cold blankets or by the use of extracorporeal cooling devices (which cool blood outside the body and reinfuse it).

Problems after anesthesia

At the termination of anesthesia and surgery another period of rapid change occurs; efforts at this time should be directed to having patients able to care for themselves to the extent of airway maintenance and adequate spontaneous respiration. In some unusual instances doing so will be impossible, and artificial airways and mechanical ventilators will then be necessary.

Perhaps the most important aspect of anesthetic management and care is a breath-to-breath, moment-to-moment observation of patients. Such observation is almost always provided in the operating room but is not so well provided in the postoperative period. Recovery rooms and intensive care facilities are now popular. These are actually attempts to provide to the recovering or acutely ill patient the same adequate observation and care to which he is entitled in the operating room.

The press of operating room schedules and other activities promotes neglect of patients in this critical period. A paradox results in that a patient may be removed from the operating room where he is the sole recipient of the attention of several physicians to the recovery area where he shares an attendant only partially trained for observation and management of his problems. These areas of acute patient care should be so managed that patients are provided comfort and safety. Since patients in these areas will be under the influence of depressant drugs and the same challenges as faced in the operating room, the same principles must be followed here as in the operating room.

CHAPTER 10

Postoperative care

RICHARD D. LIECHTY

Complications may occur after almost any operation regardless of its magnitude. Even simple, routine diagnostic procedures, with catheters or needles, drugs, or various contrast media, may be lethal.

In the study of surgical complications, *anticipation* and *early recognition* keynote successful treatment. The great majority of all postoperative complications are signaled by two signs: *fever* or *shock* (cardiovascular collapse). Pain and tenderness, so important preoperatively, are often masked by operative pain or suppressed by sedation, especially in the first few hours after operation. Because sedation dulls the patient's responses, the surgeon must develop exceptional sensitivity to the *signs* of postoperative complications.

PATTERN OF SURGICAL COMPLICATIONS
Chain reaction

Fortunately, surgical complications usually appear singly, but all too often, especially in the older, debilitated patient, they occur as *chain reactions*—one complication begets another; e.g., a prolonged ileus requires gastrointestinal suction and intravenous feeding. The patient is shackled to his bed for prolonged periods by a tube in his nose and a needle in his arm. Thus, the stage is set for thrombophlebitis (from inactivity) or pneumonitis (from irritation of the upper respiratory areas) with sepsis. These secondary and tertiary complications are serious and occasionally fatal. Any number and variety of these chain reactions may arise, but they almost invariably begin with one complication. Anticipation and prevention of these initial complications can thwart the sinister chain reaction phenomenon. Predisposing factors in surgical complications are discussed in Chapter 8.

RECOGNIZING SURGICAL COMPLICATIONS

Fever is the most common evidence of postoperative complications. *Cardiovascular collapse,* although less common, is more dramatic and emergent. Together these two signs forecast at least 90% of postoperative complications. Since early recognition is so important, I will discuss complications under these two signs that tell us something is wrong.

Fever

Mild transient fevers appear after most operations from tissue necrosis, hematoma, or cauterization. Higher sustained fevers arise with the following four most common postoperative complications:

1. Atelectasis
2. Wound infections
3. Urinary infections
4. Thrombophlebitis

These causes of fever occur frequently and should be committed to memory as the *4 W's:* "wind, wound, water, and walk." When fever occurs, the student should think first of these four common sources.

Lung problems (wind) within the first 48 hours

Lung complications commonly occur after operations for the following reasons:

1. Endotracheal tubes; oxygen and ether irritate the respiratory tree, and increased secretion results.
2. Atropine causes inspissation of bronchial secretions.
3. The position of the patient cannot be changed on the operating table and secretions tend to fill the lung and thereby encourage the growth of organisms.
4. An anesthetized patient cannot cough to clear secretions.
5. In the immediate postoperative period the patient, because of sedation or pain, cannot move or cough to clear secretions adequately; an obstruction (from secretions) and atelectasis (collapse of portions of the lung) result.

Fever, tachypnea, and cyanosis (when large portions of the lung are affected) characterize atelectasis. Pneumonitis may result from substained obstruction. Coughing, deep breathing, and moving are essential to clear the respiratory tree of these secretions. If large areas of lung are involved by pneumonia, the patient becomes confused with few other signs and symptoms. Confusion means poor oxygenation of the brain and should prompt the physician to order a roentgenogram of the chest. In the older male with chronic disease of the lung or heart, gram-negative rod pneumonia is common. In certain outbreaks in hospitals *Staphylococcus aureus* is the prime cause of pneu-

Table 10-1. The occurrence rate of wound infections

Operation	Septic wounds (%)
Gallbladder	21
Breast	15
Miscellaneous abdominal	13
Thorax	9
Hernia	7
Miscellaneous orthopedic	3
Minisectomy	0
Overall average % for England*	9.7
Overall average % for U.S.A.†	7.5

*Public health laboratory source incidence of surgical wound infection in England and Wales, Lancet 2:659, 1960.
†Howard, J. M., et al.: Postoperative wound infections, Ann. Surg. 160(suppl.): 1-192, 1964.

monia in elderly postoperative patients. Bronchoscopy or tracheal catheterization with aspiration of mucous plugs can stimulate patients who have difficulty in coughing. These procedures themselves may introduce new bacteria into the lung, bypassing all the usual host-resistance barriers.

Wound infections (wound) 5 to 7 days

Wound infections may occur after any operation. They are most common, however, after gallbladder or gastrointestinal operations and operations on the breast (Table 10-1). Drying of tissues by long exposure, operation on contaminated structures, gross obesity, or operations on the very young or very old are directly related to an increase in sepsis rate. Experiments on medical students by Elek show that the infection rate from inoculated staphylococci increases a thousandfold with a foreign body (suture).

Patients who harbor infections remote from the operative site are likely to have greater wound infection rates than those without such remote infections. Wound infection rates rise proportionately with the duration of operative procedures and with the length of prophylactic antibiotic administration. Any break in aseptic technique can contribute to wound infections during operations or with later dressing changes.

Heat, redness, and tenderness in a wound demand investigation and drainage. Wound infections involve staphylococcus alone in 60%, staphylococcus with enteric organisms in 13%, and enteric organisms alone in 17%. A prudent plan of treatment should proceed as follows: wound culture and sensitivities, anti-staphylococcal penicillin (peni-

Table 10-2. Bacteria found in wound infections*

Staphylococcus aureus	60%
S. aureus and coliforms†	13
Coliforms alone	17
Other specified organisms	4
No pathogens	6

*Data from Public health laboratory source incidence of surgical wound infection in England and Wales, Lancet 2:659, 1960.
†*Escherichia coli, Klebsiella-Enterobacter, Proteus,* and paracolon.

cillinase-resistant), change antibiotics according to the patient's response and laboratory evidence of sensitivity (Table 10-2).

Urinary infection (water) 5 to 8 days

Postoperative patients often have difficulty voiding and sometimes require catheterization. Although urinary infections occur without catheterization, the usual initiating factor is the introduction of a catheter that mechanically carries organisms into the bladder. Single catheterizations are associated even under the best of circumstances with a 4% infection rate. Irrigation of the anterior urethra with bacitracin or neomycin, frequent catheter changes, and constant irrigation with 0.25% acetic acid or neomycin-bacitracin-polymyxin mixtures help prevent sepsis. A round pad of plastic foam about 2 inches in diameter and about 1 inch thick, threaded on a Foley catheter and, pushed up to rest against the external urinary meatus, helps anchor the catheter. Subsequently the pad can be moistened with an antiseptic or with antibiotic solution or cream.*

Thrombophlebitis (walk) 7 to 14 days

We do not understand all the factors leading to spontaneous thrombosis in the deep leg and pelvic veins of certain postoperative patients. However, *stasis* and *increased coagulability* of blood are two im-

*Experimental work with *Serratia marcescens* has shown that these organisms migrate into the bladder via the fluid (urine and exudate) that forms alongside the catheter. Thus these local procedures help prevent the upward migration of organisms. Patients with infection develop dysuria, frequency, urgency, hesitancy, and fever. Systemic antibiotics can control generalized sepsis, but cannot control localized urinary infections as long as the catheter is in place. Recent experience shows that intermittent catheterization, under rigid aseptic precautions, carries less risk than continuous (Foley) catheterization.

portant factors. Obesity, birth control medications, immobility, advanced age, cardiac problems, and abdominal malignancies are associated. Thrombophlebitis is characterized by fever, pain, tenderness, and redness along superficial veins. Pain and edema occur with thromboses in deep veins. The great hazard of blood clots in deep veins rests in the possibility of the clots moving to the lungs (pulmonary emboli). About 25% of patients who develop pulmonary emboli die from one or more of the following: arrhythmias, bronchoconstriction, pulmonary edema, or inadequate return of blood to the left heart (which causes right ventricular failure). Early movement, ambulation, and wrapping of the legs help prevent stasis. Most thromboses respond to rest, elevation of the legs, and chemotherapy with heparin and fibrinolytic agents. Ligating or narrowing the lumen of the inferior vena cava can prevent subsequent emboli if patients develop emboli while on full anticoagulation with heparin (Fig. 10-1). (See Chapter 30.)

Third day fever

The "third day surgical fever" comes from inflammation surrounding intravenous catheters. Removal and antibiotic therapy bring rapid relief.

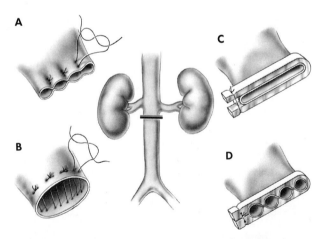

Fig. 10-1. Vena cava narrowing to prevent emboli. **A,** Multiple channel method. **B,** Suture sieve method. **C,** Slit Teflon clip. **D,** Serrated Teflon clip.

SHOCK

Table 10-3. Postoperative shock

Cause	Diagnosis	Treatment
1. *Bleeding* Usually in peritoneal or pleural cavities or retroperitoneal areas	Check wounds, drain sites, open wounds, or use diagnostic aspiration if necessary; central venous pressure is low	Blood and immediate ligation of bleeding vessel
2. *Cardiac shock* Myocardial infarction or arrhythmias, arrest	Check for pulse irregularities, electrocardiogram, absence of pulse and cyanosis suggest cardiac arrest; SGOT aids diagnosis of infarction; central venous pressure is high	Dependent on diagnosis: general measures, oxygen, sedation, cardiopulmonary resuscitation
3. *Pulmonary embolus*	No specific signs; chest pain, hemoptysis suggest diagnosis; angiography can make diagnosis; obesity, previous cardiac difficulties, cancer and pelvic operations, immobility, and increased age are associated factors	Embolectomy; fibrinolytic agents to dissolve clots are promising (see Chapters 30 and 33)
4. *Transfusion reaction* (contaminated blood)	Smears of blood show gram-negative organisms; shock rapidly follows blood administration	Discontinue blood; corticosteroids, massive doses of antibiotics intravenously
5. *Sepsis*	Culture of blood or suspicion of gram-negative bacterial source of septicemia	Massive intravenous antibiotics, fluids, corticosteroids
6. *Adrenal failure*	Must be diagnosed by suspicion or history of steroid therapy, lack of other causes	Intravenous corticosteroids (100 to 300 mg. of hydrocortisone)
7. *Anaphylactic shock*	Obscure clinical picture; history of drug sensitivities is vitally important; urticaria and edema may aid diagnosis	Epinephrine, antihistamines, corticosteroids

Cardiovascular collapse

The signs of cardiovascular collapse—a cold, clammy, pale patient, decreased blood pressure, and a rapid, thready pulse—usually occur with alarming suddenness in the postoperative patient. Table 10-3 is a helpful guide in the rapid detection and treatment of postoperative shock. The student should think of bleeding and cardiac disease (myocardial infarction) as the two most common causes.

LESS COMMON COMPLICATIONS

Acute parotiditis

Acute parotiditis is a rare complication that occurs in older, debilitated patients. An acute, painful, tender swelling of the parotid gland is an unmistakable sign. Dehydration may cause inspissation and obstruction in the duct, with a secondary staphylococcus invasion. This is one of the few instances in which roentgen-ray therapy is used for benign disease. It is effective in the early stages. Surgical incision and drainage may be necessary if roentgen-ray therapy fails to halt suppuration.

Postoperative cholecystitis and pancreatitis

Postoperative cholecystitis and pancreatitis are rarely seen; consequently they are often overlooked. Dehydration may be a factor in these conditions as in parotiditis. Treatment is conservative (fluids, gastrointestinal suction, atropine, and rest). Occasionally, cholecystostomy or cholecystectomy is required.

GASTROINTESTINAL COMPLICATIONS

A high percentage of anesthetized patients will be nauseated and vomit in the postoperative period. Such a common phenomenon cannot be considered a complication.

Aspiration of vomitus

Aspiration of vomitus is a serious complication that must be prevented by emptying the stomach prior to anesthesia (with a nasogastric tube when necessary). Turning the patient on his side with the head lowered when vomiting occurs may prevent this complication.

Paralytic ileus

A temporary cessation of peristalsis of the gastrointestinal tract will occur after anesthesia, trauma, and abdominal operations. If it becomes sustained, electrolyte imbalance, wound infections, or some metabolic disturbance (myxedema or adrenal failure) may be the cause. Nasogastric suction and fluid replacement will correct most cases.

Acute gastric dilatation

Acute gastric dilatation is an uncommon complication that may follow abdominal, chest, spine, or central nervous system procedures. The precise cause is obscure. An astonishing amount (several liters) of air and dark, foul material may collect in the stomach. Vomiting and distension are the main diagnostic points. The vomiting, which is seldom accompanied by retching, features an overflow type of regurgitation that, curiously, may not be attended with nausea.

The distension may rapidly progress to fatal cardiovascular collapse within hours. Immediate intubation of the stomach with aspiration of its contents and fluid and electrolyte replacement may be lifesaving. Aspiration of two or more liters of gas and liquid material virtually assures the diagnosis of acute gastric dilatation. Continuous decompression will usually relieve the gastric atony within 48 hours. The surgeon can safely discontinue aspiration at that time if no mechanical obstruction coexists.

Hiccup

Hiccuping in the postoperative patient may indicate some potentially serious underlying problem; this is its chief significance. Most commonly hiccups are a short-lived nuisance and nothing more. Abscesses about the diaphragm, uremia, gastric dilatation, paralytic ileus, peritonitis, anxiety, and acidosis are the more common conditions that cause these spasms of the diaphragm. Rarely hiccups may persist for days or weeks and utterly exhaust the sufferer. Correcting the associated disease is the obvious and logical treatment. Vagal pressure, rebreathing air or carbon dioxide, sedation, or tranquilization may bring symptomatic relief.

OTHER URINARY COMPLICATIONS

Retention of urine

Anesthesia, narcotics, anticholinergic drugs (atropine), operative trauma, advanced age, and diseases of the urinary system (an enlarged prostate) contribute to this common occurrence. Having the patients sit or stand to void is helpful. Sterile catheterization of the bladder must be done to prevent overdistension of the bladder, if the patient cannot void.

Acute renal insufficiency

Acute renal insufficiency is a rare condition that may occur after operative procedures. The urine output decreases despite adequate intake. Precise replacement of fluids will often be sufficient therapy, and the patients will begin excreting urine within 7 to 10 days in most cases. (See Chapter 3.)

Lavaging the peritoneum with fluids designed to collect and remove nitrogenous wastes and potassium provides a "substitute kidney" in severe cases. Because peritoneal dialysis is relatively simple, it has largely replaced the more complicated renal dialysis with the artificial kidney.

ANAPHYLACTIC REACTIONS AND SERUM SICKNESS

In addition to shock, anaphylactic reactions are characterized by urticaria, angioedema, rhinitis, conjunctival congestion, wheezing, dyspnea, or any combination of these manifestations. An injection of foreign material induces an antigen-antibody response; subsequent exposure triggers the reaction. In humans, the cardiorespiratory system (nose, glottis, pulmonary artery, bronchioles, and right ventricle), the hepatic venules, and renal glomeruli are specific targets for these reactions. A generalized urticaria often covers many patients.

Almost any organic substance such as blood proteins, enzymes, horse serum, glues, and many foods (fish, chocolate, egg whites) may cause anaphylaxis. Penicillin, dextran, local anesthetics, contrast media, and dyes are proved offenders.

Serum sickness is a close relative of anaphylaxis, but with onset 4 to 10 days after administration of the causative serum or drug. Adenopathy, arthralgia, fever, leukopenia, neuropathy, and rash characterize serum sickness.

When systemic anaphylactic symptoms appear, 0.25 ml. of 1:1,000 epinephrine is given immediately and repeated every 5 minutes until nervousness or tachycardia appears. Asthmatic symptoms may be relieved by intravenous aminophylline. Antihistamines and corticosteroids are slower acting but may curtail advancement of symptoms. Tracheostomy may be required to bypass obstructing glottic edema. Since serum sickness is much less violent than anaphylaxis, symptomatic treatment with aspirin or corticosteroids will prove adequate in most instances.

BEDSORES (DECUBITUS ULCERS)

Bedsores are caused by *pressure* over bony areas (sacrum, elbows, heels). Ischemia is induced by compression of the blood vessels that supply these areas. Since decubiti can form within hours in living tissues (but not in cadavers), some surgeons hypothesize a lytic factor arising from ischemic, compressed, viable tissue. Ischemia (arteriosclerosis) and anesthesia (paraplegia) are precedent factors in most cases. The disease affects the older, debilitated patients or the younger patient who has a neurological disease; paraplegics are extremely susceptible to bedsores.

Pressure → Ischemia → Bedsores

Protection and *frequent movement* are the key words in prevention of bedsores. The nurse plays the principal role in prevention.

POSTOPERATIVE NEUROSES AND PSYCHOSES

When a surgical procedure has been successful and nonmutilating, most patients react with mild euphoria. They feel an inner satisfaction in having overcome a hazardous experience. *Depressions* normally occur after loss of any important part of the body, whether it be functionally or cosmetically deforming. Anxiety for an uncertain future in his new state adds to the depression. Most patients, fortunately, adapt to these changes and resume a reasonably normal life. Severe depressions, marked by withdrawal, restlessness, insomnia, expressions of hopelessness, and the desire for death should arouse suspicion of suicidal intent. The surgeon's responsibility includes listening to his patient, reassuring him, and closely following a patient with symptoms of depression. Much aid can be given to the patient with a colostomy, for example. Introducing him to colostomy clubs can mean an abrupt change of attitude. When he sees others who have accepted their colostomies and lead successful, normal lives, his adjustment to his colostomy is rapid and gratifying. Similarly with amputees, early positive emphasis on physical therapy and rehabilitation is one of the most important factors in a successful recovery.

Major personality disturbances are, fortunately, uncommon in the postoperative period. The stress of the illness, the intensity of therapy, and previous emotional makeup are the important underlying factors. A sudden, acute onset of symptoms, especially when the patient seems to overreact to the stresses, often foretells a good prognosis. The immediate problem lies in physically restraining and sedating the patient. Psychiatric consultation should be obtained for these reactions as well as for severe depressions, suicidal tendencies, or any other aberrancies of behavior that may threaten a normal recovery.

Dehydration and other disturbances in fluid and electrolyte balance may cause severe personality changes. (These problems are discussed in Chapter 3.) Sepsis, uremia, alcoholism, barbiturates, and other drugs are also known offenders in producing aberrant behavior patterns. History, physical examination, or specific chemical tests can uncover most of these causes.

SPECIFIC COMPLICATIONS

The purpose of this chapter has been to discuss complications that may arise after any operative procedure. Specific complications that arise only in certain circumstances such as thyroid storm or hypoparathyroidism are discussed in later chapters.

Each of the many highly technical operative procedures has its own technical complications. In shunting procedures for hydrocephalus, for example, a variety of technical failures result from attempts to shunt excess cerebrospinal fluid from the brain through man-made conduits to other parts of the body. As new operative techniques evolve in whatever field, a new set of technical complications will follow. Of necessity, these complications must be managed by those trained to recognize and treat them.

CHAPTER 11

Malignant neoplasms

RICHARD L. LAWTON
RICHARD D. LIECHTY
A. CURTIS HASS

THE IMPACT OF CANCER

Cancer is a *group of diseases* (about 150 recognized types) of varied causes arising from many different tissues. The term *cancer* includes all *uncontrolled growth* of cells that leads to serious disability, and often death, of the host.

Cancer is the second leading cause of death in the United States (Fig. 11-1). Unless some unforeseen and providential treatment is discovered, one in four persons, or almost 52 million people living today, have or will develop cancer. In 1974, an estimated 355,000 Americans died of cancer—about 1,000 deaths each day.

In the past 30 years, the 5-year cure rate (without evidence of disease 5 years after treatment) has improved from one in four to one in three persons. Improvement in detection and treatment probably accounts for this increase. Unfortunately, the cancer incidence rate is increasing faster than the cure rate, probably because of an increasing proportion of elderly persons. The upshot of this trend is an estimated 3.5 million cancer deaths in the decade of the 70's, with 10 million people under treatment for cancer. The total cost of this problem is over $12 billion a year.

In this chapter, we discuss the chief features of this enormous medical, economic, and sociological problem. The management of specific types of cancer are outlined in following relevant chapters.

EPIDEMIOLOGY—THE GLOBAL PERSPECTIVE

Cancer is a worldwide problem with poorly understood but intriguing racial, ethnic, sex, age, and geographic differences; e.g., car-

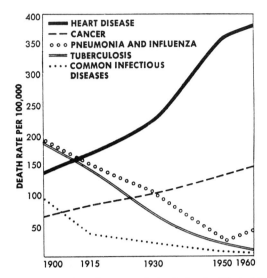

Fig. 11-1. Trends in selected causes of death in the United States, 1900 to 1966. (From Progress against cancer—1966, a report by the National Advisory Cancer Council, National Cancer Institute, Bethesda, Md.)

cinoma of the stomach has a high incidence in Japan whereas it has been decreasing in the United States. Conversely, female breast cancer so common in the United States is rare in Japan.

The Burkitt lymphoma, a curious tumor found in certain parts of Africa and largely limited to the face, appears to depend, to some degree, on environment (temperature and altitude). A virus may cause this cancer.

American Indians of both sexes have a lower (age-adjusted) cancer death rate than the white population. Chinese have an abnormally high mortality from nasopharyngeal cancer in this country and elsewhere.

Cancer of the lung, the leading cancer in men, is about five times more common in male than female Americans. But women (who started smoking after men) are beginning to catch up. Breast and uterine cancer are the most common female cancers.

Although cancer occurs at any age, the incidence of cancer increases with aging. Since older people become increasingly susceptible to and die from other diseases, the probability that they will develop

Table 11-1. Suspected factors inducing tumors

Suspected causative factors	Type of tumor
Viruses	Rous sarcomas in chickens Other animal tumors Possible leukemias Burkitt's tumor, benign warts
Sunlight overexposure	Skin cancer
Aniline dyes	Bladder cancer
Chimney soot	Carcinoma of scrotum
Cigarette smoke Air pollution	Lung cancer
Hereditary factors	Colon cancer (multiple polyposis) Retinoblastoma Breast cancer (possibly)
Ionizing irradiation	Skin cancer Thyroid cancer Osteogenic sarcoma Probably leukemias

cancer decreases slightly after 45 years of age in females and 65 years in males. The differences seen in childhood cancer are discussed in Chapter 28.

An unexplained geographic difference in cancer rates separates rural and urban areas. The risk of developing respiratory and esophageal cancer in males and digestive, genital, and respiratory cancer in females is increased in urban areas even when allowing for migration of some rural cancer patients to urban treatment centers. Other countries (Norway, Sweden, and Finland) show this same tendency.

ETIOLOGY

The 150 or more recognized human cancers are produced by, at least, a similar number of widely divergent causes. The biochemical abnormalities that somehow initiate cancer are as inscrutable as life itself. This is the basic problem of cancer research. Some of the suspected factors that have a role in inducing tumors are given in Table 11-1. These factors (physical, chemical, or viral) act within the cell to produce permanent genetic changes.

COMMON SITES OF CANCER

Although cancers can originate in any organ, certain sites are more common than others (Fig. 11-2). Skin cancer, the most common human cancer, is seldom fatal. Table 11-2 lists the seven types of cancer that are the most common *killing cancers* (Fig. 11-3). Together they account for about two-thirds of all cancer fatalities.

SPONTANEOUS REGRESSION OF CANCER

The course of almost all cancers is relentlessly progressive, but rare instances of spontaneous regression are recorded. Everson and Cole reviewed 176 cases of spontaneous regression of histologically proved

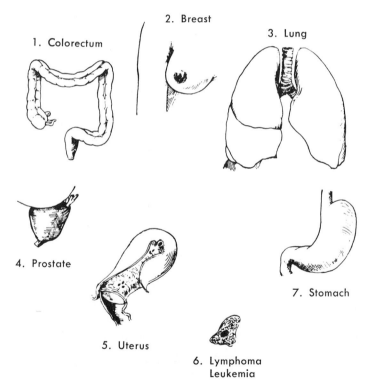

Fig. 11-2. Sites of cancer (in adults, both sexes) in frequency of occurrence.

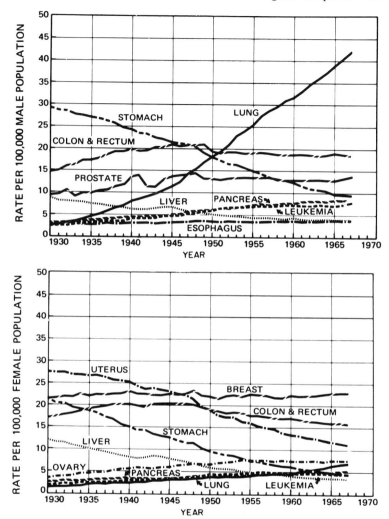

Fig. 11-3. Death rates, male and female, by site of cancer in the United States, 1930 to 1967. Rates for the male and female population standardized for age on the 1940 United States population. (National Vital Statistics Division and Bureau of the Census, United States; Statistical Research Section, Medical Affairs Department, American Cancer Society, 1971 Cancer Facts and Figures.)

Table 11-2. Most common cancers that kill

Site	Estimated new cancers (1974)
Colon and rectum	99,000
Breast	90,000
Lung	83,000
Prostate	54,000
Uterus (invasive)	46,000
Hemopoietic tissue	48,000
Stomach	23,000

cancers. The tumors that make up this group are from 20 different sites. Heading the list is hypernephroma (adenocarcinoma of the kidney), followed by neuroblastoma, malignant melanoma, choriocarcinoma, bladder sarcoma, soft tissue sarcoma, and sarcoma of bone. The reason for these miraculous regressions is one of the most provocative questions in all of medicine today. Spontaneous regression of cancer strongly suggests an *immune response* in the host. Much current research effort is directed toward identifying and intensifying this immune response.

CANCER-ENDOCRINE SYNDROMES

Some cancers have the extraordinary ability to produce hormones and thus mimic endocrine syndromes. Oat cell lung cancer, a notable example, can secrete a number of hormones (or hormone-like substances), such as ACTH, parathyroid hormone, ADH, and TSH. These curious syndromes include the following:

Syndrome	Hormone	Source
Polycythemia	Erythropoietin	Kidney cancer
Ectopic Cushing's syndrome	ACTH-like	Oat cell lung cancer
Hyperglycemia	Glucagon-like	Fibrosarcomas
Hypercalcemia	Parathyroid-like	Breast, lung cancer
Carcinoid syndrome	Serotonin	Carcinoid
Inappropriate ADH	ADH	Lung cancer

These rare syndromes tell us much about the multipotential of the living cell. All somatic cells have a complement of 46 chromosomes and have the potential to produce a wide variety of proteins, enzymes, and hormones. Many of the genes in these chromosomes are repressed ("turned off") during the process of differentiation, allowing the expression of only specific genes in each cell. The neoplastic cell, by additions, deletions, or functional changes in the genes, breaks away from these controls. By a process of derepression, some inactive genetic loci become activated in the malignant cell. These loci can produce hormones or enzymes that secondarily induce a variety of endocrine syndromes in cancer patients.

Removal of the tumor can cure the endocrine abnormality, but usually these syndromes reflect an underlying, inoperable cancer.

DIAGNOSIS

The symptoms and signs of cancer are obviously as diverse as the wide variety of cancer sites and the resultant functional disturbances. In some cases, metastases alone herald the onset of the cancer. In such cases the origin of the cancer may sometimes be determined by (1) histological appearance and (2) the pattern of lymphatic spread. About 50% of patients dying from cancer have metastatic spread to *lymph nodes,* 36% have *liver metastases,* and 30% have *pulmonary involvement.* In some cases of diffuse carcinomatosis the precise origin of the cancer remains obscure.

The cancers that metastasize to the liver most frequently are the following:

Pancreas	65%	Stomach	35%
Breast	45%	Esophagus	30%
Large bowel	40%	Uterus	10%

The *bony skeleton* is involved in at least 15% to 20% of patients with fatal cancer. The most frequent primary sites that contribute bone cancer metastases are carcinomas of the *breast, prostate, thyroid,* and *kidney.* Metastases to bone are usually multiple. The bones most frequently involved in descending order of occurrence include the vertebra, rib, skull, femur, pelvis, humerus, and sternum. Metastases from renal and thyroid cancers may pulsate. Distant spread to the *brain* occurs in about 5% of fatal cases of malignant neoplasm. Primary cancer of breast, lung, and kidney contributes most of the metastatic growths in the brain. Curiously, primary cancers in the brain rarely metastasize to other parts of the body.

Some recent developments allow more specific and early localization of metastatic disease, e.g., brain scan and liver scan using radioisotopes. Xeroradiography, a type of mammogram, localizes breast cancer.

PROGNOSIS

The 5-year cure rate for all cancer is now about one in three patients. Fig. 11-4 gives the 5-year survival rates for some common neoplasms. The importance of lymph node metastases in the prognosis of cancer is obvious from these examples.

TREATMENT

Three methods of treating cancers are widely used: (1) surgery, (2) irradiation, and (3) chemotherapy. The mode of treatment depends on the type and extent of the tumor. Immunotherapy and chemoimmunotherapy are still chiefly experimental.

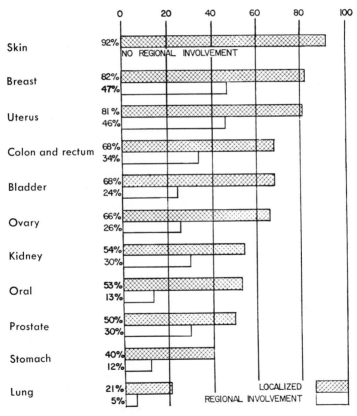

Fig. 11-4. Five-year survival rates for selected sites. Adjusted for normal life expectancy. (End results and mortality trends in cancer, National Cancer Institute Monograph No. 6; Cancer in Connecticut 1935 to 1951, Connecticut State Department of Health; from Ca **17:**1, 1967.)

Surgery

The fundamental aim of surgery is to remove all of the tumor without hopelessly disturbing the structure or function of the host. In some cases of advanced cancers palliative procedures, such as by-passing bile around a cancer of the pancreas, bring gratifying symptomatic relief. Occasionally resection of isolated metastases to lung or brain results in astonishingly long survivals.

In early cases surgical removal is the preferred primary treatment for most tumors including the common cancers: skin, colorectum, breast, lung, cervix, prostate, and stomach.

Radiation therapy

Because ionizing radiation alters the reproductive process of cells, it can destroy cancer. Although it destroys normal as well as neoplastic cells, normal cells have a greater capacity for repair and recovery. The degree of success depends on the difference in radioresponsiveness of the tumor compared to the surrounding norn.al tissues (Table 11-3). This response differential (therapeutic ratio) is extremely important, for it may enable us to control tumors whose cells have little sensitivity to radiation but are growing in tissues that will tolerate the high doses of radiation necessary for tumor control, e.g., soft tissue sarcoma in an extremity. On the other hand, some radiosensitive tumors may be surrounded by tissues that will not withstand even the lowest effective tumor dose, e.g., lymphoma in the region of the kidneys.

The primary intent of radiation therapy is to cure, the secondary intent to palliate. When evaluating a patient with cancer, the radiotherapist must first decide whether the tumor is likely to be susceptible to growth reduction by its sensitivity to radiation, as well as by its overall size and extent. He must localize the tumor precisely by radiographic studies, radioactive isotope scans, diagnostic ultrasound, and sometimes even surgical exploration. He must also spare the surrounding normal tissues from unnecessary radiation. Computers play a valuable role in complex mathematical calculations needed to plan treatment.

Radiation functions either as a primary mode of treatment or in combination with surgical removal and/or chemotherapy. For the most effective approach to the individual patient, the radiotherapist must coordinate his treatment with the patient's other physicians. Radiotherapy may be used either preoperatively or postoperatively, depending on the type, location, and extent of the tumor.

Radiotherapy and surgery, in general, are not competitive treatments. Each has its area of greatest effectiveness, although many tumors respond equally to either modality (e.g., carcinoma of the

Table 11-3. Radiosensitivity classification of normal tissues and malignant tumors

Relative radiosensitivity	Normal tissues	Primary malignancies
High	Lymphoid Hematopoietic Spermatogenic cells (testis) Follicular epithelium (ovary) Optic lens	Leukemia Lymphoma Hodgkin's disease Medulloblastoma Seminoma Dysgerminoma Retinoblastoma Anaplastic carcinoma
Medium	Skin Epithelium (mucosal linings) Endothelium (vascular) Growing cartilage Growing bone	Basal cell carcinoma Squamous cell carcinoma Adenocarcinoma Uterus Breast Bowel Prostate Liposarcoma Bronchogenic carcinoma Astrocytoma Rhabdomyosarcoma
Low	Connective tissue Muscle Fat Bone Nerve	Other adenocarcinomas Hypernephroma Teratoma Osteogenic tumors Melanoma Other sarcomas (differentiated)

lip, eyelid, larynx, or tonsil). Factors such as cosmetic results, length of treatment, and availability of facilities help the physician choose the final treatment. Whatever method is selected, the best time for cure is the first therapeutic attempt.

The list of neoplasms that may be accepted for a curative attempt by *radiation therapy alone* includes the following:

Larynx
Skin (except melanoma)
Mouth (lip, tongue)
Uterine cervix
Tonsil, palatine arch

Nasopharynx
Nasal accessory sinuses
Urinary bladder
Seminoma
Dysgerminoma

Medulloblastoma	Retinoblastoma
Lymphoma	Hypopharynx
Hodgkin's disease	Prostate
Endometrium	Esophagus
Vulva and vagina	Lung
Penis	Ewing's sarcoma
Anus	Liposarcoma (some)

Palliation

The radiotherapist often treats painful or crippling metastases regardless of whether the tumor is radiosensitive. Patients sometimes respond with gratifying relief of symptoms. Breast and lung cancers dominate the list of metastasizing tumors; accordingly, they are leading targets for palliative radiation.

Chemotherapy

The quest for a specific drug or drugs to destroy tumor cells selectively has brought some striking results, most notably, a 70% (or higher) cure rate for choriocarcinomas with methotrexate. Grossly and morphologically, cancers differ from normal tissues, but (Fig. 11-5) no distinct *qualitative* difference separates them on a chemical or molecular level. There are, however, a number of *quantitative* dissimilarities (enzymes and metabolites). If a qualitative difference is discovered, a drug or drugs could be designed to exploit this difference. Of the many thousands of antitumor agents tested in the past, only a few have proved to be useful clinically.

The same therapeutic principles apply to drugs as to surgery and irradiation. The drugs must destroy the tumor but must not irreparably injure the host. Unfortunately, the results of chemotherapy are

TISSUE

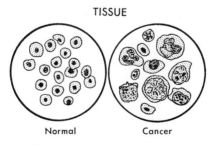

Normal   Cancer

Fig. 11-5. Microscopic appearance of most cancer cells differs markedly from normal as depicted here.

often uncertain and unpredictable. The drugs currently available have a very slight therapeutic advantage when compared to their toxicity on normal cells. Most of the drugs interfere with RNA or DNA synthesis. Many cells of the body, especially those of the *blood-forming organs, gastrointestinal tract,* and *hair follicles,* are rapidly dividing and therefore vulnerable to cytolytic agents. Newer drugs include the following: imidazole carboxamide (DTIC) acts against disseminated melanoma; the "nitroso-ureas" (BCNU, CCNU, and methyl-CCNU) cross the blood-brain barrier and palliate some brain tumors; adriamycin, an antibiotic, attacks various tumors, but especially breast cancer; bleomycin, another antibiotic, antagonizes some squamous cell tumors.

Agents in current use are classified as follows:

Alkylating agents:	Nitrogen mustard, cyclophosphamide, phenylalanine mustard, thio-tepa, nitrosoureas (BCNU, CCNU), imidazole carboxamide (DTIC)
Antimetabolites:	Methotrexate, 6-mercaptopurine, 5-fluorouracil
Antibiotics:	Actinomycin-D, adriamycin, bleomycin
Alkaloids:	Vincristine, vinblastine
Hormones:	Estrogens, androgens, corticosteroids
Miscellaneous:	Urothane, *o,p'*-DDD

Most of the drugs disrupt metabolic functions at certain phases of the cell cycle (Fig. 11-6). Nitrogen mustard and other alkylating agents can disrupt function at almost any point in the cycle, whereas other drugs are more specific. The *Vinca rosea* alkaloids produce their antineoplastic effect during the mitotic phase of the cell cycle. Actinomycin-D prevents the transcription of DNA to RNA during the G_1 phase of the cycle. Many of the other drugs including 5-fluorouracil, 6-mercaptopurine, cytosine arabinoside, and methotrexate act during the S (synthetic) phase of the cell cycle; these drugs inhibit DNA synthesis. Drugs can modify the metabolic processes in the cell either at a molecular or an organelle level.

Some drugs attack specific cells, e.g., *o,p'*-DDD versus adrenal cortical tumors; streptozotocin versus pancreatic islet cell tumors.

Some of the solid tumors that are palliated by cytotoxic agents are given in Table 11-4.

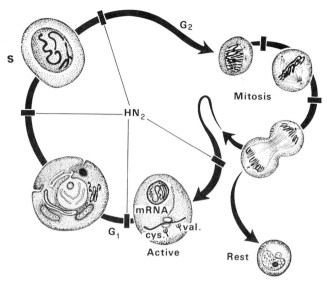

Fig. 11-6. Cell cycle and chemotherapy. Most cytolytic agents act on the cell at some point in the cell cycle. Nitrogen mustard (HN₂) can act at almost any position. Cells are usually most vulnerable during the S, or synthetic, phase of DNA synthesis. *Cys.,* cysteine; *val.,* valine.

Complications of chemotherapy

Since the therapeutic amount of these drugs approaches the toxic level, cancer chemotherapy carries a substantial morbidity. All normal, rapidly dividing cells within the organism are vulnerable to these cytolytic agents. The most serious complication of this type of therapy is *bone marrow depression*. Most drugs depress all elements of active bone marrow. An alkylating agent (cyclophosphamide) usually spares the thrombocytes. Vincristine is more selectively neurotoxic than myelotoxic (marrow toxic).

The cells in the *hair follicles* are rapidly dividing and consequently are vulnerable to these agents. With some of the drugs (5-fluorouracil), the incidence of alopecia approaches 30%. But hair regrows after cessation of therapy. Occasionally *dermatitis* may result from drug therapy, but it is usually limited to the period of drug administration.

The maximum toxicity may become manifest 5 to 7 days after discontinuing therapy. A 2 to 4% mortality is associated with the use

Table 11-4. Solid tumors palliated by cytotoxic agents

Organ	Drug
Prostate	Estrogen
Wilms' tumor	Actinomycin-D
Breast	Androgen, glucocorticoids
	Estrogen
	5-fluorouracil
	Adriamycin
Ovary	Alkylating agents (cyclophosphamide)
Endometrial carcinoma	Progesterone
Lung	Nitrogen mustard
	Cyclophosphamide
	Bleomycin
Large intestine	5-fluorouracil
Cervix	Cyclophosphamide
Melanoma	Thio-tepa
	Phenylalanine mustard
	Imidazole carboxamide (DTIC)
Adrenal cortex	o,p'-DDD
Choriocarcinoma	Methotrexate
Brain	Nitroso-urea (BCNU)

of potent cytolytic agents. If a malignant lesion is sensitive to drug therapy, it usually responds early, before toxicity becomes evident.

The cells within the *alimentary tract* also have a rapid turnover rate. Cytotoxic agents cause varying degrees of mucosal damage and attendant symptoms—melena, cramps, diarrhea, dysphagia, and sepsis.

Regional administration of chemotherapeutic agents

Widely disseminated tumors require systemic chemotherapy, but localized tumors respond best to high concentrations of drugs. *Infusion* and *perfusion* are dual techniques that increase drug concentration to the tumor, yet spare other parts of the body.

Intra-arterial infusion. Infusion is characterized by the word *continuous*. Since cells are most vulnerable during certain stages of mitosis, the anticancer drug must be present at this time. Cancer cells are "mitotically" out of step; therefore, the drug must be offered over a period of time that corresponds to the "doubling-time" of the can-

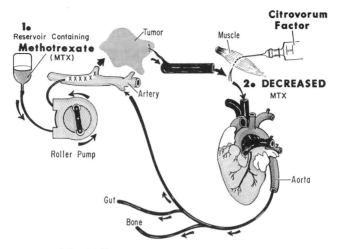

Fig. 11-7. Regional intra-arterial infusion.

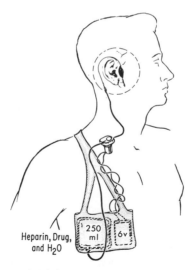

Fig. 11-8. Intra-arterial infusion. Portable unit allows full ambulation.

cer. We inject the anticancer agent through a cannulated artery supplying the tumor. The tumor receives the full force of the drug, continuously over a period of weeks or months. It is diluted and antagonized in the peripheral circulation by the normal metabolite (citrovorum factor) so that other areas of the body receive only minimal dosages of the agent (Fig. 11-7). Citrovorum factor is often used with methotrexate to antagonize its action on normal cells.

Head and neck tumors, advanced pelvic tumors, melanomas of the extremities, and hepatic metastases have been controlled by this method. Ingenious, tiny pumps supply the drug continuously through precisely placed infusion catheters (Figs. 11-8 and 11-9).

Perfusion. A portion of the body (usually an extremity) is isolated by tourniquet, and the isolated portion is made a part of an extracorporeal circuit by cannulating both artery and vein. An anticancer drug (e.g., phenylalanine mustard, actinomycin-D, or thio-tepa) in high concentration is then introduced. Perfusion is time-limited (usually 1 hour). After perfusion, the therapist washes out the isolated area and restores vascular continuity. This technique can be repeated at intervals necessary to control cancer growth. Perfusion (prophylactically) supplements primary resection of cancers, notably melanomas (Figs. 11-10 and 11-11). Following wide excision of all gross tumor (primary melanoma), the incidence of local recurrence and

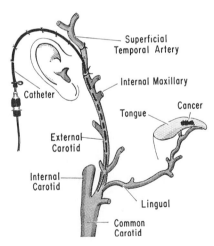

Fig. 11-9. Intra-arterial infusion. Note precise placement of catheter orifice at takeoff of lingual artery to infuse cancer of tongue.

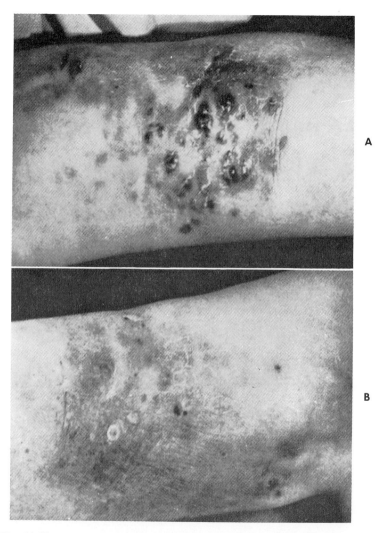

Fig. 11-10. Recurrent melanoma. **A,** Before perfusion. **B,** After perfusion (phenylalanine mustard). (From Stehlin, J. S., Jr., and others: Regional chemotherapy of cancer: experience with 116 perfusions, Ann. Surg. **151:**605-619, April 1960.)

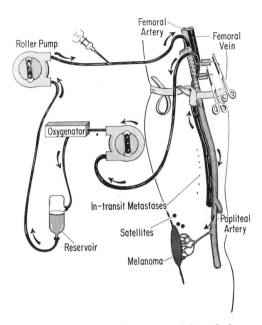

Fig. 11-11. Regional intra-arterial perfusion.

in-transit metastases (metastases between the tumor and nearest lymph nodes) averages 15 to 20%. These smaller aggregates of cells in lymphatics are probably most vulnerable to prophylactic perfusion at the time of excision of the primary tumor and its metastases. Perfusion also helps palliate far-advanced or recurrent malignant melanomas and sarcomas of the extremities.

Combined therapy

Combinations of drugs, systemically, have improved results, e.g., methotrexate, chlorambucil, and actinomycin D in the treatment of embryonal cancer of the testicle. Some regimens include as many as five drugs.

Irradiation combined with infusion have successfully palliated far-advanced cancers in the head and neck region (Fig. 11-12).

Nonspecific treatment of the cancer patient

In treating the patient suffering from advanced cancer, the physician must combine his technical skill with a vitally important sensi-

THERAPY

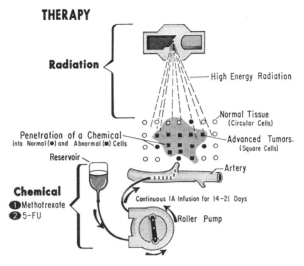

Fig. 11-12. Simultaneous radiation and chemotherapy.

tivity and sympathy. He must sustain some degree of hope for the patient, yet not mislead him. Cancer patients often go through phases of *rage* ("Why me?") and *rejection* ("I don't believe it.") on the way to eventual *acceptance*. The physician must guide the patient through these emotionally grueling periods. The patient will sense that he is in the hands of an aggressive, yet sympathetic therapist who believes, sincerely, that new cures lie just ahead. Although computers may aid treatment, they can never replace the sensitive, dedicated doctor.

Patients with cancer, even when far advanced, do not necessarily have exceptional pain. The discomfort is often a minimal physical stimulus with maximum overlay of anxiety. There are many methods of controlling pain without narcotics. When a cancer patient evinces local or regional pain, every effort should be made to use regional anesthesia. Peripheral nerve blocks with alcohol, epidural instillation of phenol, and other modifications of local and regional anesthesia can control most pain (see Chapter 40). It is too easy to addict a patient who has cancer.

In addition to the psychological and painful aspects of malignant disease, other manifestations of distant and local involvement demand treatment. Effusions of various coelomic cavities can often be controlled by systemic chemotherapy, local instillation of drugs into serous cavities, sodium restriction, and diuretics. Pleural effusions are particularly distressful because they slowly suffocate patients. The physician should aspirate these effusions and attempt to prevent their recurrence. (For direct injection into the thoracic cavity, use nitrogen mustard 0.4 mg./kg., or thio-tepa 0.8 mg./kg.) Patients who cannot tolerate cytolytic agents, because of bone marrow depression, may require quinacrine injected into the pleural space (50 mg. initially, with a similar daily increment up to 200 or 250 mg.). Ascites can be controlled similarly.

Metastasis to the central nervous system is common from lung and breast cancer and melanomas. Craniotomy may be worthwhile to remove a single mass that causes symptoms. Steroids and radiotherapy may also relieve increased intracranial pressure.

Metastasis can collapse vertebral bodies, with subsequent pressure on cord or spinal nerves. Epidural metastases may impinge on nerves without bony involvement. When symptoms of compression rapidly progress, laminectomy may prevent complete paralysis. Radiotherapy can be given postoperatively.

The superior vena cava may be selectively obstructed in patients with lymphomas and lung cancer. Simultaneous chemotherapy and radiation therapy may be palliative for these patients.

The patient with alimentary tract obstruction may benefit from a surgical procedure. Those with intra-abdominal malignancy may have a discrete area of obstruction. Operative procedures (intestinal bypass, gastrostomy, ileostomy, or colostomy) can relieve obstruction. Cervical esophagostomy (which prevents accumulation of secretions in the pharynx and bronchial aspiration) can be palliative for patients with high esophageal obstruction.

Bony metastases occasionally result in pathological fractures. The pain of bone metastasis can often be controlled with radiation therapy, and pathological fractures may show signs of healing after radiation. Fractures of weight-bearing bones often require immobilization by the use of intramedullary devices followed by radiation therapy.

The treatment of the cancer-endocrine syndromes, especially hyperparathyroid states in association with breast cancer, can prolong and improve vitality. Adrenocortical steroids, restriction of calcium, and increased fluid intake may lower hypercalcemia. Adrenalectomy or o,p'-DDD may palliate ectopic Cushing's syndrome.

IMMUNOLOGY AND CANCER

Investigators, long suspecting a link between cancer and the body's defense mechanisms, have cited the following evidence to support their suspicions: (1) some tumors have miraculously disappeared, without explanation other than some "inherent defense mechanisms"; (2) pathologists have noted that chronic inflammatory cells tend to cluster about certain cancers, and these cancers seem to run a favorable course; (3) cytological studies have revealed convincing evidence that cancer cells flood the circulation, especially during surgical procedures, yet few grow into neoplasms; (4) some defense mechanism in patients with advanced cancers resists the implantation of small, autologous tumors. Cancer immunologists have now confirmed these earlier suspicions by showing that cancer antigens coexist with virtually all cancers.

Two of these antigens have practical clinical use; their appearance in serum helps to detect underlying cancers. About 70% of patients with hepatomas show elevated serum levels of α-fetoglobulin. The hepatoma cells, reverting back to the embryonic liver tissue that normally produces this antigen during early life, secrete it pathologically. Elevated serum levels indicate hepatoma. *Carcinoembryonic antigen* (CEA), another fetal antigen, increases in the serum with gastrointestinal cancers, but unfortunately with many other diseases as well. Because CEA appears in the serum so commonly, it offers little help in cancer detection, but it acts as an excellent guide to assess patients with bowel cancers: CEA serum levels usually drop following successful resection and rise with recurrence.

The immune response

The body, sensing foreign cells through memory-cell surveillance, responds immunologically in two ways to cancer: either with (1) a *cell-mediated reaction,* or with (2) *humoral antibodies.* In either case the small lymphocyte plays the leading role. The T-cell ("killer-cell") derived from the thymus, attaches to cell membranes and lyses the cell (with the aid of macrophages). The B-cells (from bursal equivalent) produce tumor antibodies (Ab) that neutralize antigen or act as "helper cells" in the delayed sensitivity reaction. Although the cell-mediated response appears dominant, both mechanisms interact in their attempt to destroy tumors. (See Chapter 36.)

Immunotherapy

Because chemotherapy, radiation, and surgery destroy normal as well as cancer cells the oncologist must frequently "pull his punches" with these ablative therapies. Consequently, cancer cells often escape these treatments. Immunotherapy may find its greatest use following these ablative therapies because it theoretically attacks only the antigen-coated cancer cells, thus sparing normal cells. These ablative therapies reduce the main mass of tumor cells, thus helping to over-

IMMUNOLOGIC SURVEILLANCE

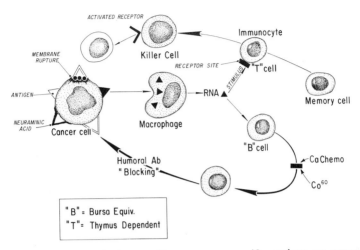

Fig. 11-13. Immunologic surveillance: tumor-specific antigen on cancer cell processed by macrophage. The product (immune RNA?) sensitizes T cells, which seek out and destroy the cancer cell if it is not protected by "blocking" substance.

ride immunotherapy's chief weakness: the overwhelming of the body's immune responses by advanced cancers. Chemotherapy may also prevent formation of "blocking" substances that interfere with immunological defenses (Fig. 11-13).

Penn discusses the methods that *suppress* the immunological responses to grafts in Chapter 36. Tumor immunologists seek just the opposite. They look for mechanisms that *enhance* the immunological response to cancer. But so far enhancement has posed greater problems than suppression. The approaches to cancer immunotherapy include: (1) active, (2) passive (adoptive), and (3) nonspecific immunotherapy.

Active immunotherapy

Researchers have tried to increase the antigenicity of tumor vaccines by coupling tumor cells with rabbit gamma-globulin (a highly antigenic protein), by irradiating or freeze-thawing cells, and by using neuoraminidase to "unmask" antigens (Fig. 11-13). To date, these attempts to fashion more potent cancer vaccines have been disappointing.

Passive immunotherapy

Antitumor antibodies, produced by patients cured of cancer, have failed to achieve clear-cut, clinical results when given to patients with similar cancers. Although laboratory work has been encouraging, clinical testing has not. Antisera therapy may neutralize blocking factors or directly encourage macrophages or lymphocytes to lyse tumor cells.

Infusion of lymphocytes or extracts from lymphocytes removed from patients with or cured from cancer have produced some tumor regressions. RNA extracts or transfer factor utilize informational molecules that transmit to homologous host lymphocytes a specific sensitization to "unwanted" cells. The recipient's own immune reaction fights the foreign cells. These extracts have definite advantages; they do not cause serum sickness, anaphylaxis, or HLA incompatibility.

Nonspecific therapy

Although the mechanism remains obscure, some substances stimulate the body's general immune defenses. Much current interest has centered on BCG, an attenuated, bovine tuberculous bacillus. This agent, injected into cutaneous melanomas, has caused regression of about 90% of the melanomas in immunologically competent patients. More astonishing, 20% of the melanomas, apart from those injected, also regressed. Unfortunately, BCG usually fails to show any effect in melanomas that invade visceral organs. Dinitrochlorobenzene (DNCB) incites a delayed sensitivity reaction in some patients with superficial, squamous, or basal cell cancers of the skin.

CHAPTER 12

The skin

DAVID W. FURNAS

The skin is the largest organ of the body and is the device that allowed our distant forebears to emerge from the sea without fear of desiccation or bacterial ambush. Composing the skin are several different structures, each giving rise to characteristic disease processes. Only those few that have surgical significance are considered here.

THE EPIDERMIS AND ITS ADNEXAL STRUCTURES

Hair follicles, sebaceous glands, and sweat glands (eccrine and apocrine) are formed by labile epithelial cells that can quickly regenerate to repair any superficial injury. (See discussion on skin grafts in Chapter 34.) Infections and tumors are common in these structures.

Infections

Furuncles or "boils" are caused by *Staphylococcus aureus* infections of hair follicles; they respond to surgical incision, drainage, and antibiotics. *Carbuncles* are staphylococcal infections of the back or of the posterior neck that burrow and branch in the deep dermis and subcutaneous tissue fat. Adequate drainage requires wide and deep incisions. *Hidradenitis suppurativa* is a chronic infection of apocrine sweat glands in the axilla or the perineum. If far advanced, this disease is treated by excision of the involved skin and repair of the resultant defect with skin grafts or pedicles. The surgical importance of *acne vulgaris*, a recurring pustular infection of the skin follicles of the face, arises from the need to improve resulting scars with excision or dermabrasion.

Benign conditions

Rhinophyma is a grotesque hyperplasia of the nasal skin, treated simply by sculpting a more desirable shape with a scalpel; it arises after years of the chronic inflammatory process *acne rosacea* (Fig. 12-1).

Epidermal cysts (sebaceous cysts or wens) occur anywhere on the body, but particularly on the face, neck, or scalp (Fig. 12-2). They

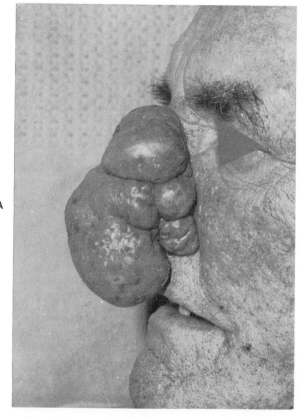

A

Fig. 12-1. Rhinophyma. **A,** Preoperative condition.
Continued.

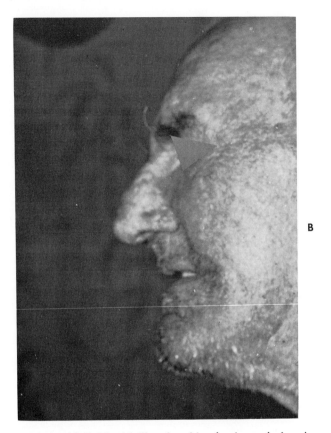

B

Fig. 12-1, cont'd. B, Nasal bulk reduced by simple surgical paring.

may result from bits of epidermis implanted in the depths of the skin by sharp objects (discussion on implantation cyst, Chapter 39), or possibly from a blocked hair follicle or sebaceous gland. They are lined by epidermis and are filled with epidermal debris. Rarely, a *true sebaceous cyst* is encountered that is lined by sebaceous cells and filled with sebum. The lining of *dermoid cysts* contains not only keratinizing epidermis but also adnexal structures. They presumably arise from primordial islands of skin that were displaced duuring embryonic development. They are common around the eyes (Fig. 12-3)

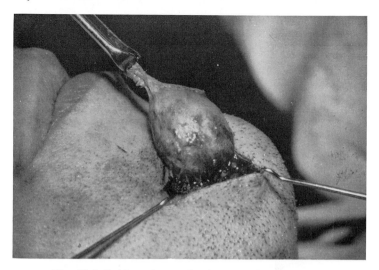

Fig. 12-2. Epidermal cyst of chin exposed at operation.

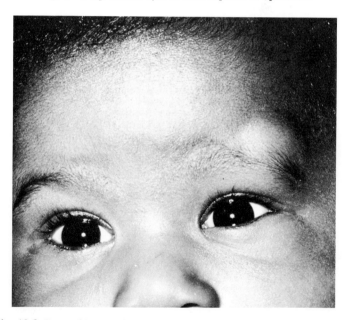

Fig. 12-3. Dermoid cyst of upper lateral part of left orbital rim. The cyst caused an indentation in the frontal bone.

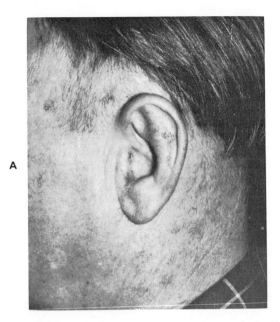

Fig. 12-4. Progress of precancerous change to cancer. **A,** Senile keratoses of left temple (just anterior to hairline) and scaphoid fossa of external ear. **B,** Frank squamous (epidermoid carcinoma of right temple of same patient with metastasis to preauricular lymph nodes—*inked circle*).

and nose, and sometimes they extend into the cranial vault; therefore, the surgeon undertaking their excision should be properly forearmed. *Seborrheic keratoses* are brownish, raised, "velvety-feeling" blotches, common in old patients. They have no potential for malignancy. Because of their superficial purchase on the skin, they can be shaved off with a knife, and the wound will epithelialize. Sometimes they are so numerous that excision is impractical. There are numerous types of *benign adenomas, papillomas, and polyps* of epidermal and adnexal origin for which excision (or dermatological removal) is performed to obtain a diagnosis and to improve appearance.

Premalignant lesions

There are numerous premalignant lesions of the skin that develop into squamous cell carcinomas or basal cell carcinomas decades after the initial inciting insult (Fig. 12-4). *Senile* or *actinic keratoses* re-

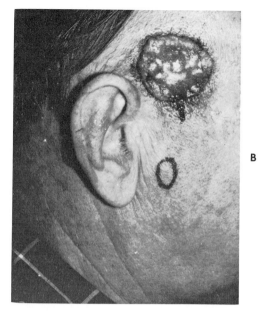

B

Fig. 12-4, cont'd. For legend see opposite page.

sult from years of exposure to sunshine (farmers and sailors). *Keratotic radiation changes* result from repeated small doses of ionizing radiation (e.g., hands of dentists) or from therapeutic doses of radiation received many years before (Fig. 12-5). Long-term treatment for syphilis or psoriasis with Fowler's solution or other arsenicals results in premalignant *arsenical keratoses,* which are found on palmar or plantar surfaces. Chronic contact with certain hydrocarbon compounds, accompanied by irritation or sunlight, may result in keratoses such as those that lead to the scrotal carcinoma of chimney sweeps. *Chronic unstable burn scars* or *chronic draining osteomyelitis* causes premalignant changes that lead to *Marjolin's ulcer,* which is a squamous carcinoma. The unfortunate children who inherit *xeroderma pigmentosum* through a recessive gene have an exquisite sensitivity to ultraviolet light, causing keratoses and ultimately multiple squamous cell carcinomas, basal cell carcinomas, and even sarcomas and mela-

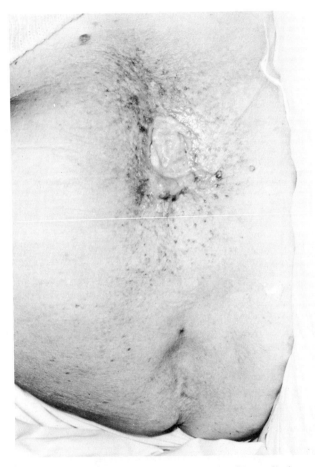

Fig. 12-5. Radiation changes in lumbar area caused by radiation received for "lumbago" 35 years previously. A central area of necrosis is surrounded by atrophic keratotic skin. Many basal cell and squamous cell carcinomas were found on microscopic examination.

nomas. They are doomed to die before adulthood. Patients with *lupus vulgaris* (tuberculosis of the skin) develop keratoses and frequent basal or squamous carcinomas (lupus carcinoma) in their later years.

Most of the skin cancers that arise from these predisposing lesions are prevented by avoiding exposure to the various inciting causes. Diagnosis is confirmed by histological examination of suspicious lesions. Either *excisional biopsy* (complete removal of suspicious lesions including margins of normal tissue on all sides), or *incisional biopsy* (removal of only a sample of the lesion) with a knife or punch is done. Premalignant lesions may be treated by excision, shaving, dermabrasion, electrodesiccation, application of chemotherapeutic agents, or careful observation.

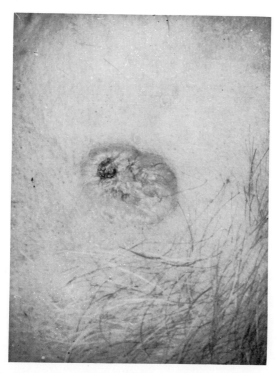

Fig. 12-6. Basal cell carcinoma. Translucency, mild lobulation, delicate vasculature, and slight ulcerations are seen.

Malignant lesions

Basal cell carcinomas and *squamous cell carcinomas* that arise in the epidermis (sometimes called *epitheliomas*) are the *most common of all malignant tumors*. They arise from the epidermis because of the above factors, or from no obvious cause. Of these predisposing factors, sunlight is by far the most important. Light-complexioned male outdoor workers in hot climates receive the most solar radiation and are therefore the most frequent victims. Hands, faces, and necks are the most common sites. The most superficial epitheliomas are *multicentric basal cell carcinoma, intraepidermal squamous cell carcinoma,* and *Bowen's disease.*

Basal cell carcinoma (basal cell epithelioma) (Fig. 12-6) of the skin is most common on the face, particularly the cheeks, eyelids, nose, and lips (nonvermilion surface). Northern European ancestry strongly predisposes to basal cell carcinoma. It has a raised, pearly, translucent appearance and a delicate capillary network, frequently without ulceration. Ulceration develops as the lesion increases in size. It almost never metastasizes, but if inadequately treated, it relentlessly erodes through soft tissues, cartilage, and bone until death ensues from invasion of arteries, brain, or airway (hence the name *rodent ulcer*). If the patient is seen early and excision and histological study are carried out properly, the cure rate should approach 100%.

Squamous cell carcinoma (squamous cell epithelioma) (Figs. 12-4, *B*, and 39-26, *F*) of the skin has the power to metastasize to regional lymph nodes; however, it is a well-differentiated carcinoma, and metastases occur late. Antecedent trauma such as radiation injury (Fig. 12-5), chronic chemical exposure (hydrocarbons, arsenic), burns from plastic or hot metal, or unstable scars (as well as sunlight) predispose to squamous cell carcinomas. They are horny, crusted lesions and frequently show rolled margins surrounding an area of ulceration. The ears, temples, upper parts of the face, and dorsum of the hands are the most common sites. Squamous cell carcinoma is almost as common as basal cell carcinoma, but it affects an older group of patients. Wide excision or radiation of early lesions yields a 5-year survival rate of over 90%. The outlook is gloomier for patients with very large lesions and those that have spread to lymph nodes. Regional lymphatic dissection is carried out when lymphatic metastases are suspected.

Keratoacanthoma (self-healing epithelioma, molluscum sebaceum) grows rapidly from a small papule to a sizable raised tumor with an umbilicated, necrotic center in 6 to 8 weeks and then subsides, leaving a scarcely visible mark. It has the microscopic picture of a well-differentiated squamous cell carcinoma. Rarely, it fails to regress, behaving like an invasive squamous carcinoma. I will not discuss the numerous types of neoplasms of the adnexal structures of the skin, because of their rarity.

THE DERMIS

Excessive proliferation of dermal fibroblasts occurs in hypertrophied scars and keloids (see Chapter 2), as well as some rare lesions such as desmoids.

PIGMENT-PRODUCING CELLS

The surgically important pigmented lesions, nevi and melanomas, arise from pigment-producing cells of neuroectodermal origin (melanocytes, Schwann cells, or both). Freckles and lentigines are pigmented but are not composed of pigment-producing cells.

Pigmented nevi

Junctional nevi (Figs. 12-7 and 12-9), in which the nevus cells are clustered at the junction of the dermis and the epidermis, are flat and hairless and can give rise to malignant melanomas. *Intradermal nevi* (Figs. 12-8 and 12-9) are formed of nests of nevus cells buried in the dermis, deep to the dermoepidermal junction. They are usually raised, may be hairy, and do not become malignant. The *compound nevus* (Fig. 12-9) has both junctional and intradermal elements and has the same malignant potential as the junctional nevus. (See Table 12-1.)

Junctional nevi are much more common in children than in adults (70% of nevi in children under 15, but only 20% in adults), yet, paradoxically, malignant melanoma is almost unknown in children. (*Juvenile melanomas,* which microscopically resemble malignant melanomas, occur in children but are not malignant.) Curiously, almost all nevi below the knee in adults are junctional nevi.

There are so many nevi and such a minute percentage of them turn into malignant melanomas that it is impractical to excise every flat, hairless mole. However, nevi at points of constant irritation (foot, belt line, neck, bearded area) and nevi that show any sort of change, such as increase in size, deeper pigmentation, itching, or bleeding, should be excised and examined microscopically.

The uncommon *blue nevus* (benign dermal melanocytoma) derives its color (sometimes a striking deep blue) from intense pigmentation plus its location deep within the dermis. Occasionally the regional lymph nodes become pigmented, but metastases are almost unknown.

The *giant hairy nevus* and *"bathing trunk" nevus* appear at birth

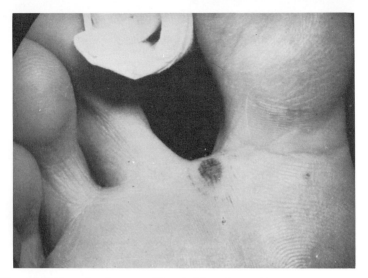

Fig. 12-7. Junctional nevus. Flat, hairless, brownish gross appearance (proposed incision line marked with ink).

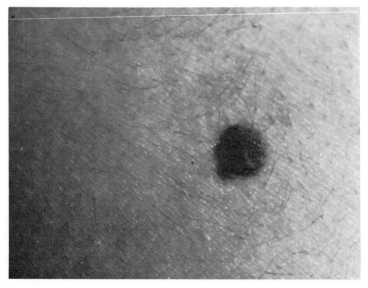

Fig. 12-8. Intradermal nevus. Note elevated contour.

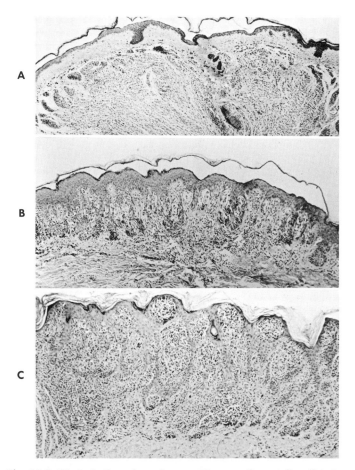

Fig. 12-9. Nevi. **A,** Intradermal nevus. Nevus cells are all well below the dermo-epidermal junction and occupy the entire lower four fifths of the pictured specimen. **B,** Junctional nevus. The nevus cells are found only in clusters at the junction area between the dermis and epidermis. **C,** Compound nevus. Nevus cells are seen in nests at the dermo-epidermal junction and also throughout much of the dermis. (Courtesy Dr. James H. Graham, Department of Dermatology, University of California, Irvine, Calif.)

Table 12-1. Description of nevi

Junctional nevus	*Compound nevus*	*Intradermal nevus*
Flat	⟵————⟶	Raised
Hairless	⟵————⟶	Often hairy
Often present below knee		Rarely present below knee
Present in most young children		80% of nevi in adults
70% of nevi in children under 15 years		Rarely present in young children
Nevus cells in clumps at dermoepidermal junction	Nevus cells at both sites	Nevus cells in nests within the dermis
Precursor to malignant melanoma	Same significance as junctional nevus	Not premalignant

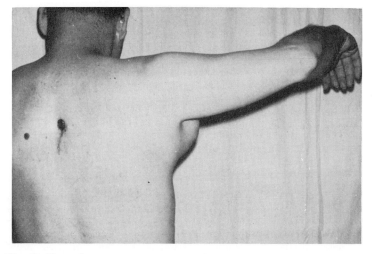

Fig. 12-10. Malignant melanoma. A malignant melanoma of the back has metastasized to the right axillary lymph nodes, causing a large axillary mass.

and may cover half of the body surface. These sometimes give rise to true malignant melanomas in childhood.

Malignant melanomas

Malignant melanomas (Fig. 12-10) are highly malignant pigmented skin lesions (rarely nonpigmented) found anywhere on the skin (and rarely on oral mucosa or anoderm). The most common sites are the head, neck, and lower limbs. They can metastasize through both the lymphatic system and the bloodstream and may spread to any organ of the body. Small islands of microlymphatic

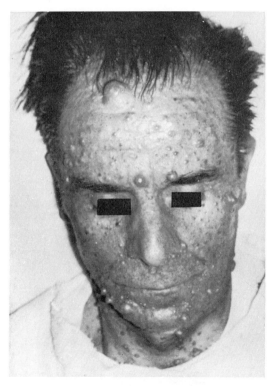

Fig. 12-11. Neurofibromatosis. Multiple neurofibromas of face in patient with von Recklinghausen's syndrome.

170 *Synopsis of surgery*

spread near the primary lesion are called *satellites*. Other foci of
spread may outline the course of regional lymphatic vessels. About
half the malignant melanomas arise from junctional or compound
nevi, and half arise anew. They occur particularly in young adults
and throughout the adult years. The blotchy *Hutchinson's spot* or
malignant lentigo, seen on the facial skin of elderly patients, is a rela-

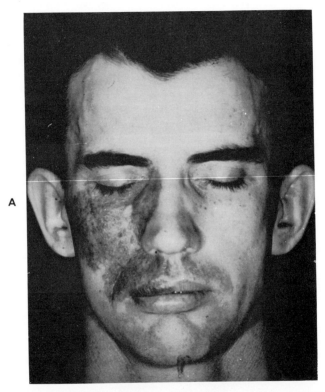

Fig. 12-12. Capillary hemangioma. **A,** Preoperative appearance of "port-
wine stain" hemangioma. **B,** Hemangioma after tattooing with light-
colored pigments. (Courtesy Dr. Herbert Conway, New York, N. Y.; case
from the Plastic Surgery Service, Veterans Administration Hospital,
Bronx, N. Y.)

tively indolent melanoma and metastasizes only at a late date. It has a proclivity to local recurrence.

Malignant melanomas are radioresistant and must be treated by wide local excision, frequently combined with removal of the regional lymphatics. Chemotherapeutic or immunological agents are sometimes useful adjuncts. (See Chapter 11.) Prognosis depends on clinical type, level of invasion, and metastasis. *Lentigo malignant melanoma* commonly afflicts the aged and has the best prognosis. *Superficial spreading malignant melanoma* and *nodular malignant melanoma* arise in youth and middle age, and carry an intermediate and poor prognosis, respectively. Clark classifies malignant melanomas in five levels: (I)

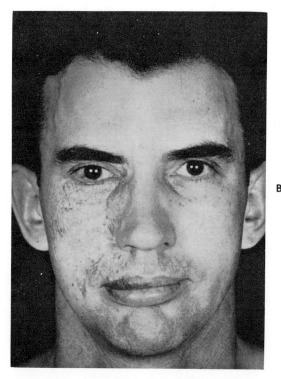

B

Fig. 12-12, cont'd. For legend see opposite page.

in situ, above basal lamina of epidermis; (II) extension through basal lamina into papillary layer; (III) tumor fills papillary level to the junction of the reticular dermal layer; (IV) invasion into the reticular layer; and (V) invasion of subcutaneous fat. Depending on type and level, the prognosis for localized malignant melanomas ranges from 20 to 100% in 5-year survivals. Lymphatic spread reduces the expected survival to 15% or less, and bloodstream seeding cuts it to practically nil.

NERVE TISSUES

A *neuroma* (traumatic neurilemoma) is an outgrowth of Schwann cells and axones, mixed with scar tissue, located at the proximal cut end of a severed nerve. (See discussion on benign tumors of the hand, Chapter 39.) A *neurilemoma* is a discrete, encapsulated, benign tu-

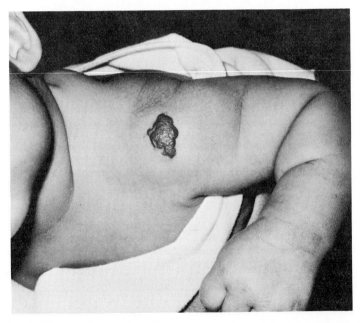

Fig. 12-13. Strawberry nevus. Lesion appeared several weeks after birth and spontaneously subsided before the age of 2 years.

mor arising from the Schwann cells of peripheral nerves. It is usually solitary, but it may occur in neurofibromatosis. A *neurofibroma* (Fig. 12-11) is a benign, nonencapsulated, diffusely infiltrating benign tumor, usually found in multiple sites. At times neurofibromas cause strikingly grotesque deformities. They are usually associated with café-au-lait spots and are part of the hereditary disorder *von Recklinghausen's syndrome*. The multiplicity and permeation of the lesions can make a mockery of ablative surgery, although often the patient's appearance can be improved. Sarcomatous degeneration is a late complication.

VASCULAR TISSUES
Capillary hemangioma

The *port-wine stain,* or *nevus flammeus,* commonly presents as a large, flat, purplish blotch on the face or neck with no disruption of normal contour (Fig. 12-12). It is present at birth, does not regress, and is important only because of its appearance. It can be camouflaged by tattooing with light-colored pigments or it can be covered with skillful makeup. *"Stork bites"* are purplish areas of delicate capillary dilatation on the nape of the neck, eyelids or glabella of newborn babies, and they subside before the child reaches 1 or 2 years of age. *Strawberry mark* (or nevus vasculosus) (Fig. 12-13) is a highly cellular capillary hemangioma that appears as a raised, bright red lesion anywhere on the body. It regresses spontaneously.

Cavernous hemangiomas

Involuting cavernous hemangiomas appear shortly after birth as a small, blue-red lesion, commonly on the face or neck, which rapidly grows into a large space-occupying mass that may cause grotesque disfigurement (Fig. 12-14). They involute and disappear before the age of 2 or 3 years, but they may leave in their wake distortion and displacement of facial features, which necessitates reconstructive surgery. Some cavernous hemangiomas in infants do not involute, but it is most difficult to distinguish these lesions except in retrospect.

Ordinary cavernous hemangiomas may be of any size, shape, or location, may be multiple, and may be associated with arteriovenous fistulas, hemorrhage, or infection. Treatment is usually excision. At times location or size may lend impracticability to surgical attack. Injection and sclerosing agents may be of help. Both capillary and cavernous hemangiomas form part of a number of specific disease syndromes.

Malignant tumors of vessels are very rare and are highly malignant.

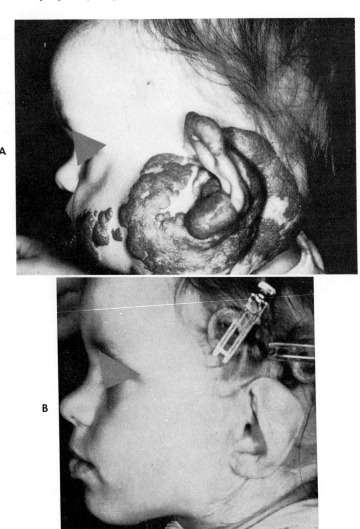

Fig. 12-14. Involution cavernous hemangioma. **A,** Appearance at height of growth cycle during first year of life. **B,** Appearance several years after spontaneous involution. (Courtesy Dr. Richard Caplan, University of Iowa Hospitals, Iowa City, Iowa.)

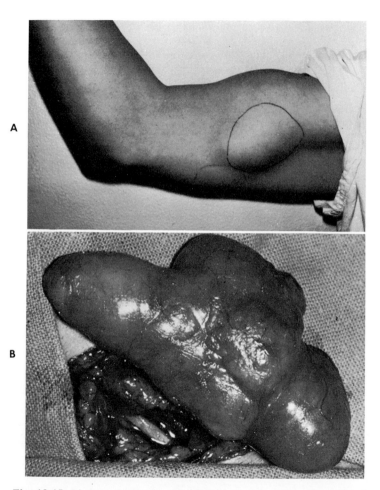

Fig. 12-15. Lipoma. **A,** Preoperative lumps on right arm, suspected to be lipomatous. **B,** Operative specimen showing fat lobulations of lipoma in contrast to pattern of adjacent subcutaneous fat.

SUBCUTANEOUS FAT

Lipomas are soft, multilobulated, benign lumps of fat that have a different color and texture than immediately surrounding subcutaneous fat (Fig. 12-15). They are treated by excisional biopsy in order to differentiate them from malignant soft tissue tumors such as *liposarcoma, fibrosarcoma,* or *rhabdomyosarcoma.* If the mass is large, hard, and truly suspicious for malignancy, an incisional biopsy with study of permanent microscopic sections is the best prelude to definitive surgery.

CHAPTER 13

The thyroid gland

RICHARD D. LIECHTY

The normal human thyroid gland weighs only 20 to 30 grams. As is true of other endocrine glands, the hormonal activity of the thyroid gland far overshadows its size.

Thyroid hormones have three vitally important functions in man: (1) they control metabolism within the cells, (2) they have a profound effect on growth and development, and (3) they strongly influence tissue differentiation.

The cellular actions of these hormones remain poorly understood, but the clinical consequences of excesses or deficits of thyroid hormones are well known and most important. The diseases of function and structure of the thyroid gland are the main concern of this chapter.

PHYSIOLOGY

The thyroid gland is the only tissue in the body with the ability to store significant amounts of iodine. It combines the trapped iodine with tyrosine to form two active hormones, thyroxine (tetraiodothyronine, T_4) and triiodothyronine (T_3).

Hypothalamic-pituitary-thyroid triangle

The pituitary gland controls the thyroid gland through its thyroid-stimulating hormone, TSH (TSH is released by TRF, thyrotropin-releasing factor from the hypothalamus), which incites thyroid cells to produce and release thyroid hormones. Without the TSH stimulus, the thyroid gland (the target gland) is absolutely powerless to function, and it consequently atrophies.

The thyroid hormones, as they increase in the blood in response to TSH, inhibit or cut off production of TSH. This negative-feedback control system monitors the amount of thyroid hormones at a steady

177

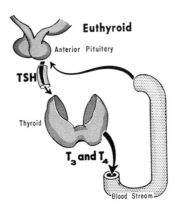

Fig. 13-1. Normal pituitary-thyroid relationship.

level. This level is "set" in brain centers (probably the hypothalamus), and TRF conveys this message to the responsive thyrotropic cells in the anterior pituitary (Fig. 13-1).

Understanding this hypothalamic-pituitary-thyroid feedback relationship is vital to understanding thyroid disease; e.g., whenever functioning thyroid tissue is ablated, thyroid hormones decrease and TSH increases (the blocking action of thyroid is removed). This increased TSH, in turn, will stimulate any remaining thyroid tissue to grow.

Conversely, when thyroid hormones are added, they block TSH and place the thyroid gland at rest. This latter effect explains the action of thyroid hormones in suppressing growth of goiters, nodules, and even some cancer, all of which theoretically arise in response to increased TSH. Exogenous thyroid hormones, acting much like a cast on an extremity, "splint" and rest the thyroid gland.

THYROID MEDICATIONS

Probably no other common drug is more misunderstood or misused than desiccated thyroid. The active substances in *desiccated thyroid* are thyroxine (T_4) and lesser amounts of triiodothyronine (T_3), purified from animal thyroids. It has a long action (up to 2 months) with peak action in 10 to 14 days. The normal daily requirement in the adult is 120 to 180 mg. Giving subnormal amounts for losing weight or "pepping up" patients is worthless; e.g., 30 mg. a day will suppress the production of TSH "30 mg. worth." The feedback sys-

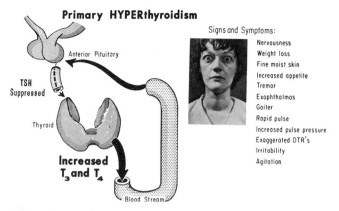

Fig. 13-2. Primary hyperthyroidism. Excess thyroid homones released by overactive thyroid gland. TSH is suppressed.

tem goes into action, TSH drops, thyroid production decreases, and the consequent level of thyroid hormones remains the same.

Synthetic thyroid substances offer more predictable physiological effects than dessicated thyroid. Triiodothyronine (Cytomel, T_3) acts rapidly (within hours) and probably is cleared from the body within a week (25 μg. of T_3 is equal to 65 mg. of desiccated thyroid). L-thyroxin (Synthroid, T_4) acts less rapidly than T_3. The usual daily dose is 200 to 300 μg.

Normal adults require full replacement doses of any thyroid drug. The only valid indication for smaller doses is in beginning treatment of myxedema. These patients are sensitive to thyroid hormones, and the dosages must be increased gradually.

DISEASES OF THE THYROID

Thyroid disease may be divided into two main types: functional diseases and anatomic or structural diseases.

Functional diseases
Hyperthyroidism (Graves' or Basedow's disease, thyrotoxicosis)

Hyperthyrodism is caused by an overproduction of T_3 and T_4 by the thyroid (Fig. 13-2). At the present time thyrotoxicosis is best thought of as a "runaway" thyroid gland. TSH is low. The onset may be preceded by sudden emotional shock, such as the death of a loved one. Thyrotoxicosis is four times as common in women as in men.

Secondary hyperthyroidism attributed to increased pituitary TSH secretion is rare.

Clinical picture. The clinical picture of hyperthyroidism includes the following: nervousness, weight loss, fine moist skin, increased appetite, tremor, exophthalmos, goiter, rapid pulse, increased pulse pressure, exaggerated deep tendon reflexes, irritability, agitation, and heart intolerance. Older patients show fewer signs and symptoms of hyperthyroidism; occasionally only refractory congestive heart failure or arrhythmias indicate thyrotoxicosis in older patients ("masked hyperthyroidism"). Severe hyperthyroidism in time may also appear paradoxically as a decrease in activity and appetite ("apathetic hyperthyroidism"). Such a state must be aggressively treated even to forced feedings.

T_3 thyrotoxicosis appears rarely (1%) as a variant of thyrotoxicosis. The usual laboratory values remain low or normal, but elevated serum T_3 levels and failure to suppress (positive Werner's test) are diagnostic.

Laboratory tests. The most dependable thyroid function tests are the serum thyroxin level (T_4) test, T_3 uptake test, and ^{131}I uptake test (Table 13-1).

The *serum thyroxin test* $(T_4$ test) measures the total serum thyroxin (by displacement with radioactive T_4 or radioimmunoassay). Increased serum proteins (chiefly thyroid-binding globulin [TBG]) cause falsely elevated T_4 values. Pregnancy and contraceptive agents are common causes of abnormally elevated serum proteins and consequently falsely increased levels of serum thyroxin.

The *T_3 uptake test* measures thyroid function based on the binding capacity of the patient's serum proteins for a known amount of radioactive triiodothyronine (T_3). The patient's serum is incubated with a measured amount of radioactive T_3. The patient's unbound proteins bind the T_3. The excess or unbound radioactive T_3 is taken up on a resin sponge, where it is measured by a radiation counter. A hyperthyroid patient, for example, will have fewer binding sites available on his TBG, thus the radioactive T_3 will be taken up in larger amounts by the resin sponge.

Conditions that cause increased serum proteins (pregnancy, contraceptive agents) will cause falsely depressed T_3 values. But these same conditions falsely elevate the T_4 test. Thus, by obtaining both T_4 and T_3 tests, the physician can evaluate a patient's thyroid function despite abnormal serum proteins.

The *^{131}I uptake test* measures the amount of radioactive iodine taken up by the thyroid in 4 hours and 24 hours. A scintillation counter records the uptake in percentages of radioactivity given. In

Table 13-1. Important diagnostic thyroid tests

Test	Normal values	Theory	Comments
Serum thyroxine	4 to 11 μg. %	Measures total thyroxine in serum	Neither inorganic nor organic iodides interfere; increased serum proteins elevate values; decreased serum proteins depress values
Radioactive iodine uptake	15 to 40% 4 and 24 hr.	Measures amount and rate that thyroid takes up ^{131}I in 4 and 24 hr.	A reliable test; not used during pregnancy; I_2 and antithyroid drugs will block this test
T_3 uptake test	25 to 35%	Measures excess radioactive T_3 that becomes absorbed on resin; in toxic patients the protein molecules are "saturated"; thus radioactive T_3 will be absorbed on resins	Radioactive T_3 is incubated with patient's blood in vitro; can be used in pregnancy; not affected by I_2 or antithyroid drugs; thus can be used to check patients treated with these drugs; low-serum proteins cause falsely increased values; increased serum proteins cause falsely depressed values
Scintiscan	Normal glands show an even distribution of ^{131}I throughout gland	^{131}I map of thyroid	Cysts, nodules, and cancer may be "cold"; little help in picking out malignant nodules; one definite asset is recording thyroid metastases to other areas (neck, bones, etc.)
Werner's test	4 and 24 hr. ^{131}I uptake is depressed by 50% (after suppression with 5-day course of T_3)	The pituitary-thyroid axis is tested by oral exogenous T_3 to suppress TSH; normal patients will suppress by 50%; toxic patients do not	Very useful in determining the borderline hyperthyroid patients, when other laboratory values are equivocal
BMR	±15%	Measures O_2 consumption	Inaccurate; false values in anxiety, starvation, tumors, metabolic defects, different body builds
Serum T_3	96-172 ng. %	T_3 may be ultimate, active product of T_4	Valuable in diagnosing T_3 thyrotoxicosis; other tests usually normal

addition to measuring thyroid activity, the radioactive iodine within the thyroid gland can be mapped by a scintillation scanner to show the size and shape of the gland, *a thyroid scan.*

Protein-bound iodine measures inorganic iodine bound to serum proteins. Because even minute amounts of iodides cause gross elevations in this test, the PBI is becoming obsolete.

Werner's test, utilizing the thyroid-pituitary feedback relationship, can often distinguish the suspected thyrotoxic patient from the anxious patient (who may appear thyrotoxic) when other laboratory tests are equivocal.

[131]I uptakes taken before and after a 5-day course of triiodothyronine (75 to 125 μg. each day) show no significant difference in the thyrotoxic patient (the TSH cannot be further depressed). Given the same test, the euthyroid patient shows a 50% depression in the ^{131}I uptakes after suppression with T_3. This test illustrates the important principle that thyrotoxic glands become autonomous; euthyroid glands remain under pituitary (TSH) control.

Treatment of thyrotoxicosis. Three methods for treatment of thyrotoxicosis are commonly employed: (1) antithyroid drugs, (2) surgery, and (3) radioactive iodine (^{131}I). Surgery and ^{131}I permanently *ablate* thyroid tissue; antithyroid drugs only *block* thyroid function (by blocking hormone synthesis by thyroid tissue) (Table 13-2). Unfortunately, thyrotoxicosis often recurs when drug therapy is discontinued. Therefore, in most instances, ablation of thyroid tissue is the preferred treatment. Many physicians do not favor using ^{131}I in young (or pregnant) women or children because of fear of irradiation. Prior to surgical removal of the thyroid gland, thyro-

Table 13-2. Antithyroid drugs—dosage and action

Drug	*Dosage*	*Action*
1. Thiocarbamides		
Propylthiouracil	100-300 mg. q.6-8 hr.	Blocks organic binding of iodine
Methimazole (Tapazole)	5-30 mg. q.6-8 hr.	
2. Potassium perchlorate	200-400 mg. q.6 hr.	Inhibits thyroid iodide transport mechanism
3. Iodine (Lugol's solution)	5-10 drops daily	Poorly understood
4. Propranolol	40-720 mg./day, divided doses	Beta-receptor blocking agent relieves toxic symptoms

toxicosis *must* be controlled by antithyroid drugs to prevent *thyroid storm*. Thyroid storm is probably caused by massive release of thyroid hormones at operation or during other stress. A frighteningly rapid pulse, high fever, and rapid fluid loss can result in death. Fluids, steroids, antithyroid drugs, hypothermia, and adrenergic blocking agents, especially propranolol, headline the current therapy. Prevention by proper patient preparation is the best treatment. Advantages and disadvantages of the three treatment methods are summarized in Table 13-3.

Table 13-3. Comparison of three common methods of treatment of hyperthyroidism

Method	Action	Advantages	Disadvantages
I. Antithyroid drugs	Block thyroid hormone synthesis	1. Avoids surgery and irradiation	1. High incidence of drug reaction, blood dyscrasias, skin reaction 2. Frequent visits to physician necessary 3. Recurrence rate high when therapy discontinued
II. Surgery	Removal of functioning tissue	1. Most rapid method of permanent control 2. Avoids irradiation	1. Complications of surgery: a. Damage to recurrent laryngeal nerves b. Damage to parathyroid glands (1%) c. Wound complications d. Permanent hypothyroidism (30%)
III. ^{131}I	Radioactive destruction of thyroid cells	1. Avoids surgery 2. Permanent control 3. Avoids drug reaction	1. Danger of irradiation 2. Hypothyroidism rate is high, 50% or more in 10 years; probably 100% in 20 years 3. Often treatment period is lengthy (up to 2 years) 4. Contraindicated in pregnancy and the very young

Prognosis. The treatment of hyperthyroidism is most gratifying. All of the signs and symptoms of thyrotoxicosis predictably diminish with treatment with the exception of exophthalmos.

Exophthalmos. Occasionally exophthalmos may become more exaggerated after treatment. The unknown etiology of exophthalmos is rendered even more obscure by the fact that exophthalmos may occur in euthyroid persons. Some ascribe exophthalmos to long-acting thyroid-stimulating (LATS) hormones, but the origin and function of this substance are still obscure. No satisfactory treatment for severe or malignant exophthalmos exists. Tarsorrhaphy and, rarely, orbital decompression may be necessary to prevent optic nerve injury and blindness.

Hypothyroidism (myxedema)

Cause. The most common cause of myxedema is *spontaneous atrophy* of the thyroid gland (Fig. 13-3). An autoimmune mechanism (a sensitization to hormone) may play a role in this process. The second leading cause of myxedema, postirradiation myxedema, occurs after treatment of hyperthyroidism with [131]I. In some series the incidence approaches 50% of those patients treated in follow-up studies of 10 years or more. TSH serum levels are usually increased. Failure of TSH production (secondary myxedema) because of pituitary failure is rare. Hypothyroidism may vary from mild signs and symptoms to the full-blown picture of myxedema.

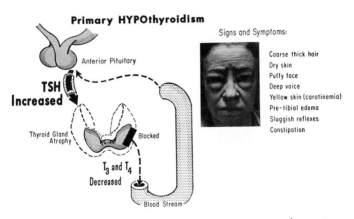

Primary HYPOthyroidism

Anterior Pituitary

TSH Increased

Thyroid Gland Atrophy

Blocked

T_3 and T_4 Decreased

Blood Stream

Signs and Symptoms:

Coarse thick hair
Dry skin
Puffy face
Deep voice
Yellow skin (carotinemia)
Pre-tibial edema
Sluggish reflexes
Constipation

Fig. 13-3. Primary hypothyroidism. Most common cause is spontaneous atrophy. Thyroid hormones are diminished. TSH is increased.

Clinical picture. The clinical picture of myxedema includes: coarse thick hair, dry skin, puffy face, deep voice, yellow skin (carotenemia), pretibial edema, sluggish reflexes, and constipation. In more severe cases ascites, pleural and pericardial effusions, paralytic ileus, hypothermia, and coma appear. The diagnosis is strongly suggested by a T_4 below 4 μg.%, a T_3 uptake below 25%, and a decreased ^{131}I uptake below 5% and 10% (4 hours and 24 hours).

Treatment. Perhaps no other disease responds to treatment more successfully than myxedema. Small doses of thyroid substances initially, increasing to full replacement doses (65 to 180 mg. of desiccated thyroid) restore normal function in almost all patients.

Anatomic or structural diseases
Goiters and nodules

A *goiter* is, by definition, an enlargement of the thyroid gland. A goiter may be diffusely enlarged (simple goiter) or nodular (nodular goiter). A nodule may occur in an otherwise normal gland; these are called solitary thyroid nodules.

The most common cause of goiter is a deficiency in iodine ingestion or metabolism (endemic goiter). The thyroid responds by increasing in size in an effort to produce the necessary thyroid hormones. Nodules and cysts may form as a consequence of thyroid enlargement.

Another cause of goiter is the ebb and tide of metabolic stress, e.g., menstrual cycles and pregnancy. This explains why women have more goiters and nodules (5:1) than men do.

Thyroiditis and malignancy also cause thyroid enlargement and will be discussed separately.

Solitary thyroid nodules (Table 13-4) suggest malignancy because they arise in a gland otherwise normal to palpation. About 50% of

Table 13-4. Clinically benign solitary nodules of thyroid (pathological diagnoses in 299 consecutive patients)

Multinodular goiters	143
Adenomas	81
Cysts	32
Thyroiditis	25
Thyroglossal duct cyst	1
Cancer	17
Total	299

these "solitary" growths are really dominant nodules in a multinodular goiter; the other nodules are too small to be palpated clinically. Some of them are "new growths"; thus all solitary nodules should be evaluated for malignancy by the only certain method, excision and microscopic study. Radioactive iodine thyroid maps (scintiscans) are of little definite diagnostic value. "Cold" nodules are most often cysts or benign adenomas rather than cancer, and cancer may arise in nodules that are "warm" or even toxic. Therefore, the student should be realistically skeptical of the value of scintiscans in diagnosing the nature of thyroid nodules.

Treatment of goiters and nodules. As a useful rule, all *solitary nodules are considered malignant* until proved benign; all *multinodular goiters are considered benign* until some evidence suggests malignancy. The incidence of malignancy in *clinically benign solitary* thyroid nodules is about 6% in our hospital. No infallible tests short of microscopic diagnosis can detect the dangerous nodules; all but the soft nodules that often occur in pregnancy should be removed. Many of these soft nodules will regress on giving suppressive doses of desiccated thyroid, or after the pregnancy is terminated.

Diffuse and multinodular goiters are not removed routinely. Small, palpable nodular goiters are very common (5 to 10% of adults); thyroid cancer is uncommon. Thus, operative mortality for routine thyroidectomy would likely exceed any saving of life from thyroid cancer. We operate only on suspicious goiters, i.e., a rapidly growing nodule, a hard or fixed lobe or nodule within the goiter, or evidence of cervical metastasis. Goiters are removed also for cosmetic reasons or for obstruction of the trachea or esophagus. Since nodules occurring in children carry a high risk of malignancy, we hasten to excise and examine all such nodules.

Thyroiditis

Thyroiditis is a general term that describes the four types of inflammatory diseases of the thyroid gland. The lymphocytic type is by far the most common.

The four types of thyroiditis and the approximate relative incidence are as follows:

	Number of cases
Lymphocytic type (Hashimoto's struma, struma lymphomatosa)	100
Viral type (subacute, granulomatous, De Quervain's)	10
Riedel's (woody)	1
Suppurative (acute, bacterial)	< 1

Clinical characteristics. Clinical characteristics of the lymphocytic, viral, Riedel, and acute suppurative types of thyroiditis are discussed in the paragraphs that follow.

Lymphocytic type. The cause is probably an autoimmune mechanism. Thyroid tissue becomes sensitized to its own hormones, resulting in an invasion of lymphocytes and fibrous tissue. A diffuse, rubbery, nontender goiter results. The thyroid antibody titre is usually, but not invariably, elevated. Although chiefly afflicting women 20 to 50 years of age, it is the most common cause of goiter in children. Many believe it eventually leads to myxedema. Biopsy and replacement of thyroid (T_3 or T_4) keynote the treatment.

Viral type. This type of thyroiditis causes a tender, diffuse enlargement or occasionally a tender nodule, mild fever, increased sedimentation rate, and general malaise. Bed rest, sedation, aspirin, and in extreme cases, steroids (to reduce inflammation) are the usual methods of treatment. Biopsy diagnosis is rarely necessary for the skilled clinician.

Riedel's type. Riedel's type is very rare. Probably the fibrous end-stage of lymphocytic thyroiditis, the gland atrophies and becomes woody-hard. Because it mimics the firmness of cancer, it should be biopsied. Treatment with replacement doses of T_3 or T_4 is indicated.

Acute suppurative thyroiditis. Acute suppurative thyroiditis is a medical oddity. We have seen only one case. We mention this entity last to emphasize its rarity. The source of bacterial thyroiditis is most often from abscessed lower teeth. Treatment, as with any abscess, includes drainage and antibiotics.

Cancer

Cancer of the thyroid has an extremely wide range of behavior. It is rivaled in this respect only by breast cancer, among the common malignancies. Most differentiated types grow slowly over years. The undifferentiated types grow rapidly and may be lethal within weeks or months. Since most undifferentiated types afflict older adults, advanced age often signals an ominous prognosis. Cancer of the thyroid may be classified as follows:

Differentiated 80%	Intermediate 5%	Undifferentiated 15%
Papillary	Medullary	Small cell
Follicular		Large cell
Mixed papillofollicular		Sarcomas

Papillary cancer occurs in children and young adults of the third and fourth decade, often with a history of prior irradiation to the neck area. It is the most common thyroid malignancy. Metastases usually appear in the neck and grow slowly. Total thyroidectomy and excision of regional metastases form the basic treatment. Total thyroidectomy accomplishes two objectives: (1) it removes thyroid tissue that competes (with tumor) for ^{131}I; (2) it removes possible multicentric foci of tumor. Some surgeons favor radical neck dissection when cervical spread has occurred, and others prefer conservative removal of just the involved tissues. The patient is allowed to become hypothyroid. If residual tumor is shown to take up iodine, ^{131}I is given in large therapeutic doses. TSH, or a thiouracil drug to increase the body's TSH, often increases the ^{131}I uptake in the metastases. Suppressive doses of thyroid are administered for the remainder of life.

Follicular cancer tends to metastasize distantly and occurs in a slightly older age group (fifth decade). Before ^{131}I treatment, total thyroidectomy prepares the patient by removing tumor and allowing any remaining metastases to more effectively pick up [131]I.

Mixed type is a commonly occurring composite of the preceding two types. Treatment is the same.

Medullary cancers contain varying amounts of amyloid and carry an intermediate prognosis. The 10-year survival rate exceeds 60% in operable patients. They tend to be familial and are associated with pheochromocytomas, hyperparathyroidism, and neurofibromatosis. Some medullary cancers produce calcitonin. Elevated levels of serum calcitonin have predicted medullary cancers, preoperatively, in family members who carry this trait.

Undifferentiated thyroid cancer is aggressively malignant. It occurs in older people and rarely takes up [131]I. Radical surgical excision and external irradiation are the only, and usually ineffective, treatment.

Sarcomas of various types are rare. Occasionally, wide excision will offer a favorable prognosis.

CHAPTER 14

Parathyroid glands

DARYL K. GRANNER
RICHARD D. LIECHTY

A multihormonal system regulates calcium, magnesium, and phosphate homeostasis in all vertebrates. The organs involved in this regulation are bone, kidney, and gut, and the major hormones are parathyroid hormone (parathormone, PTH), calcitonin (CT), and vitamin D*. In general PTH and vitamin D act in concert with (but opposing) CT to maintain serum calcium between 8.5 and 10.5 mg.%. Calcium regulates neuromuscular excitability, blood coagulation, membrane function, secretory processes, and many enzyme reactions; to maintain these vital functions, nature zealously keeps calcium within these narrow limits.

ANATOMY AND EMBRYOLOGY

Man normally has four parathyroid glands situated close to the posterior surface of the thyroid, one gland near each pole. Each gland should weigh no more than 50 mg. Their small weight and their location make the parathyroids liable to accidental removal or damage during thyroid surgery. The parathyroids, derived from the third and fourth branchial pouches, differentially migrate caudally so that the lower pair come from the third pouch and the upper pair from the fourth. About 10% of parathyroid glands are ectopically located within the thyroid, thymus, superior mediastinum, and even pericardium. Histologically, parathyroids contain cords of chief and

---

*Natural vitamin D (vitamin D_3 or cholecalciferol) is hydroxylated by the liver to 25-hydroxyvitamin D_3; then by the kidney to 1-25 hydroxyvitamin D_3, the active hormone.

oxyphilic cells. Chief cells, subdivided into water-clear and dark cells according to their content of secretory granules, secrete PTH. Most adenomas feature dark cells; hyperplastic parathyroids arise from either cell.

Calcitonin comes from "C-cells" (for calcitonin). Derived from the ultimobranchial body, these cells disperse into thyroid, thymus, and parathyroid tissues in man. They resemble adrenal medullary cells and pancreatic alpha cells, with which they probably share a common origin.

PHYSIOLOGY

PTH, a polypeptide hormone, acts primarily on *bone* leading to complete dissolution of both organic and inorganic components while inhibiting new bone formation. To facilitate a *net* increase in serum calcium, PTH acts on the *kidney* to promote calcium reabsorption and, very importantly, to inhibit tubular reabsorption of phosphate, which leads to increased phosphate excretion. This effect precedes the action on bone but is quantitatively less important. A lesser but still important third effect is on the *intestinal mucosa,* where PTH plays a "permissive" role in vitamin D–mediated calcium transport from lumen to cell. Thus the sum effect of PTH is to raise serum calcium and lower serum phosphate. CT, also a polypeptide, seems to prevent bone resorption in a manner that is independent of PTH and probably has no effect on kidneys or gut. It is not clear whether CT also increases bone formation. Vitamin D acts primarily on the intestinal mucosa to enhance calcium transport into cells. It also augments the effects of PTH on bone resorption but probably has no action on the kidney. Under normal conditions the synthesis and secretion of PTH and CT are governed by the serum calcium (and magnesium) level in a classical feedback manner. PTH and CT vary reciprocally with ionized calcium levels: as calcium decreases, PTH increases, whereas CT decreases—and vice versa.

Calcium circulating in blood and in extracellular fluid represents less than 1% of the total body content and is near its solubility maximum. About half is in an active or *ionized* form, whereas most of the rest is protein bound or *not ionized* and therefore biochemically inactive. Calcium binds chiefly to albumin; lesser amounts bind to globulins. Measurements of serum calcium should always be accompanied by a serum protein determination. About 0.9 mg. calcium is bound per gram of protein, allowing for a rough estimation of the ionized calcium level. The binding of calcium to albumin is enhanced by alkalosis (e.g., the tetany of hyperventilation) and decreased by acidosis.

HYPERPARATHYROIDISM

Clinical features of primary hyperparathyroidism. About 1 case of primary hyperparathyroidism emerges from every 1,000 carefully screened hospital admissions. This disease results from the autonomous and increased secretion of PTH, usually from neoplastic transformation (Fig. 14-1). About 80% of patients with hyperparathyroidism have as the cause a single parathyroid adenoma; hyperplasia, or multiple adenomas, or a mixture of the two (and rarely cancer) account for the rest. Most pathologists agree that distinguishing hyperplastic from adenomatous tissue, especially on frozen section, is unreliable, if not impossible.

Cancers of other organs commonly elevate serum calcium chiefly

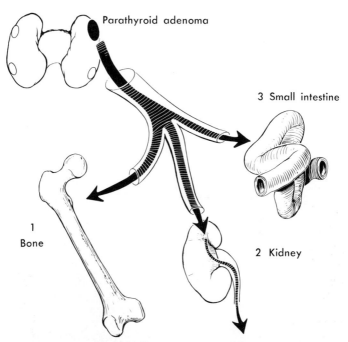

Parathyroid adenoma

3 Small intestine

1 Bone

2 Kidney

Fig. 14-1. Primary hyperparathyroidism. **1,** PTH releases calcium from bone while inhibiting new bone formation. **2,** PTH promotes renal reabsorption of calcium and inhibits tubular reabsorption of phosphate. **3,** PTH aids intestinal absorption of calcium.

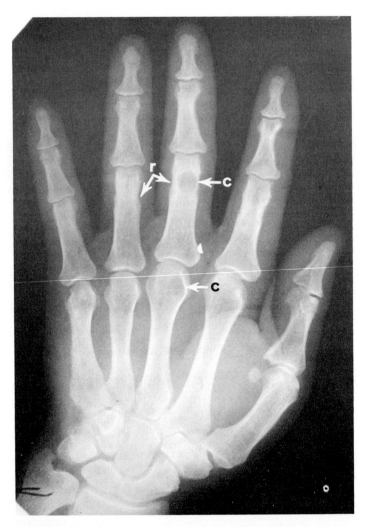

Fig. 14-2. Radiologically diagnostic lesions of subperiosteal resorption, r, and associated cysts, c. Such lesions are more likely demonstrable in patients with large adenomas.

from osteolytic metastases, but some tumors (notably lung, kidney) secrete PTH and thus mimic primary hyperparathyroidism.

The nonspecific symptoms of muscle weakness, fatigue, nausea, anorexia, constipation, mental changes, polyuria, polydipsia, renal colic and infections characterize hypercalcemia. Between 60 and 75% of patients have detectable renal involvement including stones or gravel, repeated infections, hematuria, nephrocalcinosis, and azotemia. About 5 to 10% of all patients with renal stones will prove to have hyperparathyroidism. Clinical bone involvement caused by excessive resorption is found in about 20% of patients. Most often this is diffuse and resembles osteoporosis. Less frequently seen now are the classical lesions of osteitis fibrosa cystica. Fig. 14-2 shows subperiosteal resorption, which is diagnostic. This resorption usually involves the fingers and lateral third of the clavicles.

Hyperparathyroidism, usually featuring chief cell hyperplasia or adenomata, runs in some families. Pheochromocytomas, pancreatic adenomas, medullary thyroid carcinomas, and pituitary and thyroid tumors also characterize these multiple endocrine adenomata syndromes. Peptic ulcer, pancreatitis, and hypertension increase in incidence with hyperparathyroidism and often defy therapy until the adenoma is removed. All patients with these diseases should have a serum calcium determination. Occasionally the serum calcium will become acutely and severely elevated, leading to a life-threatening aggravation of the symptoms listed above—a *parathyroid crisis*.

Diagnosis. After excluding other causes for hypercalcemia (such as malignancy, vitamin D intoxication, milk-alkali syndrome, sarcoidosis, hyperthyroidism, adrenal insufficiency, or thiazide diuretic ingestion), the physician confirms the diagnosis by detecting hypercalcemia in two or more samples. The serum phosphate is often but not invariably low and serum alkaline phosphatase increases with calcium turnover in bone. Occasionally mild metabolic acidosis, hyperchloremia, and hyperuricemia coexist. Hypercalciuria is common, but the total calcium excretion is usually less than 400 mg. per day because PTH promotes calcium reabsorption. Levels of PTH (by radioimmunoassay) rise and selective venous catheterization, with subsequent determinations of PTH on the aliquots, help localize the adenoma. The key diagnostic test is still elevated serum calcium levels.

Therapy. The unreliability of frozen section diagnosis compounds the surgeon's problems at operation. Knowing that the initial operation allows him the golden chance to evaluate parathyroid pathology, the surgeon must plan his operation methodically as follows. Because about 10% of parathyroids arise ectopically, he must attempt to identify all four glands, no matter how tedious and time consuming this may prove. He should remove the one enlarged gland if he finds three other normal or atrophic ones, and if he finds only three glands, he should resect the thyroid on the side of the missing gland. He should select subtotal parathyroidectomy (three and one-half glands removed) for (1) gross enlargement of more than one gland; (2) all glands appear normal or minimally enlarged; no evidence of fifth gland, (3) familial parathyroid disease; or (4) chronic, mild renal insufficiency. This plan offers the greatest chance (over 90%) for permanent cure with minimal risk of permanent hypoparathyroidism or recurrence.

Parathyroid crises (Ca^{++} 15 mg.% or higher) call for immediate action, including: (1) intravenous phosphates, (2) saline diuresis, (3) or calcitonin infusions. These measures aim at lowering the serum calcium prior to urgent exploration.

When operative removal is not feasible, chronic medical treatment with oral phosphate-phosphorus (2 to 5 Gm. per day) can normalize serum calcium levels in most patients.

Secondary hyperparathyroidism. Excessive secretion of PTH with associated glandular hyperplasia commonly occurs in chronic renal failure and in diseases such as rickets and renal tubular acidosis. The often associated osteodystrophy can be severely disabling. The common denominator is resistance to the action of PTH, probably because the kidney fails to hydroxylate vitamin D. Although PTH secretion is excessive, it is subject to feedback regulation but only by levels of serum calcium higher than normal. Ordinarily the serum calcium remains normal or low in secondary hyperparathyroidism and the serum phosphorus is elevated. The latter is not the primary cause of this syndrome but merely a consequence of the lack of PTH action on the kidney. Occasionally the serum calcium (or ionized calcium) will become abnormally elevated after renal transplantation and is no longer under feedback control. This so-called *tertiary* state has responded to removal of parathyroid tissue. Otherwise the treatment of *secondary* hyperparathyroidism is generally medical and aimed at the basic renal disease.

HYPOPARATHYROIDISM

Classification and clinical features. Hypoparathyroidism is characterized by hypocalcemia and hyperphosphatemia and can result from loss of glandular function or from end-organ resistance to PTH action. Hypoparathyroidism most commonly occurs after removal of the glands or damage to their blood supply during thyroid surgery. Within a few hours neuromuscular irritability emerges as muscle spasms or cramps and paresthesias, particularly of the hands, face, and feet. Tapping the facial nerve results in facial muscle contractions (Chvostek's sign), whereas application of a partially inflated blood pressure cuff leads to carpopedospasm (Trousseau's sign). Marked hypocalcemia can induce laryngeal spasm and convulsions. This syndrome can be transient or permanent. Hypocalcemia often occurs in the 24 to 48 hours immediately after removal of a parathyroid adenoma. Although usually transient, this relative hypoparathyroidism can require treatment for months, especially when the bones have suffered chronic calcium "starvation" from extensive dissolution.

Idiopathic hypoparathyroidism. This rare disease attacks in childhood or middle age. Cataracts, basal ganglia calcification, mental retardation, and cutaneous involvement such as moniliasis, brittle nails, and patchy hair loss characterize the childhood disease. Usually the glands are absent or atrophic. Symptoms often are chronic and insidious in onset, particularly in the adult.

Pseudohypoparathyroidism. Pseudohypoparathyroidism is an interesting example of end-organ (kidney) resistance to the effects of a hormone. These patients have all the chemical and clinical features of hypoparathyroidism yet have elevated PTH levels. The kidneys of these patients fail to give the normal phosphaturic response to PTH. This genetic disease also includes peculiar skeletal abnormalities (stunting, short metacarpals) that distinguish it from the idiopathic form.

Treatment. Commercially available PTH has failed to control hypocalcemia because of the rapid development of resistance, probably because of antibody formation. Current therapy consists of massive daily doses of vitamin D (50,000 to 100,000 units are commonly required because of the absence of the synergistic effects of PTH), supplemented by calcium given orally as the gluconate or lactate salt. Since the biological effect of vitamin D is measured in months, great care must be exercised to avoid vitamin D intoxication. Metabolites of vitamin D_3 (25-hydroxycholecalciferol and 1-25 dihydroxycholecalciferol), which have a rapid onset and a short biological half-life, have shown excellent clinical results.

CHAPTER 15

The adrenal glands

RICHARD D. LIECHTY

Nature has fashioned the mammalian adrenal gland in a curious way. Taking two separate embryological tissues, it has fused them, as adrenal cortex (mesoderm) and medulla (ectoderm), into one gland. Despite this anatomical merger that allows the cortex to bathe the medulla with the body's richest concentration of steroids, man and other mammals do perfectly well without the medulla. Perhaps nature, in our evolutionary past, has devalued the biological ties suggested by the anatomical fusion of adrenal cortex and medulla. Whatever the reason, most scientists today believe that the adrenal medulla (that secretes epinephrine and norepinephrine in a ratio of 4:1) has no more physiological significance than other sympathetic ganglia that secrete catecholamines. In contrast, the cortex maintains critically important functions. Together, man's two adrenal glands weigh only about 14 Gm., but without the functioning cortex or its hormones, man dies.

PHYSIOLOGY
Adrenal hormones

Three main types of hormones are secreted by the adrenal cortex: (1) glucocorticoids, (2) mineralocorticoids, and (3) sex steroids. All three originate from the cholesterol molecule. Enzymes within the cells of the adrenal cortex change the chemical structure of cholesterol to produce corticosteroids.

Hypothalamic-pituitary-adrenal triangle

Both the glucocorticoids and the sex steroids are under hypothalamic-pituitary control. ACTH (adrenocorticotropic hormone) released by the pituitary gland, in response to corticotropin-releasing factor (CRF) from the hypothalamus, stimulates the adrenal cortex to produce both glucocorticoids and sex steroids. (Mineralocorticoids are largely independent of pituitary control.) Glucocorticoids (chiefly cortisol), in turn, block ACTH secretion at the pituitary (and hypothalamic) level. This is the reciprocal, "negative feedback" mechanism (similar to the pituitary-thyroid relationship) that is vital to understanding adrenal physiology.

Corticosteroid hormones
Glucocorticoids

The chief glucocorticoid in the body is cortisol (hydrocortisone). Glucocorticoids increase glycogenolysis (breakdown of glycogen to glucose), convert proteins to glucose, and have an anti-inflammatory action. In large amounts they increase fat deposition and cause weakness (from destruction of muscle protein) and water retention. Their most important action is in protecting the body against stress. The exact mechanism of glucocorticoids in response to stress is not known. They probably act on the vascular tree by dilating small vessels, thus increasing blood volume. They make energy available in the form of glucose and free fatty acids. Some feel that protection of lysosomal membranes is a vital cellular function. Another theory relates glucocorticoid action to their inotropic effect on myocardium, which increases cardiac output.

Mineralocorticoids

Aldosterone is secreted chiefly in response to decreased blood volume mediated by renal receptors. It acts to retain sodium and water and to excrete potassium. In concert with ADH (antidiuretic hormone) and renin-angiotensin, it maintains body fluid volume at a constant level.

Sex steroids

Androgens, estrogens, and progesterone are produced by the adrenal cortex in small amounts. When they are secreted in excess they cause virilization (the adrenogenital syndrome) or, rarely, feminization. They do not suppress ACTH, and they are not essential to life.

Adrenocortical hormone similarities and differences

In the confusing welter of steroid hormones occurring in the body (more than 30 have been isolated) and the dozens of commercial steroid preparations, many students feel lost. Certain principles will help clear their understandable confusion:

1. All steroids have three basic actions: (a) "metabolic" or gluco-corticoid, (b) mineralocorticoid, and (c) sex steroids.
2. Some overlapping of actions occurs with most corticosteroids; e.g., cortisol, primarily a glucocorticoid and the "mother steroid" in the body, will show mineralocorticoid effects (water retention) and sex steroid effects (acne, hirsutism) if given in large enough amounts.
3. Suppression of ACTH is primarily a function of glucocorticoids; e.g., new, synthetic anti-inflammatory steroids with advertised "decreased side effects" means that they have less water retention and masculinizing effects—but remember, their glucocorticoid properties are very much evident, and they strongly suppress ACTH.

A "triangle of steroid activity" is a helpful device in understanding basic steroid physiology (Fig. 15-1). All steroid preparations may be placed somewhere in this triangle corresponding to their actions.

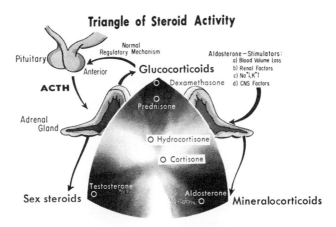

Fig. 15-1. Adrenocortical hormone activity is demonstrated by a triangle with the three main types of cortical hormones at the apices. Overlapping of functions (glucocorticoid, mineralocorticoid, and sex steroid) occurs with most steroid compounds. The approximate overlapping of functions is illustrated by several steroids placed within this triangle.

DISEASES OF THE ADRENAL CORTEX
Addison's disease (adrenocortical failure)

Any process that destroys or suppresses the adrenal cortex (or the hypothalamic-pituitary ACTH centers) will cause Addison's disease. Adrenocortical infections (meningococcosis, tuberculosis), cortical atrophy (probably of autoimmune origin), and surgical adrenalectomy can cause Addison's disease. One of the most common causes is suppression of ACTH from long-term steroid therapy. Other causes are hereditary and congenital, hemorrhage (from sepsis, from anticoagulants, or during pregnancy), or pituitary insufficiency.

Clinically, Addison's disease appears in the adult as *chronic insufficiency,* or *acute adrenal failure* or an intermediate state between these two.

Chronic addisonian patients have dark pigmentation, weakness, hypotension, apathy, nausea, vomiting, weight loss, abdominal pain, hyponatremia, hypoglycemia, and hyperkalemia. They show decreased plasma cortisol levels and urinary 17-OHCS excretion. *Inflexibility* best describes these patients. Any stress, such as an operation, or potent drugs, can throw them into shock. Infections will cause critically high fevers with subsequent shock and death unless they receive vigorous steroid replacement.

Acute adrenal failure comes on suddenly with fever, abdominal symptoms, coma, and shock. Sudden discontinuance of steroids after long-term administration is a common cause of acute adrenal failure. This critical condition demands immediate treatment with intravenous cortisol, 300 mg. (or more) the first 24 hours, with gradual tapering doses. Maintenance cortisol doses average 25 to 50 mg. per day orally.

Patients receiving steroids for long periods of time often pose problems for the surgeon. Some patients can receive large doses of steroids for several months and still maintain an effective adrenal stress response, whereas others receiving smaller doses over shorter intervals may not. In any emergency situation (lacking time to evaluate the pituitary-adrenal integrity) the surgeon should support these patients with full "stress doses" of steroids (300 mg. of cortisol each day). Little harm comes from short interval "burst" therapy, but catastrophe may follow if the surgeon overlooks the vital importance of steroid replacement in patients with marginal adrenal reserves.

Cushing's syndrome

Cushing's syndrome is caused by excess quantities of glucocorticoids, mainly cortisol. It may occur from one of the following causes:

1. Adrenal hyperplasia secondary to excess ACTH stimulation from

a pituitary tumor (either a basophilic or chromophobe adenoma) or functional pituitary overactivity probably caused by excessive hypothalamic activity. This is called *Cushing's disease.*

2. Ectopic Cushing's syndrome—some extra-adrenal cancers (cancer of the lung, pancreas, thyroid, parotid, liver, and thymus) secrete large amounts of ACTH that causes Cushing's syndrome. These cancers are usually inoperable.

3. A functioning tumor (Fig. 15-2), either an adenoma or a carcinoma, of the adrenal cortex.

4. Administration of large quantities of glucocorticoid drugs (e.g., cortisone).

The clinical picture is the same: amenorrhea, moon face, truncal obesity, muscular loss and weakness, hirsutism, acne, diabetes mellitus, skin atrophy, hypertension, abdominal striae, ecchymoses, and osteoporosis.

Laboratory tests

Diagnosing Cushing's syndrome. The *overnight dexamethasone suppression test* is the most valuable single screening test for Cushing's

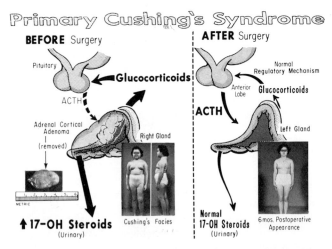

Fig. 15-2. Cushing's syndrome caused by adrenal adenoma. Note that ACTH is suppressed by excess glucocorticoids. After tumor was removed, normal pituitary-adrenal balance resumed. Insets show Cushingoid effects in a 9-year-old girl and postoperative appearance 6 months after removal of benign adrenal adenoma.

syndrome. Dexamethasone, 1 mg., taken at midnight, will lower morning plasma cortisol levels below 5 μg.% in normal people (normal values, 5 to 20 μg.%). Patients with Cushing's syndrome have values usually above 10 μg.% after suppression.

Urinary 17-hydroxycorticosteroids (17-OHCS) average 5 to 10 mg./24 hr. in normal people. High levels, especially when they fail to suppress with dexamethasone, indicate Cushing's syndrome. (See Table 15-1.)

Loss of diurnal plasma cortisol variation is a sign of Cushing's syndrome. Normal people show elevated plasma cortisol levels in morning blood samples and depressed afternoon levels. Patients with Cushing's syndrome show little or no diurnal variation.

Differentiating the cause of Cushing's syndrome. After he makes the diagnosis of Cushing's syndrome with one or more of the above tests, the physician should attempt to define the cause. Table 15-1 summarizes these tests. ACTH will invariably stimulate the normal and hyperplastic glands, but will stimulate tumors variably since their output is largely autonomous. The lower dose (2 mg./24 hr.) dexamethasone suppression test differentiates normal patients from those who have *any form* of Cushing's syndrome. The higher dose (8 mg./24 hr.) test differentiates adrenal hyperplasia from adrenal tumors.

The metyrapone test checks the integrity of the hypothalamic-pituitary-adrenal triangle, thus providing another good differentiation between adrenal hyperplasia and adrenal tumors. Metyrapone blocks the final step in cortisol production in the normal or hyperplastic cortex while allowing the precursors of cortisol to be produced. (These precursors are measured as 17-OHCS in the urine.) But these precursors cannot block ACTH; only cortisol has this ability. Thus metyrapone removes cortisol suppression of ACTH. Normal patients and those with hyperplasia respond by excreting increased amounts of urinary 17-OHCS. Patients with adrenal tumors, given metyrapone, continue to secrete excess cortisol unabated, therefore they show no variation in 17-OHCS excretion. Patients with ectopic ACTH-producing tumors continue to secrete the same excessive amounts of ACTH, despite metyrapone. Large amounts of exogenous ACTH will suppress pituitary ACTH; ectopic ACTH production acts similarly. They have lost the normal hypothalamic-pituitary-adrenal triangle. Therefore, patients with ectopic Cushing's syndrome, given metyrapone, will not produce increased amounts of urinary 17-OHCS.

Plasma ACTH measurements (by radioimmunoassay) also reliably separate the causes of Cushing's syndrome. Patients with adrenal tumors have low ACTH plasma levels; those with hyperplasia or ectopic ACTH production have high levels.

Table 15-1. Laboratory methods used to differentiate the causes of Cushing's syndrome*

	Normal	Hyperplasia	Tumor	Ectopic ACTH
1. Plasma cortisol	10-25 μGm.% Rhythmic	↑ No rhythm	↑ No rhythm	↑ No rhythm
2. Plasma ACTH	0.1-0.4 mU.%	↑	↓	↑
3. 17-OHCS In 24-hr. urine collection	5-10 mg./24 hr.	↑	↑	↑↑
4. Stimulation 25 units ACTH I.V. over 8 hr.	↑	↑↑	↑	↑
5. Suppression A. Dexamethasone P.O. 0.5 mg. q.6hr. for 48 hr.	↓ >50%	↔ or ↓	↔	↔
B. Dexamethasone P.O. 2 mg. q.6hr. for 48 hr.		↓ > 50%	↔	↔, occasionally ↓
6. Metyrapone (SU-4885) 30 mg./kg. I.V. over 4 hr.	↑	↑↑	↔	↔

24-hr. urine collections are completed:
ACTH: 24 hr. after ACTH begun
Dexamethasone: in the second 24-hr. period of dexamethasone administration
Metyrapone: 24 hr. after metyrapone begun

*Key: ↑ increased; ↓ decreased; ↑↑ greatly increased; ↔ unchanged.

Roentgen-ray examination. Skull films sometimes indicate sella turcica enlargement and intravenous pyelograms may show displacement from a suprarenal mass. Retroperitoneal air studies may demonstrate large tumors. Adrenal arteriography or venography sometimes pinpoints the lesion (Figs. 15-5 and 15-6). Elevated cortisol levels (from vena caval blood samples) help to localize its source. Radioactive iodocholesterol will selectively be taken up by overactive adrenal tissue. Scintillation scans map the uptake.

Treatment. Most experts believe that careful, high-energy pituitary irradiation is the best treatment for Cushing's disease, certainly in those patients well enough to tolerate the 6- to 12-month treatment period. Surgical resection is of course best for adenomas (or cancer) or in young women with *Cushing's disease* who wish to remain fertile. Pituitary enlargement occurs in about 10% of patients after bilateral adrenalectomy for adrenal hyperplasia. Periodic skull films should be obtained postoperatively.

Some patients have responded to o,p'-DDD, a cortical toxin. This drug is especially useful in treating adrenocortical cancers and in patients with ectopic ACTH syndrome.

Regulation of water balance—aldosterone and ADH

Aldosterone. In the normal person, the adrenal gland secretes aldosterone, the body's main mineralocorticoid, chiefly in response to decreased blood volume. The kidney's juxtaglomerular apparatus senses the volume deficit and secretes renin that in turn releases angiotensin I. Enzymes, chiefly in the lungs, rapidly convert angiotensin I to angiotensin II. Angiotensin II, a powerful vasoconstrictor by itself, stimulates the adrenal to synthesize and release aldosterone. Acting on the distal convoluted tubule, aldosterone retains Na^+ (and H_2O) and excretes K^+. Thus in normal man the kidney and adrenal gland combine two mechanisms to ensure normal blood volumes through varying states of hydration, electrolyte concentration, and position. Although low Na^+, high K^+, and ACTH also stimulate aldosterone, the most powerful influence is angiotensin II. Acting as a feedback, the aldosterone build-up and increased water volume suppress or turn off renin secretion.

Antidiuretic hormone (ADH)

The aldosterone-angiotensin mechanism has a powerful ally in the hypothalamic–posterior pituitary area. Responding chiefly to dehydration (increased osmolality), osmoreceptors in the hypothalamus stimulate release of pituitary-stored ADH. ADH, acting on the renal collecting ducts, causes reabsorption of H_2O. Severe volume deficits (sensed in the heart and large arteries) also elevate ADH, as nature attempts to protect volume at all costs even in the face of hypo-osmolality. Coupled to the osmoreceptor cells, a thirst center signals severe thirst synchronous with water conservation. Thus two main neurohormonal centers, in the brain and paravertebral gutters, protect the body's water balance.

Aldosteronism

Hyperplasia or tumors can arise from any of the three cortical cell types. Although the glomerulosa layer may become hyperplastic, it usually forms single adenomas that secrete excess aldosterone. Hypertension results that, although uncommon, is surgically curable.

Hyperaldosteronism and hypertension coexist in two clinical situations: (1) *primary aldosteronism* that usually responds to adrenalectomy, and (2) *secondary aldosteronism* from extra-adrenal causes.

Primary aldosteronism. Primary aldosteronism begins with cortical tumors or hyperplasia that produces aldosterone (Fig. 15-3). If the student understands the physiology of aldosterone he can predict the

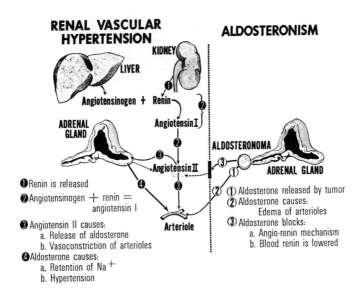

Fig. 15-3. Comparison of mechanisms causing renal vascular hypertension and primary aldosteronism.

classical clinical picture: hypertension and headaches—from Na^+ and water retention; polydipsia and polyuria—from kaluresis; muscle weakness and EKG change—from hypokalemia. Laboratory tests show elevated serum Na^+ and alkalosis, depressed K^+, increased serum and urine aldosterone, and low serum renin. The feedback mechanism of increased volume and aldosterone suppress serum renin.

Secondary aldosteronism. Any disease that stimulates renin also elevates aldosterone: renal artery stenosis, intrinsic renal ischemia, juxtaglomerular hyperplasia, etc. Secondary aldosteronism always involves increased renin levels; pure primary aldosteronism, never. Thus renin and aldosterone determinations provide us with valuable tools to help select those patients (from the millions of hypertensives) who have potentially curable, aldosterone-induced hypertension. The diagnostic steps should proceed as follows: observe hypertension, then hypokalemia, then suppressed renin, and, finally, elevated aldosterone production (Table 15-2).

Radiographic diagnosis and treatment of primary aldosteronism. Any of the radiographic techniques that localize cortisol-secreting adrenal tumors can also point to aldosteronomas. Aldosterone levels assayed from vena caval blood (like cortisol) often lateralize the guilty adrenal gland. The surgeon should expose both adrenals, removing the gland with a solitary tumor, or excising one gland and three-fourths of the other with multiple tumors or hyperplasia.

Adrenogenital syndrome

In the steps of cortisol synthesis a branching chain is responsible for the formation of the sex steroids (Fig. 15-4). In some children a defective enzyme system allows the sex steroids to be produced while cortisol production is blocked. One can anticipate the chain of events that ensues. In the absence of cortisol, the main inhibitor of ACTH from the anterior pituitary, the anterior pituitary produces excess amounts of ACTH and thus stimulates the secretion of more sex ste-

Table 15-2. Serum renin and urinary aldosterone relationships in 3 main types of hypertension*

Cause of hypertension	Serum renin	Urinary aldosterone
Renovascular	↑	↑
"Essential"	↔	↔
Aldosteronism	↓	↑

*Key: ↑ increased; ↓ decreased; ↔ unchanged.

206 Synopsis of surgery

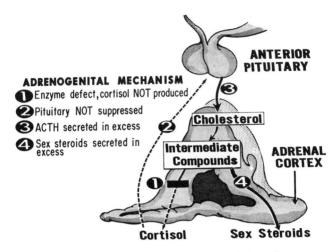

ANTERIOR PITUITARY

ADRENOGENITAL MECHANISM
❶ Enzyme defect, cortisol NOT produced
❷ Pituitary NOT suppressed
❸ ACTH secreted in excess
❹ Sex steroids secreted in excess

Cholesterol

Intermediate Compounds

ADRENAL CORTEX

Cortisol   **Sex Steroids**

Fig. 15-4. Mechanism of the adrenogenital syndrome.

roids (that cannot suppress ACTH). The overall result is a masculinizing effect. In children, the treatment is simply giving cortisol or other glucocorticoids that supply bodily needs while blocking the secretion of excess ACTH. This cuts off all stimulation to the abnormal pathway for sex steroid production. Virilizing symptoms that appear in adult life strongly suggest an adrenal or ovarian tumor.

Pheochromocytoma

Pheochromocytoma is a rare tumor arising from the nervelike tissue of the adrenal medulla. Bilaterality, malignancy, and extra-adrenal location each occur in roughly 10% of the cases. Thus, it has been called the "10% tumor." Extra-adrenal pheochromocytomas usually arise from the abdominal sympathetic ganglia, but they may originate within the chest, cranium, or even the bladder wall. Increased production of epinephrine and norepinephrine is responsible for the clinical picture that features two main types of symptoms—*hypermetabolic* and *neurologic*. These symptoms (and signs) are nervousness, sweating, palpitation, headache, weakness, weight loss, syncope, psychic disturbances, and hypertension. The tumors have been reported in all age groups from the newborn to the aged. The patients are usually thin, and about 50% will show abnormal glucose tolerance curves or glycosuria. Neurofibromas coexist in some patients with pheochromocytomas. The symptoms come in "attacks" in about half the cases.

Pheochromocytoma

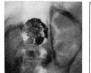

SYMPTOMS:
BP 280/160
Headache
Nervousness
Sweating
Personality Changes

Retroperitoneal Air Outlines
Tumor on X-ray Film

Fig. 15-5. Left adrenal pheochromocytoma outlined by retroperitoneal air insufflation

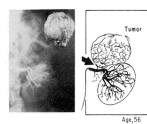

Tumor

Age,56
ADRENAL TUMOR (Pheochromocytoma)
Outlined by Selective Renal Arteriography

Fig. 15-6. Left adrenal pheochromocytoma outlined by dye injected into left renal artery.

Pheochromocytomas tend to be familial. Coappearing with medullary thyroid cancers, parathyroid adenomas and a Marfan-like body build, they form a multiple endocrine adenopathy with autosomal dominant transmission.

Diagnosis. The most difficult problem is diagnosis. Among the thousands of patients with hypertension, the patient with a pheochromocytoma is sometimes hopelessly obscured. Diagnostic work-ups are costly and time consuming. Thus, suspicion and selection are vital diagnostic requisites. Hypertension associated with childhood, glycosuria, pregnancy, postural hypotension, neurofibromas, paroxysmal sweating and headaches, and wide variations in blood pressure recordings should evoke our suspicions.

Laboratory tests. Elevated urinary metanephrines and vanilmandelic acid (VMA) levels provide a diagnostic accuracy of over 90%. Quantification of these metabolic products of the epinephrines have largely replaced the more hazardous histamine provocative test and the adrenergic blockade test. Intravenous pyelograms, tomography, and retroperitoneal air insufflation may localize these tumors (Fig. 15-5). Selective renal arteriography and venography have proved to be excellent diagnostic aids (Fig. 15-6).

Treatment. Surgical excision is usually curative. Because 10% of these tumors are bilateral and 10% extra-adrenal, most surgeons prefer the abdominal approach. Preoperative preparation (for 10 to 14 days) with alpha-blocking agents (Dibenzyline) that decrease blood pressure, increase blood volume, and reverse myocardial damage, provides a smoother operative and postoperative course.

CHAPTER 16

The breast

RICHARD D. LIECHTY

Diseases of the breast originate from four basic pathological processes: disturbances of hormonal activity, irritant effects of retained secretions, infections, and tumors. These processes produce a variety of symptoms, including a large measure of anxiety. From a clinical standpoint the most frequent complaint, by far, is that of a mass. The overwhelming significance of any breast mass to the anxious patient and to the concerned physician is the potential threat of cancer. The differential diagnosis and treatment of the three common types of breast masses (mammary dysplasia, fibroadenoma, and cancer) are our major concerns in this chapter.

ANATOMY

The glands of the breast arise from the skin and are similar to sweat or sebaceous glands. About 15 to 25 branching epithelial channels form in early life (Fig. 16-1, *A*). At puberty a resurgence of growth results in the formation of lobes with each main duct emptying into the nipple. Lymphatics within the breast drain into the axillary nodes, internal mammary nodes, supraclavicular nodes, and the nodes in the second and third intercostal spaces (Fig. 16-1, *B*).

Supernumerary breasts or nipples occur along the milk line (Fig. 16-2). Cancer has been known to originate in extra breast tissue occurring in the axilla. Extra breast tissue should be removed for diagnostic or cosmetic reasons.

Physiology

Most women develop some swelling, mild pain, and tenderness of the breasts in a cyclical fashion at the time of menstrual flow. Estro-

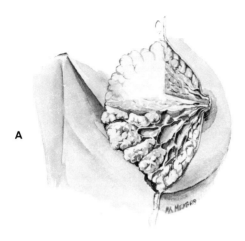

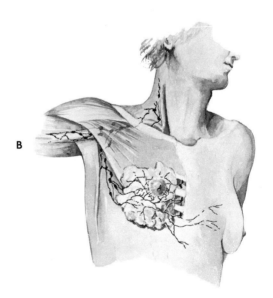

Fig. 16-1. **A,** Cross-section of breast illustrating lobes and ducts. **B,** Main lymphatic channels of breast.

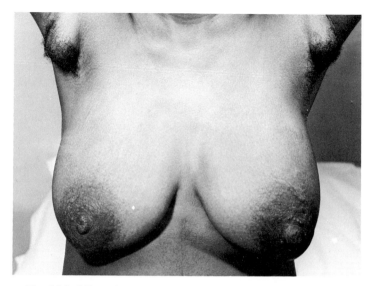

Fig. 16-2. Bilateral breast tissue in axillae of 22-year-old woman.

gens stimulate duct cells the first 2 weeks of the cycle. Progesterones stimulate acini (glandular structures) the last 2 weeks. In pregnancy this process is repeated but in terms of months rather than weeks. Estrogens stimulate the duct cells for the first 4 to 5 months, and progesterones continue until delivery. Prolactin (from the pituitary) induces lactation after delivery.

GYNECOMASTIA

Gynecomastia (enlargement of the male breast) is often seen in pubertal boys, probably from sensitized breast tissue overresponding to a changing hormonal environment. It is usually unilateral, transient, and *never* malignant. Gynecomastia in the adult male is characterized by a firm, discrete subareolar disc of breast tissue that is less often unilateral. It usually results from similar functional endocrine disturbances and only rarely from testicular tumors or hyperfunctioning adrenal or pituitary tumors. Severe liver disease (failure to metabolize estrogens), long-term estrogen therapy (for prostatic cancer), digitalis, methyldopa, and starvation may induce gynecomastia. In teenagers, the surgeon excises gynecomastia for cosmetic (psychological) reasons;

in the adult, to rule out cancer (especially when the lesion is unilateral).

HYPERTROPHY

Neonatal hypertrophy commonly occurs in both male and female infants secondary to maternal estrogenic stimulation. It usually subsides within 6 months.

Virginal hypertrophy occurs as normal bilateral enlargement of the breasts during puberty. Excessive growth occasionally causes painful and disfiguring enlargement; reduction mammoplasty is necessary in the extreme cases. Precocious breast hypertrophy, seen in the first 5 years of life, is almost always caused by estrogen-producing tumors of the endocrine system.

BREAST MASSES

Which *masses are significant?* Many breasts have granular or nodular tissues that blend into a "background." The significant masses are "three-dimensional" and appear to stand apart from this "background" breast tissue. Such distinct masses should be removed and studied histologically (Fig. 16-3).

Diagnosis. The finding of these masses depends almost entirely on the examiner's palpatory skill. The early breast cancers present only as a lump. When obvious skin retraction, fixation, or ulceration appears, the tumor is far advanced. Transillumination is of no help.

Self-examination is often helpful, but difficult because the woman who examines her breast has no basis for comparison or interpretation. Even among nurses, self-examination is fraught with doubts and anxieties that only an experienced physician can resolve.

Mammography. Radiographs of the breast have proved effective in diagnosing breast cancer. Radiographic signs of malignancy are ragged, tentacled borders, finely stippled calcifications, and thickened overlying skin (Fig. 16-4). Unfortunately this procedure is time consuming and costly, and demands highly skilled personnel. Many physicians use mammography to screen high-risk patients (those with family history of breast cancer; those with cancer of opposite breast) or exceptionally anxious patients, but mammography's most appealing potential lies in screening all patients *before* they develop palpable masses. Recent studies confirm that these radiographically detectable, early cancers have less nodal metastases and less 5-year mortality. Xeroradiography features a charged plate that forms an electrical image corresponding to the x-ray image. This image, captured on special paper, shows finer details than x-ray film. Experts report over 95% accuracy with xeroradiography. Because of dense breast tissue,

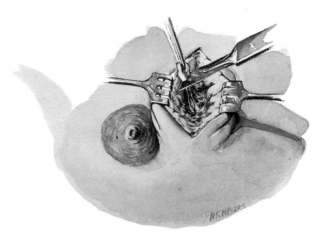

Fig. 16-3. Open excision biopsy of breast mass. Frozen section microscopy done immediately for specific diagnosis.

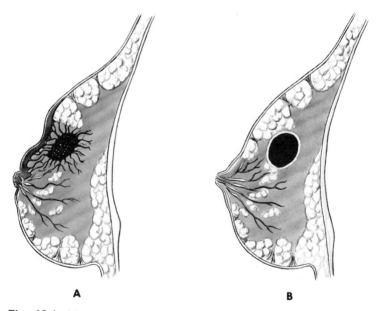

A   **B**

Fig. 16-4. Mammography. **A,** Malignant mass—ragged borders, skin thickening, stippled calcifications, and nipple retraction. **B,** Benign mass —smooth borders, no calcifications, and normal skin.

young women defy reliable diagnosis (except for calcifications) by
either method.

Thermography. Thermography depends on sensitive heat-measuring sensors to detect increased metabolic activity (thus increased heat) over cancers. Thermography may someday be a valuable diagnostic aid, but currently it remains chiefly an investigative procedure.

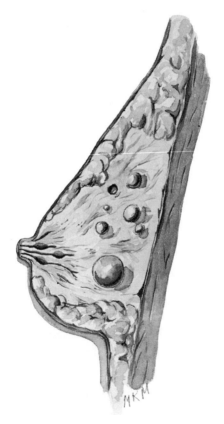

Fig. 16-5. Cross-section of breast with mammary dysplasia, showing multiple cysts and excessive fibrous tissue.

The big three (mammary dysplasia, fibroadenoma, and cancer)

Mammary dysplasia (chronic cystic mastitis)

Mammary dysplasia occurs in at least one-third of all women (Fig. 16-5). The cause is an abnormal reaction of the breast tissue to cyclical stimulation and withdrawal of hormones. The *symptoms* are bilateral breast pain, tenderness, nodularity, and fullness that is maximal just prior to menstrual flow. Cysts and fibrous or epithelial tissue hyperplasia form masses that resemble cancer. In years past clinicians debated the malignant potential of mammary dysplasia, but this controversy has largely been resolved. Current evidence suggests that it is associated with a higher incidence of breast cancer than is normal breast tissue, especially the types with predominant proliferation of ductal epithelium.

Treatment. *Pain and tenderness* occur in women just before their menstrual periods. Firm supports help most. Androgens may benefit extreme cases, but usually sympathetic counseling is all that is required.

Three-dimensional, solid *masses* should be excised and studied microscopically. Cysts should be aspirated (Fig. 16-6). At least 80% will disappear permanently after aspiration. This simple and safe

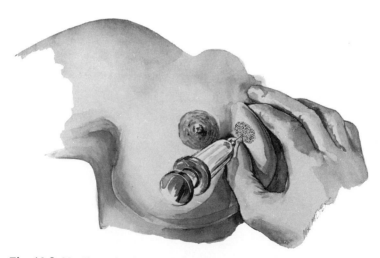

Fig. 16-6. Needle aspiration of breast cyst; typical cloudy, greenish fluid aspirated with small-bore needle.

office procedure avoids the psychologically traumatic effects of hospitalization (often repeated) for biopsy diagnosis. If the cysts refill, excision biopsy will rule out cancer. In rare instances, after multiple recurrences and biopsies, simple mastectomy may be indicated to allay permanently the fears of breast cancer in exceptionally anxious patients, or if the biopsies show excessive epithelial ductal hyperplasia. *Subcutaneous mastectomy,* through inframammary incisions, features removal of virtually all breast tissue while preserving skin and nipples. Younger women especially benefit from this procedure and subsequent insertion of prosthetic implants.

Nipple discharge is often a frightening symptom to women who have been made cancer-conscious by articles in lay periodicals. If a dominant mass occurs concurrent with the discharge, the mass should be biopsied. If the discharge is not bloody and no mass is present, the patient should be reassured and have periodic examinations. Cytological studies have been unrewarding in our experience.

If the discharge is bloody, probing of the duct and excision of the lobule of breast tissue draining into the involved duct will allow histological examination to determine the need for more extensive resection (Fig. 16-7). Bleeding is usually caused by an intraductal papilloma, which is *not* a premalignant tumor. If the patient is past the menopause and no intraductal papilloma is found to account for the bleeding, a simple mastectomy will effectively rule out cancer. The

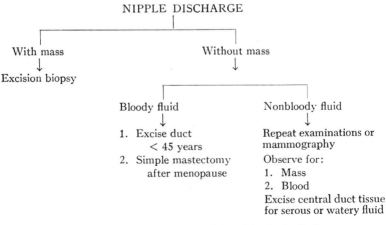

Fig. 16-7. Management of the patient with nipple discharge.

likelihood of bloody nipple discharge being caused by cancer increases after the menopause.

Fibroadenoma

Fibroadenoma, a firm, freely movable lesion (Fig. 16-8), occurs in women most frequently in the early twenties. Fibroadenomas are usually smooth walled and solitary, although 10 to 15% are multiple. Because they are dominant lumps and also may evolve into *cystosarcoma phylloides,* a bulky tumor that rarely metastasizes, fibroadenomas should be excised.

Cancer

Incidence. One out of 18 women (5.5%) who lives to age 72 will develop breast cancer. About 90,000 new cases of breast cancer in the United States are estimated for 1976. The age-adjusted mortality has remained almost the same for the past three generations, despite

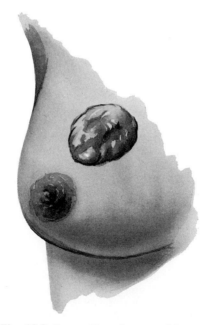

Fig. 16-8. Large fibroadenoma of breast.

aggressive new treatment methods. This inexorable fact has stimulated current reappraisals of breast cancer therapy.

Epidemiology and etiology. The epidemiology of breast cancer includes many factors, some of which are endocrine, heredity, geography, economic status, race, preexisting pathology, and possibly diet.

Endocrine and heredity. Unmarried women, nulliparous women, and parous women who have never nursed run a higher risk of breast cancer. But early pregnancy (before age 20) or early artificial menopause apparently decrease this risk. Breast cancer shows a definite familial tendency. Daughters whose mothers have had breast cancer have at least a threefold increase in their risk of developing it.

Geography and economic status. Japanese women have the world's lowest incidence of breast cancer, Danish women the highest. Some relate this to decreased subcutaneous fat in the Japanese, others to more iodine in the Japanese diet. Some evidence links hypothyroidism to breast cancer, but definite proof of this relationship (whether in Japan or elsewhere) remains elusive. Caucasian women of higher socioeconomic status seem more vulnerable to breast cancer than their opposites. This vulnerability may be related to both fertility and nursing.

Infections. Viruslike particles have been traced from the mother's milk of mice to infant mice that subsequently developed breast cancer. Since similar particles have appeared in human milk from patients with breast cancer, a history of breast cancer should interdict women from nursing.

Contraception. We have recently treated five young women (below 30 years of age) with breast cancer and a history of contraceptive medication, but the overall incidence of breast cancer in young women over the past 20 years has remained the same (University Hospitals Tumor Registry 1950-1975). Data from other centers also fail to confirm, as yet, a relationship between the "pill" and breast cancer.

Sex and age. The 100:1, female:male sex ratio of breast cancer is well known. This ratio probably relates to high levels of female estrogens. Breast cancer incidence rises with age, although a slight leveling of the rate marks the menopausal years. Although 75% of all breast cancer strikes patients 40 years of age and over, *breast cancer remains the leading killer of the young mother.*

Trauma. Trauma probably plays no causative role in breast cancer.

Besides providing many interesting facts about breast cancer, epidemiological research may prove most useful in pointing to those areas where other types of research can explore most effectively.

Patterns of growth. Some patients with breast cancer die in just a few months; others survive for years with advanced disease. We have followed one patient in whom this disease has smoldered for almost

30 years. This wide range in activity probably represents a varying relationship between tumor and host. Studies based on the time required for breast tumors to double in size reveal the astonishing fact that three-fourths of the life of an average breast cancer (8 years) is preclinical (before it reaches 1 cm. in diameter). Thus, before it is palpable, the future course of breast cancer is probably established. The type of cancer and the resistance of the host ("host-tumor relationship") are the decisive factors in prognosis. Metastasis to the axilla, even to one node, is a grim portent of decreased host resistance or perhaps increased malignant potential of the tumor.

Pathology. The breast is composed of ducts and glands (acini) along with fibrous tissue and fat; 95% of breast cancer arises in the ducts, and 5% is of acinar origin.

Location. Cancer of the breast originates most often in the upper outer quadrant (40%) and in the subareolar area (25%). Breast cancers probably arise from multicentric areas of neoplastic change. Premalignant changes are not uncommonly seen throughout a breast removed for one locus of malignancy. Lobular cancer is often bilateral.

Types of cancer. Table 16-1 illustrates the types of cancer of the breast. Most cancers of the breast cannot be precisely "pigeonholed" into any certain histological type. About 80% will have profound sclerosing changes (desmoplasia), which give breast cancer its typically hard and gritty (scirrhous) characteristics (Fig. 16-9).

Although breast cancer can be classified into prognostic patterns, any of these types of cancer may metastasize and kill. *Inflammatory*

Table 16-1. Types of breast cancer

Pathological types	% of all breast cancers	Patients with positive nodes; % at diagnosis	Prognosis
Infiltrating ductal with fibrosis	78	60	Usually poor to variable
Infiltrating lobular	9	60	Variable
Medullary	4	44	More favorable
Colloid	3	32	
Comedo carcinomas	5	32	
Papillary infiltrating	1	17	
Paget's Inflammatory	Variants of ductal cancers (see text)		

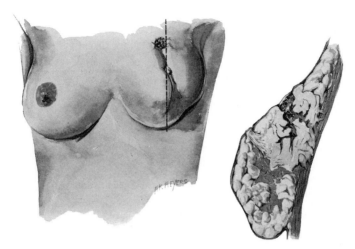

Fig. 16-9. Advanced breast cancer showing skin ulceration, nipple retraction, deformity of breast contour, and fixation to chest wall.

cancer is singled out only because of its astonishing ability for rapid growth and spread that mimics inflammation—thus its name. *Paget's disease* features a chronic eczematous lesion of the nipple usually with extension to adjacent skin. A duct carcinoma, of relatively low malignancy, underlies the skin changes. The Paget cells, seen microscopically, appear to be metastatic tumor cells.

Grading. Attempts to predict the course of breast cancer from histological appearance of the cells, except for the favorable types (Table 16-1), are unreliable and unrewarding.

Metastasis. Regionally, breast cancer spreads most commonly to (1) axillary nodes, (2) internal mammary nodes, (3) supraclavicular nodes, and (4) skin. Distant metastases occur in descending order to (1) chest (lungs, pleura, ribs), (2) bones, (3) liver, (4) adrenal glands, (5) brain, and (6) ovaries.

Staging. Staging defines the extent of the disease and thus determines both treatment and prognosis. Clinical staging is important since this determines what kind of treatment each patient will have.

Clinical staging for cancer of the breast follows:

> Stage I.   Limited to breast
> Stage II. Regional node involvement
> Stage III. Distant metastases

Many errors between the palpating hand and the microscope appear after the breast is removed and examined pathologically. Small axillary nodes invaded by tumor may be impossible to palpate, and, conversely, in about 1% of cases involved, axillary nodes may appear before the cancer in the breast is palpable (occult breast cancer). Size alone does not determine operability nor prognosis; e.g., medullary cancers may grow to a large diameter while remaining localized to the breast. They often have an excellent prognosis. Similarly, the location of the cancer (whether in the upper-outer quadrant or elsewhere) has little prognostic significance.

Clinical staging is only a crude attempt to determine whether an operation will benefit the patient. Edema of the skin, large axillary metastases, ulceration, fixation, or a very rapid growth rate are all gloomy harbingers of prognosis. Only the surgeon, weighing all these factors and considering the overall condition of the patient, can make the final decision of whether an operation will benefit the patient.

Treatment and prognosis. Medical literature bulges with reports and statistical studies of operations designed to treat breast cancer. The student is soon hopelessly submerged in conflicting data. Operative procedures ranging from partial mastectomy ("lumpectomy") and simple mastectomy (removal of breast to the fascia) to superradical mastectomy (in which breast, pectoral muscles, axillary nodes, internal mammary nodes, and overlying chest wall are removed) are advocated with varying degrees of enthusiasm. Proponents of simple mastectomy or "lumpectomy" cite the immunological importance of regional lymph nodes in protection against the spread of cancer and the psychological benefits of preserving some breast tissue. Advocates of the superradical operation justify this enlarged procedure by logically attempting (following the concepts of Halsted) to extirpate more completely the cancer-bearing tissue. Thus, they propose inclusion of the internal mammary nodes in the standard radical mastectomy dissection. To add to this dilemma, studies have shown that no significant difference in the 5-year survival rate is evident in comparing conventional radical mastectomy with simple mastectomy and lymph node irradiation.

Some help in understanding this problem is gained from study of national data showing that survival and death rates in breast cancer patients have remained stable over the past 30 years in spite of unquesioned improvement in diagnostic and therapeutic skills and advancement of technical (including radiotherapy) facilities.

Some inexorable factor seems to control in large measure the survival of patients with breast cancer. This factor appears to be the all-important *host-tumor relationship* that ultimately determines the

222 Synopsis of surgery

Table 16-2. Survival rate comparison in treated and untreated patients

Years of survival	Untreated patients (percent)	Radical mastectomy (percent)	
		Negative nodes	Positive nodes
5	20	80	50
10	5	65	30

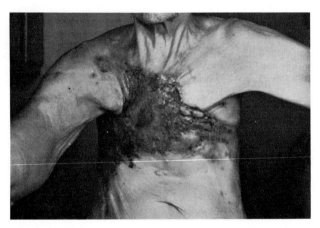

Fig. 16-10. Far-advanced, untreated, ulcerating breast cancer in an elderly female.

course of most breast cancers. This biological fatalism must temper but not dominate our thinking. We know that conventional treatment (radical mastectomy) will more than double the 5-year survival rate in operable cases (Table 16-2). The course of some breast cancers, we must remember, is favorable. In these tumors surgical and radiotherapeutic treatment has been unquestionably effective. Surgical treatment of breast cancer can also prevent (in almost 80% of the patients) the noxious effects of local ulceration and infection that often make life unbearable (Fig. 16-10). This factor alone would justify mastectomy in most instances. Most studies show that prophylactic roentgen-ray therapy either before or after radical mastectomy adds nothing to the 5-year survivals.

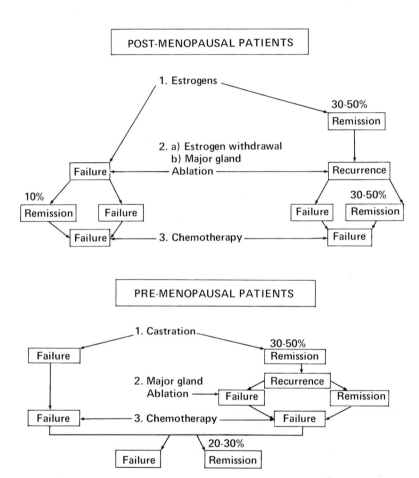

Fig. 16-11. Therapeutic steps in sequential treatment of advanced breast cancer in pre- and post-menopausal women.

Many surgeons prefer modified radical mastectomy (with preservation of the pectoral muscles) to the classical radical mastectomy.

If the student understands that the host-tumor relationship is a vital prognostic factor in breast cancer, and if he develops a healthy skepticism toward all present-day forms of treatment, he will be prepared to accept whatever future therapeutic measures shatter this 30-year stalemate.

Palliation of advanced breast cancer. About 70% of all breast cancer patients, including operable cases, have or will develop metastases from their cancer. Palliation, therefore, is a most important concern to both patient and physician.

Radiotherapy. Radiotherapy is most effective in treating *localized* lesions of bone or soft tissue. If the metastatic tumor can be arrested in this manner, systemic therapy with hormones or chemical agents is held in reserve. Some metastases have been controlled for over 10 years with roentgen-ray therapy alone.

Hormone therapy. Hormone therapy (Fig. 16-11) is utilized to treat diffuse metastases. Remission rates average about 30 to 35%. The exact mechanisms of hormonal response are unknown, but two factors seem pertinent and helpful in planning hormonal treatment: (1) the menopausal age of the patient and (2) the addition to, or subtraction from, these patients of estrogens. Premenopausal patients respond best to estrogen withdrawal (oophorectomy). Post-menopausal patients respond best to estrogens. Both androgens and estrogens are produced by the adrenal cortex, and they can be suppressed by cortisone administration or ablated by hypophysectomy or adrenalectomy. Each of these therapies changes the internal hormonal environment of the patient. Theoretically, this change in turn alters the growth pattern of the cancer.

In general, slower growing tumors, tumors that involve bone or soft tissues, tumors that occur just before menopause, or tumors that occur at least 4 years after menopause respond better to hormone manipulation. Tumors that grow rapidly or involve brain or liver respond poorly. Therapy should be continued for at least 3 months, because evidence of objective remission is delayed in some patients. Patients who respond will survive about 3 to 4 times longer than nonresponders.

Except for rare instances, the physician should advise major gland ablation only for hormonally responsive cancers. In assessing each patient, he must weigh the chance for remission against operative risk and the hormonal consequences after hypophysectomy or adrenalectomy (thyroid, steroid, and vasopressin replacement). Ideally, the candidates for major ablations should have responded to castration

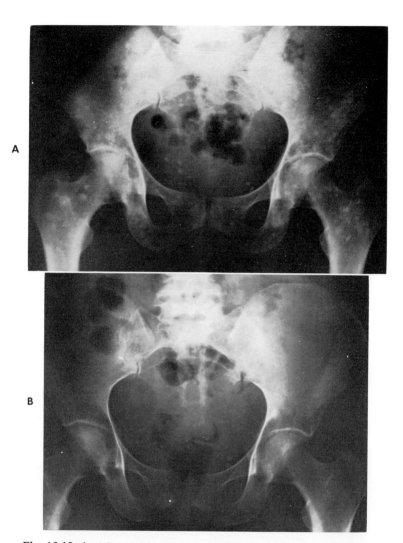

Fig. 16-12. A, Advanced breast cancer (52-year-old female). Note extensive metastases to pelvis. **B,** Same patient 2½ years later after steroid therapy. Metastases have almost vanished. Patient died 1 year later.

or estrogen, or their cancers should take up (at estrogen binding sites) radioactive estrogens. Some patients respond well to steroids alone (Fig. 16-12).

Chemotherapy. Cyclophosphamide (Cytoxan), prednisone, vincristine, methotrexate, and 5-fluorouracil in combination have induced responses in up to 68% of patients. Combination treatment, compared to any one drug, increases the precentage of patients responding as well as the average length of response (21 months in one series).

LESS COMMON BREAST DISEASES
Male breast cancer

Male breast cancer accounts for less than 1% of all breast cancers. It advances somewhat more rapidly in the male, but the 5-year cure rate is about the same as in the female. Mastectomy, hormone therapy, and irradiation are also used in the male. Orchiectomy followed by estrogen therapy (and adrenalectomy) have produced some remissions in advanced stages.

Infections

Acute infections usually occur during lactation and are treated like any other infection, with incision, drainage, and antibiotics when indicated. Less commonly, breast infections occur in the newborn, presumably secondary to maternal hormone stimulation of breast tissue.

Tuberculosis and other chronic granulomatous lesions are curiosities that must be diagnosed by biopsy or culture.

Traumatic fat necrosis

Traumatic fat necrosis occurs after injury and can usually be diagnosed by history or signs of hemorrhage. Subsequent fibrosis may require biopsy to differentiate these firm areas from cancer.

Plasma cell mastitis

This rare disease mimics inflammatory breast cancer because it produces pain, skin induration, and erythema. It usually occurs in women below the age of 40 years and responds to radiation therapy. Biopsy and histological diagnosis are essential for the diagnosis.

Mondor's disease

Mondor's disease is a phlebitis of the superficial veins, usually in the outer quadrants of the breast. This uncommon condition usually begins with pain and terminates in venous thrombosis that slowly resolves.

CHAPTER 17

Liver and biliary tract

ROBERT T. SOPER
LAWRENCE DEN BESTEN

The liver and biliary ducts form a functional unit directing numerous metabolic and excretory processes that are essential to life. The liver has many unique features:

1. It is the largest internal organ in the body, weighing 1.5 kg. in the adult.
2. It is the chemical center regulating at least 40 to 50 metabolic processes ranging from detoxification to synthesis and excretion, and probably many others that are presently unknown.
3. Its unusual blood supply provides inflow of both arterial (hepatic) and venous (portal) blood from two different vascular systems (systemic and portal, respectively).
4. The liver therefore is the only organ that has large inflow arteriovenous shunts, an admixture that occurs in the hepatic sinusoids.
5. It is composed of two lobes, right and left, with a different boundary line separating the anatomic lobes (at the falciform ligament) from the functional lobes (entirely within the right anatomic lobe, at about the position of the gallbladder fossa).
6. It possesses an enormous functional reserve and prodigious regenerative capability. In the experimental animal, 80% of the liver can be removed without detectable impairment of function, with regeneration virtually to normal size occurring in 3 to 4 weeks.

These unusual features make the liver and biliary tract one of the organ systems most vital to life and largely dictate the role played by the surgeon in caring for patients with hepatic disease.

ANATOMY
Liver

The liver, one of the best protected organs in the abdominal cavity, is guarded anteriorly and laterally by the lower rib cage and superiorly by the muscular diaphragm. Furthermore, it is anchored superiorly and inferiorly by the ramifying vascular and ductal structures that pass vertically through it. Quite dense peritoneal ligaments attach the superior and posterior surfaces of the liver to the inferior surface of the diaphragm, encompassing a large triangular area of liver devoid of peritoneum and known as the "bare area"; the bare area is attached directly to the diaphragm by areolar tissue and also contains the efferent hepatic veins that return blood to the inferior vena cava. The falciform ligament, which contains the ligamentum teres and divides the liver into its anatomic right and left lobes, anchors the liver to the anterior abdominal wall down to the umbilical level. The lesser omentum connects the inferior surface of the liver with the duodenum and stomach, and the hepatorenal ligament attaches the inferior and posterior surfaces of the liver to the right kidney, adrenal gland, and inferior vena cava. All these ligaments and tubular structures tend to anchor the liver securely to the surrounding structures and prevent rapid dislocation during trauma.

The blood supply to the liver comes from two sources (Fig. 17-1). Venous blood returns from the entire gastrointestinal tract through the tributary veins that converge to form the portal vein; this blood constitutes 80% of the inflow of blood to the liver, it is delivered with a relatively low pressure (5 to 15 cm. water) and oxygen content, but it is rich in products of digestion. The arterial inflow comes via the hepatic artery under high arterial pressures and rich in oxygen, but delivering only 20% of the afferent blood to the liver. Both of these vessels enter the inferior surface of the liver in juxtaposition to the major bile duct (Fig. 17-1, *A*), constituting a triad of structures of extreme importance to the surgeon during operations on the duodenum, stomach, and biliary system. Each of these structures divides into a right and left branch to service the two functional lobes, the dividing line of which lies entirely within the right anatomic lobe in the neighborhood of the gallbladder fossa.

The microscopic anatomy of the liver is epitomized by the smallest functional hepatic unit or lobule (Fig. 17-2). It is composed of a central vein that contains venous blood efferent from the liver to the inferior vena cava and thence to the right heart. Surrounding the central vein are radially arranged polygonal hepatic cells that perform most of the chemical and excretory work of the liver. The hepatic sinusoids lie between the radiating cords of liver cells; these

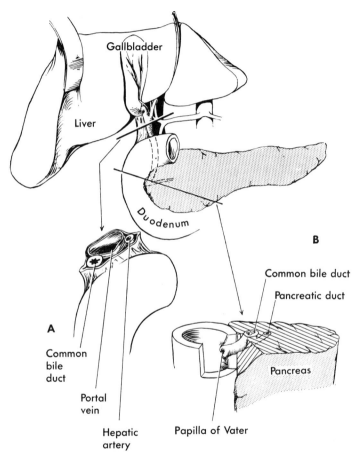

Fig. 17-1. Gross anatomy of liver, biliary ducts, and duodenal loop area. Inset **A** shows the intimate relationship of the common bile duct, portal vein, and hepatic artery. Inset **B** shows relationships of the common bile duct, pancreatic duct, pancreas, and duodenum.

Central vein
Hepatic cells
Hepatic sinusoid   Bile duct

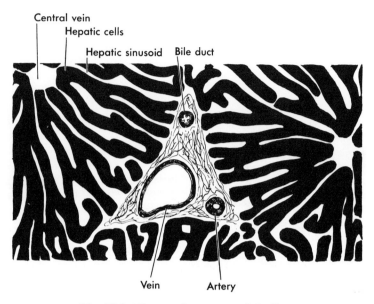

Vein   Artery

Fig. 17-2. Microscopic anatomy of the liver.

sinusoids are lined by endothelial and specialized Kupffer cells of the reticuloendothelial system; the sinusoids are thought to contain an admixture of both the incoming portal venous blood and the hepatic arterial blood; these sinusoids are supplied by tiny lobular end branches from both the portal and hepatic vessels. The bile canaliculi likewise are juxtaposed between the cords of liver cells and coalesce in the peri-lobular spaces into cholangioles and tiny biliary ductules. These in turn converge to form the right and left hepatic ducts that emerge from the inferior surface of the liver with the hepatic and portal vessels.

Biliary ducts

The two main biliary ducts emerging from the inferior surface of the liver join to form the common hepatic duct, which becomes the common bile duct when joined by the cystic duct from the gallbladder (Fig. 17-1). The common bile duct then enters the head of the pancreas and empties into the medial or concave surface of the duodenum through a thickening in the muscle of the duodenal wall known as the sphincter of Oddi (Fig. 17-1, *B*). The ampulla of Vater is a dilatation of the terminal portion of the common bile duct just proximal to the sphincter of Oddi, and it is the site of entry of the main pancreatic duct when a so-called "common channel" (of bile and pancreatic juice) exists. The main pancreatic duct may empty independently into the duodenum.

The common bile duct is 6 to 8 mm. in diameter and occupies the free edge of the lesser omentum, lying anterior to the aperture into the lesser sac known as the foramen of Winslow. The hepatic artery lies medial to the common duct, its right hepatic branches crossing posterior to the common hepatic duct in transit to the right lobe of the liver. The cystic artery is a branch of the right hepatic artery. The portal vein lies posterior and between the common duct and hepatic artery. Abnormalities of positions and relationships of these ducts and vessels are common, requiring meticulous dissection and absolute identification during operations in this area.

The gallbladder is a pear-shaped hollow organ with a normal capacity of approximately 50 ml. It lies within the depression on the inferior surface of the right lobe of the liver known as the gallbladder fossa, roughly marking the division between the *functional* right and left hepatic lobes. The rounded fundus of the gallbladder protrudes below the sharp edge of the right liver lobe and is continuous with the slightly larger body, which then narrows into the neck of the gallbladder. Often the neck of the gallbladder is sacculated into a structure known as *Hartmann's pouch,* where stones are commonly sequestered.

The cystic duct connects the gallbladder to the common bile duct and is characterized by a tortuous and narrow channel filled with spiraling mucosal folds known as the valves of Heister. It is understandable why gallstones so frequently become impacted in the cystic duct when one considers its tortuous and relatively small lumen.

The gallbladder wall has serous, fibromuscular, lamina propria, and mucosal layers from without inward. The biliary duct walls are thinner and contain few, if any, muscular elements. The bile duct serves as a simple conduit. Bile flow is the result of pressure produced by elaboration of bile from the hepatocytes plus contractions of the gallbladder. The colicky pain of obstruction results from distention of the bile duct. Veins and lymphatics of the gallbladder may enter the liver directly.

PHYSIOLOGY
Liver

The polygonal liver cell is responsible for the vast majority of the important metabolic, detoxifying, and secretory functions of the liver.

The Kupffer cells, members of the reticuloendothelial system, are mainly concerned with manufacture of bilirubin in the degradation of red blood cells.

Bile formation

Bile is excreted by the liver at an irregular rate, averaging approximately 40 ml./hr. Liver bile is a dilute, slightly alkaline, and only mildly pigmented material composed largely of water (97%), bile salts (2%), bile pigment, cholesterol, phospholipids, and minute amounts of calcium and other electrolytes.

The bile pigments are manufactured by the Kupffer cells by a conjugation of the bilirubin-globin complex delivered to the sinusoids after degradation of worn-out red blood cells in the spleen and bone marrow (Fig. 17-3). After conjugation with glucuronic acid, the

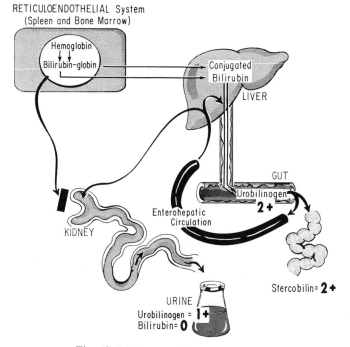

Fig. 17-3. Normal bilirubin metabolism.

water-soluble bilirubin diglucuronide is excreted into the bile canaliculi and passes downstream to the biliary ducts.

Bile salts are water-soluble substances formed by liver cells from cholesterol, and are conjugated to glycine or taurine. Cholesterol is excreted into bile by the liver cells. Cholesterol is totally insoluble in aqueous systems and would immediately precipitate were it not acted upon by the bile salts and phospholipids. Lecithin, the chief phospholipid in bile, combines with cholesterol to form liquid crystals. In turn, bile salts exert a detergent-like effect to break these insoluble liquid crystals into small soluble aggregates called mixed micelles. The hepatic secretion of cholesterol, lecithin, and bile salts in ideal ratios prevents cholesterol from precipitating in bile as stones. Bile salts are conserved by their reabsorption from the intestine (mainly distal ileum) into the portal system where they are re-excreted into the bile (enterohepatic circulation).

If the ductal system is obstructed, bile is regurgitated into the general circulation. Conjugated bilirubin is excreted by the renal glomerulus to lend the golden yellow color to the urine so characteristic of obstructive jaundice. Unconjugated bilirubin cannot pass the glomerular endothelium; therefore the jaundice associated with excessive breakdown of red blood cells (hemolytic jaundice) is acholuric (colorless urine). Excessive levels of bile salts in the serum are precipitated in the skin, causing pruritus associated with obstructive jaundice and biliary cirrhosis.

Carbohydrate metabolism

Monosaccharides enter the portal circulation after intestinal digestion and absorption and are transported to the liver sinusoids. Liver cells polymerize monosaccharides to glycogen (glycogenesis), which is then stored. As metabolic needs dictate, glycogen is broken down to glucose (glycogenolysis) for delivery to the bloodstream and tissues. Heparin is manufactured from glucose in the liver. Galactose is hydrolyzed, and some of the carbohydrates are metabolized in the production of proteins and fats.

Fat metabolism

Fats are metabolized by liver cells to their basic fatty acid and glycerol constituents; a small fraction is stored within the liver, but the majority is converted into carbohydrates, oxidized to ketone bodies and burned, or used in the synthesis of cholesterol and phospholipids.

Protein metabolism

Amino acids are transported from the intestine to the liver where new protein molecules are formed and different amino acids are created; some of the amino acids are deaminized and converted into carbohydrate or fat. Serum albumin, prothrombin, and fibrinogen are three important proteins manufactured by the liver cell. The amine groups resulting from deaminization are synthesized to urea and uric acid for excretion by the kidney. Hyperammonemia ("ammonia intoxication") results when the liver is incapable of handling the amine load, leading to CNS depression and ultimate coma in terminal phases of liver failure.

Steroid synthesis and metabolism

Steroids containing the phenanthrene ring (cholesterol, estrogen, cortisone, bile acids) are synthesized (cholesterol, bile acids) and metabolized (estrogen, cortisone) to inert metabolites by the liver.

Detoxification

Ammonia from protein metabolism is converted to urea. Morphine and barbiturates are metabolized to inactive forms and excreted by the liver.

The bile is the major excretory pathway for iodinated phenolphthalein compounds (Telepaque or Cholografin), certain dyes (Bromsulphalein, rose bengal), and some enzymes (alkaline phosphatase) to form the basis for diagnostic tests of hepatic and biliary tract function.

Biliary ducts

Approximately one liter of bile is produced each day by the liver at a pressure of 25 to 30 cm. of water (Fig. 17-3). The sphincter of Oddi, a thickening in the muscular wall of the duodenum at the ampulla of Vater where commonly the bile and pancreatic juice enter the duodenum, maintains this head of pressure by tonic contraction. During periods of fasting, much of the bile is diverted into the cystic duct for storage within the gallbladder. Here the bile is concentrated 10 to 15 times by absorption of water and electrolytes such that the solid content of the gallbladder bile approaches 10 to 15% as contrasted with 2 to 3% in the bile as it is excreted by the liver. With the entrance of hydrochloric acid and food into the duodenum during a meal, the hormone cholecystokinin is excreted which causes the sphincter of Oddi to relax and the gallbladder to contract, emptying its bile into the common duct for delivery to the duodenum.

Bile is important to normal digestion principally because it emulsifies and saponifies ingested fats to improve their digestion and absorption from the intestine; fat-soluble vitamins A, E, D, and K require emulsification for normal absorption. Lipolytic and proteolytic enzymes within the succus entericus are activated by bile. Bile increases the absorption of iron and calcium, increases intestinal motility, and is bacteriostatic for many gastrointestinal tract organisms.

After reaching the intestine, colon bacteria reduce bilirubin to urobilinogen and then to stercobilin, to give the brownish pigmentation characteristic of normal stools. Some of the urobilinogen and more than 95% of bile salts are reabsorbed into the portal circulation from the intestine (so-called enterohepatic circulation) where much of it is conserved to produce more bile, and a fraction enters the general circulation; small amounts of urobilinogen are normally excreted in the urine.

Obstruction of the biliary tract (obstructive jaundice) prevents bile from reaching the intestine, producing gray-colored stools that are bulky and fatty because of the poor digestion and absorption of dietary fat; reduced absorption of the fat-soluble vitamin K will cause a hemorrhagic tendency if existing for a long enough period of time. Anorexia, weight loss, osteoporosis, and an iron deficiency anemia are commonly seen with long-standing absence of bile from the intestine.

Tests of liver and biliary tract function

Literally dozens of different tests on blood, urine, duodenal drainage, and stool measure, directly or indirectly, different aspects of hepatic and biliary tract function (Table 17-1). Because of the enormous functional reserve of the liver, widespread and far-advanced liver disease may occur before distinctive changes are seen in many of these tests. Furthermore, the results of the tests vary from time to time as the disease waxes and wanes, and some functions of the liver may be severely curtailed while others proceed normally, at least according to our limited ability to measure them.

Liver function tests are most commonly performed to differentiate among the three major types of jaundice: parenchymal hepatic disease, extrahepatic biliary ductal obstruction, and hemolytic jaundice. They help in measuring advanced degrees of hepatic insufficiency and indicate the trend of hepatic disease or the residual liver damage after recovery. Tests of liver function help in evaluating the risk that liver or biliary surgery imposes on the patient. A few of the more commonly employed tests are described in some detail in the paragraphs that follow.

Tests of liver excretory function

Serum bilirubin. Total serum bilirubin normally varies from 0.4 to 1 mg. per 100 ml. The direct-acting (immediate) fraction represents bilirubin that has been conjugated with glucuronic acid in the

Table 17-1. Liver function tests

Liver function tests		Normal	Hemolytic jaundice	Parenchymal jaundice	Obstructive jaundice
Bilirubin	Serum — Direct	0.2–0.5 mg.%	Normal	Increase	Marked increase
	Serum — Indirect	0.2–0.5 mg.%	Increase	Increase	Normal early
	Urine — Urobilinogen	1+	3+	2+	0
	Urine — Bilirubin	0	0	2+	4+
	Stool stercobilin	3+	4+	3+	0
Serum alkaline phosphatase		120 mμ./ml.	Normal	Increase	Marked increase
Serum albumin		4–5 Gm.%	Normal	Decrease	Normal early
Prothrombin time		12–14 sec. or 85–100% of normal control	Normal	Prolonged	Normal early Prolonged late
Bromsulphalein		3–5% remains in 45 min.	Normal	Increase	Increase
Serum glutamic oxaloacetic transaminase (SGOT)		7–40 mμ./ml.	Normal	Increase	Normal to slight increase

liver, and the indirect (delayed, 30-minute value) represents bilirubin tied to its globin molecule prior to conjugation. A normal total value is dependent on normal rates of red blood cell breakdown, normal conjugation and excretion by the liver, and normal passage through the biliary ducts to the intestine. Abnormalities of any one of these three steps involved in bilirubin metabolism might alter these levels. *Extrahepatic* obstruction classically produces an elevation of the total and direct bilirubin whereas hemolytic jaundice will elevate the total and indirect fraction. *Parenchymal* liver disease is associated with elevation of total bilirubin and generally both its direct and indirect fractions.

Serum alkaline phosphatase. The normal value of this enzyme is from 3 to 13 King-Armstrong units or 1 to 4 Bodansky units, or less than 120 mμ./ml. in most automated methods of analysis. The enzyme is released by rapidly metabolizing cells in many organ systems of the body, especially in bone and liver. It is excreted by the liver into the bile and is ultimately lost from the body in the stool. Elevation of serum alkaline phosphatase occurs with extrahepatic biliary tract obstruction and to lesser degrees with hepatic cellular disease, liver metastases, hyperparathyroidism, bone tumors, and Paget's disease of bone.

Urine and stool bile and urobilinogen. Urobilinogen, formed by the action of colon bacteria on bilirubin, is partially reabsorbed in the enterohepatic circulation and partially excreted in the stool; small amounts are normally present in both the stool and the urine. Urobilinogen may be measured by simple gross or fairly sophisticated quantitative tests. Extrahepatic obstruction of the biliary ducts is associated with no urobilinogen or bilirubin in the stool (acholic stool) and no urobilinogen but increased amounts of conjugated bilirubin in the urine. With increased hemolysis, the amounts of both urobilinogen and bilirubin are increased in the stool whereas in the urine the urobilinogen is increased; there is no bilirubin in the urine, since unconjugated bilirubin is not excreted by the kidney.

Metabolic function tests

Serum albumin. Serum albumin is one of the proteins manufactured by the liver cells. The normal serum albumin level is 4.5 to 5 Gm. per 100 ml. of serum, and the albumin:globulin ratio in the serum is generally above 1. Chronic liver cellular damage is associated with a lowering of the serum albumin and a decrease or reversal of the albumin:globulin ratio.

Prothrombin time. Prothrombin is manufactured by the liver cells when adequate amounts of vitamin K are present. A deficiency of vitamin K occurs with prolonged obstructive jaundice (no bile to emulsify and aid in the absorption of the fat-soluble vitamin K) or chronic hepatocellular disease, resulting in inadequate production of prothrombin and elongation of the prothrombin time. Normal prothrombin time is about 12 to 14 seconds. An elevated prothrombin time signals the need for parenteral vitamin K administration in the preoperative patient, a return to normal indicating adequate liver cell reserve and perhaps a less bloody operation.

Bromsulphalein test. Bromsulphalein, a dye, is metabolized by the liver cell and excreted in the bile very rapidly; only 3 to 5% remains in the serum 45 minutes after intravenous administration. Elevation of the amount of Bromsulphalein present 45 minutes after administration is a rather sensitive indicator of hepatocellular damage.

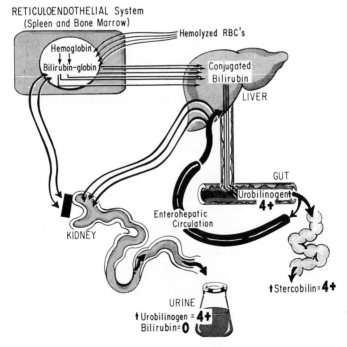

Fig. 17-4. Bilirubin metabolism in hemolytic jaundice.

Serum glutamic oxaloacetic transaminase (SGOT). This enzyme is present in liver, heart muscle, skeletal muscle, kidney, and pancreas, and may be elevated after injury to any of these organs. In reference to the liver, greatest elevations of this enzyme occur with hepatocellular injury (parenchymatous jaundice), and very slight elevations accompany hemolytic or obstructive jaundice.

Jaundice

Jaundice is a yellowish discoloration of the skin, sclera, body surfaces, and secretions. It can be detected on clinical examination when the serum bilirubin rises above 2.5 mg.%. Three major classifications of jaundice are based on the nature and site of the disturbance of bilirubin metabolism:

1. *Excessive hemolysis* of red blood cells (hemolytic, acholuric, prehepatic jaundice)
2. *Hepatocellular (parenchymatous) disease,* which inhibits bilirubin conjugation (hepatocellular, retention, intrahepatic, or medical jaundice)
3. *Obstruction* of bile flow occurring anywhere from the canaliculi on down the biliary tract into the intestine (obstructive, regurgitation, posthepatic, extrahepatic, or surgical jaundice)

In *hemolytic jaundice* (Fig. 17-4) an excessive lysis of red blood cells causes increased production of bilirubin by the reticuloendothelial cells in the spleen and bone marrow; more bilirubin is produced than can be excreted by the normally functioning hepatic excretory mechanisms. The excess of nonconjugated bilirubin in the serum cannot be excreted in the urine (acholuria) but elevates the *indirect* (or delayed) fraction of bilirubin in the serum, with normal *direct*-acting (one-minute) fraction. The tests for hepatocellular function are normal, but excessive amounts of *urobilinogen* in the urine and stool and bilirubin (stercobilin) in the stool are diagnostic. Hemolytic jaundice is seen in congenital spherocytosis, Mediterranean anemia, Cooley's anemia, septicemia, transfusion with mismatched blood, and after certain venomous snake bites. Treatment is directed at the cause of the hemolysis rather than the jaundice per se, and it is nonsurgical except for the definitive treatment of congenital spherocytosis (splenectomy).

Intrahepatic or *parenchymatous jaundice* (Fig. 17-5) is seen with liver infections (hepatitis), exposure to hepatotoxic agents (chloroform, arsenicals, occasionally chlorpromazine), and in the terminal stages of liver failure. Acute viral hepatitis is characterized by elevated SGOT and SGPT in the serum, but with chronic hepatic disorders the liver function tests are seldom diagnostic. There is a mod-

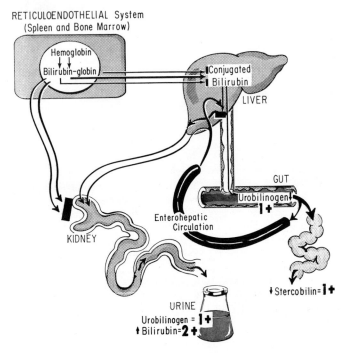

Fig. 17-5. Bilirubin metabolism in intrahepatic jaundice (hepatitis).

erate elevation of both the direct and indirect serum bilirubin with decreased serum albumin levels, a mild increase in the alkaline phosphatase, prolongation of the prothrombin time (with a poor response to vitamin K), and disturbances of the flocculation tests. Treatment is nonsurgical and largely supportive until the disease has run its course.

Obstructive jaundice (Fig. 17-6) results from interference of bile flow somewhere within the biliary ductal system. Most of these obstructions occur within the extrahepatic ducts and are amenable to surgical bypass or removal of the obstruction; therefore, differentiation from the other two major types of jaundice becomes very important. In obstructive jaundice the stool is clay colored or very lightly pigmented, the stool and urine urobilinogen are diminished or absent, and the bilirubin (chiefly the direct fraction) is elevated. The hepatocellu-

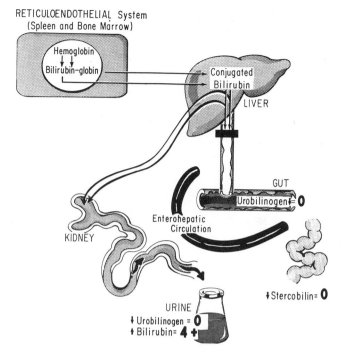

Fig. 17-6. Bilirubin metabolism in obstructive (surgical) jaundice.

lar tests are normal early, but with increasing duration of jaundice liver cellular damage occurs.

Stones within the common bile duct (choledocholithiasis) are the most common cause of extrahepatic obstructive jaundice, generally associated with pain and fluctuation in the intensity of the jaundice. Strictures of the bile ducts most commonly result from duct injury during cholecystectomy. The resulting jaundice tends to be fluctuating, essentially painless, and is often associated with fever and ascending cholangitis. Cancers of the bile ducts, ampulla of Vater, and head of the pancreas characteristically produce a progressively deepening and painless jaundice. Congenital atresia of the bile ducts is one of the two chief causes of *jaundice in the newborn.* It must be distinguished from neonatal hepatitis by early laparotomy.

Occasionally with the administration of certain drugs (chlorpromazine, arsenicals) and during the acute course of hepatitis, the intra-hepatic cholangioles become obstructed by edema and inflammation to produce a variety of obstructive jaundice indistinguishable (except at laparotomy) from extrahepatic obstructive jaundice. Furthermore, the longer obstructive jaundice from any cause persists, the more damage to liver cells will ensue from back pressure, regurgitation of bile, and infection; tests of hepatocellular function become progressively altered, and the laboratory tests therefore become less helpful in distinguishing obstructive jaundice from parenchymatous jaundice.

The type of jaundice can be diagnosed correctly in 75 to 80% of patients by a carefully taken history, complete physical examination, and a few simple tests performed on the patient's urine, stool, and blood. In the remaining 20%, the more sophisticated liver function tests, percutaneous cholangiography or liver biopsy, or even exploratory laparotomy are necessary to make a correct diagnosis.

Although not an emergency, the work-up of a jaundiced patient should proceed expediently, and a decision regarding the need for surgical exploration should be made as early as possible. The complications of untreated and long-standing jaundice are biliary cirrhosis, ascending (suppurative) cholangitis, bile nephrosis, and ultimately both hepatic and renal failure. All have high morbidity and mortality.

SURGICAL DISEASES OF THE LIVER

Although the liver is often *damaged* by surgical disease (extrahepatic obstructive jaundice) or becomes secondarily involved by surgical disease (liver metastases from a primary intestinal neoplasm), and although liver disease can produce secondary changes that require surgical treatment (splenectomy, esophageal varices ligation, and portasystemic shunts for portal hypertension), few diseases *of* the liver are treated by operations *upon* the liver.

Trauma

The liver is commonly injured by penetrating wounds of the abdomen and chest (stabbings, high velocity missiles), and it ranks third among the intra-abdominal organs injured by nonpenetrating abdominal trauma. Even minor trauma may severely damage a liver enlarged by disease. The right anatomic lobe of the liver is larger and more exposed than the left and is therefore more frequently traumatized. Associated injuries to the right rib cage and other intra-abdominal organs often overshadow the hepatic injury.

Traumatic rupture of the liver results in intra-abdominal spillage of blood and bile with signs of shock and peritoneal irritation proportionate to the volume and speed of extravasation. Pain is initially localized to the right upper abdominal quadrant, which then becomes more generalized and often is referred to the right shoulder tip. Abdominal tenderness and guarding follow the pain, with percussion dullness and occasionally a palpable (hematoma) mass. Paralytic ileus with abdominal distention occur late.

Flat and decubitus plain radiographs of the chest and abdomen and four-quadrant abdominal paracentesis are helpful in suggesting the diagnosis of liver injury. Early exploratory laparotomy is indicated when shock is severe after abdominal trauma, for both diagnostic and treatment purposes.

Treatment of minor degrees of hepatic trauma is nonsurgical with bed rest, analgesics, and supportive care. Occasionally delayed subscapular liver hematomas may rupture; thus observation of the patient for 1 to 2 weeks is advisable. The more serious liver lacerations are treated by debridement of damaged tissue, ligation of exposed bile ducts or blood vessels, and extensive drainage to prevent intra-abdominal collection of blood and bile during the postoperative period. Liver tissue holds sutures poorly, and great care must be taken in placing and tying down sutures. Massive trauma, largely confined to one functional lobe of the liver, is sometimes treated by surgical excision of the involved lobe after careful identification and ligation of all vessels and ducts to this lobe. High mortality rates after formal lobectomy for liver trauma have reversed the trend toward lobectomy and reemphasized the place of extensive debridement, ligation of the hepatic artery branch to the injured part, careful ligation of exposed ducts and blood vessels, and extensive drainage to the damaged area. The administration of antibiotics, albumin, and parenteral vitamin K are indicated after major liver injury.

Surgical infections of the liver
Pyogenic liver abscess

Better diagnosis and treatment of infections have markedly reduced the incidence, morbidity, and mortality of pyogenic liver abscesses. Most begin as small microabscesses in the portal triads, which then progress to destroy liver cells and coalesce into gross abscesses. Selective antibiotic therapy administered during the microabscess stage probably reverses the infection and is the best explanation for the lowered incidence of frank abscesses.

The origin of at least one half of the pyogenic liver abscesses is unknown; the majority of the remainder originate in some portion of the gastrointestinal tract with spread via the portal vein (septic pylephlebitis) to secondarily involve the liver. Acute suppurative appendicitis is the chief offender; diverticulitis, ulcerative colitis, and enteritis are less common contributors. Ascending infection from a partially obstructed extrahepatic biliary tree (cholangitis) is the next most common source. Coliform organisms understandably are responsible for most pyogenic liver abscesses. Staphylococcal liver abscesses arise from systemic infections (osteomyelitis, carbuncles) and reach the liver via the hepatic artery.

The early clinical features are dominated by signs and symptoms of the causative extrahepatic infection. Right upper quadrant distress heralds hepatic abscess progressing to pain, spiking temperature elevation, sweating, shaking chills, and a palpably enlarged and tender liver. Mild jaundice may complicate the picture late in the clinical course.

The laboratory tests show anemia and leukocytosis with a shift to the left in the differential white blood cell count. Radiographs reveal an elevated and relatively immobile right hemidiaphragm with an enlarged hepatic shadow. Blood cultures are positive unless antibiotics have been given. Liver scintiscans taken about 1 hour after the intravenous injection of radioactive material (Au 198) will disclose a filling defect provided that the abscess is more than 2 or 3 cm. in size and is located fairly near the surface. Angiograms taken through the portal vein (umbilical vein injection) or hepatic artery inflow tract (selective abdominoaortic injection of dye) will disclose large abscesses as areas within the liver not perfused by the intrahepatic tributaries of these vessels.

Treatment and prognosis. Diffuse bacterial insults to the liver are critical diseases. Antibiotics and supportive care are always indicated. With progression or failure to improve rapidly, surgical drainage is necessary, although occasionally simple aspiration of smaller abscesses is sufficient.

Amebic abscess

Acute amebic colitis is common in tropical and less developed countries; about 10% of cases will be complicated by amebic liver abscesses if not properly treated. Trophozoites of the parasite *Entamoeba histolytica* gain access to the portal venous tributary through the involved colon wall and migrate to the liver, where liquefactive necrosis of liver tissue occurs with coalescence into larger cavities. These abscesses are composed of necrotic liver tissue of a chocolate-red color often likened to *anchovy paste*. The offending parasite can usually be found in the wall of the abscess cavity, and with proper treatment it becomes encapsulated and calcified in time. If untreated, the abscesses may enlarge and perforate into the abdominal cavity or burrow through the diaphragm and empty into the thoracic cavity.

The clinical and laboratory findings resemble those of pyogenic liver abscesses except that the white blood cell count is lower, with less of a shift to the left in the differential count. Eosinophilia may be present. The liver complication may occur weeks after the colonic phase, which is often minor and unrecognized. Sigmoidoscopic examination and scrapings from the superficial mucosal ulcerations and warm stool examinations will usually reveal the amebas.

When the diagnosis of amebic hepatitis is suspected, a trial course of emetine hydrochloride (65 mg. subcutaneously for 5 days) or chloroquine (0.5 to 1 Gm. daily with tetracycline) should be started. A dramatic improvement in the patient's condition confirms the diagnosis and is therapeutic as well. If the signs of liver infection worsen, laparotomy is necessary for confirmation of diagnosis; aspiration of the amebic abscess is preferable to open drainage for fear of a more general contamination of the peritoneal cavity by external drainage.

Cysts and tumors of the liver
Simple cysts

Liver cysts may be associated with cysts of the kidneys and may be multiple and small or single and large. They are thin-walled and filled with watery, colorless fluid. The larger cysts are treated by total or partial excision. Their main importance lies in distinguishing them from neoplasms, primary or metastatic to the liver.

Echinococcus cysts

Echinococcus cysts of the liver are common in sheep-growing countries of the world where man serves as the intermediary host in the life cycle of the dog tapeworm *(Taenia echinococcus)*. The tapeworm within the dog intestine sheds eggs that are excreted and ingested by sheep or man (especially children), with secondary involvement of the liver and lung from intestinal migration. Echinococcus liver cysts, usually slow-growing, may reach a large size with rupture into the free peritoneal cavity, lung, or bile ducts.

Eosinophilia occurs frequently, and complement fixation tests are specifically diagnostic. Plain radiographs often reveal calcification in the cyst wall. Surgical treatment consists of excision after careful evacuation of the cyst contents by aspiration and injection of 2% formalin.

Malignant tumors of the liver

The most common malignant tumor of the liver is *metastatic* from primary neoplasms occurring in the stomach, colon, breast, and pancreas. The gastrointestinal tract metastases reach the liver via the portal vein, and others reach the liver via the hepatic artery. Direct spread from primary malignancies of the gallbladder, stomach, and other organs adjacent to the liver also occurs.

The majority of liver metastases are multiple and involve both lobes; only rarely are metastases localized so that resection can be considered. The exceptions to this treatment rule are liver metastases from malignant carcinoids, or the Zollinger-Ellison type of pancreatic neoplasms, in which partial resection of the liver metastases are indicated to palliate the functional hormonal effects of the metastases. Radiotherapy of hepatic metastases is rarely indicated because of the severe symptoms (anorexia, nausea, vomiting) that occur when liver tissue is irradiated and because of the relentless (and hopeless) course of liver metastases. Chemotherapeutic agents occasionally produce palliation, especially when delivered directly into the portal or hepatic vascular circuits by indwelling catheters.

Primary malignant lesions of the liver are rare in the United States but are common among certain ethnic groups such as the Chinese and the African Bantu. Hepatomas arise from the liver cells and are almost invariably preceded by years of cirrhosis or hemochromatosis or some other such chronic primary inflammatory liver disease. Cholangiocarcinomas arise from the intrahepatic bile duct cells and are not necessarily sequelae of chronic liver disease.

Symptoms of primary malignant liver tumors are insidious and nonspecific at first, including weight loss, anorexia, and low-grade fever. Liver enlargement (nodular or localized) follows with ultimate development of ascites and jaundice. The serum alkaline phosphatase is characteristically high. Treament is usually futile. Although cholangiocarcinomas, localized to one lobe, are amenable to hemihepatectomy, the prognosis is poor. Chemotherapeutic agents may offer some palliation.

Benign tumors of the liver

Hemangiomas, fibromas, and hamartomas occasionally arise in the liver and must be distinguished from metastatic or primary malignant neoplasms. Large hemangiomas of the liver are removed if they are traumatized (hemorrhage) or sequester large amounts of blood.

Portal hypertension

The pressure within the portal vein varies between 5 and 15 cm. of water, depending on position, exertion, and other variables. Portal venous pressure consistently above 20 cm. of water pressure indicates portal hypertension. Portal hypertension occurs whenever the flow of blood within the portal vein is impeded or obstructed; such obstruction can occur at three major sites:

1. *Intrahepatic obstruction:* This is the most common cause of portal hypertension and is almost always caused by cirrhosis (of varying types) of the liver. Alcoholism generally precedes cirrhosis among adults in this country, although among non-drinkers and children previous severe hepatitis with *postnecrotic cirrhosis* is the most likely precursor. The fibrosis and scarring that occur with any type of cirrhosis inhibit the transport of blood into the central veins of the hepatic lobules, leading to stasis and increased pressure within the portal venous system.

2. *Subhepatic obstruction:* Obstruction of the portal vein is the most common cause of portal hypertension among children and very young adults. Portal vein obstruction may result from the following: (a) an extension of the normal postnatal obliterative mechanisms in the umbilical vein and ductus venosus, (b) neonatal septic pylephlebitis (from omphalitis), (c) sepsis of other origin, or (d) occasionally a congenital malformation (cavernous transformation) of the portal vein. Whatever the cause, portal vein obstruction inhibits passage of its blood *to* the liver.

3. *Suprahepatic obstruction:* Obstruction within the hepatic veins or the vena cava itself results in stasis of blood within the liver that is transmitted to the portal venous system leading into the liver. The obstruction may result from thrombosis *(Budd-Chiari syndrome)* or from tumors. It is the least common of all causes for portal hypertension, accounting for about 1% of cases.

Regardless of the site of the block in the venous drainage, the increasing volume and pressure of blood within the portal venous system produce a nonspecific group of secondary clinical disorders that are grouped together under the title of *portal hypertension.*

The most serious symptoms are caused by enlargement and collateralization of the vessels that connect the portal with the systemic venous systems. Normally these collateral veins are small and carry minute amounts of blood under low pressure. The naturally occurring portasystemic venous shunts are as follows: *esophageal veins* (which carry portal blood into the azygos system), *hemorrhoidal veins* (which carry portal blood into the pudendal and iliac veins), and *umbilical veins* (which carry portal blood to the anterior abdominal wall veins). There are innumerable other unnamed collaterals in the retroperitoneal spaces adjacent to the kidneys and spleen. The dilatation and increase in venous pressure within all of these systems may then result in:

1. *Esophageal varices:* Esophageal varices protrude into the lumen of the esophagus, where ulceration results from irritation of food, tubes, or acid-peptic factors. Massive and potentially lethal upper gastrointestinal bleeding is a dreaded result. Diagnosis is confirmed by esophagram (Fig. 22-2) and esophagoscopy.

2. *Hemorrhoids:* Hemorrhoids may prolapse and bleed.
3. *Caput medusae:* In this condition the abdominal wall collaterals may increase in size, radiating outward from the umbilicus.

A second major effect of portal hypertension is upon the spleen (discussed in Chapter 19). It is characterized by splenomegaly and hypersplenism and may produce a reduction in some or all of the formed elements of the blood with anemia, leukopenia, and thrombopenia.

The final effect of portal hypertension is increased production of ascitic fluid, associated with the suprahepatic or intrahepatic blockage. Poor drainage of the lymphatics of the liver capsule with "bleeding" of this lymph fluid into the free peritoneal cavity is the probable cause. Additional causes for ascites often accompany portal hypertension associated with primary liver disease and include hypoalbuminemia and sodium and water retention because of endocrine and renal factors.

Portal hypertension attributed to primary liver disease may be complicated by hepatic coma from liver decompensation. This is especially prone to occur when large amine loads are thrust upon a poorly functioning liver (by massive gastrointestinal tract hemorrhage, usually bleeding esophageal varices). The liver cells are incapable of handling the amine load imposed by the absorption of blood proteins from within the gastrointestinal tract, or these amines are shunted via the portasystemic collaterals into the systemic circulation without passage through the liver. Resulting hyperammonemia is responsible for many of the central nervous system manifestations of hepatic failure (coma, liver flap).

Clinical features. Massive and spectacular hematemesis and upper gastrointestinal tract bleeding are the most frightening manifestations of portal hypertension. Consequent hypovolemia and hyperammonemia superimposed on severe liver disease may be lethal. Bleeding from esophageal varices in patients with subhepatic obstruction (normal liver function) is tolerated much better. Caput medusae is an interesting diagnostic adjunct to the diagnosis of portal hypertension but is not clinically significant. The enlarged and bleeding hemorrhoids, often a nuisance, are not a serious threat to the patient's life and are seldom treated surgically.

Signs of impending liver failure often occur after gastrointestinal tract bleeding in patients with liver disease; concurrent jaundice is a grave prognostic sign. Ascites may be the outstanding clinical feature of patients with suprahepatic obstruction.

Diagnosis and differential diagnosis. Massive upper gastrointestinal tract bleeding from esophageal varices must be distinguished from blood originating within the stomach and duodenum (Chapter 22). Peptic ulcer of the stomach or duodenum is the most common lesion to be differentiated, although carcinoma of the stomach in the older patient must also be ruled out. Distinguishing a bleeding peptic ulcer from esophageal varices is difficult, especially if the patient has cirrhosis, since cirrhotic patients have a 7 to 10 times greater incidence of peptic ulcer than does the general population. To complicate the picture further, peptic ulcer and esophageal varices may coexist.

If most of the blood is effortlessly vomited and little appears per rectum, esophageal varices are likely to be the site of bleeding; on the other hand, bleeding that presents mainly as tarry stools with little blood in the stomach is most likely to be duodenal (and peptic) in origin. Hemorrhage originating in the stomach may present with significant hematemesis and tarry stools concomitantly. Differentiation among these three sites of bleeding is important because of the different approaches in management.

Careful attention to the history of previous acid-peptic diathesis plus a history of current or previous alcoholism or hepatitis is important. Children and nondrinkers who have never had hepatitis most likely have subhepatic blockage. Physical examination should be directed toward finding stigmas of liver disease such as jaundice, reddened palms, spider hemangiomas, caput medusae, ascites, hepatosplenomegaly, and hemorrhoidal varices.

Prothrombin time, Bromsulphalein retention, and serum ammonia tests may be diagnostic. If they are abnormal, the diagnosis of cirrhosis can be presumed, and treatment with vitamin K is begun. Gastric intubation and lavage are helpful in assessing the volume of blood loss. Emergency upper gastrointestinal barium studies and emergency esophagoscopy and gastroscopy are often indicated. Central venous pressures should be monitored.

Emergency treatment. The initial treatment of bleeding esophageal varices must be aimed at stabilization of the circulating blood volume with fluid and blood. Fresh blood is preferable to bank blood because of its higher platelet content and other support of the blood coagulation mechanism.

A triple-lumen rubber tube, *Sengstaken-Blakemore tube* (Fig. 22-3), is helpful in both differential diagnosis and treatment of bleeding esophageal varices. The tube is passed into the stomach, and the gastric balloon, inflated with air, is pulled up snugly against the esophagogastric junction. Compression of the gastroesophageal collaterals by this maneuver commonly arrests bleeding from esophageal varices. The inner lumen of the tube allows continued gastric aspiration and lavage. If bleeding ceases, its origin from esophageal varices

is confirmed. Also, if blood continues to well up into the hypopharynx
with the gastric balloon in place, esophageal varices are probably responsible. These can be tamponed temporarily by inflating the esophageal balloon with air to a pressure of 30 to 40 mm. Hg. The Sengstaken-Blakemore tube is left inflated for 24 to 36 hours. This respite
allows time for diagnostic work-up and stabilization of the patient.
The esophageal and gastric balloons must be deflated gradually and
the tube removed. Pressure necrosis of gastric or esophageal surfaces
may result if the Sengstaken-Blakemore tube remains in place for
longer than 48 to 72 hours.

Treatment of the patient during the period of tube inflation should
include blood transfusions, vitamin K, neomycin to reduce the bacterial flora (responsible for liberating the amines from the blood proteins), and vigorous laxation and enemas to remove the residual blood
from the gastrointestinal tract. Intravenous glucose and vitamin B

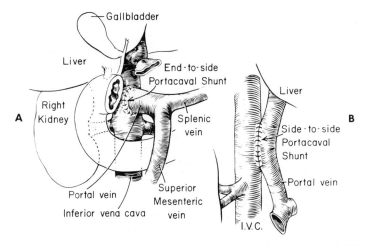

Fig. 17-7. The three major types of shunting operations performed for
portal hypertension and esophageal varices bleeding. **A,** End-to-side
portacaval shunt (end of divided portal vein anastomosed to side of
inferior vena cava). **B,** Side-to-side portacaval shunt (portal vein not
divided, some blood flows retrogradely from liver into inferior vena
cava). **C,** Side-to-side splenorenal shunt (splenic vein anastomosed to
left renal vein). **D,** Mesocaval shunt (superior mesenteric vein connected
to the inferior vena cava by a knitted Dacron graft 18 to 20 mm. in
diameter, 5 to 8 cm. in length).

support the diseased liver. Peritoneal dialysis or exchange blood transfusions may be helpful if liver failure seems imminent.

If bleeding from the esophageal varices resumes after deflation of the tube, the gastric and esophageal balloons are quickly reinflated. Placement of a catheter in the superior mesenteric artery for the constant infusion of vasopressin is extremely effective in controlling variceal bleeding during preparation for definitive surgery, and sometimes is followed by long-term cessation of bleeding.

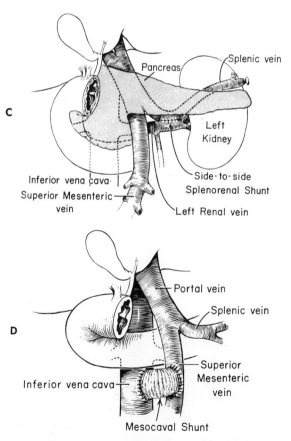

Fig. 17-7, cont'd. For legend see opposite page.

Emergency portasystemic venous shunting procedures carry a high mortality, and every effort is made to control acute bleeding, followed by intensive medical treatment, in preparation for elective portasystemic shunting.

Definitive treatment. Surgical procedures are available for prophylactic and more definitive treatment of good-risk patients with hypersplenism and portal hypertension. Patients with serious liver disease who have already had one episode of major hemorrhage from esophageal varices run a 50% risk of being dead within a year from a second massive hemorrhage. On the other hand, patients with subhepatic portal obstruction almost never die from major esophageal hemorrhage provided that adequate blood replacement and supportive care are available.

The mortality for the major portasystemic venous shunt operations (Fig. 17-7) is about 10%; the highest mortality is seen in patients with intrahepatic block with a serious degree of liver impairment. Good-risk patients have a serum bilirubin less than 3 mg.%, serum albumin greater than 3 Gm.%, BSP retention less than 30%, and prothrombin time more than 50% of normal after the administration of vitamin K; they will not have ascites and should be less than 60 years of age. These are useful guidelines in selecting candidates for portasystemic shunt procedures.

Work-up of a patient who is a candidate for operation includes careful esophagogastroscopy to verify the presence of varices and the absence of concomitant peptic ulcer, selective arteriography with careful attention to the venous phase to visualize vascular anomalies and the patency of the portal system, and percutaneous splenoportography in selected patients in whom the question of portal pressure or the state of the portal venous system is unclear. This information is vital in both timing and selecting the proper shunting operation.

Definitive operations. The only portacaval shunts possible for patients with subhepatic obstruction are the splenorenal or mesocaval shunts (Fig. 17-7). Splenectomy is often done at the time of side-to-side splenorenal shunt (Fig. 17-7, *C*), but is seldom indicated as the sole treatment of portal hypertension because the thrombosis of the splenic vein that inevitably occurs obviates later splenorenal shunt should that become necessary. After successful portasystemic shunting, the spleen diminishes in size and returns to a normal function.

Four types of portasystemic venous shunts are commonly used in patients with intrahepatic portal block. The end-to-side (Fig. 17-7, *A*) or side-to-side (Fig. 17-7, *B*) anastomosis of the portal vein just below the liver to the inferior vena cava is a commonly used shunt. When the portal vein is thrombosed, the splenorenal shunt may be performed (Fig. 17-7, *C*). The mesocaval shunt (Fig. 17-7, *D*) has the advantage of relative technical simplicity (as compared to side-to-side splenorenal and portacaval shunts) and maintains portal blood flow to the liver.

Prognosis. The benefit of any of the shunting procedures depends on maintained patency of the anastomosis, since thrombosis is followed by a recrudescence in the portal hypertension and its serious sequelae. A postoperative complication of portacaval shunt, not seen after a successful splenorenal anastomosis, is *postprandial hyperammonemia* (drowsiness and stupor after ingesting a meal with a high nitrogen load). This syndrome occurs because the absorbed amine radicals are shunted directly into the systemic circulation without passage through the liver.

After a successful portasystemic shunt, the prognosis in patients with subhepatic block is excellent, whereas that in patients with intrahepatic obstruction and cirrhosis is dependent on the liver disease itself.

SURGICAL DISEASES OF THE BILIARY DUCTS AND GALLBLADDER

Operations on the gallbladder and biliary tree rank next to hernia repair and appendectomy in frequency of abdominal operations performed in the United States. Most of the biliary tract disorders arise from the complications of gallstones. Postmortem studies show that approximately 10% of Americans harbor gallstones at autopsy, adequate explanation for the large number of operations performed upon these structures in this country.

Meticulous dissection in a bloodless operative field and absolute identification of anatomic structures are laudable principles in any surgical procedure, but never are they so vital as in gallbladder and biliary tract operations (Fig. 17-1). The close approximation to the portal vein, hepatic arteries, and other structures vital to life, the propensity for congenital anatomic variations, and the obliteration of landmarks imposed by inflammation combine to emphasize the need for strict adherence to these general principles. Biliary tract surgery in the infant and young child is further complicated by a different spectrum of diseases than that in the adult, plus the additional technical problems imposed by size.

Congenital anomalies

The liver and biliary tree arise embryologically as a diverticulum from the second part of the duodenum at the 3-mm. embryo stage, from which the gallbladder branches; the lumen early becomes solidified by cellular accumulations, but later recanalizes. Liver cells and supporting mesenchymal tissue proliferate beneath the developing diaphragm. Abnormalities in development are common, thus explaining the many anatomic variations of the biliary ducts and their relationship to the hepatic artery, portal vein, and pancreatic ducts that are encountered at operation.

Neonatal jaundice is clinically apparent in about 50% of term babies and 80% of premature babies. In almost all of them, fortunately, it is transient and insignificant. The age of onset of jaundice has some bearing on cause and prognosis:

1. Jaundice beginning on the first day of life generally results from intrauterine hemolysis, most often with Rh incompatibility (erythroblastosis fetalis) and less frequently with major ABO blood group incompatibility between the fetus and the mother.

2. Jaundice that is first apparent on the second or third day of life is almost always "physiological," with rapid and spontaneous resolution.

3. Jaundice arising on days 3 to 7 of life is most commonly caused by infections (sepsis, syphilis, toxoplasmosis, cytomegalic disease) and drugs (vitamin K, sulfa drugs), but occasionally it may result from hematoma absorption and thrombocytopenic purpura.

4. Jaundice becoming apparent at or beyond 2 weeks of life may be caused by neonatal hepatitis, infections (sepsis, syphilis, herpes, toxoplasmosis), metabolic storage disorders (Gaucher's disease, Niemann-Pick disease), or galactosemia. Extrahepatic obstructive jaundice occurs less often and results from bile inspissated within the ducts, atresia of the ductal system, or choledochal cyst.

Differential diagnosis of jaundice arising at 2 to 3 weeks of age rests between hepatitis and obstructive jaundice. The other medical causes for jaundice can generally be diagnosed or ruled out. Differentiation between hepatitis and extrahepatic obstructive jaundice is difficult (if not impossible) by physical examination or laboratory tests; therefore, if the jaundice persists for 4 to 6 weeks, exploratory laparotomy is required. Open liver biopsy with frozen section evaluation will quickly establish the diagnosis of hepatitis, and no further exploration is necessary. If the liver biopsy is not diagnostic, the surgeon must determine ductal patency by cholangiograms and surgical dissection.

The *inspissated bile syndrome* results from a plug of tenacious and thick bile somewhere within the ductal system. Some cases are associated with previous hemolytic disorders, and others complicate neonatal hepatitis. Cholangiograms obtained after flushing the ductal system with saline introduced through a needle or catheter in the fundus of the gallbladder are both diagnostic and therapeutic.

Congenital atresia of the bile ducts is marked by partial or complete obliteration of some portion of the biliary tree. In only about 10% will the obstruction be found distal to a dilated and bile-distended proximal segment of bile duct with normal liver connections. Surgical bypass is carried out by means of choledochojejunostomy. Until recently, the other 90% of babies with biliary atresia died of liver failure within 2 years. However, Japanese surgeons have recently developed an operation (hepatic portoenterostomy) that cures 20% to 40% of these patients. A button of tissue is removed from the liver hilum where the intrahepatic bile ducts converge, to which jejunum is anastomosed. The operation succeeds if there are bile-containing ducts within the liver hilum, but not if the intrahepatic ducts are sclerosed or nonexistent.

Choledochal cyst is a cystic dilatation of the supraduodenal portion of the common bile duct containing stagnated bile (and often stones). A tiny and poorly functioning connection to the duodenum at the ampulla of Vater is usually seen. Whether the cyst is truly congenital (because of developmental difficulties) or whether it arises secondary to impeded drainage of bile into the duodenum is unknown. In any event, the complications of gallstone formation, cholangitis with biliary cirrhosis, and perforation have all been reported.

Choledochal cyst commonly presents as a right upper quadrant abdominal mass in a child or young adult with recurrent bouts of mild jaundice and attacks of right upper abdominal pain. Oral cholecystography reveals displacement of the gallbladder; upper gastrointestinal tract barium studies reveal a downward and medial displacement of the duodenum. Anastomosis of the cyst to the duodenum or jejunum is usually curative.

Gallstones

Gallstones produce the majority of surgical diseases of the gallbladder and biliary ducts (Fig. 17-8). The incidence of gallstones varies with different races, geographic location, and dietary habits, being highest at autopsy in Australia and the United States (10 to 13%) and lowest in Japan and Russia (2%). A distinct relationship to age is seen in the United States; 20% of the people over the age of 40 and 30% over the age of 70 years have gallstones. A striking sex relationship is also noted; women harbor stones three times as often as men, and at a younger age. Gallstones almost invariably arise within the gallbladder and only secondarily involve the common bile

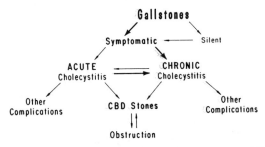

Fig. 17-8. Natural history of gallstones. *CBD,* Common bile duct.

duct. At the age of 80 years, 50% of gallbladder stones are associated with common bile duct stones. A higher than normal incidence of gallstones occurs with pregnancy, diabetes, pancreatitis, cirrhosis, and hypothyroidism. About 10 to 15% of gallstones are radiopaque.

Two main types of gallstones are recognized:

1. *Cholesterol* stones: Stones containing 60 to 95% cholesterol by dry weight are numerically the most common type of gallstones. The noncholesterol component of such gallstones is predominately inert material with small amounts of bile pigment and calcium. They are generally multiple, faceted by indentations crested by their neighbors, firm, and contain concentric laminations suggesting periodic deposition. Occasionally cholesterol stones present as a single, large, smooth, soft, yellow-white stone containing almost pure cholesterol arranged in a radiating manner. *Cholesterosis of the gallbladder* is a specific pathological entity in which tiny plaques of cholesterol are present within heaped-up mucosal folds in the gallbladder; there are generally myriads dotting the interior lining of the gallbladder, and since they resemble the seeds of a ripe strawberry the term *strawberry gallbladder* is often used. Cholesterol stones are often associated with hypercholesterolemia. Hypercholesterolemia alone does not seem to be associated with an increased incidence of cholesterol gallstones.

2. *Pigment* stones: Pigment stones are multiple, soft, black in color, and resemble fine particles of sand. They are composed of bilirubin or biliverdin and commonly follow hemolytic disorders of one kind or another. Whereas cholesterol stones are most common in Western civilizations, pigment stones are more frequent in countries where Cooley's anemia, congenital spherocytosis, sickle cell anemia, and certain parasitemias are common.

Etiology. Although the precise cause of gallstones is poorly understood, four etiological factors are present, to varying degrees, in most patients with cholelithiasis.

1. *Metabolic:* Cholesterol stones are commonly associated with diabetes mellitus, obesity, pregnancy, and hypothyroidism. Although these same conditions are associated with increased levels of cholesterol in blood, hypercholesterolemia itself has not been clearly established as the cause of cholesterol stones in these patients. Pigment stones are associated with hemolytic disorders such as Cooley's anemia, congenital spherocytosis, and sickle cell anemia.

2. *Chemical:* Cholesterol is insoluble in water and is held in emulsion by combining with lecithin and bile salts to form tiny soluble micelles. Thus the concentration of bile cholesterol, lecithin, and bile salts control cholesterol solubility. Chronic elevation of bile cholesterol (as seen in the American Indian or the morbidly obese) or reduction of bile salts (as seen in ileal resection and inflammatory bowel disease) frequently result in cholesterol gallstone formation. Once a nidus of cholesterol is present, additional cholesterol will be precipitated during those periods of each day when bile is supersaturated with cholesterol even in normal individuals.

3. *Stasis:* Stagnation of bile flow favors precipitation of the emulsified solids. Stasis of bile occurs during pregnancy as well as proximal to tortuous or narrowed portions of the ductal system.

4. *Inflammation:* Inflammation is almost always associated with cholelithiasis. The inflammatory exudate of mucus, cellular debris, and fibrin is thought to be incorporated within the substance of developing stones; inflammatory edema also can narrow the ducts, thereby encouraging stasis and obstruction to perpetuate the cycle.

Acute cholecystitis

Acute cholecystitis is triggered by *obstruction* to the outflow of bile from the gallbladder (Fig. 17-9). The point of obstruction is commonly within the tortuous cystic duct, most often because of stone impaction. Less common causes of cystic duct obstruction are inflammatory edema, neoplasm, and rarely volvulus of an abnormally formed gallbladder suspended from a mesentery. Acute cholecystitis is basically a *chemical* inflammation. Bacterial inflammation may occur secondarily from organisms within the bile (coliform in type) or organisms that reach the gallbladder via lymphatics and vessels.

Early in the course of acute cholecystitis the gallbladder becomes

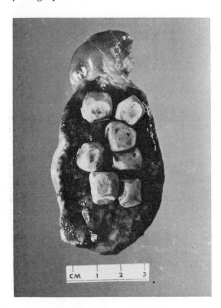

Fig. 17-9. Large gallstones causing acute cholecystitis.

distended with bile, to which is later added inflammatory exudate. Its wall becomes thickened, edematous, and injected, and an acute cellular inflammatory reaction develops rapidly. The cycle is self-perpetuating until and unless the obstruction to outflow is relieved. Migration of the omentum and adjacent organs to the inflamed gallbladder occurs, with fixation of the serosal surfaces to each other by vascular adhesions. These serve as tampons to prevent the inflammation from reaching the general peritoneal cavity. *Empyema of the gallbladder* is a descriptive term applied to the acutely inflamed, totally obstructed gallbladder to which bacterial contamination (with a purulent exudate) has been added. Complications will occur rapidly unless the obstruction is relieved.

Complications of acute cholecystitis occur in 10 to 15% of cases if treatment is inadequate or delayed. Increasing intraluminal pressure of the inflamed gallbladder produces ischemia, ulceration, necrosis, and perforation of its wall. Pericholecystic collections of bile or pus will result if the walling-off forces are adequate, or contamination of the general peritoneal cavity will result if progression is unduly rapid or if the defense mechanisms are lacking.

10. (4+5)
11 - 6
15 7,8
16 9, super

17-25 Trauma) Genip
                    Rev;

26 - oral notes + oral exam
27 -) Real   written test 12-2:30
28 -) Rev;
         "   "   "

96 - 132
268 - 275
385 - 404
958 - 966
998 - 1003

1 hr.

100
103-7

CeP

DIFFERENTIATE	DEAL WITH... MEDICALLY	DEAL WITH... SURGICALLY	DISASTERS!

In the other 85 to 90% of patients with acute cholecystitis, the cystic duct obstruction is relieved spontaneously (by a "ball valve" disimpaction of the stone) to abort the current attack. However, the stage is set for subsequent recurrences.

Clinical features. Acute cholecystitis is often preceded by a rather nondescript history of postprandial bloating, indigestion, selective fatty food intolerance, and varying degrees of right upper abdominal quadrant pain.

The acute attack begins suddenly, often a few hours after ingestion of a large or fatty meal. The chief symptom is pain, initially colicky but later sustained. It is located in the right subcostal or epigastric region but is frequently referred to the tip of the right scapula. The pain is aggravated by pressure, but, contrary to many other inflammatory intra-abdominal conditions, the patient is often more comfortable when up and about walking. Nausea, vomiting, abdominal distention, and belching or flatulence are commonly associated. Later in the attack, fever and mild jaundice are often noted.

Physical examination reveals an acutely ill patient with upper abdominal tenderness and guarding, most pronounced in the right subcostal area with aggravation upon inspiration (positive *Murphy's sign*). The tender, globular gallbladder can be palpated in almost one third of the patients with adequate relaxation and analgesia.

Urinalysis is normal unless dehydration with ketosis is present. The white blood count is elevated to 15,000/cu. mm. or above, with a pronounced shift to the left in the differential count. The serum bilirubin level may be elevated to 2 to 3 mg.%, the borderline of scleral icterus. Plain radiographs of the abdomen often show a localized paralytic ileus and calcified stones in 10 to 15% of patients.

Differential diagnosis. The differential diagnosis of acute cholecystitis may be difficult. Acute appendicitis must be considered, but in this disease the evolution of the acute episode is slower, and the maximal signs of inflammation are anatomically lower than in acute cholecystitis. Right lower lobe pneumonia and pleurisy are extremely difficult to differentiate. Rales, a pleural friction rub, or radiographic evidence of pneumonia suggest pulmonary disease. Acute pancreatitis can be especially confusing and occasionally is associated with acute cholecystitis. Radiation of pain to the back, elevated serum amylase level, maximal tenderness in the epigastrium or left upper abdominal quadrant, marked tachycardia, and shock favor the diagnosis of pancreatitis. Duodenal ulcer, pyelonephritis, and myocardial infarction are sometimes confused with acute cholecystitis.

Treatment. The treatment of acute cholecystitis is initially conservative: nasogastric suction, intravenous fluid and electrolyte replacement, analgesia (with drugs that do not produce smooth muscle sphincter spasm, as does morphine), bed rest, and antispasmodics. Antibiotics are not given early, since this is primarily a chemical infection. When improvement is prompt (6 to 8 hours), conservative treatment is continued. In most cases the acute episode subsides. Cholecystectomy is planned in 3 to 4 weeks when inflammation has resolved and a more complete work-up (including cholecystography) has been done.

If the acute symptoms persist or worsen with conservative therapy, exploratory laparotomy is indicated. In the very elderly, obese, or poor operative risk patient, simple evacuation of the distended gallbladder contents via trochar suction is performed, with removal of the obstructing stones and tube drainage of the gallbladder *(cholecystostomy)*. Cholecystectomy is carried out on a nonemergent basis some weeks later after complete recovery.

In the good-risk patient immediate cholecystectomy can be done provided that the inflammatory reaction is limited enough to allow meticulous and orderly anatomic dissection of the ductal structures. Common bile duct exploration is undertaken if a common duct stone is suspected. Should the acuteness of the inflammatory reaction make dissection difficult, simple cholecystostomy is preferable to cholecystectomy even in the good-risk surgical candidate.

Chronic cholecystitis

Over 90% of patients with chronic cholecystitis have stones in the gallbladder. The gallbladder is generally rather small and invariably has fibrosis and other evidence of chronic inflammation in its wall. Many previous episodes of indigestion, selective fatty food intolerance, and acute or subacute attacks of right upper abdominal pain characterize chronic cholecystitis. The typical patient is "fair, fat, forty, and fertile with flatulence." With advancing age, the sex incidence (favoring females) becomes less and less apparent.

Occasionally the cystic duct becomes totally obliterated by fibrous scar tissue. In the absence of infection, the bile pigment is absorbed during the ensuing weeks, and the gallbladder becomes slowly and progressively more distended with secreted mucus *(white bile)*. This phenomenon is called *"hydrops of the gallbladder"* and may be thought of as the "sterile" and slowly evolving counterpart of empyema of the gallbladder. It is the only variety of chronic cholecystitis in which the gallbladder is palpable on physical examination. *"White bile,"* devoid of pigment, is characteristic of any long-standing and complete obstruction of the biliary tree.

Physical examination of the patient with chronic cholecystitis is seldom diagnostic. Blood and urine studies are of little help. Oral cholecystography commonly fails to visualize the gallbladder. If the gallbladder is still functioning, the nonradiopaque stones will stand out as filling defects (Figs. 17-10 and 17-11). Because the majority of the patients are middle-aged or elderly, barium studies of the upper and lower gastrointestinal tracts are often performed to rule out peptic ulcers, gastric and colonic neoplasm, hiatus hernia, and other conditions that may mimic the nondescript clinical features of chronic cholecystitis. Electrocardiographic examination should be performed in patients with a history of heart disease.

Treatment of symptomatic chronic cholecystitis is clearly surgical. Cholecystectomy is curative and gives the surgeon the opportunity to palpate the common bile duct carefully or evaluate it by means of dye injected through the cystic duct at the time of the operation *(operative cholangiography)* to rule out common bile duct stones.

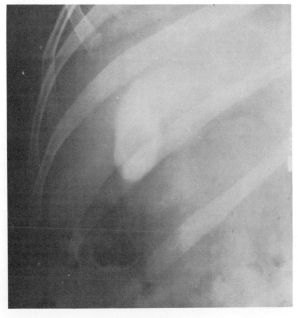

Fig. 17-10. Large, solitary gallstone producing a filling defect in a functioning gallbladder on oral cholecystography.

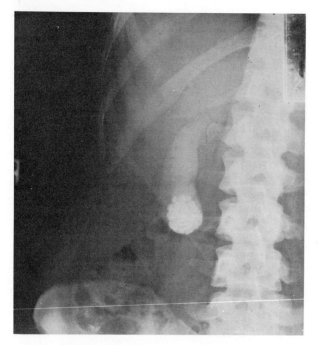

Fig. 17-11. Multiple, calcified gallstones.

Silent gallstones

People who are incidentally found to harbor gallstones without symptoms are said to have "silent gallstones." The incidence of silent gallstones is increasing as our population ages and as screening examinations become routine. They pose a treatment dilemma, inasmuch as they are potentially dangerous and yet not immediately or invariably so. Each patient with silent gallstones must be evaluated individually, the low risk of elective operation being balanced against such factors as the patient's general health, longevity, wishes, and the potential hazard of the gallstones themselves as measured by their size, number, and location. The trend in this country favors prophylactic surgical treatment because an estimated 50% of patients with silent gallstones will ultimately develop serious trouble from them.

Common bile duct stones (choledocholithiasis)

Overall, about 10% of patients with gallbladder calculi also have stones within the common bile duct, although over 80 years of age this association will be found in nearly 50%. They are thought to originate within the gallbladder, with subsequent passage into the common duct. Therefore, common duct stones found months or even years after cholecystectomy were probably overlooked at the time of the initial operation. Since repeat operation upon a jaundiced patient has a formidably high mortality and morbidity, exploration of the common bile duct at the time of cholecystectomy is preferred should any doubt exist about the presence of choledocholithiasis. In other words, it is better to explore the common bile duct unnecessarily at the time of elective cholecystectomy than to overlook retained stones. Even the most experienced surgeons will overlook an occasional common bile duct stone, and despite the strictest criteria for choledochostomy, the common bile duct will contain no stones when explored in approximately 25% of cases.

Relative indications for common bile duct exploration (choledochotomy) at the time of cholecystectomy are (1) existing or recent jaundice, (2) a dilated and thickened common bile duct, (3) palpable stones within the duct, (4) small stones in the gallbladder with a large cystic duct, and (5) filling defects or other abnormalities in the operative cholangiogram.

Common bile duct stones cause symptoms from impaction within the distal duct at the ampulla of Vater. A "ball valve" effect produces intermittent obstruction with stagnation and increase in pressure of the bile, colicky pain (from hyperperistalsis), and a regurgitant type of obstructive jaundice. As the obstruction abates, so do the symptoms and signs. During total obstruction, the stool is acholic or only lightly pigmented and the urine is dark. Secondary infection may produce cholangitis with shaking chills and fever (Charcot fever) and intrahepatic abscesses. Biliary cirrhosis results if the obstruction is chronic.

The clinical features of choledocholithiasis wax and wane with the obstruction. Occasionally a patient harbors a common bile duct stone with no obvious symptoms (silent stone). If the gallbladder is present, cholecystitis may dominate the physical findings. *Courvoisier's sign* is negative; the gallbladder is usually not palpable with extrahepatic obstructive jaundice caused by gallstones since a chronically inflamed gallbladder is contracted.

The work-up of the jaundiced patient should include evaluation of the stool for bilirubin and the urine for urobilinogen and bilirubin. The serum bilirubin is elevated, mainly the direct fraction, as well as the serum alkaline phosphatase. Plain abdominal radiography may reveal a radiopaque stone. If the serum bilirubin is above 2 mg.%, oral cholecystography is futile because the biliary tract will not visualize. Intravenous cholangiography may concentrate enough dye proximal to the stone to reveal common bile duct dilatation.

Percutaneous cholangiography (Fig. 17-12), with injection of radiopaque dye through a long needle inserted into the liver after aspiration of bile, will clearly show the biliary duct anatomy and point of obstruction. Because of the dangers of extravasation of blood and bile into the peritoneal cavity, this diagnostic procedure is performed just prior to laparotomy.

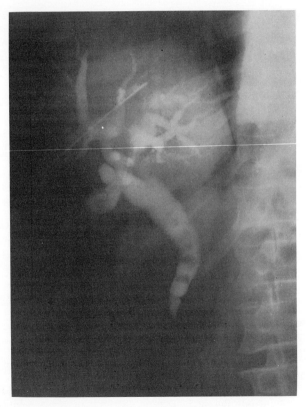

Fig. 17-12. Percutaneous cholangiogram showing multiple stones (filling defects) in dilated common bile duct.

Peroral ampullary cannulation. The advent of the fiberoptic duo-
denoscope has made it possible to cannulate the ampulla of Vater in
the awake patient. Contrast material injected through the cannula
will identify the cause of jaundice.

Differential diagnosis. Choledocholithiasis must be differentiated
from the other causes of obstructive jaundice: ductal strictures and
carcinomas of the extrahepatic biliary duct, ampulla of Vater, and
head of the pancreas. Progressive and unrelenting jaundice associated
with fatty stools, hyperglycemia, and an enlarged gallbladder (Courvoisier's sign) suggest carcinoma of the pancreas. Intermittent jaundice associated with occult blood in the stool and a filling defect in
the duodenal concavity on upper gastrointestinal tract barium studies

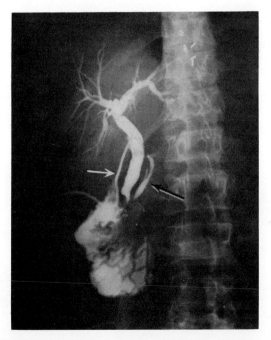

Fig. 17-13. Operative cholangiogram. Dye injected by the T-tube *(white
arrow)* fills the entire biliary system and pancreatic duct *(black arrow)*
and enters the duodenum inferiorly. A faint shadow in the center of the
common bile duct is a retained stone.

favor carcinoma of the ampulla of Vater. Unrelenting jaundice with
an enlarged gallbladder, but with no evidence of pancreatic exocrine
or endocrine dysfunction, suggests carcinoma of the extrahepatic
biliary tree. Intermittently painful and repeated episodes of jaundice
with no palpable gallbladder indicate choledocholithiasis. Strictures
of the common bile duct occur after accidental injury to the duct
structures at the time of cholecystectomy; the jaundice is obstructive
in type, generally painless, and associated with ascending cholangitis.
The history of preceding biliary surgery sets this apart clearly from
other causes of obstructive jaundice. Since laparotomy is necessary
for diagnosis and treatment of all these conditions, it should not be
delayed.

The treatment of choledocholithiasis is surgical removal of stones
and temporary drainage of the common bile duct. If the patient is
seriously ill, preoperative treatment with vitamins K and B complex,
intravenous fluids, electrolytes, and glucose and other supportive measures for a short period of time may be needed. If the gallbladder is
present, cholecystectomy should be performed in addition to choledochotomy and removal of all the common bile duct stones. The common bile duct is explored both proximally and distally and is irrigated
with saline until the bile is free of debris. A probe is passed through
the ampulla and into the duodenum, and the duct is carefully palpated around this probe to be certain that no stones remain. The duct
should be closed snugly around a T-tube, the short limbs of which
are placed into the common bile duct and the long limb exteriorized
through a separate stab wound. Operative cholangiograms should
then be done through the T-tube (Fig. 17-13) to be certain that the
common bile duct contains no additional filling defects and that it
empties freely into the duodenum. The T-tube serves as an external
vent for drainage of bile during the first few postoperative days.
Cholangiograms are repeated through the T-tube prior to its removal
on the tenth postoperative day to assure once again that the biliary
ducts are free of stones.

Postcholecystectomy syndrome

In about 5 to 10% of patients who have had cholecystectomy,
some or all of the symptoms that the patient had prior to operation
(originally ascribed to cholelithiasis) persist or recur. This is referred
to as the "*postcholecystectomy syndrome*." This syndrome has a number of causes, including an erroneous original diagnosis, an unduly
long and dilated cystic duct stump, residual common bile duct stones,
biliary dyskinesia, or conditions outside of the biliary tract with similar
symptoms (hiatus hernia, duodenal ulcer, pancreatitis). Intravenous

or percutaneous cholangiography is helpful in sorting out this problem, often accompanied by barium studies of the upper gastrointestinal tract. Repeat operation is necessary should a dilated cystic duct remnant or residual common duct stone be found.

Carcinoma of the gallbladder and biliary ducts

Carcinomas of the gallbladder and common bile ducts are generally associated with cholelithiasis and chronic inflammatory disease of the gallbladder and ducts, but no good evidence indicts inflammatory factors in the etiology of these neoplasms. The cancers arise from the mucosal surfaces as adenocarcinomas.

Neoplasms of the gallbladder spread early to the liver by direct invasion and also spread to the periportal lymph nodes. Jaundice is often the heralding sign, and surgical cure is possible only when the carcinoma is an incidental finding at the time of cholecystectomy carried out for benign disease.

Neoplasms of the bile ducts are even more rare than those of the gallbladder, but because they cause earlier symptoms, the prognosis is better. The duct lumen is abruptly narrowed at the point of the neoplasm with proximal dilatation, stagnation, and ultimately obstructive jaundice. Spread occurs locally to the contiguous viscera and to the liver via the periportal lymph nodes and portal vein.

Neoplasms of the extrahepatic bile ducts comprise a small fraction of the patients with total obstructive jaundice. When localized to the distal ductal system and if spread has not occurred, they are amenable to treatment by pancreaticoduodenectomy (Whipple procedure, Chapter 18). The 5-year cure rate with this operation in treatment of carcinomas of the distal biliary ducts (15%) is better than that for carcinoma of the head of the pancreas (5%) but not nearly so good as that for carcinoma of the ampulla of Vater (40%). If incurable surgically, bypass of the obstructed bile duct is carried out by anastomosis of the duct to jejunum when possible.

CHAPTER 18

The pancreas

KENNETH J. PRINTEN

EMBRYOLOGY AND ANATOMY

The pancreas begins as dorsal and ventral buds of duodenal ectoderm in the 4-week-old fetus. As the fetus develops these anlages and their ducts fuse, so that the tail, body, and part of the head are formed by the dorsal pancreas, and the remainder of the gland by the ventral pancreas. The ventral duct and the distal dorsal duct form the main pancreatic duct (of Wirsung), while the proximal dorsal duct becomes the accessory pancreatic duct (of Santorini). Because of their common origin, the main pancreatic duct and the common bile duct maintain close but not consistent anatomic relationships as they enter the duodenum (Fig. 18-1). Both pancreatic acini and islets of Langerhans appear at about 3 months of fetal development.

The pancreas is a finely lobulated pink-white structure that extends transversely behind the stomach from the sweep of the second portion of the duodenum to the splenic hilus. Because of its retroperitoneal position, the pancreas lies in close proximity to a number of structures. The duodenum lies lateral and superior to the head of the pancreas, while posterior are the inferior vena cava, right renal vein, and the right crus of the diaphragm. The common bile duct passes through a groove in the head of the pancreas. The pancreatic neck overlies the superior mesenteric vessels and the portal vein. The body of the pancreas overlies the aorta and the junction of the neck and body is directly over the vertebral column at the L2-L3 level. The tail of the pancreas overlies the splenic hilus, the left adrenal gland, and the superior portion of the left kidney. These complex anatomic relationships make surgery of the pancreas technically difficult. The duct of Wirsung provides the main drainage of the pan-

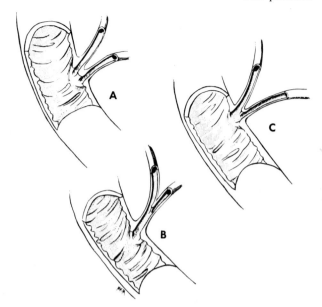

Fig. 18-1. The common bile and pancreatic ducts may, **A,** enter the duodenum separately (40%), **B,** join to form an ampulla (15%), or, **C,** enter the duodenum together at the papilla of Vater (45%). Configurations **B** and **C** (60%) represent a "common channel" entrance into duodenum.

creas in 90% of cases. The accessory duct of Santorini usually drains only the head of the gland and enters the duodenum approximately 2 cm. proximal to the ampulla of Vater.

Pancreatic blood supply is derived from branches of both the celiac axis and the superior mesenteric artery. The lymphatic drainage parallels the blood supply.

Visceral afferent innervation of the pancreas is through the vagus and splanchnic nerves. Vagal fibers end in parasympathetic ganglia within the pancreas from which postganglionic fibers innervate the acini, islets, and ducts. Sympathetic fibers pass into the celiac plexus to synapse with postganglionic fibers, which innervate the vasculature of the pancreas. Visceral efferent impulses from the pancreas are probably mediated through the splanchnic nerves.

PHYSIOLOGY

Pancreatic exocrine secretion, usually a colorless alkaline (pH, 8) fluid, averages about 1,500 ml. per day. It is rich in protein, chiefly proteolytic, amylolytic, and lipolytic enzymes, as well as bicarbonate, which is secreted by active transport in exchange for chloride. Sodium and potassium concentrations approximate plasma levels.

While proteolytic enzymes are secreted in inactive form, lipase and amylase are secreted in active form. Lipase splits dietary triglycerides, while amylase hydrolyzes starch. Both require Ca^{++} for optimal activity. A physiological hallmark of the pancreatic enzymes is the rapidity with which they are synthesized. Under normal conditions this requires a relatively large and constant supply of amino acids, so that systemic protein deficiencies are usually associated with defects in pancreatic exocrine function.

Control of pancreatic exocrine function is almost as complex as the anatomy of the pancreas (Table 18-1). The ultimate stimulus to pancreatic secretion is the presence of food in the duodenum and upper jejunum, although many agents modify the final pancreatic response. The vagus mediates a "cephalic phase" of secretion, analogous to that of stomach, producing a small volume of enzyme-rich pancreatic juice. Secretin and cholecystokinin (pancreozymin), both released by the duodenal mucosa, increase both the volume and enzyme content of pancreatic juice. Secretin is released by the action of H^+ ions on the duodenal mucosa, while cholecystokinin is secreted in response to fat or amino acids in the intestine. The exact effects of gastrin upon pancreatic secretion have not yet been documented, although it can influence both volume and enzyme content of pancreatic juice.

The islets of Langerhans produce three pancreatic endocrine secretions: insulin, glucagon, and gastrin. Although they are numerous (about 1 million in number), the islets form only about 2% of weight of the pancreas and are located primarily in the body and tail of the gland.

Table 18-1. Effects of various pancreatic stimulants on volume and enzyme output of pancreas

Stimulant	Flow	Enzyme output
Vagus	+	++++
Secretin	++++	+
Cholecystokinin (CCK)	+	++++
Gastrin	++	++

Insulin is synthesized and released from the beta cells of the pancreas in response to hyperglycemia, protein ingestion, and intravenous administration of amino acids. Other hormones such as ACTH, thyroxin, secretin, CCK, and gastrin are also capable of increasing insulin release through various mechanisms.

The alpha cells of the pancreas and intestinal mucosa secrete glucagon in response to stimulation by CCK, insulin, or amino acids. Glucagon in turn causes hepatic glycogenolysis and transient hyperglycemia.

Gastrin has recently been detected in islets of Langerhans. Though its exact origin is unclear, the gastrin-producing ulcerogenic tumors of pancreas may arise from C and delta cells in the islets.

TRAUMA

Serious pancreatic trauma is relatively infrequent, occurring in only about 1 to 2% of abdominal wounds. However, because of intricate anatomical relationships with other organs, penetrating trauma to the pancreas is almost never an isolated injury but adds significant morbidity to associated injuries of the duodenum, liver, stomach, and major abdominal vessels. In addition, because of relative inaccessibility, minor penetrating pancreatic injuries may be overlooked at initial laparotomy with subsequent development of postoperative pancreatitis, pancreatic fistula, or pseudocyst.

Pancreatic trauma occurs more commonly following blunt than penetrating abdominal trauma, and understandably is more difficult to diagnose. It may occur as an isolated entity and its symptoms may span the spectrum from vague epigastric distress to peripheral vascular collapse, depending upon the magnitude of the injury. The retroperitoneal fixation of the pancreas with its neck and body draped across the vertebral column predisposes to fracture of the gland when it is impinged by a blow. This realization should provoke suspicion of pancreatic injury with any blunt trauma to the upper abdomen.

Elevated serum amylase levels are the most useful laboratory test to detect pancreatic damage early after injury. Urinary amylase is often elevated up to 4 days postinjury. Markedly elevated levels of amylase may also be found in paracentesis fluid. This procedure should be performed without hesitation in cases of suspected pancreatic trauma. Celiac and superior mesenteric arteriograms are rarely useful and should be reserved for diagnostic dilemmas.

Suspected pancreatic injury demands laparotomy because of the complications of untreated injury, including pancreatic abscess, fistulization, and pseudocyst.

CONDITIONS OF THE PANCREAS

Congenital lesions

Annular pancreas is a rare embryonic defect in the fusion of the dorsal and ventral pancreatic anlage. A ring of pancreatic tissue encircles and obstructs the second part of the duodenum. If the obstruction is severe it may cause vomiting of bile-stained material in infancy. Upright abdominal roentgenograms show the "double bubble" gas pattern typical of duodenal obstruction. However, annular pancreas is often asymptomatic until late childhood or adulthood. Duodenojejunostomy or duodenoduodenostomy will effectively bypass the obstruction. Since postoperative pancreatitis and pancreatic fistula may complicate resection of the annular pancreas, this form of therapy is contraindicated.

Ectopic pancreas is a rare anomaly characterized by aberrant or ectopic deposits of pancreatic tissue, occurring most frequently in the stomach, duodenum, jejunum, ileum, or Meckel's diverticulum. Pancreatic rests usually contain a duct communicating with the area of the intestinal tract with which it is associated. Inflammation, ulceration, or intestinal intussusception of, or intestinal obstruction by, the ectopic tissue brings the patient to the doctor. The treatment is local excision.

For a discussion of *meconium ileus,* see Chapter 28.

Pancreatitis

The main forms of pancreatitis are *acute* and *chronic.* Chronic relapsing pancreatitis represents recurrent attacks of acute pancreatitis superimposed on the course of chronic pancreatitis.

Acute pancreatitis is characterized by the sudden onset of severe, constant epigastric pain occurring typically after an intemperate evening of alcohol and food. The patient rapidly develops generalized, diffuse, and prostrating abdominal pain accompanied by nausea, vomiting, and abdominal distention. Characteristically the pain is described as constant and boring straight through to the back. Abdominal tenderness and rigidity, mainly epigastric but sometimes generalized, are the important physical findings. In addition, the patient is uncomfortable in any position and may constantly thrash around in bed.

Examination of the pancreas at operation or autopsy reveals a spectrum of findings from edema and congestion at one extreme to hemorrhage, suppuration, and necrosis at the other. The principal factor responsible for these changes is escape of pancreatic enzymes into the parenchyma of the gland and adjacent tissues. Although the severity of the clinical picture usually parallels the pathological findings, many times it is impossible to clinically distinguish between these forms of pancreatitis (edematous, hemorrhagic, and suppurative).

Patients with acute pancreatitis fall into the following three general groups, with about equal frequency: (1) one-third have associated biliary tract disease, (2) one-third have associated alcoholism, and (3) a miscellaneous one-third have so-called idiopathic pancreatitis or associated hyperlipemia, hyperparathyroidism, viral infection, autoimmune mechanisms, vascular factors, drug toxicity, and other conditions. The majority of patients with pancreatitis in large county or city hospitals have a history of excessive alcoholic intake. In contrast, most patients with pancreatitis in private hospitals have associated biliary tract disease.

High serum or urine amylase levels with appropriate history and physical findings establish the diagnosis. However, other acute abdominal conditions may also elevate serum amylase: e.g., perforated peptic ulcer, intestinal obstruction, and acute cholecystitis. Serum bilirubin is mildly elevated, perhaps because of swelling around the intrapancreatic portion of the common bile duct. Amylase-containing peritoneal fluid (from peritoneal tap) provides additional diagnostic support.

Treatment of acute pancreatitis is determined by the patient's clinical state. Management includes (1) administering colloid- and crystalloid-containing solutions to replace fluid and electrolytes sequestered in the lesser sac and retroperitoneum, (2) closely monitoring vital signs, central venous pressure, hourly urine output and specific gravity, and serial microhematocrits to assess the patient's hemodynamic state and adequacy of fluid replacement, (3) nasogastric intubation to diminish gastric secretion and associated paralytic ileus, and administering adequate doses of anticholinergic drugs to reduce pancreatic secretions, (4) awareness that most patients (except those with the mildest form of pancreatitis) require broad-spectrum antibiotics even though bacteria play an insignificant role early in the course of this disease, (5) withholding analgesics until the surgeon decides whether the patient has pancreatitis or a surgically correctable cause for the abdominal findings, and (6) close monitoring of blood sugar and serum electrolytes, especially potassium and calcium.

Recurrent bouts of pancreatitis may destroy the gland (and islet cells) with consequent diabetes mellitus. Hypocalcemia and hypomagnesemia (with tetany) are complications of acute pancreatitis. Hypocalcemia may be caused by saponification of intra-abdominal fat (fat necrosis) or to increased secretion of glucagon. Serum calcium levels should be monitored as closely as the patient's condition demands and the patient examined for a positive Chvostek's sign. Intravenous calcium should be given prior to the onset of tetany; if tetany persists after adequate intravenous calcium, parenteral magnesium sulfate should be given.

Exploratory laparotomy is indicated if there is (1) uncertainty of the diagnosis in a deteriorating patient, (2) evidence of an acute pancreatic abscess, (3) correctable biliary tract disease, or (4) pancreatitis unresponsive to nonsurgical therapy. The overall mortality in patients with acute pancreatitis is 10 to 20%.

Chronic pancreatitis results when the pancreas is irreversibly damaged by inflammation. The distinction between acute and chronic pancreatitis rests on the absence of residual damage, anatomical or functional, after a bout of acute pancreatitis. Chronic pancreatitis is characterized clinically by epigastric pain, frequently radiating to the back, and weight loss. Patients with chronic pancreatitis frequently have associated alcoholism, drug addiction, and diabetes mellitus. Physical signs may include moderate abdominal tenderness, a mass in the epigastrium, and jaundice. The serum amylase is seldom elevated unless a pancreatic cyst coexists. Abdominal radiographs may reveal calcification in the area of the pancreas.

Etiology of chronic pancreatitis is obscure. The factors associated with acute pancreatitis are probably operative in producing chronic pancreatitis with a pathological picture of chronic inflammation, fibrosis, and calcification within the parenchyma and/or duct system.

Treatment is nonoperative except for patients who develop intractable pain, pancreatic pseudocyst, or pancreatic abscess. Since no single operation is applicable to all forms and stages of this disease, the surgeon must utilize the procedure that best fits the pathological, anatomic, and functional situation of each patient. Current procedures include plastic operations on the ampulla of Vater, drainage procedures anastomosing the main pancreatic duct to jejunum, and resection of involved portions of the gland, including total pancreatectomy.

Pseudocysts of the pancreas may occur with acute or chronic pancreatitis, or subsequent to trauma. An epigastric mass, occasionally tender, with an elevated serum amylase suggests a pseudocyst. Pseudocysts develop as a result of pancreatic necrosis with escape of pancreatic enzymes that become encapsulated by the resulting inflammatory reaction and contiguous anatomic structures. The cyst may communicate directly with the pancreatic ductal system; however, there is usually no connection with the main duct. Treatment consists of draining the cyst into the stomach, duodenum, or jejunum by anastomosing the cyst wall to a neighboring segment of the gastrointestinal tract. When the cyst wall is thin and immature it may require external drainage by means of sump drains; however, this procedure is followed by a high rate of recurrent pseudocysts.

Neoplasm of the pancreas

Benign tumors of the pancreas are relatively rare. Cystadenoma, the most common, must be differentiated from cystadenocarcinoma by the pathologist.

Periampullary carcinomas

Carcinoma of the head of the pancreas and malignant tumors of the periampullary areas (ampulla of Vater, duodenum, and lower common bile duct) are often indistinguishable clinically. In 75% of the cases, carcinoma of the head of the pancreas will be the cause. The next most common is carcinoma of the ampulla of Vater. The remainder are primary tumors of either the duodenum or common bile duct. Carcinomas of pancreatic origin have a poorer prognosis than the other histological types.

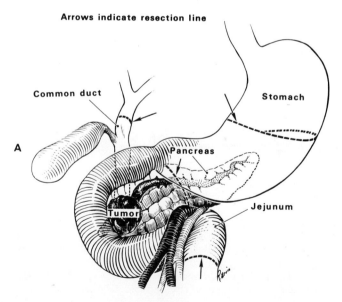

Arrows indicate resection line

Fig. 18-2. Pancreaticoduodenectomy. **A,** Anatomic resection lines.
Continued.

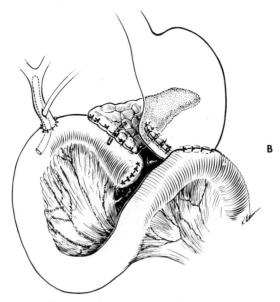

Fig. 18-2, cont'd. B, Completed operation. Three anastomoses: pancreato-jejunostomy, choledochojejunostomy, gastrojejunostomy.

Classically these tumors occur in patients 50 years of age or older. Progressive, unremitting, painless jaundice, anorexia, weight loss, and a palpable gallbladder (Courvoisier's sign) dominate the clinical findings. However, this classic picture is uncommon. Most patients experience varying amounts of vague upper abdominal pain, and the majority, for various reasons, do not have a palpable gallbladder. Occasionally intermittent jaundice is seen, probably because tumor necrosis temporarily unblocks the common bile duct. Laboratory tests and roentgenographic examinations are seldom helpful early in the disease. When roentgenographic findings suggest pancreatic tumor, the disease is usually beyond the stage of surgical curability. Hypotonic duodenography has helped to discover relatively small tumors of the ampulla of Vater. Although selective celiac angiography may detect pancreatic tumors, most diagnosed in this manner are surgically incurable.

Surgical exploration establishes diagnosis and resectability of the tumor. Extension of pancreatic cancer to the portal vein, superior mesenteric, gastric, splenic, or hepatic arteries, or distant metastases preclude curative operations in 85 to 90% of patients. The resectability rate for carcinoma of the ampulla of Vater is greater than 65%.

Resection of tumors of the head of the pancreas or periampullary area requires pancreatoduodenectomy, always a formidable operative procedure (Fig. 18-2). The operation has appreciable morbidity and mortality, and should be performed by experienced surgeons. Patients with unresectable carcinoma of the head of the pancreas or periampullary area survive for about 6 months but rarely over 1 year. However, relief of pruritus associated with the jaundice is well worth palliative biliary bypass (Fig. 18-3).

Although splanchnicectomy has been advocated for relief of pain in patients with inoperable lesions, it is rarely successful. Celiac ganglion block often relieves pain temporarily.

Carcinoma arising in the body or tail of the pancreas produces signs and symptoms late and is one of the most lethal of all tumors. No 5-year cure has been reported after resecting a carcinoma of the body of the pancreas.

Insulinoma

Insulinoma is a rare neoplasm of the pancreas arising from the beta cells of the islets of Langerhans (Fig. 18-4). Patients report bizarre symptoms including irritability, confusion, disorientation, visual disturbances, coma, and convulsions. The diagnosis is established by Whipple's triad: (1) signs and symptoms of insulin shock induced by exercise or fasting, (2) repeated fasting blood sugar levels below 50 mg.%, and (3) relief of symptoms by oral or parenteral glucose. Reliable blood insulin assays have simplified diagnosis. The tolbutamide tolerance test (stimulating insulin release) is also very useful. Ten to twenty percent of the tumors are malignant and about 12% are multiple. The majority are less than 1.5 cm. in diameter. Most of these tumors (over 90%) arise within the substance of the pancreas; ectopic pancreatic tissue accounts for the remainder. Preoperative selective angiography occasionally pinpoints their location within the gland (Fig. 18-5). Other methods of preoperative location of the tumor, such as selenomethionine (^{75}Se) pancreatic scans have been disappointing.

Superficially located tumors are usually treated by simple enucleation. Distal pancreatectomy is required for adenomas within the body and tail of the gland and pancreatoduodenectomy for adenomas within the head of the gland. If the surgeon cannot find a tumor (primary or ectopic), he performs a blind distal pancreatectomy. Symptoms

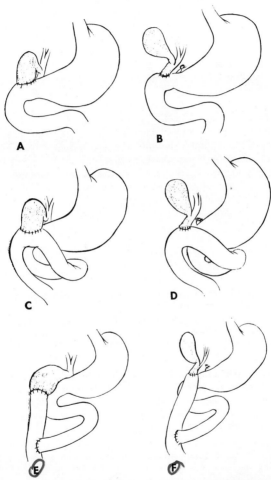

Fig. 18-3. Methods used to bypass inoperable carcinomas of the head of the pancreas. **A,** Cholecystoduodenostomy. **B,** Choledochoduodenostomy. **C,** Cholecystojejunostomy loop. **D,** Choledochojejunostomy loop. **E,** Cholecystojejunostomy, Roux-en-Y. **F,** Choledochojejunostomy, Roux-en-Y.

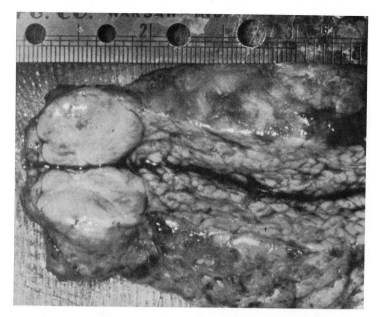

Fig. 18-4. The islet cell neoplasm found in a patient with classic clinical findings.

persisting after this procedure require pancreatoduodenectomy or total pancreatectomy. If the tumor is malignant, the primary tumor should be resected as well as all the metastases possible, in order to reduce the insulin-secreting mass. Diazoxide and streptozotocin are helpful in controlling hypoglycemic symptoms. The mechanism of action of diazoxide is obscure. Streptozotocin exhibits selective toxicity to the pancreatic beta cells. The overall cure rate for surgically treated patients is greater than 75% and the operative mortality is about 5%.

Zollinger-Ellison syndrome

Nonbeta islet cell tumors of the pancreas associated with a fulminating ulcer diathesis were first described in 1955 (see the discussion on Zollinger-Ellison syndrome in Chapter 23). Originally, the syndrome was defined as the following triad: (1) fulminating peptic ulcer diathesis, (2) recurrent ulceration despite intensive medical and surgical treatment, and (3) a nonbeta islet cell tumor of the pancreas. Variations of the syndrome have since been described, includ-

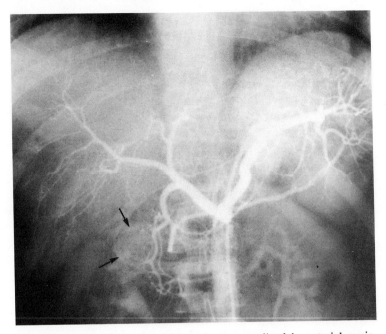

Fig. 18-5. Insulinoma. *Arrows,* Round tumor outlined by arterial angiographic dye.

ing profuse diarrhea with or without an ulcer diathesis, and multiple endocrine tumors (Wermer's adenomatosis).

The Z-E tumor secretes a gastrinlike substance that stimulates excessive secretion of hydrochloric acid and pepsin. A characteristic history coupled with gastric analysis (increased volume and acidity) and elevated serum and urine gastrin levels confirm the diagnosis. Roentgenograms are nonspecific. Most of these tumors are of low-grade malignancy, and metastases have been reported to regress after total gastrectomy. A third of the benign tumors are multiple. Because these tumors are dispersed (i.e., multiple and/or metastatic), removal of a "single" tumor is seldom curative. Total gastrectomy is required to remove the target organ responsible for the symptoms.

CHAPTER 19

The spleen

ROBERT T. SOPER
SIROOS SAFAIE-SHIRAZI

The spleen is part of the reticuloendothelial system, filtering blood rather than lymph. In the adult, it is not vital to life, and the only operation ordinarily performed on this organ is its removal, splenectomy.

ANATOMY

The anatomic peculiarities of the spleen dictate much of its importance to the surgeon (Fig. 19-1). Thus it is held loosely in the depths of the left hypochondrium by dense vascular ligaments to surrounding organs (greater curvature of stomach, splenic flexure of colon, inferior surface of left diaphragm). When these ligaments are retracted during operations (on adjacent organs) or stretched suddenly when the spleen is rapidly displaced by external trauma, the fragile splenic capsule may tear. The splenic vein receives many short branches from the adjacent pancreas, anatomic features that generally require splenectomy when the distal pancreas is removed. A portion of the lymphatic drainage of the stomach is through nodes in the splenic hilum, and splenectomy is necessary when curative gastrectomy is performed for carcinoma of the body of the stomach. Finally, the splenic vein contributes about one-fourth of the portal blood; since this is a two-way street, any increase in portal pressure is transmitted to the splenic pulp. This results in splenomegaly and hypersplenism, at times the earliest and most serious manifestations of portal hypertension.

FUNCTION

The splenic capsule contains elastic fibers that allow considerable fluctuation in size of the organ. The spleen therefore acts as a blood

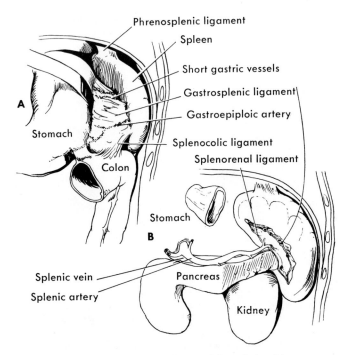

Fig. 19-1. Gross anatomy of the spleen and its relationships to surrounding organs. **A,** Note the intimate attachments of the spleen to the diaphragm, stomach, and colon. **B,** Cutaway section showing relationship of the spleen to the pancreas.

reservoir in lower animals; it stores up to one-third of the blood volume for release back into circulation when additional blood is required, as in response to stress or epinephrine release. This is not an important function of the human spleen.

Red blood cells are destroyed in the spleen as they approach the end of their 120-day life-span, with degradation of hemoglobin and salvage of iron. This destruction probably occurs because of increased osmotic and mechanical fragility of the cells with aging. Red blood cells that are excessively fragile for other reasons (spherocytosis) also are trapped and destroyed in the spleen. It is a curious paradox that red blood cells can also be manufactured (extramedullary hematopoiesis) in the spleen, normally during fetal life and abnormally in the

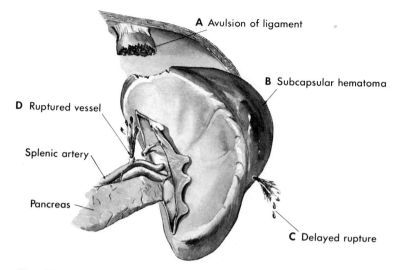

Fig. 19-2. Four types of splenic trauma. **A,** Avulsion of supporting splenic ligament, as with surgical traction; **B,** subcapsular hematoma with, **C,** delayed rupture and, **D,** massive bleeding from major hilar vessels of spleen.

adult with chronic bone marrow failure (fibrosis). Extramedullary hematopoiesis produces splenomegaly; bone marrow smears are done prior to elective removal of a large spleen to rule out marrow failure as the cause for splenomegaly.

As part of its reticuloendothelial function, the spleen produces antibodies, lymphocytes, and plasma cells. The spleen seems to be an especially important source of antibodies in the infant and young child, with many reports indicating a high and serious infection rate after splenectomy in the very young. For this reason, splenectomy should be avoided if possible for the first few years of life, or if unavoidable, prophylactic antibiotics should be administered postoperatively.

SURGICAL DISORDERS OF THE SPLEEN
Splenic rupture and its causes

The most common indication for splenectomy is hemorrhage secondary to rupture (Fig. 19-2). In descending order of importance, splenic rupture is caused by (1) trauma, (2) surgical traction, and

(3) diseased condition of the spleen, which then ruptures spontaneously.

Trauma

Despite the relatively small size of the spleen, its mobility, and the protection afforded by the left lower rib cage, the spleen is the intra-abdominal organ most susceptible to rupture by trauma. The trauma may be direct or indirect, by a penetrating or a nonpenetrating force. Associated injury to surrounding organs (stomach, colon, pancreas, left kidney) is common, and often splenic rupture is seen with multiple injuries to other parts of the body. The signs and symptoms of splenic injury may be masked by these other injuries. Splenic penetration by missiles is often seen in combat military practice. Nonpenetrating multiple system injury is more common in civilian automobile accidents or falls.

Surgical traction

Iatrogenic tears in the splenic capsule by excessive traction on the tough capsular ligaments are occasionally produced during operations on adjacent organs. Downward traction on the stomach (transabdominal vagotomy or hiatus hernia repair) injures the spleen in about 5% of cases. Better exposure and more gentle traction reduce the frequency of this misadventure.

Spontaneous rupture of a diseased spleen

An enlarged spleen from any cause will be more exposed and therefore subject to rupture by lesser degrees of trauma. A spleen softened by disease, such as malaria or lymphomatous involvement, on occasion ruptures spontaneously. Awareness of this possibility, especially in children subjected frequently to minor trauma, justifies early treatment of the primary disease.

Clinical manifestations. Multiple injuries to other parts of the body commonly complicate and mask splenic injury. The signs and symptoms of splenic rupture in turn will depend on the amount and rate of blood loss (Fig. 19-2). Thus, a complete rupture of the major artery or vein in the splenic hilum produces massive blood loss signaled by profound shock. Lesser degrees of blood loss, as with rupture of the splenic pulp, are associated with gradually appearing signs of shock, often accompanied by abdominal pain, tenderness, percussion dullness, and an expanding hematoma mass in the left upper abdominal quadrant. The pain is more severe with breathing and may be referred via the phrenic nerve to the left shoulder tip (Kehr's sign, noted in 15% of cases). The left hemidiaphragm is elevated and restricted in its movement. Free blood in the peritoneal cavity may cause loin bulging and shifting dullness and is suggested on rectal examination by a fullness in the rectovesical space. Deepening pallor, rising pulse rate, narrowing pulse pressure, and serial diminution in the hemoglobin and hematocrit reflect the resultant hypovolemia.

In about 15% of patients with traumatic rupture of the spleen, the bleeding is controlled by intrinsic tamponade by the omentum or diaphragm to produce a perisplenic hematoma, or else the hemorrhage is confined beneath the splenic capsule. In this situation the signs of hypovolemia may be minimal or lacking and the abdominal signs may be more localized to the left upper abdominal quadrant. In time this hematoma may resolve entirely and remain as a splenic cyst, or occasionally it may rupture secondarily into the free peritoneal cavity with a return of the progressive signs of hypovolemia and spreading hemoperitoneum. Delayed rupture has been reported up to 50 days after injury.

Exploratory laparotomy is the safest and most decisive way to confirm the diagnosis of splenic rupture. Abdominal paracentesis may help confirm the diagnosis of intraperitoneal hemorrhage prior to laparotomy. Transfusion therapy should begin immediately, followed by laparotomy.

When bleeding is slower, additional diagnostic study of the patient is possible. A leukocytosis of 15,000 to 20,000/cu. mm. is an early but nonspecific sign of splenic rupture. Serial hemoglobin and hematocrits, which reflect dilution of circulating blood with extracellular tissue fluid to compensate for lost blood, are sometimes helpful. Plain radiographs show elevation of the left hemidiaphragm, medial displacement of the gastric air bubble with serration of its greater curvature, and inferior displacement of the air within the splenic flexure of the colon associated with a "ground-glass" tissue density in the left upper abdominal quadrant. When diagnosis is doubtful, splenic angiography may confirm presence of splenic laceration or hematoma.

Treatment. Splenectomy is the preferred treatment for splenic rupture. Successful suturing of minor tears in the splenic capsule has been reported, but this procedure is hazardous. The operation is not complete without a meticulous and orderly search for other intra-abdominal injuries, once the spleen has been removed and hemostasis achieved.

Hypersplenism

The term *hypersplenism* is nonspecific and implies abnormal splenic sequestration of one or more of the formed elements of the blood (RBCs, WBCs, or platelets) (Table 19-1). It is almost always

Table 19-1. Primary hypersplenism*

Disease	Blood	Marrow	Benefit by sple-nectomy
1. Idiopathic thrombocyto-penic purpura	↓ Platelets	↑ Megakaryocytes	80%
2. Congenital spherocytosis	↓ RBCs	↑ Erythroid elements	100%
3. Primary neutropenia	↓ Neutrophils	↑ Myeloid elements	80%
4. Primary pancytopenia	↓ Formed ele-ments	↑ All precursor ele-ments	80%

*Key: ↑ elevated; ↓ lowered.

associated with splenomegaly, a depression of the sequestered blood elements, and increased bone marrow production of those elements that are diminished in the peripheral blood.

Hypersplenism may be primary or secondary. In *primary hypersplenism* no other known disease process induces the exaggerated splenic function. Examples include idiopathic (primary or essential) thrombocytopenic purpura, idiopathic (primary) splenic neutropenia and/or pancytopenia, and congenital spherocytosis. Splenectomy is generally quite effective in the treatment of primary hypersplenism.

In *secondary hypersplenism* the overactivity is caused by another disease process involving the spleen and other portions of the reticuloendothelial system (leukemia, lymphomas, Hodgkin's disease, sarcoidosis, tuberculosis, and the metabolic storage diseases). Splenectomy may temporarily improve the hematological picture in secondary hypersplenism, but it does not affect the course of the primary disease per se. Hypersplenism secondary to portal hypertension is the most common form of secondary hypersplenism.

Idiopathic thrombocytopenic purpura

Idiopathic thrombocytopenic purpura is characterized by marked diminution in circulating platelets with a resultant bleeding diathesis. It must be distinguished diagnostically from thrombopenia and purpura secondary to toxic bone marrow depression (and diminished platelets) caused by a wide variety of agents such as tuberculosis, excessive radiation, leukemia, widespread bony metastases, and bone marrow sensitivity to drugs such as sulfonamides, chloramphenicol, arsenicals, and benzol. Secondary thrombocytopenic purpura is not helped by splenectomy.

Idiopathic thrombocytopenic purpura is more common in females, children, and young adults. As the name suggests, the basic cause is unknown. Some theories incriminate a hormone from the spleen that prevents platelet release from the bone marrow; others suggest a globulin that agglutinates platelets to increase their splenic sequestration and destruction.

Clinically the disease is characterized by periodic exacerbations of abnormal bleeding manifested by the appearance of petechiae, ecchymoses, and hematomas, which appear either spontaneously or after minor trauma. Surface bleeding can occur into the intestinal or urinary tracts, and menometrorrhagia is seen in the menstruating female. Hematomas in the intestinal wall can produce obstruction or can serve as the lead point in intussusceptions. The most crippling and lethal bleeding occurs intracranially, and its prevention compels early treatment of this disorder. Large hematomas or hemarthroses are uncommon. This is the only form of hypersplenism that is not commonly (in only about 20% of cases) associated with splenomegaly; furthermore, if thrombopenia and splenomegaly are associated, it is likely that one is dealing with a secondary type of thrombocytopenic purpura.

The diagnosis of idiopathic thrombocytopenic purpura is suggested by a positive Rumpel-Leede test: petechiae are produced distal to a sphygmomanometer cuff inflated above venous pressure. The bleeding time is prolonged and the clot retraction is poor, although the coagulation time is normal. Platelet count in the peripheral blood is below 40,000/cu. mm., and the bone marrow smear contains increased numbers of platelet precursors (megakaryocytes).

Initial treatment often consists of transfusion of platelets or fresh blood collected in a siliconized container; this temporarily prevents additional bleeding. Remissions occur spontaneously and are often induced by steroid therapy, especially in children. The remissions may be permanent.

Splenectomy is indicated if a remission is not achieved or if the disease exacerbates while under steroid maintenance therapy. Splenectomy generally produces a thrombocytosis that reaches its peak between 2 and 12 days postoperatively, followed by a return of the platelet count to near normal ranges. Improvement in clot retraction and bleeding time will likewise occur promptly. Some patients are relieved of their bleeding tendencies even though the platelet count is unchanged.

Splenectomy is curative in about three-fourths of patients with idiopathic thrombocytopenic purpura. It will prevent further serious bleeding episodes or will make steroid management easier in the majority of the other patients, even though the platelet counts remain low.

Idiopathic splenic neutropenia and pancytopenia

In these rare *primary* disorders there is a deficiency in one or all of the formed blood elements within the peripheral blood, associated with an increase in marrow activity in the element or elements deficient peripherally. Further, no other diseases contribute to these changes. Splenectomy is curative.

Much more commonly, these varieties of hypersplenism are *secondary* to other primary disorders including infections (malaria, sarcoidosis), neoplasms (leukemia, lymphosarcoma, Hodgkin's disease), metabolic storage diseases (Gaucher's disease, Niemann-Pick disease, Hand-Schüller-Christian disease, Letterer-Siwe disease), and portal hypertension. Progressive splenomegaly is characteristic of secondary splenic pancytopenia, and treatment should be directed at the primary disease rather than the spleen. Occasionally splenectomy is indicated when the massive size of the spleen itself produces symptoms or poses a threat to life because of ease of injury. Splenectomy is also done to improve the hematological picture when the latter changes are extreme. Portal hypertension is the most common cause of secondary splenic pancytopenia; the hypersplenism improves with lowering of the portal pressure by portasystemic venous shunts (Chapter 17).

Hemolytic anemias

Hemolysis of red blood cells associated with anemia can be produced in many ways, including transfusion of mismatched blood, septicemia, and exposure to various hemolysins, as certain snake venoms. Apart from these is a group of disorders in which the spleen is instrumental in destroying red blood cells to cause anemia and splenomegaly. Sickle cell anemia and Mediterranean (Cooley's) anemia are not often benefited by operation and will not be considered further.

Congenital spherocytosis

Congenital spherocytosis is the best understood of these so-called hemolytic anemias. In this disorder, the red blood cells are morphologically altered to a spheroid rather than a biconcave disc shape. This is genetically determined as a mendelian dominant trait transmitted by either parent. About 20% of cases seem to arise spontaneously, presumably by mutations, but the remainder show a strong family history of anemia and jaundice. However, the gene responsible for the hemolysis exhibits varying degrees of penetrance. Some members of the family have spherocytosis with little evidence of anemia or splenomegaly, whereas others have the full-blown clinical picture with the same degree of spherocytosis. The mechanical and osmotic fragility of the spherocytes is increased, thus making them more susceptible to entrapment and hemolysis by the spleen.

Characteristically, mild anemia and jaundice with a slightly enlarged spleen are apparent in the first decade of life. Patients with mild forms of the disease may live a normal life-span, although a significant proportion (25%) ultimately develop gallstones because of the chronic hyperbilirubinemia.

Aplastic crises. Patients with more severe forms of spherocytosis will develop intermittent crises, sometimes precipitated by infections. Such crises are marked by abdominal pain, fever, nausea and vomiting, progressive anemia, acholuric jaundice, and splenomegaly. The peripheral blood reveals spherical erythrocytes on smear with an anemia that reflects the severity of the disorder. Reticulocytosis is expected during the recovery period after a crisis, but the reticulocyte count may fall to zero during a crisis. Recent theory ascribes the crisis to cessation of red blood cell formation in the bone marrow rather than to an increase in hemolysis within the spleen. A splenic hormone may be involved in this mechanism.

The red blood cell fragility test (preferably interpreted after 24 hours' incubation) is the single most diagnostic study. Hemolysis of the spherocyte begins in 0.75% saline rather than in the 0.45% saline concentration necessary to lyse normal red blood cells. Hemolysis is completed at 0.4% rather than 0.3% saline in the normal individual. The indirect serum bilirubin level is elevated and stools are more darkly pigmented than normal, although no bile is present in urine in keeping with the conjugated nature of the bilirubin. Coombs' test for immune globulin is negative, and a bone marrow smear reveals erythroid hyperplasia.

Initially treatment is directed at tiding the patient over the acute crisis by cautious blood transfusions. Splenectomy cures the serious hemolysis and prevents future crises but does not alter the red blood cell shape or fragility. All patients who are symptomatic should have splenectomy as an elective procedure since there is no known medical treatment, and spontaneous remissions do not occur when symptoms are marked. Cholecystectomy should be carried out at the same time if the patient's condition allows and if cholelithiasis is present.

Acquired anemias. The *other hemolytic anemias* are acquired (or secondary) and are not of primary surgical interest. Idiopathic acquired hemolytic anemia is a condition that belongs among the autoimmune family of disorders with spontaneously arising agglutinins and hemolysins that damage otherwise normal red blood cells. Splenomegaly, hemolysis, and anemia result. Coombs' immune globulin test is usually positive, the morphological appearance of the red blood cell is generally normal (although cases are reported that do have some spherocytosis), and there is no family history of hemolytic anemia. Steroids are the preferred treatment. Splenectomy is indicated only for those who fail to respond to nonoperative treatment.

Miscellaneous

Primary neoplasms of the spleen are extremely rare and generally of mesenchymal tissue origin. Secondary splenic involvement is common in the leukemias and lymphomas, but metastases from carcinomas are almost unheard of.

Cysts of the spleen are rare and may be congenital, secondary to liquefaction of old hematomas or parasitic infestations such as hydatid cyst, or caused by a solitary dermoid cyst.

Accessory spleens are miniature duplications of splenic tissue found on routine postmortem examination in about 10% of the population. They are usually located near the splenic hilum or the gastrocolic ligament and are darker than lymph nodes. Interestingly enough, accessory spleens are found in 20% of people with hypersplenism. Hypertrophy probably allows easier detection in hypersplenism. Accessory spleens must be removed at the time of splenectomy for hypersplenism—if left behind they may undergo hyperplasia and assume the function of the parent spleen. Missed accessory spleens are occasionally a reason for failure of splenectomy in the treatment of hypersplenic conditions.

CHAPTER 20

The peritoneum and acute abdominal conditions

RICHARD D. LIECHTY

Peritonitis is the leading cause of death on surgical wards despite modern antibiotic agents. Understanding the role of the peritoneum in response to injury or contamination is a cardinal requisite for all physicians.

DESCRIPTION AND FUNCTION

The peritoneum is composed of a single layer of mesothelial cells overlying a loose connective tissue layer. The *parietal* peritoneum lines the abdominal cavity and is reflected onto the abdominal viscera and mesenteries as the *visceral* peritoneum or *serosa*. It encompasses about the same relative surface area as the skin. The peritoneal cavity is a closed sac except for the fimbriated ends of the fallopian tubes in females.

The functions of the peritoneum are essentially two in nature. First, the mesothelial cells secrete small amounts of serous fluid, which moistens the peritoneal surfaces and allows gliding movements of the viscera. Second, it reacts rapidly against insults by bacteria, intestinal contents, bile, urine, etc. to eliminate or localize the resulting inflammation. It accomplishes this by vascular dilatation, hyperemia, and increased capillary permeability, thus permitting an influx of peritoneal fluid, white blood cells, and fibroblasts into the area. The omentum and loops of adjacent bowel also move into the site and localize or "wall off" the infection. Localization is further aided by inhibition of bowel motility secondary to paralytic ileus.

The peritoneal cavity has two main weaknesses: (1) it is a continuous cavity through which contamination can spread, and (2) it readily absorbs toxins from its extensive surface.

PERITONITIS

Inflammation of the peritoneum may be divided into two major classes: (1) primary, which is infection of the peritoneum from a distant source, and (2) secondary, which is caused by involvement from some other primary cause such as perforated ulcer, penetrating abdominal wounds, or a ruptured appendix.

Primary peritonitis

Primary peritonitis is a rare bacterial inflammation, constituting only about 1% of all cases. It does not have an intra-abdominal source, and most cases occur in young children, females, nephrotics, or patients taking steroids. The offending organisms, usually hemolytic streptococci or pneumococci presumably gain access to the peritoneum via the fallopian tubes or are blood borne.

The differentiation between primary and secondary peritonitis may be difficult, but important because of the difference in management. Peritoneal aspiration with smear of the exudate that shows pure streptococci or pneumococci is diagnostic, and appropriate antibiotics, fluids, rest, and nasogastric suction comprise accepted treatment.

Tuberculous peritonitis is also considered a form of primary peritonitis. This disease is now rare because of better control of tuberculosis in general and pasteurization of milk and inspection of dairy herds.

Secondary peritonitis

Secondary peritonitis, the usual form of peritonitis, accounting for 99% of all cases, is caused by acute bacterial inflammation secondary to contamination. This contamination may result from a breach in intestinal integrity (ruptured appendix, gunshot wound, brokendown anastomosis) or penetrating abdominal trauma carrying in pathogens from outside. The two most common pathogens found are *Escherichia coli* and *Streptococcus pyogenes*. Others of importance are staphylococci, pneumococci, Friedländer's organisms, *Pseudomonas aeruginosa,* and *Clostridium perfringens*. These organisms, virulent human pathogens, usually present as a mixed flora. As in all infectious processes, the extent of the resulting infection depends on the virulence of the organisms, the extent and duration of contamination, the resistance of the host, and the therapy. The balance achieved between these antagonists often determines the life or death of the patient.

Clinical characteristics

The signs and symptoms of peritonitis vary widely with the intensity and extent of the inflammation. Abdominal pain, fever, and malaise invariably accompany peritonitis. Vomiting often occurs early, but it may be totally absent. The patient resists movement and tends to flex his hips in an effort to relax and splint his abdomen. Tenderness, rebound tenderness, and rigidity on palpation are the most significant findings. The abdomen may be silent (paralytic ileus).

Peritonitis also produces a shift of fluid, electrolytes, and protein into the "third space," i.e., the peritoneal cavity, retroperitoneal tissues, and the atonic gastrointestinal tract. This shift of fluid may cause shock as may bacterial endotoxic effects (on heart and vessels), hepatorenal failure, and occasionally adrenal failure.

Laboratory aids

The white blood cell count is elevated with a "shift to the left." Plain films of the abdomen may show air within the large and small bowel, typical of an adynamic ileus. Upright or decubitus films may show free air in the peritoneal cavity from perforation of a "hollow viscus."

Treatment

Therapy of peritonitis is directed against all the factors that cause and sustain the peritonitis. The definitive treatment, surgical intervention, aims directly at stopping the source of contamination. Closure, exteriorization of the perforation, or a short-circuiting technique (colostomy) may be required, depending on the cause and location of the trouble. Drainage of a specific contaminated area is often indicated. The following therapeutic steps help prepare the patient for operation. Gastrointestinal intubation and decompression decrease the contamination by draining and resting the gastrointestinal tract. Antibiotics offset the virulence of the pathogens. (Culture and sensitivities should be obtained.) Blood, fluid, and electrolytes restore fluids lost in the third space and help prevent hypovolemic shock.

Bile, gastric juice, pancreatic juice, and free blood produce chemical reactions of the peritoneum. Bacteria, like scavengers following predators, often follow chemical injury to the peritoneum. Surgical intervention is usually necessary to close the "leak" and to drain a specific portion of the peritoneal cavity such as the gallbladder bed.

ACUTE ABDOMINAL DISEASES

The panoramic view of the problems of acute abdominal diseases is presented here. The vital question concerning the patient with an acute abdomen is whether an operation is necessary. Fortunately clinical evaluation and laboratory study provide the surgeon with valuable assistance in making his final decision. The broad concepts underlying this decision concern us here. More specific features of acute abdominal diseases are discussed in subsequent chapters.

Classification. The term *acute abdominal disease* describes any abdominal disease that demands immediate surgical evaluation. From the students' viewpoint a breakdown of the acute abdomen into three descriptive clinical categories is helpful: the *"hot abdomen,"* which is exquisitely painful and tender, the *"warm abdomen,"* which is painful but minimally tender, and the *"cold abdomen,"* which is often neither painful nor tender but which may be lethal (gastrointestinal bleeding).

The "hot" abdomen, which indicates peritonitis, and the "cold" abdomen, which results from G.I. bleeding, often require immediate operative treatment. The patient with a "warm" abdomen must be watched carefully and reassessed regularly because a "warm" abdomen can suddenly become "hot" or "cold"; e.g., early appendicitis may produce some pain and only minimal tenderness and then subside. With progression, however, evidence of peritoneal irritation signals the need for immediate appendectomy. A painful peptic ulcer may suddenly hemorrhage. Acute abdominal disease is a dynamic, changing situation. The physician who treats the patient with an acute abdominal disease must recognize these changes. The two most important points in this recognition are (1) the overall condition of the patient (fever, pulse, pain, blood pressure, vomiting, etc.) and (2) abdominal tenderness, which reflects underlying peritoneal inflammation, and other abdominal signs (distension, bowel sounds, mass).

Table 20-1 lists some of the common diseases that produce an acute abdominal condition. Although they have been separated into three descriptive categories, they may dramatically shift from one to another. They are listed in the approximate frequency of occurrence. These categories are admittedly arbitrary, but we believe they help the student to understand a complex problem.

The combination of shock, bloody vomitus, and bloody or tarry stools invariably means gastrointestinal hemorrhage (the cold abdomen). This is discussed in the next section. Differentiation of the hot abdomen from the warm abdomen is the purpose of this section. It is a very common clinical problem.

History. A careful history should be taken, relating the acute abdomen to the past history.

Character of the pain. Colicky pain usually denotes an obstruction;

Table 20-1. Diseases producing an acute abdominal condition

"Hot" abdomen (pain and tenderness)	"Warm" abdomen (pain but minimal if any tenderness)	"Cold" abdomen (shock—often no pain or tenderness)
1. Appendicitis	1. Early bowel obstruction	1. G.I. bleeding
2. Cholecystitis	2. Viral enteritis	
3. Perforated peptic ulcer	3. Gastritis	
4. Pancreatitis	4. Peptic ulcer	
5. Pelvic inflammatory disease	5. Renal stones	
6. Diverticulitis	6. Mesenteric adenitis	
7. Ruptured ectopic pregnancy	*Mimics of the "warm" abdomen*	
8. Acute renal infections	(Extra-abdominal causes)	
9. Regional enteritis	1. Myocardial disease	
10. Ulcerative colitis	2. Respiratory disease	
11. Dissecting or ruptured aneurysm	3. Crises (sickle cell, diabetes, syphilis, Schönlein-Henoch purpura)	
12. Mesenteric arterial occlusion	4. Spinal cord tumor	
	5. Glaucoma	

smooth muscle hyperperistalsis attempts to push fluid past the obstruction (ureteral colic, gallbladder colic, intestinal colic). The pain subsides between episodes. With infection or abscess, however, the pain never completely subsides (appendicitis, empyema of the gallbladder). A sustained pain occurs and may become episodically more severe.

The *onset* of the pain is often a valuable clue to the cause. Rupture of an aneurysm or perforation of a peptic ulcer produces sudden, frighteningly painful catastrophies. Gastritis is usually more gradual and often occurs after heavy alcoholic intake.

The *location* of abdominal pain is helpful but not infallible since pain may be referred to the abdomen from other areas. Lower lobe pneumonias, cardiac disease, or glaucoma may cause referred abdominal pain. Similarly, abdominal pain may be referred elsewhere. Renal colic is commonly referred to the inguinal area; gallbladder pain may be referred to the right shoulder area. Pancreatic disease is often accompanied by back pain. Referred pain is explained by a common nerve root origin of sensory nerves supplying separate anatomic areas. The sensory areas of the brain misinterpret the source of the pain.

The importance of relating the acute abdomen to the past history seems obvious yet is frequently forgotten in the excitement of the emergency situation. The history of a previous duodenal ulcer, gallstones, cirrhosis, renal stones, menstrual abnormalities, and alcoholism often suggest the correct diagnosis.

Physical examination. Physical examination should include general signs, abdominal examination, pelvic examination, renal examination, paracentesis, and rectal examination.

General signs. Fever, pain, rapid pulse and respirations, nausea and vomiting, and changes in bowel function often keynote the diagnosis of "hot abdomen." Shock and hematemesis or melena are often the only signs of the "cold abdomen."

Abdominal examination. Tenderness is the key to differentiating the "hot" from the "warm" abdomen. Peritoneal inflammation (from pus, gastric juice, bile, pancreatic juice, intestinal contents, or blood) causes the nerves of the parietal peritoneum to become sensitive to touch. Sudden removal of hand pressure from the abdomen causes immediate pain from movement of these inflamed surfaces *(rebound tenderness).* The area of maximal tenderness will often localize the point of insult. Coughing jars the inflamed peritoneum and causes localized pain, thus simulating this rebound phenomenon.

The *location* of the tenderness is most helpful in diagnosing the cause. In localized abdominal peritonitis the point of maximal tenderness usually overlies the area of inflammation. Tenderness, in contrast to pain, is rarely referred to the abdomen from other areas.

Pelvic examination. Exquisite tenderness of the cervix signals pelvic inflammatory disease (P.I.D.), which may begin with vague lower abdominal pain and tenderness. A careful pelvic examination should be routine in the evaluation of acute abdominal disease in females— bimanual rectal examination will substitute in the young or when routine pelvic examination is impossible.

Renal examination. Checking for tenderness at the costovertebral angles is often helpful in ruling out kidney disease as the source of pain.

Paracentesis. A highly valuable and rapid aid in diagnosis of acute abdominal disease when bleeding or perforation into the peritoneal cavity is suspected is *peritoneal aspiration* (paracentesis) or *peritoneal lavage.* Recovery of blood, pancreatic fluid, bile, pus, or fecal material (a positive tap) is often diagnostic and confirms the need for immediate laparotomy. A negative tap should be viewed with skepticism, however, as isolated areas of peritoneal fluid may be missed by needle aspiration. Routine four-quadrant taps or peritoneal lavage with sterile saline are less likely to yield false negative results.

Rectal examination. Rectal examination is always indicated, especially when the tenderness is in the lower abdomen. Sigmoidoscopy can screen out intrinsic lower bowel lesions (cancer, amebiasis, colitis, etc.).

Laboratory tests. The following laboratory tests and the roentgen-ray tests discussed in the next section are commonly used in evaluating patients with acute abdominal pain. These aids will be all that is necessary in over 95% of the patients. More sophisticated procedures are discussed in later chapters.

White blood count. An elevated white blood count usually indicates inflammation from many sources (chemical, bacterial, neoplasia). Viral inflammations often depress the white blood count. Thus, this is an important test to differentiate viral enteritis or mesenteric adenitis from bacterial peritonitis. A differential count will show a predominance of juvenile forms ("shift to the left") in acute inflammation. Overwhelming infections may result in normal or depressed white blood cell counts. *Hemoglobin and hematocrit* are often depressed with tumors, chronic infections, or bleeding.

Urine. Pyuria or hematuria strongly suggests a renal cause of abdominal pain. Contiguous organ disease (an inflamed appendix overlying the ureter) may rarely cause these abnormalities.

Amylase. Pancreatitis will, in its early stages, cause an increased serum amylase (above 500 units), which may be transient. Biliary tract disease, perforated duodenal ulcer (the duodenum contains pancreatic juice), intestinal obstruction, or mumps, may cause a lesser elevation in serum amylase.

SGOT. Serum glutamic acid oxaloacetic transaminase is helpful in distinguishing necrosis of liver cells (infections or tumors) or myocardial infarction from surgical diseases of the abdomen. Values may be elevated above 1,000 units in massive liver necrosis (normal 10 to 40 units).

Other tests. An EKG is helpful in assessing cardiac status. A BUN gives a reliable indication of renal function. Electrolytes are obtained when vomiting, diarrhea, or inadequate intake is encountered.

Roentgen-ray examination. Roentgen-ray examination may include: plain and upright films, intravenous cholangiogram, renography, chest roentgenograms, and G.I. barium studies.

Plain and upright films. A plain film of the abdomen may show calculi in the biliary tract, kidneys, ureters, bladder, or rarely in the appendix (appendolith). Bowel obstruction is evident from air or air-fluid levels in the small bowel (best seen on upright films).

Free air in the peritoneal cavity indicates perforation of a hollow viscus.

Intravenous cholangiogram. Intervenous injection of cholografin is very helpful in diagnosing biliary tract disease. If the dye outlines the common bile duct but not the gallbladder, the diagnosis of cholecystitis is strengthened.

Renography. Urinary tract disease is diagnosed by dye injected intravenously that shows the kidneys and ureters and, less accurately, the bladder (intravenous pyelograms). Retrograde pyelography utilizes contrast material injected into ureteral catheters. This procedure necessitates cystoscopy.

Chest roentgenograms. Chest roentgenograms are helpful in ruling out pneumonitis but are less accurate in diagnosing pulmonary embolus. (The chest film may be normal early in the course of pulmonary embolism.) Fluoroscopy to check diaphragm movement is often helpful in diagnosing abscesses below the diaphragms.

G.I. barium studies. When a large bowel obstruction is suspected, *barium enema* may localize the area and suggest the cause. In cases of intussusception the barium enema is diagnostic, and often used therapeutically as well.

Upper gastrointestinal barium studies are seldom indicated (or possible) in the "hot" abdomen because of vomiting. They are often helpful in localizing upper gastrointestinal bleeding.

Diagnostic laparotomy. In acute abdominal disease no apologies are required if a precise diagnosis is not made preoperatively. Spreading peritonitis or massive gastrointestinal bleeding are singularly immune to contemplation. The surgeon, reinforced with as much preoperative information as he can safely obtain, must often make the final diagnosis at the operating table.

CHAPTER 21

Intestinal obstruction

RICHARD D. LIECHTY

Intestinal obstruction is defined as an interference in the normal movement of the bowel contents through the intestinal tract. Two main types of obstruction occur: (1) *paralytic ileus,* which arises from a failure of the neuromuscular propulsive action of the bowel wall, and (2) *mechanical obstruction,* which arises from structural lesions (adhesive bands, stones, tumors, etc.) that block the bowel lumen. The distinction between these types is vitally important because mechanical obstruction, if unrelieved, may progress to *strangulation* (shutting off of the blood supply to the obstructed segment) or *perforation.* Both of these complications pose a serious threat to life. Paralytic ileus, on the other hand, rarely threatens life and is treated conservatively with gastrointestinal decompression and correction of the factors causing the bowel wall paralysis.

Simple obstruction, in contrast to *strangulation obstruction,* occurs when the blood supply to the obstructed bowel is adequate. *Vascular obstruction* occurs when an impedance to the arterial flow or venous return sets the stage for bowel infarction. In *partial obstruction* the signs and symptoms of bowel obstruction occur, but some passage of bowel contents continues.

MECHANICAL OBSTRUCTION
Site of mechanical obstruction

The small bowel is about 20 feet in length, and the large bowel is 5 feet in length. This 4:1 ratio parallels the ratio of mechanical obstructions that occur in the small and large bowel; 80% occur in the small bowel, and only 20% involve the large bowel. The student can recall the relative incidence favoring small bowel obstruction by this helpful question: Given a certain amount of traffic, will more accidents occur along a 20 mile two-lane curving highway or along a 5 mile four-lane straighter highway?

Etiology

The "big three" in causation of adult mechanical intestinal obstruction are hernias (incarcerated or strangulated), adhesions, and tumors (Fig. 21-1). Hernias and adhesions together account for about 70% of *all* bowel obstruction. Tumors cause about 15% of all intestinal obstruction, but they are, by far, the most common cause of *large bowel obstruction*. Volvulus, intussusception, inflammatory lesions, vascular obstruction, and obturation (fecal impactions, gallstone ileus) make up the remaining causes of adult intestinal obstruction. Intestinal obstruction in the child, limited primarily to congenital defects and intussusception, is discussed in Chapter 28.

Hernias

The various sites of hernias (including incisions) should be inspected and palpated carefully (Fig. 21-1, *C*). Hernias in obese people are often difficult to detect through thick paddings of fatty tissue. Richter's hernias (a knuckle of bowel in the defect) may be deceptively small. If a hernia becomes tense, tender, and nonreducible, the surgeon must assume that it is strangulated. He should operate immediately, reducing it surgically, with resection of any necrotic bowel.

Adhesions

The incidence of intestinal obstruction caused by adhesions appears to be increasing (Fig. 21-1, *A* and *B*). *Lower abdominal incisions* are more likely to produce adhesive obstructions than *upper abdominal incisions* because the omentum shields the small intestine from the incision in the upper abdomen. About 15% of obstructions caused by adhesions are strangulating. *Closed loop* obstructions, in which a portion of bowel is closed at both ends, threaten perforation from increasing gas pressure (from putrefaction) within the bowel lumen. Early operative release of the obstructing bands can prevent these complications.

Tumors

Neoplasms of the *small bowel* (carcinoma, carcinoid, lymphoma, and benign tumors) are rare causes of obstruction. In contrast, neoplasms cause most obstructions of the colon (Fig. 21-1, *D*) (diverticulitis is next in incidence). Left colon lesions may cause tremendous dilatation of the proximal colon when the ileocecal valve is competent. Because the proximal colon wall is thinned from dilatation and the bowel cannot be prepared preoperatively, decompressive colostomy or cecostomy usually must precede resection of the tumor. In certain cases the obstructing tumor, with bowel and mesentery,

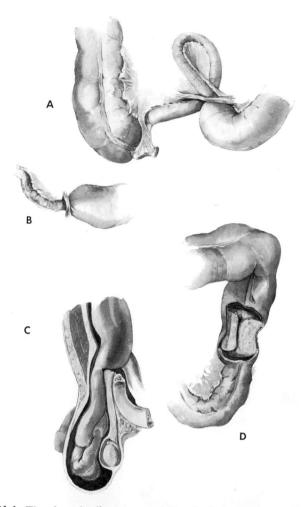

Fig. 21-1. The three leading causes of intestinal obstruction—adhesions, hernias, and tumors. Adhesions causing bowel obstruction. **A,** Fibrous band causing obstruction and volvulus about the band. **B,** Fibrous band obstructing a segment of small bowel. Note proximal dilatation. **C,** Inguinal hernia with loop of obstructed small bowel. Note that obstruction occurs at the internal inguinal ring. **D,** Cancer of the colon causing bowel obstruction.

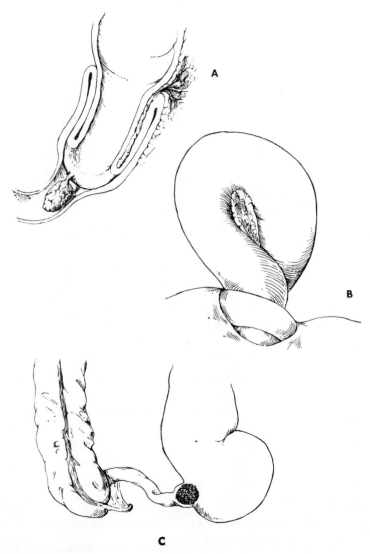

Fig. 21-2. **A,** Polyp of the bowel "leading" an intussusception. **B,** Volvulus of the bowel. **C,** Gallstone ileus. Large gallstone obstructing distal ileum.

can be exteriorized and removed (obstruction resection). (See Chapter 25.)

Other causes of mechanical obstruction
Intussusception

This condition, common in children (Chapter 28), is rare in adults. Polypoid tumors often "lead" the adult intussusception (Fig. 21-2, *A*). Because of these mechanical lesions underlying adult intussusception, we never attempt hydrostatic reduction as in children, but immediately explore and resect the involved bowel.

Volvulus

Volvulus is a twisting of a portion of the gastrointestinal tract on its mesentery. The blood supply is always threatened, if not completely occluded, in this situation (Fig. 21-2, *B*).

Sigmoid volvulus (Fig. 21-3) is the most common type of volvulus because the sigmoid mesentery is long and redundant. In eastern European and some Asian countries sigmoid volvulus is one of the most common causes of bowel obstruction. The high cellulose diet in these areas may be an etiological factor. In western areas sigmoid

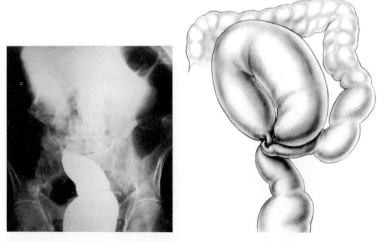

Fig. 21-3. Sigmoid volvulus. Radiograph shows large fluid-filled mass and typical bird-beak deformity outlined by barium in distal sigmoid colon. Diagram shows the twist.

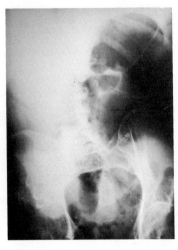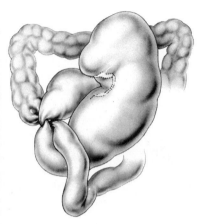

Fig. 21-4. Cecal volvulus. Note dilated, gas-filled cecum in left upper quadrant on radiograph. Diagram shows the twist.

volvulus usually occurs in older, debilitated patients. Barium enema will often outline the twist. Sigmoidoscopy with insertion of a soft rubber rectal tube usually effects decompression amidst a rush of gas and liquid feces. Operative treatment (detorsion or sigmoid resection) is utilized for recurrence, strangulation, or failure of decompression by a rectal tube.

Cecal volvulus (Fig. 21-4) occurs when the cecal mesentery is long, allowing the cecum free movement within the peritoneal cavity. The twisted cecum containing gas usually (and paradoxically) appears in the left upper abdomen on roentgen-ray examination. Barium enema confirms cecal volvulus and differentiates the contained gas from air within the stomach.

Volvulus of the stomach is rare. It is usually associated with paraesophageal hernias. *Small intestinal volvulus* almost invariably results from adhesions. Adhesions pathologically join two portions of the small bowel that form the base of the loop. Volvulus results from a twisting of this loop about the base. *Midgut volvulus,* which occurs almost exclusively in children, involves an abnormality in the embryological rotation and return of the developing intestine (Chapter 28).

Obturation

Obturation results when materials *within* the gut occlude the lumen. *Fecal impaction* and *gallstone ileus* (Fig. 21-2, *C*) are the most common causes of intraluminal obstruction in more advanced countries. Parasitic infections (chiefly *Ascaris lumbricoides,* which may produce a ball of worms) cause intestinal obstruction in less advanced areas. Bezoars of various types are common in patients who are mentally defective.

Inflammatory causes

Tuberculosis, regional enteritis, ulcerative colitis, and amebiasis are the more common causes of intestinal obstruction secondary to inflammation. The diagnosis is usually obscure and depends on biopsy and culture specimens.

Clinical features

Symptoms. Pain, obstipation, distension, and vomiting keynote the patient's symptoms in intestinal obstruction.

Pain is typically crampy and intermittent, resulting from forceful contraction of the bowel wall musculature attempting to push fluid and gas past the obstruction. Continuous pain usually signifies strangulation or perforation. Vomiting temporarily relieves the pain from upper gastrointestinal obstructions as bowel distension is ameliorated. In colon obstruction the crampy pains occur at longer intervals than with small bowel obstruction.

Because intestinal obstruction may be only partial or intermittent, *obstipation* is not absolutely necessary to make the diagnosis of intestinal obstruction. Gas or feces in the bowel segment distal to the obstruction may pass in small amounts, especially in response to enemas. However, complete obstruction usually produces eventual failure to pass either gas or feces.

Distension, to some degree, always accompanies obstruction. In high (proximal small bowel) obstruction distension is minimal. In lower obstructions distension is massive because of the greater amount of bowel that is filled with gas and liquid.

In high obstruction *vomiting* occurs as an early symptom because the upper small bowel receives bile and pancreatic and gastric juice (in addition to its own secretions) and is poorly absorptive. In obstructing lesions of the low ileum or colon, *feculent vomiting* results from stagnation and bacterial putrefaction and strongly suggests the low site of obstruction. In obstruction of the colon with a competent ileocecal valve, vomiting seldom occurs as a "backup" phenomenon, but it does result on a reflex basis.

Laboratory diagnosis

Roentgen-ray examination. Plain films of the abdomen taken with the patient in the upright (or decubitus) and supine positions are the most important aids in diagnosing intestinal obstruction. Small intestinal gas and fluid levels in the adult patient invariably indicate mechanical intestinal obstruction (Fig. 21-5). This pattern usually appears within 12 hours of the onset of symptoms. Air and fluid levels throughout both large and small bowel indicate adynamic (paralytic) ileus.

Plain films of the abdomen may also show free air in the peritoneal cavity (from perforation of a hollow viscus), calculi in the biliary or renal areas, fecaliths, tumors, or radiopaque foreign bodies. Barium enemas help to localize the area of colon obstruction. In suspected cases of obstruction, radiologists use oral barium cautiously because of the threat of inspissation of the barium above the obstruction.

Blood studies. Elevations in the hemoglobin and hematocrit commonly indicate dehydration and hemoconcentration. The white blood count is usually elevated, with a shift to the left, especially with strangulation obstruction.

Urinalysis. A high specific gravity and ketonuria indicate a common complication of intestinal obstruction: dehydration and metabolic

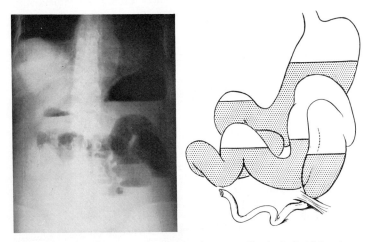

Fig. 21-5. Mechanical bowel obstruction. Localized air-fluid levels seen on upright film of abdomen. Diagram shows dilated proximal bowel and stomach, air-fluid levels, and adhesive band causing the obstruction.

acidosis. Adynamic ileus may be caused by *diabetic acidosis* or *primary renal disease.* Glycosuria or proteinuria (with abnormal cellular elements in the urine) should always suggest the possibility of these diseases.

Blood chemistry. Amylase may be slightly elevated in intestinal obstruction. Usually, electrolyte determinations guide preoperative fluid replacement. (See Chapter 3.)

PARALYTIC ILEUS (ADYNAMIC ILEUS, NEUROGENIC ILEUS)

In evolutionary terms *paralytic ileus* is a protective mechanism that "splints" the gastrointestinal tract after abdominal injury. It prevents the muscular contractions of the gastrointestinal tract from continuously pouring out noxious bowel contents into the peritoneal cavity after a hollow viscus is perforated, thus allowing the perforation to seal.

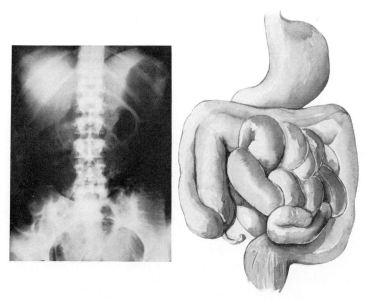

Fig. 21-6. Paralytic ileus. Upright film of abdomen shows dilated small and large intestine. Gas is scattered diffusely throughout intestinal tract. Diagram shows the diffuse intestinal dilatation.

Etiology

Four general causative mechanisms for paralytic ileus are:

1. *Direct peritoneal irritation* from any source: acute cholecystitis, pancreatitis, appendicitis, perforation of a hollow viscus, or any abdominal operation; this is the commonest cause.

2. *Extraperitoneal irritation* such as: pneumonitis, hemorrhage, fractured ribs or spine, trauma to retroperitoneal nerves, renal lesions.

3. *Systemic imbalances:* infections, electrolyte imbalance, shock, myxedema, Addison's disease, uremia, diabetes, or porphyria.

4. *Neurogenic disorders:* spinal cord lesions, severe strokes, or CNS trauma.

Bowel sounds are absent, and gas appears scattered throughout the gastrointestinal tract (Fig. 21-6). Nasogastric suction, correction of the mechanisms causing the paralytic ileus, and parenteral fluid replacement keynote the treatment.

DIFFERENTIAL DIAGNOSIS
Simple versus strangulation obstruction

Since strangulation obstruction requires immediate operative treatment, the physician must constantly look for these five diagnostic points: (1) when intermittent, colicky pain becomes steady and unrelenting, (2) when abdominal tenderness (and rebound) become evident, (3) when a mass becomes palpable, (4) when the temperature and pulse increase, and (5) when laboratory studies suggest acute inflammation. In brief, the warm abdomen changes dramatically to the hot abdomen when strangulation of the bowel occurs. Diagnostic laparotomy is a certain method for determining strangulation obstruction in the difficult diagnostic case.

Mechanical obstruction versus paralytic ileus

In *paralytic ileus* an obvious cause of the ileus is usually evident, such as acute peritonitis from appendicitis, pancreatitis, cholecystitis, gastroenteritis, abdominal surgery, pneumonitis, or trauma (Figs. 21-5 and 21-6). The abdomen is silent. When the cause of the ileus is not associated with peritonitis, the abdomen is painless and nontender. The radiograph of paralytic ileus shows gas distributed evenly throughout the large and small bowel (Fig. 21-6). Radiographs of the abdomen are not infallible, however. Because any condition that causes peritonitis also causes some degree of paralytic ileus, these hot abdominal disorders mimic strangulation obstruction. The abdominal roentgen-ray films are usually the only objective method, other than a diagnostic laparotomy, for differentiating paralytic ileus (secondary to peritonitis) from strangulation obstruction (Table 21-1).

Table 21-1. Comparison of paralytic ileus and mechanical obstruction

	Paralytic ileus	*Mechanical obstruction*
Cause	Peritoneal irritation Extraperitoneal irritation Neurogenic disorders Metabolic disorders	Hernia Adhesions Tumors Volvulus Intussusception Obturation Inflammation
Site	Entire bowel is dilated	Dilatation proximal to obstruction
Clinical	Distension, vomiting, obstipation Silent abdomen Abdomen may or may not be tender	Crampy pain, distension, vomiting, obstipation, hyperactive bowel sounds at first; later bowel may be silent
Roentgen ray	Gas throughout bowel (Fig. 21-6)	Gas and fluid proximal to obstruction No gas distal to obstruction (Fig. 21-5)
Treatment	Conservative with treatment of the cause of the ileus	Operative release or bypass of the obstruction
Prognosis	Usually good after correction of cause Strangulation and perforation are *not* a threat	Strangulation or perforation constant threat until obstruction relieved

Small versus large bowel obstruction

Differentiating colon from small bowel obstruction depends on radiographic evidence, either plain abdominal radiographs or barium enema demonstration of an obstructing lesion of the colon. Differentiation is important so that the patient (and his family) can be prepared for a colostomy, if it is necessary. Clinical localization, although less accurate, is also possible. Obstruction in an older patient, with no hernia or history of previous abdominal operations, and with distension and no vomiting, suggests a carcinoma of the large bowel. Sharp frequent abdominal cramps, severe vomiting, and early fluid and electrolyte imbalance suggest small bowel obstruction.

PATHOPHYSIOLOGY

Simple intestinal obstruction causes death, if untreated, because of two factors: (1) *distension* of the bowel proximal to the obstruction and (2) *dehydration*.

Distention of the proximal bowel constantly threatens ischemia of the involved bowel wall. Violent contractions of the proximal bowel wall attempting to force bowel contents past the obstruction ultimately cause edema of the bowel wall. An edematous bowel wall loses some of its absorptive capacity while secretions (and edema fluid) increase. Anxiety, pain, and nausea cause increased aerophagia (air is mostly nitrogen, which is poorly absorbed). Thus, intraluminal pressure (both gas and fluid) builds up to the point where it compresses the small vessels in the bowel wall, and eventually it exceeds the capillary perfusion pressure. Consequent ischemia causes further edema and eventuates in bowel wall necrosis, perforation, and peritonitis. As this final phase approaches, the edematous, stretched, and thinned bowel wall loses its power to contract. The patient no longer complains of cramping pains, and the abdomen is forebodingly silent. Thus, every case of "simple" obstruction will ultimately become "self-strangulating" obstruction if proximal bowel distension is not relieved.

Dehydration occurs rapidly because oral intake is impossible and water and electrolytes are lost by (1) vomiting, (2) increased net secretions from the gastrointestinal tract (because the reabsorptive power of the mucosa is impaired), and (3) edema of the bowel wall with transudation into the peritoneal cavity.

As strangulation approaches, bacteria and their toxins escape into the peritoneal cavity, causing edema of the parietal peritoneum, venous thrombosis with more anoxia, and eventually endotoxic shock. When strangulation precipitates the bacterial phase of intestinal obstruction, all the lethal effects of diffuse peritonitis are suddenly superimposed on an already critically ill patient. The mortality is understandably high.

TREATMENT OF MECHANICAL BOWEL OBSTRUCTION

The treatment of bowel obstruction is keyed to the pathophysiological developments, but *in reverse order*. *Dehydration* and *proximal bowel distension* initiated by the obstruction must be treated first, and the *obstruction* is relieved subsequently.

Dehydration

Severe dehydration poses the serious threat of hypovolemia and shock; this threat is heightened by the vasodilator effect of anesthetics, which causes further decrease in circulating blood volume. Thus, replacement of these abnormal fluid losses is a vital first step in the treatment of bowel obstruction. In estimating the amount of replacement fluids, the physician must realize that obstructed patients lose fluids from (1) increased net secretion into the bowel lumen, (2) transudation, (3) edema (bowel wall, mesentery), and (4) vomiting. When signs of shock appear in advanced stages of bowel obstruction in the adult, the patient has lost at least 5 or 6 *liters* of fluid.

Proximal bowel distension

Intestinal intubation with suction to remove gas and fluid accumulation keynotes the treatment of bowel distension. Surgeons use nasogastric tubes, long intestinal tubes, or tubes inserted directly (at laparotomy) to decompress the distended gastrointestinal tract.

Nasogastric versus long-tube decompression

In proximal small bowel obstruction nasogastric suction is adequate to relieve intestinal distension. In lower obstructions many surgeons cite the advantage of the long intestinal tube in more completely decompressing the dilated loops of bowel, thus decreasing pressure on the stretched and edematous bowel wall. Subsequent operative correction of the obstruction is aided by the flattened, decompressed small bowel. Several long and trying hours may be required to pass a long tube into the lower small bowel; thus other surgeons favor nasogastric intubation with immediate operative decompression and removal of the obstruction.

Intestinal intubation as definitive treatment

In a minority of instances long-tube decompression may relieve intestinal obstructions completely (usually those caused by adhesions). This treatment requires several days of suction and intravenous feedings (and immobility) to be certain that the obstruction is relieved. During this treatment the threat of recurrent obstruction constantly plagues both surgeon and patient alike. Because of the hardship and uncertainty of this treatment, most surgeons lack enthusiasm for the conservative treatment of mechanical bowel obstruction.

Removal of the obstruction—operative treatment

The final goal in treating mechanical bowel obstruction is removal of the obstruction. Strangulating or potentially strangulating lesions (hernia, volvulus, intussusception in older patients, and complete obstruction because of adhesions or closed-loop obstructions) demand emergent operative treatment. With partial or early obstructions, the surgeon has valuable time for diagnostic studies.

SMALL BOWEL OBSTRUCTIONS

Since most small bowel obstructions are extrinsic, the surgeon can easily lyse adhesions or reduce hernias. If the small bowel is necrotic, he can safely resect it since the small bowel is relatively sterile. By-pass operations (enteroenterostomies or enterocolostomies) are useful in complicated situations such as multiple dense adhesions in critically ill patients. To prevent recurrent obstructions, some surgeons pass a long tube with an inflatable balloon (Baker tube) into the proximal jejunum and manipulate it to the cecum. It serves as an internal stent to allow adhesion to form without sharp kinking of the small bowel.

LARGE BOWEL OBSTRUCTIONS—CAUSE AND TYPE

The vast majority of large bowel obstructions (in contrast to those of the small bowel) are caused by intrinsic lesions (cancer or diverticulitis). Most obstructions of the colon occur in the sigmoid area because (1) this is the most common site for both cancers and diverticulitis, and (2) the sigmoid lumen is smaller and the feces are more solid than in the more proximal colon.

Closed loop obstructions

Because the ileocecal valve is competent in about 50 to 60% of all people, *closed loop* bowel obstructions occur in a similar percentage of all large bowel obstructions. Radiographs of the abdomen show gross dilatation of the colon between the one-way cecal valve and the obstructing lesion. Immediate operative decompression keynotes the treatment. Foolish reliance upon long-tube decompression of the small bowel may cause a deadly delay. Mounting gas pressure from putrefaction within the closed loop will eventually burst through the thinned bowel wall (usually the cecum), contaminating the peritoneal cavity with toxic bowel contents.

Incompetent ileocecal valve obstruction

When the ileocecal valve permits regurgitation, the distal obstruction differs very little clinically from a low small bowel obstruction. Barium study of the distal colon will usually detect the colonic site of obstruction.

Large bowel decompression

Because the large bowel teems with bacteria and the weakened colonic wall holds sutures poorly, primary anastomosis is always hazardous (Chapter 25). (Infection jeopardizes any anastomosis.) Proximal colostomy is a safe and simple procedure, decompressing the bowel and totally bypassing gas and feces through the abdominal wall. Cecostomy differs from colostomy in providing only a vent through the abdominal wall; it does not provide a bypass for *all* the cecal contents.

In certain cases when sufficient mesentery provides adequate mobility, the colon lesions may be *exteriorized* and removed (obstructive resection). The proximal and distal portions of the colon remain above the skin and may be subsequently reunited.

VASCULAR OBSTRUCTION

Vascular obstruction is the reverse, pathologically, of *strangulation obstruction; primary* blood vessel blockage precedes and causes bowel obstruction. (See Chapter 24.)

The final clinical picture is identical to strangulation obstruction. The early stages of vascular obstruction feature extreme abdominal pain that comes on abruptly (with crescendos) before becoming steady, and vomiting and diarrhea. Many patients, perhaps one-third, give a prior history of crampy pains following meals.

The diagnosis of vascular obstruction is difficult especially in older patients, in whom it occurs frequently. The onset may be deceptively subtle with minimal symptoms. In younger patients the onset is frequently sudden and confusing. A thorough knowledge of the patient and of the possible antecedent causative factors gives the physician the best opportunity to make this diagnosis.

Etiology

Embolism (cardiac or arteriosclerotic), *increased venous pressure* (abdominal tumor, cirrhosis, congestive heart failure), *hypercoagulability* (polycythemia, some cancers), or *vascular diseases* (collagen diseases, vasospastic diseases, prolonged infections, or trauma) should be considered in the differential diagnosis. Arteriograms will often pinpoint the obstructed artery. Immediate operation, with embolectomy when possible, and bowel resection (often massive) are the only therapeutic options. In older patients the mortality is extremely high.

CHAPTER 22

Gastrointestinal hemorrhage

ROBERT J. CORRY
ROBERT T. SOPER

Massive hemorrhage from the gastrointestinal tract continues to represent a major diagnostic and therapeutic challenge, enlisting the cooperative efforts of surgeon, endoscopist, and radiologist. Bleeding that is either small in volume or occurs abruptly and then stops, although not life-threatening in itself, may be the harbinger of more serious gastrointestinal tract disease such as cancer. Although massive bleeding is more common from the upper gastrointestinal tract, its management is sometimes even more challenging when it occurs from a colonic source.

Regardless of the cause, location, or rate of gastrointestinal hemorrhage, the patient must be approached in a logical, step-wise manner, the immediate goal being to stop the bleeding and the ultimate goal to eliminate its cause. For the patient with a massive hemorrhage, the first priority is to prevent exsanguination. Precise diagnosis and definitive management remain important but are less urgent considerations.

Three fundamental evaluations are required for each patient with gastrointestinal hemorrhage: (1) the volume and rate of blood loss, (2) the location and specific lesion producing the bleeding, and (3) the general condition of the patient.

The *volume and rate of blood loss* must be determined with a fair amount of accuracy since therapy will have to be instituted immediately in the patient with massive bleeding. The triad of hematemesis, hematochezia, and hypovolemia indicate massive gastrointestinal bleeding and require urgent treatment, as discussed later in this chapter. Signs and symptoms of hypovolemia including weakness, pallor, sweat-

314

ing, dizziness, tachycardia, and extreme thirst signify massive bleeding. A nasogastric tube should be immediately passed so that the rate of continuing blood loss can be measured. If the rate of bleeding slows as measured by vital signs, hematocrit determinations, the number and character of stools, and the volume of nasogastric aspirate, a more elaborate diagnostic work-up can be instituted. In patients with slow gastrointestinal bleeding, serial hematocrit determinations are probably the most reliable measurement of the rate of blood loss.

The *location* and the *specific lesion* producing the bleeding should be ascertained as soon as possible in the patient with massive hemorrhage. Most patients with brisk upper gastrointestinal bleeding have hematemesis and thus the differential diagnosis between lower and upper gastrointestinal bleeding is made by history. When hematemesis has not occurred in the presence of massive hematochezia, aspiration of bile from the stomach usually indicates a source of bleeding below the ligament of Treitz. As discussed in detail later, endoscopy or angiography is usually necessary to determine the precise source of hemorrhage preoperatively.

The *general condition of the patient* should be assessed as quickly as possible, because the so-called poor-risk patient will require a more precise diagnostic and therapeutic approach than the good-risk patient without cardiovascular disease or diseases of other systems.

For the purpose of clarity this chapter will deal first with upper and second with lower gastrointestinal bleeding and will emphasize general principles, rather than attempting to either deal thoroughly with the basic disease processes or outline a complex formula to manage gastrointestinal hemorrhage.

UPPER GASTROINTESTINAL HEMORRHAGE

Massive upper gastrointestinal hemorrhage produces signs of acute hypovolemia following closely on the heels of both hematemesis and hematochezia. For all practical purposes, this type of bleeding is equally distributed among peptic ulceration, gastritis, and ruptured esophageal varices, with the bleeding ulcer being slightly more common than the other two.

Unusual causes of massive upper gastrointestinal hemorrhage are worthy of brief mention so that they will not be forgotten in the haste of the moment. *Oronasopharyngeal bleeding* may be suspected if the patient appears to be swallowing blood; bleeding can be quite massive, but usually stops with direct tamponade. *Hematobilia* can be diagnosed only by angiography or choledochotomy, but should be suspected when there are symptoms and signs of hepatobiliary disease. Bleeding as a complication of a *cholecystoduodenal fistula* is an unusual entity usually diagnosed at laparotomy. The *Mallory-Weiss syndrome* is most commonly diagnosed at gastroesophagoscopy. *Bleeding disorders* should be considered in all cases and an accurate history, inspection for cutaneous bleeding, and laboratory bleeding studies should be carried out. (See Chapter 4.)

General considerations of diagnosis and management

Massive blood loss from peptic ulcer eroding into the left gastric or gastroduodenal artery, hemorrhage from gastritis, or a ruptured esophageal varix can all result in hypovolemic shock. Usually a history of ulcer pain or previous bleeding from an ulcer can be elicited from the patient or his family, which enables the physician to place high priority on peptic ulcer as a source of hemorrhage. However, a patient may bleed from an acute duodenal ulcer without a previous history.

Similarly, a history of cirrhosis, chronic alcoholism or remote hepatitis alerts the physician to consider bleeding esophageal varices, particularly if physical signs point to evidence of hepatic dysfunction such as caput medusae, jaundice, spider angiomata, ascites, etc. It must be emphasized, however, that the patient with liver disease is also prone to develop gastritis.

The patient who has been generally well but who has had a recent history of ingesting alcohol, aspirin, or Indomethacin may have hemorrhagic gastritis. Physical examination usually does not help differentiate duodenal ulcer from gastritis.

The first priority in the patient with massive upper gastrointestinal hemorrhage is intravenous insertion of two 15-gauge needles or plastic cannulas for rapid transfusion of volume expanders followed by blood. A No. 36 F Ewald tube is then passed into the stomach for gastric lavage with iced saline. Occasionally, the bleeding will stop with vigorous lavage and evacuation of stomach blood clots.

The most important diagnostic maneuver in the patient with massive upper gastrointestinal bleeding is endoscopy, preferably with a flexible fiberoptic esophagogastroscope. If the bleeding continues during endoscopy, its source, location, and magnitude may be determined simultaneously.

Once diagnosis is established, definitive therapy is instituted, as shown schematically in Fig. 22-1. It is unusual for hemorrhage from the gastroduodenal or left gastric artery to stop with iced saline lavage; in that situation, the patient should be taken directly to the operating room for surgical control of the bleeding. On the contrary, bleeding from minor or small vessels often justifies a period of intensive iced saline lavage. If the bleeding stops as a result of this

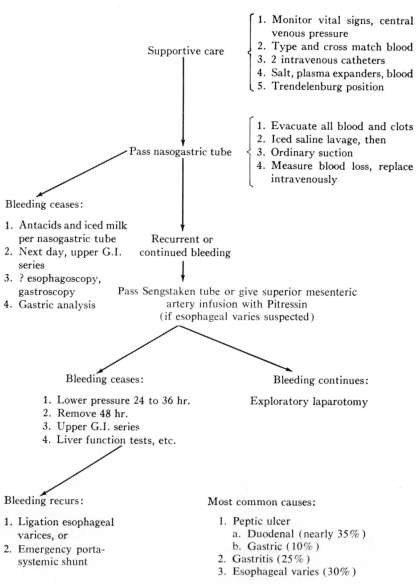

Supportive care
1. Monitor vital signs, central venous pressure
2. Type and cross match blood
3. 2 intravenous catheters
4. Salt, plasma expanders, blood
5. Trendelenburg position

Pass nasogastric tube
1. Evacuate all blood and clots
2. Iced saline lavage, then
3. Ordinary suction
4. Measure blood loss, replace intravenously

Bleeding ceases:
1. Antacids and iced milk per nasogastric tube
2. Next day, upper G.I. series
3. ? esophagoscopy, gastroscopy
4. Gastric analysis

Recurrent or continued bleeding

Pass Sengstaken tube or give superior mesenteric artery infusion with Pitressin (if esophageal varies suspected)

Bleeding ceases:
1. Lower pressure 24 to 36 hr.
2. Remove 48 hr.
3. Upper G.I. series
4. Liver function tests, etc.

Bleeding continues:

Exploratory laparotomy

Bleeding recurs:
1. Ligation esophageal varices, or
2. Emergency porta-systemic shunt

Most common causes:
1. Peptic ulcer
   a. Duodenal (nearly 35%)
   b. Gastric (10%)
2. Gastritis (25%)
3. Esophageal varies (30%)

Fig. 22-1. Management of massive upper gastrointestinal hemorrhage.

maneuver, gastric suction for 24 to 48 hours with a No. 18 Levin tube should be followed by institution of hourly milk and antacid therapy.

Angiography

Although the flexible fiberoptic esophagogastroscope has substantially increased the diagnostic accuracy of bleeding lesions of the esophagus, stomach, and duodenum, angiography has added yet new dimensions to both diagnosis and therapy. Commonly the endoscopist is uncertain of the diagnosis, mostly because of inadequate evacuation of stomach blood clots or persistent hemorrhage that floods the field. If bleeding persists and the definitive diagnosis is not made, or if the diagnosis is made and the patient is a poor operative risk, emergency angiography should be carried out. Angiography is not only a diagnostic maneuver but is therapeutic. The skilled angiographer can selectively cannulate the left gastric artery, infuse Pitressin, and frequently stop the bleeding of hemorrhagic gastritis; he can cannulate the gastroduodenal artery and either infuse preformed blood clot or Pitressin to stop duodenal ulcer bleeding, and he can cannulate the superior mesenteric artery and infuse Pitressin to lower portal pressure and stop variceal bleeding. When the bleeding is at a rate of 30 ml. per hour, angiography will frequently show bleeding from shallow lesions not easily seen endoscopically.

Peptic ulceration

When hemorrhage occurs from a peptic ulcer, whether the source is in the stomach or the duodenum, the immediate aim is to control the bleeding. The diagnosis can usually be made by history unless bleeding is occurring for the first time as the presenting symptom of an acute stress ulcer. Physical examination and laboratory studies are usually of little help.

If the bleeding stops as a result of gastric lavage or if bleeding has stopped prior to admission to the hospital such that a nasogastric tube aspirate yields only old or changed blood, gastroscopy may be deferred and angiography will not be helpful. The patient should be managed with gastric suction to reduce gastric acidity and decompress the stomach. An upper gastrointestinal contrast radiographic study may be safely performed if bleeding has not recurred for 12 hours. If bleeding recurs, then endoscopy and angiography should be carried out to identify the precise source of bleeding.

Once the diagnosis of peptic ulcer is made by any of the above measures, it is treated either medically or operatively depending on the previous history of bleeding, pain, and chronicity. A second episode of bleeding while in hospital on intensive medical therapy usually justifies an operation. The choice of operation, discussed in Chapter 23, is designed to reduce gastric acidity and prevent recurrence of peptic ulcer disease.

Esophageal varices

The diagnosis of bleeding from a ruptured varix is suggested in the patient with upper gastrointestinal hemorrhage who has a history of chronic alcoholism and/or chronic liver disease. Frequently the patient presents in a precomatose state and physical examination reveals mild jaundice, ascites, and muscle wasting. Definitive diagnosis of variceal hemorrhage is made by esophagoscopy. A barium swallow that will outline the extent of the varices is more useful when the patient is not bleeding (Fig. 22-2). Occasionally patients with portal hyper-

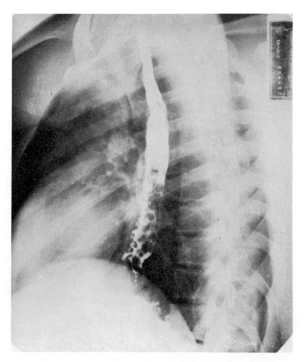

Fig. 22-2. Barium in esophagus outlining large esophageal varices.

tension bleed from hemorrhagic gastritis rather than from varices, although its frequency is probably exaggerated; endoscopy and angiography may help make this decision.

Emergency management of the patient with bleeding varices is directed toward stopping the hemorrhage as soon as possible. In addition to the deleterious effects of blood loss and shock common to all patients with upper gastrointestinal bleeding, hepatic coma is a superadded complication that is unique to patients who bleed with com-

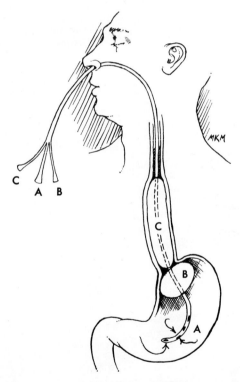

Fig. 22-3. Sengstaken-Blakemore tube. Triple-lumen tube: **A,** gastric suction; **B,** balloon in gastric fundus; **C,** balloon in lower esophagus. The tube is passed into the stomach, inflated gastric balloon is snugged up to the esophageal junction, and the esophageal balloon is then inflated to compress the varices.

promised hepatic function. Immediate efforts are made to rid the gastrointestinal tract of blood by vigorous catharsis and to eradicate intestinal bacterial flora coincident with attempts to control the hemorrhage.

The therapy for bleeding esophageal varices is controversial. If the bleeding is massive and does not stop by the usual measures of gastric lavage, balloon tamponade usually controls the acute hemorrhage (see Fig. 22-3 and Chapter 17).

The high morbidity and complication rate associated with balloon tamponade has led to the increased use of pharmacological control of hemorrhage from varices. Some centers report good success with selective infusion of vasopressin into the superior mesenteric artery, reducing portal venous pressure by reducing splanchnic arterial inflow and portal venous drainage. In addition to acting as a pressor, the drug stimulates intestinal peristalsis to help empty the gut of blood, thereby further limiting ammonia production and consequent encephalopathy.

If the bleeding stops by one of these emergency measures, an intermediate-risk patient can be converted over a period of a few weeks to a good-risk patient for definitive surgical therapy. If the bleeding does not stop, either ligation of the varices or emergency portasystemic shunt must be carried out. Both of these operations have a mortality rate approaching 50% in the patient with poor liver function (hypoalbuminemia, jaundice, ascites, and incipient coma). If the liver function is good and the patient has little ascites he will tolerate a direct portacaval shunt. Splenorenal and mesocaval shunts result in less postoperative hepatic encephalopathy than a direct portacaval shunt, but are poor operations when done at the time of bleeding since they produce less decompression of the splanchnic venous system. All the shunt procedures are better performed at a time of election after intensive medical management has improved the patient's liver function and nutritional status.

Gastritis

Until recently, massive hemorrhage from gastritis has represented somewhat of a surgical dilemma. The history is frequently helpful in diagnosis, the patient commonly having ingested aspirin, Indomethacin, or alcohol. Gastroscopy confirms diagnosis, but rarely shows the bleeding to be localized enough for a modest gastric resection to encompass. More commonly, hemorrhagic gastritis is diffuse and operative management demands a high subtotal resection with vagotomy to control bleeding that does not spontaneously cease.

Recently, selective cannulation of the left gastric artery with infusion of Pitressin has been reported to stop hemorrhage from acute gastritis with gratifying regularity. Continuous infusion of Pitressin for 24 and even 48 hours allows healing of the superficial erosions and temporary cure. When the gastritis has a specific cause that can be eliminated or avoided in the future, operative intervention is obviated.

Other causes of upper gastrointestinal hemorrhage

Aberrant blood vessels, tumors undergoing necrosis, aorticoduodenal fistulas, and lesions of the small intestine including vascular malformations and Meckel's diverticulum are managed with ad hoc operations applicable to the particular lesion. Recurrent slow bleeding from chronic peptic ulcer disease is usually diagnosed by contrast studies of the upper gastrointestinal tract and is managed by the operation appropriate to the disease entity.

LOWER GASTROINTESTINAL BLEEDING

Rarely, colonic bleeding is massive and life-threatening, but more commonly it is slow and intermixed with stool. Persistence of chronic rectal bleeding warrants an immediate and thorough investigative work-up to establish its cause. In this situation the bleeding is not the problem, but its cause can be serious and life-threatening.

Massive colonic bleeding

It must be emphasized at the outset that an upper gastrointestinal source of bleeding should be eliminated as a possibility in the patient who presents with massive rectal bleeding. Aspiration of clear bile from the stomach for all practical purposes establishes the source of bleeding as being located at least below the ligament of Treitz.

As with upper gastrointestinal bleeding, plasma expanders followed by blood transfusions should be instituted immediately while diagnostic measures are undertaken. Anoscopy and sigmoidoscopy with adequate facilities to aspirate blood should be undertaken as soon as possible. If the bleeding arises above the end of the sigmoidoscope and is persistent and massive, selective arteriography should be immediately carried out. Inferior mesenteric artery followed by superior mesenteric artery injection of contrast material frequently identifies the source of bleeding. When the bleeding point is identified and is localized to either the left or the right colon, continuous intra-arterial infusion of Pitressin is begun. Some centers are reporting success with this procedure and consequent laparotomy with colon resection is avoided. If bleeding is not controlled or if it recurs, resection of the appropriate segment of bowel is carried out.

Prior to the development of skilled angiographic techniques, surgical management of massive lower gastrointestinal bleeding was far less than optimal. Emergency barium enema might reveal diverticulosis, but would not indicate which one of the numerous diverticula was bleeding. At laparotomy it was frequently necessary to apply clamps to segments of the colon to see which segment filled with blood; experience with this method has been dismal. Colotomies and endoscopic examination of the colon at laparotomy have the disadvantage of spilling feculent material within the peritoneal cavity and are frequently not definitive. Usually, subtotal colectomy with ileorectal anastomosis was performed when extensive diverticulosis was found. With localized sigmoid diverticulosis, a sigmoid resection was carried out with relatively good results. Occasionally, rare causes of bleeding (superficial erosions of the cecum) were frequently overlooked if they were not suspected preoperatively.

Although diverticula of the colon are the most common cause of massive lower gastrointestinal bleeding, numerous other conditions can produce brisk rectal bleeding such as *internal hemorrhoids,* an ulcerating *colonic neoplasm, ischemia* of a segment of colon, *ulcerative colitis,* and in rare instances *superficial erosions* of the colonic mucosa.

History is not usually as helpful as it is in upper gastrointestinal bleeding, and the physical examination is equally unrevealing. Although it is said that diverticulitis does not bleed, we have noted on at least four occasions massive hemorrhage coincident with acute diverticulitis in which the patients presented with severe left lower quadrant tenderness, localized peritoneal irritation, fever, and massive rectal bleeding.

Chronic lower gastrointestinal bleeding

Slow and recurrent or persistent colonic bleeding is suggested by history of blood passed per rectum in a patient with chronic anemia. Bright red rectal blood indicates a point of origin within the anus or rectum, especially when it coats the outside of stool. Anal fissures, hemorrhoids, and low-lying carcinomas are the most likely sources of this type of slow rectal bleeding. Tarry-appearing material or dark blood intermixed with stool suggests a right colonic or small bowel origin. Bloody diarrhea mixed with mucus suggests *ulcerative colitis, granulomatous enterocolitis,* or *amebic colitis.* The diagnostic work-up is performed with dispatch but not as an emergency. Careful rectal examination, anoscopy, and sigmoidoscopy should be carried out when the patient is first seen. These procedures will confirm the diagnosis of numerous conditions including hemorrhoids, fissures, ulcerative colitis, and about three-fifths of the colonic neoplasms. The next diagnostic maneuver should be a barium enema, usually with air contrast.

This procedure will confirm the diagnosis of colonic diverticulosis, neoplasms above the reach of the sigmoidoscope, chronic ulcerative colitis, and colonic polyps.

If these procedures fail to reveal the diagnosis of the bleeding, colonoscopy should be carried out. In the hands of an experienced operator, diagnostic colonoscopy carries little morbidity. Furthermore, transcolonoscopic removal of polyps may make obsolete the endless debate about the neoplastic state of polyps.

CHAPTER 23

The stomach and duodenum

RICHARD D. LIECHTY

Three diseases of the stomach and duodenum completely over-shadow all other diseases that involve these important digestive or-gans: *peptic ulcer, gastric cancer,* and *hypertrophic pyloric stenosis.* The main concerns of this chapter are peptic ulcer and gastric cancer. Hypertrophic pyloric stenosis is discussed in Chapter 28. The less com-mon diseases of the stomach and duodenum are mentioned at the end of this chapter.

PEPTIC ULCER

Peptic ulcer by definition is any gastrointestinal ulcer caused by contact with acid-pepsin secretions. Without question the most com-mon disease of the stomach and duodenum, peptic ulcer afflicts only *Homo sapiens.* It occurs in males more often than in females and in all age groups, and it virtually limits itself to civilized societies. About 10 to 20% of all Americans will suffer from peptic ulcers sometime dur-ing their lifetime, and some 40,000 of these sufferers miss work each day because of their distress. Peptic ulcers, as the name suggests, re-quire acid and pepsin to form. Patients with pernicious anemia (total anacidity) never get peptic ulcers. Although acid-pepsin secretions link together the three main types of peptic ulcers, important differ-ences separate them. The student should envision these three main classifications as follows:

1. Duodenal ulcer diathesis (duodenal, pyloric channel, and syn-chronous gastric and duodenal ulcers)
2. Gastric ulcer
3. Acute gastric mucosal ulcerations

Gastric physiology

Vagal-antral phase

A combined vagal-antral phase increases gastric secretion as follows. Stimuli from the brain (hunger, smell of food) travel along the vagus nerves to (1) incite the gastric parietal cells to secrete acid and pepsin, and (2) stimulate the antral cells to release gastrin, a secretory hormone that also stimulates the parietal cells. Thus, nervous stimuli trigger a dual mechanism that heightens gastric secretion. Distension of the antrum (by food) also stimulates these vagal responses. Various secretogogues (peptones and amino acids from food) directly stimulate antral gastrin release that further augments gastric secretion. These overlapping mechanisms of gastric secretion potentiate one another.

Intestinal phase

The acid contents of the stomach, as they flow into the duodenum, trigger release of a hormone (secretin) that inhibits both gastric secretion and motility. Acid, fat, and hypertonic solutions, as they enter the duodenum, all have the ability to suppress gastric secretion (possibly by release of enterogastrone). In addition, antral acidity in the empty stomach slows gastric activity. Thus in normal people a remarkable mechanism stimulates gastric secretion during hunger and food intake and shuts it off as the food leaves the stomach.

The mucosal barrier

The answer to the question: "Why doesn't the corrosive gastric content digest the stomach wall?" rests on the concept of a gastric mucosal barrier; a secreting, dynamic "containing wall" capable of maintaining an H^+ gradient (stomach to blood) of about 2,000,000:1.

This wall features a layer of mucus acting chiefly as a lubricant and weak buffer, and most important, a layer of highly specialized columnar cells, tightly joined, that prevent back diffusion of acid. A rich blood supply supports both of these layers and allows the mucosal cells to replace themselves within 48 hours, if injured. Much current research has centered on this mucosal layer and its blood supply. From these studies new theories have emerged to explain how gastric ulcers arise in tandem with low gastric acids and why acute gastric mucosal ulcers accompany shock and stress.

Duodenal ulcer

Cause. Excess gastric secretion and hypergastrinemia keynote the pathogenesis of duodenal ulcer. Some researchers believe that defective absorption of acid from the duodenum may play a minor role in inciting duodenal ulcers, but at present this theory lacks clinical verification.

Most experienced clinicians accept psychological factors as the most common link in the genesis of duodenal ulcers. Chronic psychic stress (e.g., the hard driving, ambitious person) undoubtedly augments gastric secretion through brain centers and the vagus nerves. Duodenal ulcer traits run through families, especially those members sharing blood group O. Several investigators have shown an increased parietal cell mass (perhaps inherited) in patients with this disease. The role of diet (e.g., coffee drinking) remains debatable, but excess alcoholic intake definitely increases gastric secretion and the incidence of duodenal ulcers. For unknown reasons, patients with pulmonary emphysema suffer a threefold increase in duodenal ulcers but cirrhotic patients, contrary to previous opinion, show no special tendency for duodenal ulcers.

Clinical examination. The classic symptoms of duodenal ulcer are a gnawing pain in the upper abdomen an hour or two after meals (sometimes described as heartburn), radiating occasionally to the back and relieved by food. Acute episodes are often seen, for unex-

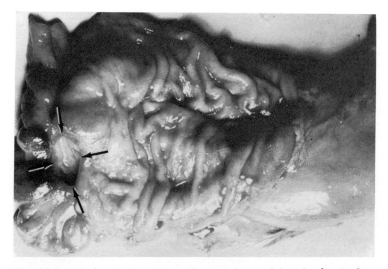

Fig. 23-1. Duodenal ulcer. Opened stomach on right; duodenal ulcer with sharply demarcated edges on left.

plainable reasons, in spring and fall. Some patients complain only of vague discomfort—a feeling of hunger or cramps. Pain that awakens patients from sleep, that eases with milk or other buffers, or that radiates to the back is likely to be ulcer pain. An occasional patient will bleed severely yet deny any prior pain. The only common physical finding is mild tenderness in the right upper abdomen.

Laboratory examination. Overnight collections of gastric secretions show a twofold to fivefold increase in volume and concentration of acids. Barium roentgen-ray studies of the stomach and duodenum will usually show an ulcer crater or scarring in the proximal portion of the duodenum (duodenal bulb). Gastroscopy and serum gastrin assays add valuable evidence in some problem cases.

Treatment. Initial treatment is almost always a four-point conservative regimen:

1. *Change of environment:* Bed rest in a hospital; change jobs, if possible, when tension is excessive.
2. *Sedation:* Barbiturates or tranquilizers are given to calm anxiety.
3. *Antacid therapy:* A bland diet with interval feedings and antacid medicine is designed to neutralize the high gastric acidity.
4. *Anticholinergic drugs* such as belladonna or atropine to depress vagal activity.

Most duodenal ulcers heal on this program. Surgical therapy is indicated only for the four *complications* of duodenal ulcer, as follows in order of frequency seen:

1. *Intractability:* Failure of medical management, or failure of the patient to adhere faithfully to the treatment.
2. *Bleeding:* Surgical treatment is indicated when bleeding cannot be controlled medically or when episodes of moderate hemorrhage have recurred. The decision for surgical therapy depends on such factors as the patient's age, blood type, reliability, and general health. (See Chapter 22.)
3. *Obstruction:* Chronic duodenal ulcers may cause obstruction of the pyloric area attributed to edema and scarring, with symptoms of nausea and vomiting. Obstruction causes stasis and excites the antral phase to further increase gastric secretion. A vicious cycle results, which often must be interrupted by surgical correction.
4. *Perforation:* An ulcer may perforate the duodenal wall, releasing caustic duodenal contents into the peritoneal cavity. Severe peritonitis with a boardlike abdomen and shock results, requiring emergency closure of the perforation. Surgical treatment of the ulcer is usually deferred.

In general, duodenal ulcers need *not* be removed. If the conditions

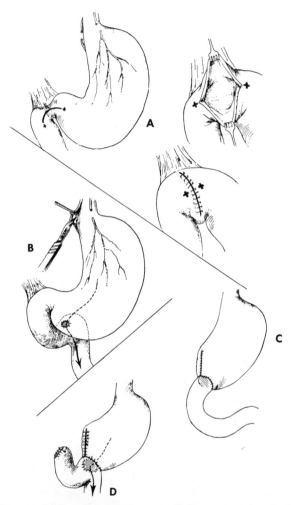

Fig. 23-2. Surgical treatment of peptic ulcer. **A,** Vagal nerve division and pyloroplasty. **B,** Vagal nerve division and gastrojejunostomy—arrow shows new exit for gastric contents. **C,** Billroth I partial gastric resection—stomach is anastomosed to duodenum. **D,** Billroth II partial gastric resection—duodenal stump is closed and stomach is anastomosed to jejunum.

causing duodenal ulcers are corrected by the surgical procedure, the ulcers will heal.

Theoretically, the ideal surgical treatment for duodenal ulcer is (1) control of the vagal-antral phase of gastric secretion by division of the vagus nerves, and (2) antrectomy. Experience has shown that opening the gastric outlet can substitute effectively for antrectomy.

Three commonly employed operations designed to improve gastric emptying are as follows:

1. Pyloroplasty (longitudinal division of the pyloric muscle with transverse closure) will effectively widen the pyloric channel at the gastroduodenal junction (Fig. 23-2, *A*).
2. Gastrojejunostomy (anastomosis of the stomach to the jejunum) will provide an alternative means of egress of food from the stomach into the small bowel (Fig. 23-2, *B*).
3. Gastroduodenostomy (anastomosis of stomach to duodenum, Jaboulay procedure).

None of these emptying procedures sacrifices any of the stomach, so that its reservoir capacity remains unaltered.

Vagotomy plus antrectomy, or one of the emptying procedures, have largely replaced the older surgical approach to the control of duodenal ulcers, which involved removal of large portions (up to 80%) of the stomach. The newer procedures are as effective, yet safer and technically easier to perform than extensive gastric removal. Extensive gastric resections may produce gastric cripples (failure to gain weight, diarrhea, debilitation). This complication occurs uncommonly with lesser gastric procedures.

Highly selective vagotomy (HSV), or parietal cell vagotomy, is a new procedure that involves cutting vagal fibers to the upper stomach, thus denervating the parietal cells only, while leaving lower gastric motility intact. Extensive clinical experience, chiefly from England and Denmark, appears promising.

Recurrence. Recurrent or stomal ulcerations usually indicate incomplete vagotomy or inadequate drainage. The *Hollander test,* based on insulin (hypoglycemic) stimulation of vagally-mediated gastric secretion, assays vagal integrity. Insulin (20 units intravenously) should elevate gastric acidity by 10 mEq./L. over basal levels if the vagus nerves are intact. Two 15-minute basal samples are compared to 15-minute samples (collected consecutively) after insulin. The 10 mEq./L. rise should come within 45 minutes after insulin. Recurrent ulcers, attributed to incomplete vagotomy, respond well to transthoracic vagotomy. Sluggish gastric drainage, detected by barium studies, often necessitates refashioning of the gastric outlet. The Zollinger-Ellison syndrome also causes recurrences.

Gastric ulcer

Cause. About 80% of gastric ulcers appear in stomachs that secrete normal or decreased acids. Evidence now points to a defective mucosal barrier and a back diffusion of acid (from stomach lumen into the mucosa) as the immediate cause. A defective pyloric sphincter allows bile to reflux into the stomach and disrupt the vital mucosal barrier; the resulting chronic gastritis precedes almost all gastric ulcers.

The other 20% of gastric ulcers usually occur just inside the pylorus or are associated with duodenal ulcers in proximity to the pylorus, causing pylorospasm or obstruction. These ulcers, arising in a hyperacidic environment, belong in the duodenal ulcer group.

Clinical examination. The clinical picture of gastric ulcer is similar to that of duodenal ulcer. Gastric ulcers tend to occur in a slightly older age group and in patients of lower social status than duodenal ulcers. The pain localizes more often to the left upper quadrant and sometimes is provoked by food or hot or cold liquids. Gastric ulcers are more worrisome than duodenal ulcers because about *10% of gastric ulcers are malignant; duodenal ulcers are virtually never malignant.*

Laboratory examination. Overnight collections of gastric secretions show a decrease in both volume and concentration of acid in gastric as compared to duodenal ulcer (Table 23-1). Barium roentgen-ray studies often show an ulcer crater in the stomach (Figs. 23-3 and 23-4). Gastroscopy and biopsy or gastric washings with careful cytological studies give the clinician vital information.

Treatment. The same conservative treatment is tried for gastric ulcer as for duodenal ulcer, with exception of anticholinergic drugs that cause stasis. However, because gastric ulcers may be malignant, the physician must recommend operation if the ulcer fails to heal after 4 weeks of treatment. About 50% of benign gastric ulcers fail to re-

Table 23-1. Approximate average values of volume and acidity in 12° collection of gastric juice for conditions listed

	12° nocturnal aspiration of stomach	
	mEq. of HCl	*Volume of secretion*
Normal	20	200 ml.
Duodenal ulcer	60	500 ml.
Gastric ulcer	12	150 ml.
Zollinger-Ellison syndrome	100 or more	1,000 or more
Gastric cancer	8	100 ml.

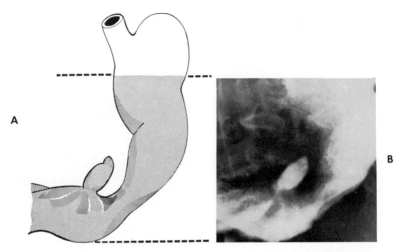

Fig. 23-3. Benign gastric ulcer. **A,** Diagram of roentgen-ray findings. **B,** Upper G.I. series showing gastric folds radiating away from ulcer and sharp margins that are not elevated.

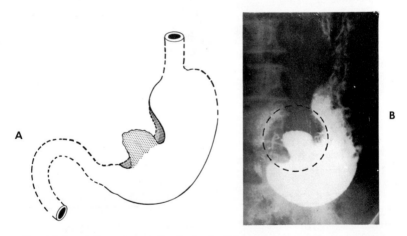

Fig. 23-4. Malignant gastric ulcer. **A,** Diagram of roentgen-ray findings. **B,** Upper G.I. series showing no radiating folds and heaped-up ulcer margins.

Table 23-2. Comparison of duodenal and gastric ulcers

	Duodenal ulcer	*Gastric ulcer*
Cause	Increased acid secretion; increased gastrin; defect in acid disposal	Abnormal pyloric sphincter; bile reflux; gastritis; increased back diffusion of hydrogen ion
Location	Duodenum	Stomach
Age	Younger (40 to 50 years)	Somewhat older
Sex	Men > Women	Men > Women
Incidence	7 to 10	1
Symptoms	Much the same	
Malignancy	Rare	10%
Free HCl (12-hr. night secretion)	60 mEq. (average)	12 mEq. (average)
Medical treatment	Excellent (successful in 80-90%)	Poor (successful in 50%)
Surgical treatment	Vagotomy and antrectomy or emptying procedure; parietal cell vagotomy	50% gastrectomy

spond satisfactorily to medical treatment and must ultimately be treated surgically. If surgical treatment of gastric ulcer becomes necessary, the ulcer should always be biopsied to rule out cancer (Table 23-2).

Over the years, removal of the distal half of the stomach has given excellent results for gastric ulcer. (The antrum is of course removed in this procedure.) Some surgeons add vagotomy when they suspect the ulcer is related to hyperacidity.

Hyperparathyroidism

Because hypercalcemia increases gastric secretion, patients with hyperparathyroidism develop a higher than normal incidence of duodenal ulcers. These ulcers usually fail to respond to medical therapy but subside with treatment of the hyperparathyroidism.

Multiple endocrine adenopathy

Two main syndromes involving adenoma of endocrine glands have been described: M.E.A. I (parathyroid, pituitary, and pancreas), and M.E.A. II (parathyroid, adrenal medullary, and thyroid C cells). But the boundaries of these syndromes are currently not nearly as distinct as previously described. Both entities are associated with duodenal ulcerations, probably because of hyperfunctioning parathyroid (parathormone) and pancreatic (gastrin) tissues.

Drugs

The exact cause of drug-induced gastric ulcerations is unknown. They may disrupt the mucosal cell barrier or the protective mucus. Aspirin, phenylbutazone, Indomethacin, cinophen, colchicine, and steroids are the chief offenders.

Acute gastric mucosal ulcers (AGM ulcers)

Cause. AGM ulcers arise after varied insults including shock, burns, sepsis, operations, and drugs. *Ischemia* and a *damaged mucosal barrier* are the common denominators underlying these superficial erosions. Almost all patients in severe shock will show AGM ulcers. Ischemia disrupts the vital mucosal barrier; ileus, with reflux of bile, adds to the mucosal damage. Gastric acids diffuse through the impaired mucosa, and ulcers—often multiple—result.

Clinical. Upper gastrointestinal bleeding that develops in a critically ill patient with no prior history of peptic ulcerations should indicate AGM ulcerations. Because of clots within the stomach and the superficial nature of AGM erosions, diagnostic barium studies often fail to detect them. But gastroscopy and celiac arteriography often help to localize the bleeding site.

Treatment. Prevention is probably the most important measure. The physician should anticipate these ulcers in any critically ill patient. Continuous nasogastric suction with instillation of antacids helps in neutralizing gastric acidity. Concurrent treatment of shock, sepsis, etc., will relieve gastric ischemia. If, despite these measures, the patient bleeds, arteriographic localization of the bleeding points followed by vasopressin, a potent arterial constrictor, may stem bleeding at least temporarily. (A paradoxical treatment, since the cause is ischemia, but vasopressin has proved effective in some desperately ill patients). If these conservative means fail, most surgeons rely on vagotomy with gastric resection or pyloroplasty (and oversewing the bleeding sites) to stop the bleeding. Total gastrectomy remains the final therapeutic resort.

PEPTIC ULCERS FROM OTHER CAUSES
Zollinger-Ellison syndrome

This rare syndrome of recurrent, severe ulcer disease is of special interest because it emphasizes the importance of gastrin in gastric secretion and because it explains the frustrating phenomenon of recurrent ulceration in some patients who have had adequate previous treatment.

The cause is a gastrin-secreting tumor of the pancreas. Gastric secretion is enormous (12-hour volume is over 1,000 ml., and free HCl is over 100 mEq.). Serum gastrin levels in these patients average over 600 pg./ml. (normal < 200 pg./ml.). Also the basal acid secretion is high, usually 60% or more of maximal acid output (after stimulation with Histolog). The ulcer trait almost totally defies cure unless the tumor can be removed (80% are either malignant or multiple) or a total gastrectomy performed to remove the target organ.

CARCINOMA OF THE STOMACH

Stomach cancer is the seventh leading malignancy in this country today. Although decreasing in incidence for unknown reasons, gastric cancer still kills about 24,000 people each year.

Pathology. Three types of stomach cancer occur in terms of gross physical characteristics, with about equal frequency. They are the *polypoid, ulcerating,* and *infiltrating* varieties, in order of ascending malignant activity.

The histological types are adenocarcinoma, colloid carcinoma, carcinoma simplex, and undifferentiated carcinoma, also in ascending order of malignant activity.

Local spread. Spread occurs submucosally and subserosally for surprising distances even though it cannot be palpated. Gastric cancer may also spread throughout the peritoneal cavity. It may form deposits in the pelvic floor, *Blumer's shelf.* Deposits to the ovary, from colloid carcinoma, bear the eponym *Krukenberg tumor.*

Lymphatic spread. Lymphatic spread is very common. Because of its rich lymphatic system, cancer of the stomach is often inoperable. Four zones of metastasis have been described: superior gastric nodes, suprapyloric nodes, pancreatico-splenic nodes, and the inferior gastric subpyloric nodes. Rarely the left supraclavicular nodes are involved (Virchow's nodes), presumably via the thoracic duct.

Staging. The following is a system of clinical staging that is helpful in treatment and prognosis:

Stage A: No metastasis—cancer limited to stomach
Stage B: Regional lymph nodes involved
Stage C: Distant metastases

Invasion. A system for classifying according to invasion is similarly employed:

Stage I: Superficial growth—confined to mucosa or muscularis
Stage II: All gastric layers including serosa are involved
Stage III: The tumor has extended to neighboring organs

These systems can be combined to give a reasonably accurate prognosis; e.g., stage A-I gives an excellent prognosis; stage C-III is a far-advanced, inoperable situation.

Clinical characteristics. Specific or early *symptoms* are notoriously lacking in cancer of the stomach. Epigastric pain, weight loss, anorexia, fatigue, and anemia occur insidiously and are often ignored. Males outnumber females about 3:1. Diseases that may precede and predispose to cancer of the stomach include pernicious anemia (achlorhydria), gastric polyps, and chronic atrophic gastritis.

Diagnosis. Cancer of the stomach is suspected from roentgenographic evidence, gastroscopy findings, histamine-fast achlorhydria, and cytological evidence of malignant cells in the gastric aspirate. These lesions are usually located on the greater curvature, on the prepyloric portion of the lesser curvature, or in the fundus.

Treatment. Surgical excision of the lesion and involved nodes is the only treatment of definite value. Radiation therapy offers little help and is seldom used.

Prognosis. If all the tumor can be removed, with no spread beyond the stomach, up to 50% of these patients will live 5 years. However, because of the lack of early symptoms, the rich lymphatic supply, and the aggressiveness of these tumors, less than 15% of all patients with gastric carcinoma survive 5 years.

SARCOMA OF THE STOMACH

Sarcomas account for about 2% of all malignancies of the stomach.

Lymphosarcoma is the most common type and is, fortunately, quite radiosensitive. It may occur primarily in the stomach or as a manifestation of a generalized process. Grossly it appears as mucosal thickening, multiple nodules, or a single polypoid growth. Since lymphosarcoma is radiosensitive and gastric carcinoma is not, biopsy of gastric tumors for specific diagnosis is often indicated even when the tumors appear far advanced.

Leiomyosarcoma and fibrosarcoma are less commonly encountered. Excision is the treatment of choice.

MISCELLANEOUS CONDITIONS OF STOMACH AND DUODENUM
Gastric polyps

Polyps in the stomach are rare but often troublesome. Malignant potential increases with the size of the polyps. Polyps over 1.5 cm. are likely to be malignant and should be removed.

Multiple benign polyposis (Peutz-Jeghers syndrome) is hereditary and may involve the stomach as well as other parts of the gastro-intestinal tract. It is associated with melanin spots of the lips and buccal mucosa. Conservative treatment is usually indicated.

Duodenal diverticula

Duodenal diverticula are outpouchings in the duodenum. They usually cause no symptoms and should be left alone unless they are a suspected cause of bleeding or inflammation.

Gastritis

Inflammation of the stomach wall may occur after dietary in-discretions, especially after an increased intake of alcohol. Atrophic, hypertrophic, and erosive gastritis are all terms that have been used to describe various forms of gastritis. Gastritis, in general, is poorly understood and difficult to diagnose. The treatment is conservative with operative intervention held in reserve for complications.

Mallory-Weiss syndrome

Mallory-Weiss syndrome is an uncommon complication of severe vomiting that results in a laceration across the esophageal-stomach junction. By definition the laceration occurs only through the mucosa. Surgical ligation of the laceration is sometimes necessary to stop bleeding.

Dumping syndrome

Dumping occurs to some extent in about 10 to 20% of patients who have gastric operations. This syndrome features two general types of symptoms, *gastrointestinal* and *hemodynamic*. *Gastrointestinal symptoms* include nausea, vomiting, abdominal pain (fullness, cramps), and diarrhea. *Hemodynamic symptoms* are weakness, fatigue, pal-pitations, sweating, pallor, and sensation of warmth. These symptoms begin during or within 30 minutes after a meal; they usually last less than 60 minutes. The intensity of dumping symptoms varies widely.

Although the precise cause remains unknown, the basic trigger seems to be rapid *distension of the jejunum* from hyperosmolar fluid rushing (or dumping) into it. Investigators are less certain about the hemodynamic aspects of dumping. Older theories cite the importance of hypovolemia from plasma elements pouring into the jejunum to neutralize the sudden hyperosmolar load. Newer theories, focused on chemical mediators released from the distended mucosa, have indicted both serotonin and bradykinin. Some patients have responded to cyproheptadine, a serotonin antagonist. Others report good responses

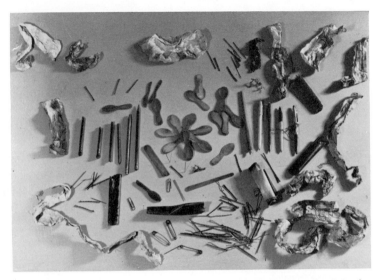

Fig. 23-5. Foreign bodies removed from stomach of mentally defective patient.

from procaine, which presumably blocks release of bradykinin from the jejunal mucosal cells.

Until some rational chemical treatment emerges from a precise understanding of basic mechanisms, we must rely on the time-honored therapy. High protein–low carbohydrate diet, recumbency after meals, and withholding fluids during meals highlight the conservative treatment. Narrowing of wide anastomoses and interposition of reversed segments of jejunum (both designed to slow down the rush of fluid into the jejunum) keynote the operative treatment. Symptoms improve with time as patients adjust to their postgastrectomy state; less than 5% of patients have protracted dumping. Thus operative treatment should be reserved for patients with severe and chronic dumping symptoms.

Foreign bodies

Children or mental incompetents may swallow an astonishing variety of foreign bodies (Fig. 23-5). Most foreign bodies pass through the gastrointestinal tract in 3 to 4 days without symptoms or complications. *Trichobezoars* are hair balls that may accumulate in the stomach from chronic hair ingestion. *Phytobezoars* are balls of accumulated indigestible food fibers. Patients with such foreign bodies in the stomach are usually incapable of giving any reliable history. Thus detection is based on radiographic or operative evidence.

CHAPTER 24

The small intestine

ROBERT T. SOPER
SIROOS SAFAIE-SHIRAZI

The small intestine is the longest segment of the gastrointestinal tract, extending from the pyloric sphincter to the ileocecal sphincter or valve. Curiously enough, although the small bowel is frequently operated upon (resection, bypass, decompression, lysis of adhesions, placement of indwelling catheters for suction or feeding purposes), few of these operations are done *upon* the small bowel for diseases that originate *within* the small bowel. Thus, duodenal ulcer is caused by acid-peptic factors originating within the stomach with the major effect upon the duodenum; mesenteric vascular occlusion infarcts and perforates the small bowel but originates primarily as a vascular lesion; small bowel obstruction is most commonly caused by extrinsic factors (hernias, adhesions) not of primary origin from the small bowel itself. Numerically, few surgical diseases primarily arise *within* the small intestine itself.

ANATOMY

The small intestine measures 7 to 8 meters in the adult, and a surprisingly long 200 cm. in the newborn infant. Its subdivisions (duodenum, jejunum, and ileum) are continuous, and only the duodenojejunal junction is marked clearly (by the ligament of Treitz).

The duodenum begins at the pylorus, measures roughly 25 cm. in length, and is largely retroperitoneal. It receives the contents of the stomach proximally, and the bile and pancreatic enzymes in the concave mesenteric surface of its second portion, which is occasioned by embryological rotation. It can be mobilized partially by the *Kocher maneuver*, which divides the peritoneal attachments to its convex surface. The juxtaposition of large vessels, pancreas, and vital duct structures makes surgical manipulations of the duodenum hazardous and necessitates removal of the distal stomach, common bile duct, and pancreatic head if the duodenum must be resected (see discussion on Whipple procedure, Chapter 18).

In contrast, the jejunum and ileum are suspended freely in the peritoneal cavity by the dorsal mesentery and are therefore easy to inspect, manipulate, and resect at laparotomy. The jejunum encompasses the proximal 40% of the bowel from the ligament of Treitz to the ileocolic valve, and the ileum makes up the remainder. The junction between the two is not clearly defined. In general, the jejunum has (1) a larger lumen, (2) thicker walls, (3) larger and more numerous transverse mucosal folds *(valvulae conniventes),* and (4) a better blood supply delivered through fewer vascular arcades than the ileum.

Arterial blood to the small intetsine is supplied entirely from the superior mesenteric artery, and largely via end arteries. There is little collateral blood flow to the small bowel, in striking contrast to the stomach and colon, and therefore vascular occlusion is more likely to produce bowel infarction.

Venous blood from the small bowel carries fluid end-products of digestion to the liver via the portal vein. The small bowel lymphatics, or *lacteals,* travel in the mesentery and collect retroperitoneally into the *cisterna chyli;* they transport products of fat digestion (chyle) into the systemic venous system through the thoracic duct.

The nerve supply to the small bowel is entirely from the autonomic nervous system. The efferent nerves ensure coordinated aboral peristaltic waves to carry intestinal contents downstream during digestion. The sensory afferents localize and discriminate pain of small bowel origin very poorly as a dull, vague aching in the epigastrium or periumbilical area of the abdomen.

The wall of the small intestine is composed of four layers:

1. The inner mucosa is composed of simple columnar epithelium with innumerable intestinal glands, the absorptive surface being increased enormously by the presence of villi, plus the mucosal folds known as the *valvulae conniventes.*

2. The submucosa consists of fibrous and supporting tissue and is richly supplied by the intrinsic vascular and nervous elements of the intestine.

3. The outer longitudinal and inner circular muscle layers contribute the peristalsis necessary to propel intestinal material downstream.

4. The outer serosa is visceral peritoneum that, in its pristine state,

allows free motion of the intestine, provides an impermeable barrier to the passage of bacteria to the peritoneal cavity, and adds considerably to the suture-holding qualities of the bowel wall.

PHYSIOLOGY

During intrauterine life the intestine functions as an integral part of normal amniotic fluid circulation. Amniotic fluid is swallowed by the fetus and a portion is absorbed, utilized, and then excreted as urine back into the amniotic fluid. Interruption of this cycle at any stage results in retention of abnormal amounts of amniotic fluid, a condition known as *hydramnios;* 50% of babies born of mothers with polyhydramnios will have major congenital anomalies that interfere with this circulatory system, including hydrocephalus, anencephaly, myelomeningocele, upper gastrointestinal tract obstruction, and congenital hydronephrosis.

In postnatal life the small intestine has digestive and absorptive functions. In the adult, 8 to 10 liters of digestive secretion are produced daily in the oral cavity, stomach, small bowel, pancreas, and liver to aid enzymatic breakdown of ingested food to molecules small enough to be absorbed. The small bowel adds somewhat to the digestive secretions and propels the succus entericus downstream in an orderly and relatively slow manner. After digestion has been completed, the mucosal surface of the small intestine absorbs water, electrolytes, and the basic breakdown products of the food. Fat travels via the lacteals and lymphatic ducts to the superior vena cava, and the bulk of the remaining products is conveyed to the liver via the portal venous system for further metabolic alteration. Normally up to 98% of the liquid volume of the succus entericus is absorbed, largely from the lower portion of the small intestine.

Resection or bypass of up to 50% of the small intestine is generally followed by an initial period of diarrhea and weight loss, but is compatible with perfectly normal subsequent growth and development, regardless of age at the time of operation. Chronic diarrhea, anemia, osteomalacia, and varying degrees of malnutrition, at least temporarily, occur after loss of more than half of the small intestine.

SURGICAL DISEASES OF THE SMALL INTESTINE

The majority of operations performed upon the small bowel are done because of peptic ulcers, intestinal obstruction (including those of congenital origin), or as a necessary part of operations primarily upon the colon; these entities are properly discussed in their own specific chapters and will not be considered further here. The remainder of this chapter is therefore devoted to that small fraction of surgical diseases arising primarily within the small intestine.

Neoplasms

The small intestine is singularly free of neoplasms, both benign and malignant, as compared with the esophagus, stomach, and colon. The reasons for this discrepancy are unknown. They comprise well under 5% of all primary neoplasms of the gastrointestinal tract. Benign tumors include polyps, villous adenomas, myomas, fibromas, lipomas, and aberrant gastric or pancreatic tissue. They commonly are asymptomatic and are found incidentally at autopsy or laparotomy. They become symptomatic by ulcerating the overlying mucosa with bleeding, or by acting as the leading point for small bowel intussusception; the

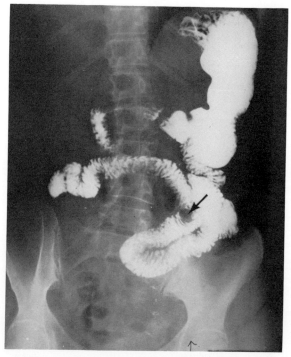

Fig. 24-1. Small bowel polyp designated by arrow.

larger tumors may obstruct the lumen. Diagnosis is made at laparotomy, but occasionally the tumors show as filling defects in the barium column during small-bowel roentgenograms (Fig. 24-1). Treatment is surgical excision (Fig. 24-2).

The *Peutz-Jeghers syndrome* is the association of intestinal polyps with melanin spots on the mucosa of the lips, mouth, and anus. The disorder seems to be inherited on a genetic basis. The polyps are generally localized to the small intestine and are from one to five in number; occasionally they are more numerous and are located within the stomach or colon. Malignant degeneration is extremely unusual with the Peutz-Jeghers type of polyp, and surgical treatment is undertaken only when the polyps produce symptoms.

The most common malignant neoplasm of the small intestine is the *adenocarcinoma,* about one half of which are primary within the

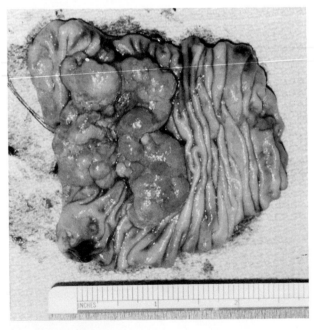

Fig. 24-2. Benign villous adenoma resected from the third portion of the duodenum; seen preoperatively by fiberoptic endoscopy.

duodenum. Bleeding and obstruction are the most common signs and often occur late in the evolution after metastasis has already occurred. *Lymphosarcomas* are the next most common variety, generally occurring in children and young adults and often in association with widespread disease.

The signs of small bowel malignancy are those of intestinal obstruction, gastrointestinal tract bleeding, an abdominal mass, and perforation in roughly descending order of frequency. Diagnosis is made at laparotomy, but plain and barium contrast studies of the intestine may be helpful. Treatment is wide surgical resection of the involved bowel and its draining lymphatic pathways when possible and if distant metastasis has not already occurred. Roentgen-ray therapy is useful in additional treatment of lymphomas. Local resection or bypass occasionally palliates incurable neoplasms. The overall 5-year survival rate is from 10 to 15%, the prognosis for lymphosarcoma being materially better than that for primary small bowel adenocarcinoma.

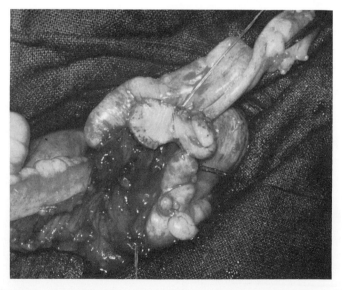

Fig. 24-3. Carcinoid tumor at base of appendix. The probe (upper white line) points to the yellow-white tumor, which has been sectioned. The appendix is retracted toward the upper right of the field.

Carcinoid tumors (Fig. 24-3) arise from argentaffin cells near the base of the intestinal glands. They are most commonly found in the appendix, with the small intestine next in frequency. However, they can arise anywhere within the gastrointestinal tract, and pulmonary carcinoids have occasionally been reported. Carcinoid tumors are yellow or gray in color; the cells have a columnar arrangement and stain with chromic acid to allow a specific histological diagnosis.

Carcinoid tumors may be either benign or malignant, probably related more to the time at which they are discovered than to any inherent difference in malignant potential. This supposition is supported by the observation that although 60% of carcinoid tumors arise within the appendix, they are never malignant in this location; they probably produce early obstruction of the very small appendiceal lumen that initiates signs of appendicitis leading to prompt surgical excision and cure. On the other extreme, carcinoid tumors arising in the small intestine are almost always malignant by the time of discovery. The larger lumen of the intestine allows years of undetected growth to occur before symptoms are produced and surgical treatment carried out. Metastasis occurs via the portal venous system to the liver.

The *carcinoid syndrome* is seen only when malignant carcinoids have *metastasized* widely to the liver or other extraportal sites such as the lungs; it is present in about 25% of reported malignant carcinoids. The clinical features of the *carcinoid syndrome* are periodic attacks of (1) colicky abdominal pain with diarrhea and weight loss, (2) flushing of the face, neck, and torso, and (3) asthmatic wheezing. Late in the course of the carcinoid syndrome, pulmonic or tricuspid valvular stenosis develops gradually, leading to cardiac failure and death.

Argentaffin cells normally produce minute amounts of hydroxytryptophan (as an intermediate in the biosynthesis of serotonin), which is thought to play a role in hemostasis and maintenance of smooth muscle tone in blood vessels and intestine. Carcinoid tumors synthesize enormous amounts of serotonin that, however, are altered and "detoxified" by the liver so long as the venous drainage goes into the portal system. However, large hepatic or extraportal metastases secrete serotonin directly into systemic blood to induce the smooth muscle contractions responsible for the characteristic signs and symptoms previously related. The reason for the periodicity of attacks is unknown. Diagnostic confirmation is provided by demonstrating excessive levels of serotonin in the serum (5-hydroxytryptamine or 5-HT) or its degradation products (5-hydroxyindoleacetic acid or 5-HIAA) in the urine. Serotonin is also excreted by the lungs into expired air, explaining why valvular disease is limited selectively to the valves on the right side of the heart.

Malignant carcinoids are the exception to the rule that the metastases of incurable primary intestinal neoplasms should not be resected. Malignant carcinoids grow slowly, and removal of portions of the metastases may provide gratifyingly long relief from the distressing and ultimately serious (or fatal) effects of hyperserotoninemia.

Trauma

The small intestine is damaged by both *penetrating* and *nonpenetrating* abdominal trauma, often in association with other visceral injuries. The penetrating missile may perforate intestine or produce mesenteric vascular injury, ranging from a minor hematoma confined to the mesentery to massive hemorrhage into the free peritoneal cavity with shock and serious compromise to the blood supply of the involved segment of intestine. Plain supine and decubitus abdominal radiographs will often show free air and will locate the missile if it has been retained in the body to help map out the pathway traversed. Laparotomy is almost always indicated, with a painstaking and orderly inspection of the entire peritoneal cavity for injury. The missile need not be removed, but damage to the viscera must be repaired. Minute or sharply demarcated puncture wounds of small intestine may be turned in, but large or ragged lacerations and severely contused or devascularized bowel require resection and anastomosis. Mesenteric bleeding must be controlled by pressure or ligature. Because of the chemically irritating and septic content of the small intestine, the peritoneal cavity should be lavaged, suctioned, and drained and appropriate antibiotics administered postoperatively if spillage has occurred.

The mortality for nonpenetrating abdominal trauma is approximately three times that for penetrating injuries, probably because there are less compelling indications for exploratory laparotomy in the former. The intestine ranks fourth behind the spleen, kidneys, and liver in frequency of damage by nonpenetrating abdominal trauma. The jejunum and ileum are relatively mobile and tend to slide away and escape injury from a nonpenetrating blow, although sudden dislocation may indeed lacerate the small bowel mesentery. The duodenum and duodenojejunal junction are anchored retroperitoneally and cannot escape, resulting in a much higher incidence of injury. This is especially true for the fourth part of the duodenum, trapped between the wounding blow anteriorly and the rigid second lumbar vertebra posteriorly. Intramural hematoma and laceration are the common duodenal injuries incurred in this manner. If the duodenum is lacerated beneath its peritoneal cover, extravasation of duodenal contents occurs retroperitoneally.

Intramural *duodenal hematomas* produce symptoms by obstructing the lumen, which may take several hours or even days to complete. Diagnosis is suggested by narrowing of the lumen and a "coil spring" appearance of the duodenal mucosa on upper G.I. barium roentgenograms. Surgical treatment consists of evacuating the hematoma through a serosal incision, careful inspection for a break in the mucosa, and drainage.

The diagnosis of retroperitoneal laceration of the duodenum may be extremely difficult to establish, although the plain abdominal radiograph often shows obliteration of the right kidney profile and small bubbles of gas above the kidney. In view of the subtle clinical signs and the disastrous results of untreated duodenal laceration, any patient with a nonpenetrating abdominal injury must be hospitalized and observed very closely. Diagnostic laparotomy should be carried out if his condition does not promptly improve. The laparotomy is not complete without performing a Kocher maneuver to allow inspection of the retroperitoneal duodenum and exploration of the lesser sac to look for associated pancreatic injury. Duodenal lacerations are closed in two layers, and the area is generously drained.

People involved in automobile accidents while wearing abdominal seat belts suffer a peculiar type of subtle injury to their abdomen that deserves special mention. Rapid deceleration whips the upper part of the torso forward, and if the seat belt is above the pelvic bony girdle (where it generally is), it momentarily traps the viscera against the vertebral column and imposes many different shearing and compression injuries to gut and mesentery. The abdominal injuries most commonly seen are mesenteric hematoma, devascularization of bowel, severe damage leading to rupture of the bowel wall, and delayed ecchymosis and hemorrhage of the abdominal wall in a beltlike area. Symptoms are likely to be slow in onset and often are overshadowed by other injuries. Any automobile accident victim who bears the ecchymotic imprint of a seat belt injury on his abdomen and who develops late abdominal pain, distension, paralytic ileus, or slow return of gastrointestinal function is a prime candidate for serious visceral injury. Repeated abdominal examinations, roentgenograms, and paracenteses are often helpful in confirming this diagnosis, but laparotomy often must be the final arbiter.

Infections

None of the primary infections of the small intestine or its mesentery is treated primarily by surgical means, but often the symptoms produced by them mimic surgically treated diseases (appendicitis) or are complications of hospitalized patients (pseudomembranous enterocolitis).

Acute gastroenteritis

Acute gastroenteritis is generally caused by food poisoning or virus infections, and in this country it is less commonly caused by dysentery *(Shigella, Salmonella)* or paratyphoid infection, and very rarely by typhoid fever. Profuse vomiting and diarrhea are associated with colicky abdominal pain, diffuse abdominal tenderness, and hyperactive bowel sounds. Attention to these features on physical examination will in most cases adequately distinguish gastroenteritis from appendicitis. The temperature is often elevated, but tachycardia is not seen until the late stages of the disorder when the patient becomes dehydrated. Stool culture and serum agglutination tests are helpful in the diagnosis, and leukopenia is a characteristic finding with both typhoid and viral infections.

Primary intestinal tuberculosis

Primary intestinal tuberculosis is extremely rare in this country, with the elimination of bovine tuberculosis and with better control of the human pulmonary tuberculous infection. Intestinal tuberculosis involves the distal small bowel and cecum with a granulomatous mass and is best treated by chemotherapy in a tuberculosis sanatorium; obstructive complications of the tuberculous mass may require surgical bypass.

Tuberculous peritonitis

Tuberculous peritonitis is a bland form of peritonitis that is self-limiting in its course; it is characterized by yellowish deposits on the mesenteric surface that are composed of typical tubercles. The diagnosis is confirmed by biopsy of one of the tubercles. Intestinal tuberculosis is often the source of peritoneal involvement, although hematogenous spread may be responsible.

Mesenteric lymphadenitis

Mesenteric lymphadenitis is a hyperplastic enlargement of mesenteric lymph nodes, generally seen only in children and young adults, which produces pain difficult to distinguish from that of appendicitis. It is probably caused by a viral enteritis (adenovirus) with secondary mesenteric lymph node involvement. The clinical picture is characterized by central and right lower quadrant abdominal pain in a mildly febrile child who commonly has evidence of pharyngitis or tonsillitis. Abdominal tenderness is maximal in the right lower abdominal quadrant or right paraumbilical area without sharp localization or signs of peritoneal irritation. The enlarged nodes can be palpated as irregular, tender nodules if the patient is adequately relaxed. Treatment is supportive, and the patient is observed to be certain that signs of appendicitis do not supervene. Exploratory laparotomy is indicated when appendicitis cannot be ruled out, at which time prophylactic appendectomy is recommended to avoid subsequent confusion should the disease recur.

Acute necrotizing enterocolitis

Acute necrotizing enterocolitis (pseudomembranous enterocolitis) (Fig. 24-4) is a fulminating infection of the small bowel and/or colon that is sometimes caused by an overgrowth of staphylococci but that may also occur in the absence of any cultured pathogen. The clinical settings favoring the development of acute enterocolitis are chronic low-grade intestinal obstruction (children with Hirschsprung's disease) or cases in which treatment with broad-spectrum antibiotics has upset the balance of the intestinal flora to allow overgrowth of bacteria in the gastrointestinal tract. There is widespread denudation of the intestinal mucosa, especially in the small bowel, with edema and inflammation of the wall and pooling of large amounts of fluid within the bowel lumen.

Acute enterocolitis is characterized by the sudden onset of profuse diarrhea containing desquamated mucosa and blood that is associated with a high fever, tachycardia, nausea and vomiting, abdominal pain,

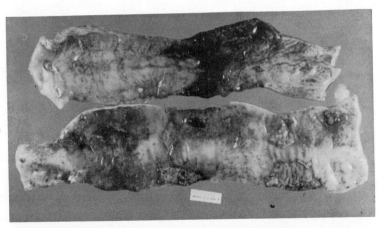

Fig. 24-4. Acute necrotizing enterocolitis. Note the hemorrhage, edema, superficial ulceration, and exudation of the mucosa.

and tenderness. Dehydration, electrolyte imbalance, and shock quickly occur from the massive amounts of fluid entrapped in the bowel lumen, which may not become evident as diarrhea for several hours because of a dynamic ileus. Hypovolemic and septic shock is the most common cause of death.

Treatment must be heroic, with rapid replacement of fluids, electrolytes, and blood. Nasogastric suction is begun, and cleansing enemas are given to expel the fluid retained within the bowel lumen. Antibiotics to which staphylococci are sensitive (penicillinase-resistant penicillin, vancomycin) should be given if stool smear and culture suggest an overgrowth of staphylococci. Steroids and fecal enemas are sometimes helpful. In patients harboring chronic intestinal obstruction, the obstruction should be relieved as soon as possible.

Granulomatous (transmural) enterocolitis

The term *granulomatous (transmural) enterocolitis* includes regional enteritis, regional ileitis, regional ileocolitis, and Crohn's disease. It is preferable to the older terms of Crohn's disease or regional enteritis because a granulomatous reaction is the most characteristic microscopic feature of the disorder, and it can indeed involve all layers of any or all portions of the intestine. It was first described in 1932 by Crohn and his associates as a specific entity distinct from tuberculous enteritis and other less specific infectious disorders of the intestine.

Granulomatous enterocolitis is an uncommon disease that affects principally young adults. It is rare among Negroes and has an equal sex incidence. The cause of the disease is unknown, although allergic, infectious, and autoimmune factors have been suggested as contributing factors.

Granulomatous (transmural) enterocolitis either originates in, or is totally confined to, the distal ileum in the majority of cases. Spread commonly occurs proximally and occasionally distally to the colon; during the latter stages it often has multiple sites of involvement with uninvolved "skip areas" intervening. In early phases the bowel mucosa ulcerates and the wall becomes grossly thickened, erythematous, and edematous, with thickening of the adjacent mesentery and rubbery enlargement of the mesenteric lymph nodes. At this stage the outstanding histological features are mucosal ulceration, submucosal lymphoid hyperplasia, and transmural lymphangiectasis, infiltrates of inflammatory cells and eosinophils, sclerosing lymphangitis, and granulomas without caseation. Involvement of all layers of the bowel wall justifies the descriptive term *transmural* and, when this peculiar disease attacks primarily the colon, serves to distinguish it from the primarily mucosal inflammation of chronic ulcerative colitis.

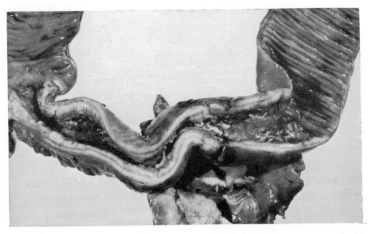

Fig. 24-5. Chronic granulomatous enterocolitis (regional ileitis) with scarring, rigidity, and thickening of the bowel wall and narrowing of the lumen. (From Anderson, W. A. D., and Scotti, T. M.: Synopsis of pathology, ed. 7, St. Louis, 1968, The C. V. Mosby Co.)

If limited to the ileum, the early stages of acute granulomatous enterocolitis often mimic appendicitis and are distinguished only at laparotomy; if the cecal base is not involved, prophylactic appendectomy may be safely performed at this time, along with confirmatory biopsy of a mesenteric lymph node. Approximately 50% of such cases will have spontaneous subsidence of the small bowel inflammation, with lengthy periods of remission.

In later stages of the disease, the edema and erythema of the involved bowel wall is replaced by fibrous tissue with rigidity, contracture, and narrowing of the lumen (Fig. 24-5). A moderately tender mass can usually be palpated at this stage, which is clinically manifested by periodic bouts of crampy abdominal discomfort and diarrhea associated with weight loss and anemia caused by occult blood loss in the stool. Fever and leukocytosis parallel the activity of the disease, and for unknown reasons perianal abscesses and fistulas are common.

The later stages of transmural enterocolitis are characterized by abscess formation and inflammatory involvement of adjacent viscera leading to both external and internal fistulas. The viscera more commonly involved in these fistulas are small bowel, bladder, and sig-

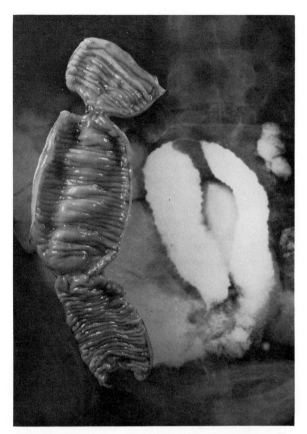

Fig. 24-6. Granulomatous enterocolitis (regional ileitis). "String sign" and uninvolved "skip areas" illustrated in distal ileum superimposed on barium study.

moid colon, with varying symptoms related to the fistulas. The signs and symptoms of chronic low-grade intestinal obstruction (caused by the extreme narrowing of the lumen) are often superimposed.

The course of granulomatous enterocolitis is characterized by chronicity and periods of remissions and exacerbations. Generally speaking, the younger the age and the more acute the onset, the more guarded must the prognosis be in terms of later recurrences and complications.

The diagnosis of transmural enterocolitis is generally confirmed by contrast (barium) roentgenograms; the early radiographic signs include a modest degree of narrowing of the lumen associated with flattening and a raggedness of the mucosal pattern with puddling of barium. Later stages are extreme narrowing of the lumen, referred to as the *string sign* (Fig. 24-6), with dilatation of the proximal loops according to the degree of intestinal obstruction present. Occasionally fistulas or extravasation of barium into abscess cavities is seen. Barium enema with retrograde filling of the distal ileum occasionally is helpful in diagnosing transmural ileitis.

Treatment of granulomatous enterocolitis is nonoperative until and unless complications occur. Indications for operative treatment are the development of intestinal obstruction, fistulas, intra-abdominal abscesses, and hemorrhage, or if the patient's general well-being is severely compromised by chronic malnutrition, anemia, pain, and debility. Malignant degeneration rarely occurs. In large series of cases, over one-half will ultimately require surgical intervention.

Specific treatment for granulomatous enterocolitis is nonexistent. Evaluation of different forms of therapy is difficult because of the unpredictable and remitting course of the disease. Corticosteroids or ACTH, a nutritious and low-residue diet, supplements of vitamins and iron, systemic antibiotics, ingestion of nonabsorbed sulfonamides (Azulfidine), rest, and symptomatic treatment for diarrhea are all employed in the nonoperative treatment of granulomatous enterocolitis. Operative treatment is directed to the specific complication or indication for surgery, including resection or total bypass of the involved intestine. Recurrence of the disease in previously uninvolved bowel can be expected in fully one-fourth to one-third of patients who are followed for many years after surgical treatment. Repeated resections and bypassing procedures are fraught with nutritional and metabolic disturbances in themselves, thus warranting intensification of nonoperative treatment and avoidance of operative therapy when possible.

Vascular diseases
Superior mesenteric vascular occlusion

Occlusion of the superior mesenteric artery and vein may occur singly or together, because of a host of disparate influences. Trauma, stagnation of flow, compression, a state of hypercoagulability, and atheromatous plaques favor thrombosis. Occlusion also may occur from emboli originating within the left side of the heart, generally associated with auricular fibrillation. Rarely is the superior mesenteric vein alone thrombosed, but venous thrombosis predictably occurs after occlusion of the arterial inflow. The inferior mesenteric vessels are rarely involved.

Occlusion of the superior mesenteric vessels produces vascular compromise of that segment of small intestine distal to the point of occlusion; the more proximal the occlusion, the longer the segment of bowel that will be involved. Primary venous occlusion is associated with a "wet gangrene" type of reaction with marked cyanosis, hemorrhage, and edema of the involved bowel and an effusion of sanguineous fluid from its surface. Arterial occlusion produces initial blanching of the intestine with venous stagnation subsequently inducing a blue-red discoloration. The intestine becomes slightly distended and hypotonic because of paralytic ileus that, with continued ischemia, progresses to perforation and peritonitis. Bowel infarction is generally limited to the jejunum, ileum, and right colon, even when the superior mesenteric artery is occluded at its takeoff from the aorta, because of collateral arterial blood flow to duodenum and colon.

Clinically, acute occlusion of the superior mesenteric vessels is characterized by rapid onset of abdominal tenderness and distension associated with vomiting, shock, and later the passage of blood-tinged stool. Signs of peritoneal irritation ensue as transudation of fluid and bacteria into the peritoneal cavity occurs.

Prime candidates are the very elderly with advanced generalized arteriosclerosis, patients with thrombocytosis (postsplenectomy) or who are recuperating from operations upon the aorta or portal vein, and patients with recent fibrillation (often associated with mitral stenosis).

Physical examination reveals a distended abdomen with dullness to percussion and generalized tenderness, often with guarding and rebound. Bowel sounds are absent and rectal digital examination reveals bloody stool. Often a vague central abdominal mass is palpable. Plain flat and decubitus roentgenograms of the abdomen are not very helpful in the diagnosis.

Diagnosis and treatment are made at early laparotomy after nasogastric suction and rapidly administered supportive treatment in the form of intravenous fluids, electrolytes, blood, and antibiotics. Thrombectomy, embolectomy, endarterectomy, and arterial bypass are indicated if frank necrosis has not occurred, but generally the surgeon's efforts are limited to resection of frankly necrotic intestine. Prognosis is poor unless the length of infarcted intestine is short, or the occlusion can be corrected before bowel necrosis occurs.

"Abdominal angina" and *"postprandial intestinal angina"* are terms used to describe a clinical syndrome associated with gradually develop-

ing superior mesenteric artery insufficiency generally caused by atheromatous plaques. Intestinal ischemia follows the stimulus to intestinal secretion and activity provoked by ingesting a large meal. Retrograde aortic angiography demonstrates narrowing at the takeoff of the superior mesenteric artery from the abdominal aorta. Direct arterial reconstructive surgery relieves symptoms and may avert the later development of total occlusion.

Superior mesenteric artery syndrome

The superior mesenteric artery syndrome consists of obstruction of the distal duodenum where it is compressed by the superior mesenteric artery against the unyielding second lumbar vertebral body posteriorly. The obstruction may be acute, or chronic and intermittent. Epigastric distension and bilious vomiting parallel the degree and acuteness of the duodenal compression. Diagnosis is suggested by a very carefully performed barium upper gastrointestinal tract roentgen-ray series demonstrating a dilated stomach and duodenum with abrupt narrowing at the point where the duodenum crosses under the vessel. Normal small bowel is seen distal to this point. Differentiation from other types of duodenal obstructions (intrinsic stenotic membrane) is made at the time of laparotomy, and the obstruction is bypassed by a side-to-side duodenojejunal anastomosis.

Diverticula
Meckel's diverticulum

Meckel's diverticulum (Fig. 24-7) is the most common type of small bowel diverticulum, occurring in 2% of the general population. It represents a persistence of the atavistic structure known as the vitellointestinal tract (omphalomesenteric duct), which connects the distal ileum to the yolk sac early in embryonic life. The vitellointestinal tract normally obliterates and disappears entirely by the seventh week of gestation. Persistence of the entire tract is rare but is manifested early in life by drainage of ileal content at the umbilicus; diagnosis is confirmed by injecting the fistula with radiopaque material to show a connection with the distal ileum. If the lumen of the retained tract is obliterated, the anomaly presents as a fibrous cord between the ileum and the umbilicus; the diagnosis is made incidentally at laparotomy, or when small bowel obstruction occurs because of external compression by the fibrous cord.

The most common remnant of the vitellointestinal tract is persistence of its proximal end, known as Meckel's diverticulum. It is represented by a blind diverticulum situated on the antimesenteric border of ileum, which in the adult is located about 2 feet proximal to the

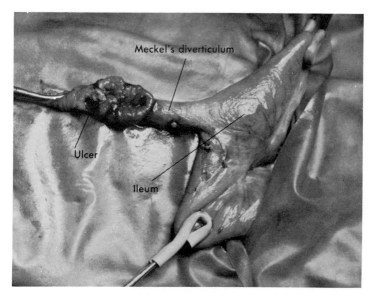

Fig. 24-7. Meckel's diverticulum opened to show bleeding peptic ulcer.

ileocecal valve. The majority of these common types are asymptomatic and are discovered incidentally at autopsy or laparotomy.

The symptoms of Meckel's diverticulum are produced by peptic ulceration, intussusception, or diverticulitis. About 50% of the symptomatic diverticula (and about 15% of all Meckel's diverticula) contain ectopic gastric mucosa that secretes hydrochloric acid directly upon unprotected adjacent ileal mucosa; peptic ulceration occurs with pain, bleeding, inflammation, or sometimes perforation. Dark red to tarry blood passed per rectum is the most common complaint prompting surgical consultation. The diverticulum may become inverted into the lumen of the ileum to provide the leading point of an ileoileal intussusception, with ultimate symptoms of intestinal obstruction and currant jelly type of bloody stools. Most Meckel's diverticula are wide necked and drain readily, but occasionally the neck is narrow with poor drainage of intestinal material producing primary diverticulitis.

The diagnosis of Meckel's diverticulum is virtually impossible by barium contrast roentgenograms. Abdominal scan after infusion of ^{99m}Tc may show a "hot spot" of uptake in Meckel's diverticulum, providing it contains functioning ectopic gastric mucosa. Asymptomatic Meckel's diverticula are discovered incidentally at exploratory laparotomy carried out for other purposes, and the symptomatic ones are found at laparotomy undertaken for symptoms produced by the various complications. Appendicitis is the most common presumptive diagnosis when pain, inflammation, and perforation are the presenting symptoms. Treatment is complete surgical excision.

Other small bowel diverticula

Diverticula of the small bowel unrelated to the viteollintestinal tract remnant usually arise from the mesenteric surface and are much more common in the duodenum than in the jejunum or ileum. Duodenal diverticula are said to be present in 6% of patients who have upper gastrointestinal tract barium studies performed, but they are present in about 20% of cadavers at autopsy. Duodenal diverticula commonly arise at our near the ampulla of Vater, are generally single, and are rarely symptomatic. They must be distinguished clinically from other and much more common, symptom-producing lesions of the pancreas, stomach, and biliary tract. Jejunal and ileal diverticula are likely to be multiple. Large diverticula may cause diarrhea, weight loss, and malabsorption-like states attributed to stagnation of contents producing inflammation, infection, and ulceration. Small bowel diverticula are diagnosed from barium roentgen-ray series as sacculations that readily fill with barium.

Symptomatic diverticula of the jejunum and ileum are uncommon, but they are treated surgically with ease by resection of the involved segment of the bowel. Duodenal diverticula are more frequent, less commonly symptomatic, and dangerous to approach surgically because of the relative inaccessibility of the duodenum. Resection or inversion of duodenal diverticula must be done with infinite care and meticulous dissection, with the common bile duct protected by cannulation when necessary. For these reasons, conservatism is the rule in the treatment of duodenal diverticula.

CHAPTER 25

The large intestine

RICHARD D. LIECHTY
CHARLES A. BUERK

Throughout the world, surgeons share a common respect for the colon and its septic contents. Intra-abdominal infections destroy suture lines; they may induce ileus, perforation, abscess, and fistulas, or progress to lethal peritonitis. To compound this problem, cancers of the colon and rectum, the *most common internal cancers* in humans, arise within this hostile environment. In contrast to the small bowel, in which both sepsis and cancer are uncommon, the large bowel teems with microorganisms and its mucosal cells can change into a variety of tumors.

Despite antibiotics, postoperative infections may occur after any operation on the colon. Understanding surgical management of colonic disease (especially surgical bypass procedures) requires a clear comprehension of the treacherous nature of the large bowel content.

Diseases of the large bowel are almost evenly divided between *neoplasms* (cancers and polyps) and *inflammations* (appendicitis, diverticulitis, ulcerative colitis). Since cancers can masquerade as infections (cecal cancer as appendicitis; sigmoid cancer as sigmoid diverticulitis), the surgeon must be prepared for either eventuality.

GENERAL PRINCIPLES

Sigmoidoscopy. The only indication required for performing a sigmoidoscopy is an *adult patient*. No adult physical examination is complete without one. Sigmoidoscopy discloses more potentially serious human health problems than any other routine diagnostic procedure.

The procedure is performed as follows:

1. Sigmoidoscopy may be performed in the Sims or jack-knife position or on a table folded at the hips.

2. A prepackaged enema 30 minutes before the examination provides a clean field. (If a patient has had a bowel movement within 2 to 3 hours, an enema is not always necessary.)

3. Constant reassurance by the examiner immensely aids relaxation and the ease of the examination.

4. Rectal examination followed by pressure from within the rectum toward the perineal body for several seconds relaxes the anal sphincters.

5. The scope is introduced and, under *direct vision,* advanced. After advancing as far as possible it is withdrawn slowly, and the entire bowel wall circumference is methodically scanned.

6. This procedure may be uncomfortable, but it should *never be painful!* One painful experience may, unfortunately, destroy a patient's enthusiasm for subsequent examinations. The lower 10 to 15 cm. (where roentgen-ray examination is the least accurate) is the most important area to be visualized. Painful (and dangerous) forcing of the sigmoidoscope beyond 10 to 15 cm. (where a natural curve often impedes progress) is indefensible.

Diagnostic value. About 60% of both polyps and carcinomas of the large intestine arise within reach of the sigmoidoscope (25 cm.). Sigmoidoscopy allows inspection of the mucosa, biopsy of suspicious growths, smear and culture of ulcers, and introduction of tubes to decompress the bowel. It is helpful in the diagnosis of benign and malignant neoplasms and inflammatory disorders that involve the distal large bowel. Endoscopy for diseases of the anal canal is discussed in the next chapter.

Colonoscopy. New fiberoptic colonoscopes permit visualization of the entire colon in up to 90% of patients and allow biopsy of larger lesions or removal of pedunculated, smaller ones.

Colonic bypass procedures. Colostomies divert the fecal stream through the abdominal wall and away from areas of the distal colon that are *obstructed, perforated, severely traumatized, infected* (diverticulitis), or the site of *difficult, tenuous anastomoses.* Note that in all these conditions *perforation* or *erosion* exists or threatens. Perforation of the colon engenders *continued contamination,* which may eventuate in generalized peritonitis and death. Colostomies are not done if resection and primary anastomosis of the lesion can be performed safely.

Three main options in designing colostomies are available (Fig. 25-1 and Table 25-1): (1) the *loop colostomy,* (2) the *divided limb colostomy,* and (3) *exteriorization* of the diseased portion of the colon.

Loop colostomy. Loop colostomies are technically simple procedures in which a segment of colon (usually transverse colon) is brought out through a small incision in the abdominal wall (Fig. 25-1, *A*). A small rod or tube under the loop supports it until healing takes place. If the

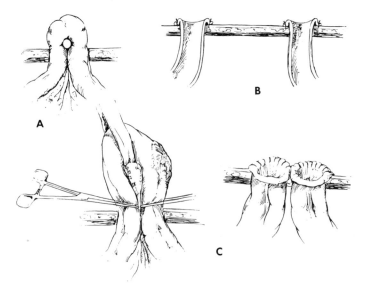

Fig. 25-1. Types of colostomies. **A,** Loop colostomy unopened. **B,** Divided limb colostomy. **C,** Exteriorization of the diseased portion of the colon; *left,* segment of colon with tumor is brought out through abdominal wall incision—specimen is removed above clamps; *right,* clamps are later removed—colon ends sutured to skin.

proximal portion is distended with gas, aspiration with a needle or a small rubber catheter will immediately decompress it. This is essentially a sterile procedure since the bowel lumen is not entered until the wound is closed. The exteriorized loop is opened in 24 or 48 hours. Although subsequent "spillover" may result, excessive gas pressure in the distal limb is immediately and permanently relieved. Loop colostomies should be considered temporary, with anticipated closure at a later date. Loop colostomy closure is technically simple.

Divided limb colostomy. Divided limb colostomies (Fig. 25-1, *B*) prevent "spillover" of fecal material, but since the colon must be divided, some operative contamination invariably results. With careful technique, however, contamination is minimized. The divided bowel ends are exteriorized through separate incisions. Divided limb colostomies require more dissection than loop colostomies, but the resultant proximal stoma is smaller, more esthetic, and easier to fit with a colostomy appliance. Divided limb colostomies are preferred when per-

Table 25-1. Comparison of types of colostomies

Type	Advantages	Disadvantages
Loop (proximal to lesion)	Sterile procedure; rapid and simple; easy closure	Fecal "spillover"; large cumbersome stoma; in perforations, feces in distal limb may continue peritoneal soilage; more stages to surgical treatment
Divided limb (proximal to lesion)	No fecal "spillover"; small stoma, easily cared for	Contaminated field; later colostomy closure is more difficult; technically more difficult; in perforations, feces in distal limb may continue peritoneal soilage; more stages to surgical treatment
Exteriorization of lesion itself	Well adapted to perforations (no fear of continued fecal contamination); double-barreled colostomies simplify closure; removed lesions allow histological diagnosis; fewer operations required	Technically often difficult; limited to mobile areas of colon; cancer operations are often compromised; double-barreled stoma is clumsy

manent fecal diversion is desired or when complete sterility of the distal limb is important.

Exteriorization procedures (Fig. 25-1, C). After the diseased colon is exteriorized, the remaining proximal and distal bowel ends can be brought out together as a *double-barreled colostomy,* or they can be divided and brought out separately. Closure of the colostomy is carried out later. The major disadvantage of exteriorization-resection is inadequacy of mesenteric lymph node dissection should the lesion be malignant.

INFLAMMATORY DISEASES
Appendicitis

For a full description of appendicitis, see Chapter 28. Some of the features associated with adult appendicitis are mentioned briefly here.

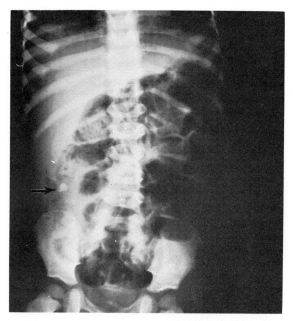

Fig. 25-2. Arrow marks fecalith in appendix.

Although appendicitis chiefly afflicts the young, no age is immune. The basic initiating factor in most adult appendicitis is *obstruction* secondary to a fecalith (Fig. 25-2), impacted within the appendiceal lumen. Obstruction of the left colon from carcinoma has been cited as a precipitating factor in adult appendicitis, presumably because of increased intraluminal pressure in the colon. Perforation of the appendix is less common in adults than in children. (It is most common below 2 years of age.) In the aged patient the response to appendicitis may be deceptively mild. In some older patients, for example, the white blood cell count and temperature remain normal with acute suppurative appendicitis. However, pain and tenderness are remarkably constant factors in appendicitis, regardless of the age. In the adult patient a fistula occurring after appendectomy should always suggest distal colonic obstruction. The obstruction must be relieved before the fistula will close.

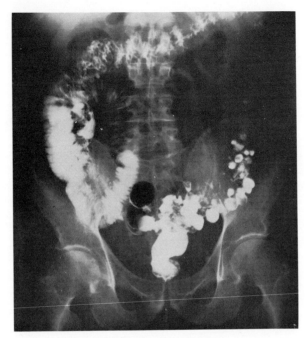

Fig. 25-3. Sigmoid diverticulitis. Globular collections of barium within diverticula.

Diverticulosis and diverticulitis

Incidence. Diverticulosis occurs in about one-third of all adults. (This incidence increases with age.) About one-sixth of all persons with diverticulosis will develop symptoms of diverticulitis. When operative treatment is required, one-third of all patients operated upon will have complications. Thus, diverticular disease is a common and serious surgical problem.

Site. Diverticulosis has a predilection for the sigmoid and distal descending colon (about 80% of patients) (Fig. 25-3). The reason for this relationship is not clear (firmer feces and increased pressure in the sigmoid loop may be important). Diverticula are usually (1) acquired and (2) appear where blood vessels penetrate the colonic wall. Since vessels normally course through the bowel wall in the mesenteric border and beneath appendices epiploicae, diverticula most commonly appear in these areas, although no part of the bowel wall is immune. Diverticula rarely occur in the rectum.

Epidemiology. Diverticulosis chiefly afflicts civilized societies. Lack of dietary roughage may play a leading role in causation. Other factors include: aging, obesity, genetic trait, and chronic constipation.

Pathology. Although the area of diverticulitis is usually less than 10 inches in length, it may extend to include the entire colon. Obstruction of the neck of the diverticulum (by feces or barium) initiates diverticulitis. Inflammation and consequent edema in the bowel wall may constrict adjacent diverticula, inducing "secondary diverticulitis." This process may continue as a chain reaction limited only by the extent of diverticulosis. Massive *lower* gastrointestinal bleeding (the most common cause is diverticulosis) results from anatomic proximity of the diverticulum and the blood vessel that accompanies it through the bowel wall.

The inflammatory process causes some degree of bowel narrowing and may progress to complete bowel obstruction that mimics carcinoma. Abscesses, fistulization to adjacent structures, or perforation often complicate the course of diverticulitis. Pericolitis and edema of the mesentery invariably accompany the inflammation. Muscular hypertrophy of the bowel wall usually coexists with the above findings. Most evidence points to this hypertrophy as secondary to the inflammation and not a primary cause of the diverticula.

Clinical course. Clinical signs and symptoms vary with the pathological stages and complications that have been described. Left lower quadrant pain, fever, and altered bowel habits (small caliber stools or diarrhea) are common. Symptoms of pyuria (frequency, dysuria, urgency) characterize fistulas to the bladder. A mass is sometimes palpable in the left lower quadrant or on pelvic or rectal examination.

Barium enema examination may show normal mucosa in the typically funnel-shaped constricted area, but this seldom, if ever, absolutely rules out carcinoma. (Some sigmoid cancers may also cause pain, fever, and a mass.) Sigmoidoscopy often helps to rule out cancer. Diverticulitis usually runs an intermittent course of remissions and exacerbations over periods of months or years, but we have seen acute perforation with *no* previous warning signs or symptoms.

Treatment. Medical treatment with bed rest, antibiotics, nasogastric suction, and sedation usually results in subsidence of all symptoms. Bulk-forming laxatives and bulky diets may help prevent progression of the disease. Surgical treatment (as in peptic ulcers, regional enteritis, and ulcerative colitis) is usually reserved for the *complications* of diverticulitis: *perforation, hemorrhage, fistulization, obstruc-*

tion, or *abscess formation.* With complete obstruction a three-stage plan is the safest treatment:

1. The obstruction is relieved by a *proximal colostomy.*
2. After the inflammation subsides (4 to 6 weeks), the *diseased segment is resected.*
3. After subsequent healing of the anastomosis, the *colostomy is closed* as the final stage.

With hemorrhage, the offending segment is resected or exteriorized. The surgeon should drain abscesses, but resect fistulous bowel loops (after protective colostomy). He later closes the colostomy after barium studies ensure an intact anastomosis. In uncomplicated cases (after the inflammation has subsided), most surgeons prefer single stage resection of the involved colon with primary anastomosis. Some surgeons advocate cutting the bowel musculature longitudinally to prevent recurring attacks; although limited, their results are encouraging.

Mucosal (ulcerative) colitis

Idiopathic ulcerative colitis, or *mucosal colitis,* is a strange disease of unknown etiology. Viral, bacterial, autoimmune, and various other theories of origin all lack verification. Marked psychological aberrations that almost universally accompany this disease have also been cited as causative, but again, no unequivocal evidence confirms these clinical observations.

Pathology. The pathological findings, most marked in the mucosa, feature inflammatory cells, ulcerated areas, and many small abscesses (Fig. 25-4). The submucosa is edematous with evidence of fibroplasia. The seromuscular layers show significantly little pathological reaction except in areas of perforation or abscess formation. The origin of ulcerative colitis lies clearly within the mucosal layer. The pathological findings vary with the clinical course. In the *fulminant variety* little mucosa remains, and the outer colon layers are edematous and infiltrated with inflammatory cells (Fig. 25-5). In the *chronic form* the colon is contracted, the mesentery fibrotic, shortened, and edematous. Ulcerations run in a longitudinal direction and may coalesce, leaving intervening islands of intact mucosa known as *pseudopolyps.*

In 80 to 90% of the cases the upper rectum is involved with or without retrograde involvement of the remainder of the colon. A "backwash" involvement of the terminal ileum occurs in about 10% of all cases of mucosal colitis.

Cancer is about 10 times more common in patients with chronic ulcerative colitis than in normal people; the longer the disease per-

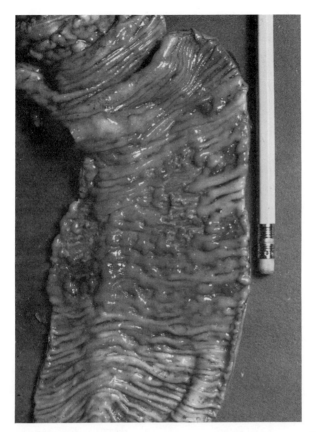

Fig. 25-4. Ulcerative colitis. Note shallow ulcers oriented longitudinally and areas of edematous mucosa.

sists, the greater the risk of cancer. Cancers associated with mucosal colitis have an extremely poor prognosis.

Clinical course. Chronic ulcerative colitis usually begins in young adulthood (20 to 30 years of age). The disease may be *fulminant* (toxic megacolon) or *chronic* with exacerbation and remissions recurring over a period of years. Bloody diarrhea with 10 to 30 stools per day, fever, abdominal cramps, weakness, and weight loss characterize *acute episodes*. In toxic or fulminating cases the symptoms progress

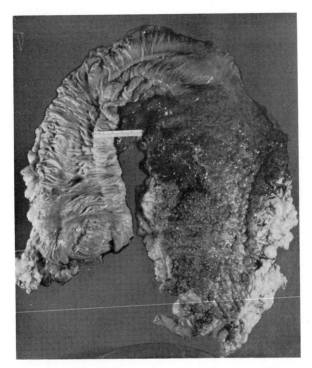

Fig. 25-5. Ulcerative colitis. Note diffuse involvement of half of the specimen; marked pseudopolyposis.

and the colon dilates, threatening perforation. Plain abdominal films show the immensely dilated colon. The periodicity of recurrences in the *chronic form* varies with each patient and the intensity of treatment. Barium enema studies show a contracted, shortened colon with loss of haustral markings—the typical "stove pipe" deformity (Fig. 25-6). Abnormalities of other organs such as uveitis, arthritis, stomatitis, cirrhosis, and biliary duct fibrosis accompany many chronic cases of mucosal colitis. The precise causal relationship of these associated ailments remains obscure.

The diagnosis of mucosal colitis is confirmed by (1) the course just described, (2) sigmoidoscopy, which shows a diffusely edematous, hyperemic mucosa, and (3) negative cultures and histology for specific diseases.

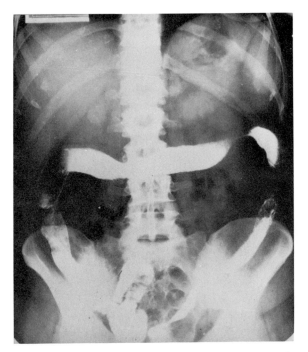

Fig. 25-6. Ulcerative colitis. Barium enema shows contraction, fore-shortening, ragged mucosa, and loss of haustral markings.

Treatment. As in other diseases of unknown etiology, the treatment is empiric. Rest, sedatives, bland diet, vitamins, fluids, Azulfidine, ACTH, and corticosteroids are temporarily effective in most cases. Over 30% (and up to 65%) of the cases will require eventual operative treatment in the following circumstances: (1) unremitting toxic megacolon, (2) massive hemorrhage, (3) fistulization, perforation, or abscess formation, (4) failure of medical treatment, and (5) when cancer is suspected. Note that all of these indications represent *complications* of mucosal colitis. Some surgeons favor a diverting ileostomy for the acute fulminant variety of mucosal colitis. Others resort to immediate abdominal colectomy and ileostomy. In the chronic form most surgeons, fearing cancer (that occurs at a rate of 4% per year after 10 years), recommend total proctocolectomy and ileostomy. Retention of the rectosigmoid segment with later anastomosis to the ileum has been generally disappointing because of recurrence of the proctitis.

Transmural colitis (granulomatous colitis, Crohn's disease) (see Chapter 24)

We know now that transmural colitis involves the colon in up to 50% of all cases previously thought to be exclusively mucosal colitis. Patients with transmural colitis have much the same symptoms as those with mucosal colitis, i.e., diarrhea, abdominal cramps, and fever. We cannot differentiate between the two diseases from symptoms, but we can get help from clinical findings as outlined in Table 25-2.

The symptoms of mucosal and transmural colitis are identical; the medical treatment is also the same. Why should we bother to distinguish them? Because a precise diagnosis helps the clinician to anticipate complications, including cancer, plan the operation, and justify radical procedures (total colectomy and ileostomy) when necessary.

Table 25-2. Comparison of mucosal and transmural colitis

Diagnostic features	Mucosal colitis	Transmural colitis
Preoperative findings		
Usual location	Rectum, left colon	Right colon, ileum
	Rectum involved about 100%	Rectum involved about 20%
Rectal bleeding	Common, continuous	Rare, intermittent
Fistulas	Rare	Common
Ulcers	Shaggy, irregular, continuous	Linear (cobblestone mucosa), patchy distribution
Colon shortening	Frequent	Extremely rare
Bowel stricture	Rare (suspect cancer)	Common
Carcinoma	Common (12% or more)	Rare
Segmental distribution	Never	Frequent
Toxic megacolon	Common	Rare
Bowel perforation	Common	Rare
Operative findings		
Serositis	Absent	Always
Inflammatory masses	Never	Frequent
Enlarged mesenteric lymph nodes	Infrequent	Usual

Diagnosis (See Table 25-2). These findings highlight the differential diagnosis. Mucosal colitis features grossly *bloody stools, rectal involvement* (in almost all patients), and occasionally episodes of *toxic megacolon* and *cancer* (12%). *Perianal and internal fistulas* and *bowel strictures* commonly accompany transmural colitis, but only rarely mucosal colitis.

Occasionally, under emergent conditions, the surgeon lacks adequate preoperative information to pinpoint the diagnosis. The appearance of the colon at the operative table almost invariably makes the diagnosis (Table 25-2).

Treatment. Transmural colitis responds more slowly to medical treatment and is less apt to undergo complete remission. It rarely evolves into the often lethal toxic megacolon and even more rarely into cancer. Therefore, the physician can treat strictures as such without the constant fear of cancer that bowel narrowing in mucosal colitis evokes.

Total colectomy with ileostomy usually cures the patient who has mucosal colitis; it removes the risk of cancer and allows only a slight chance of recurrent postoperative ileitis.

The tendency for transmural colitis to recur, often involving the small bowel (skip areas), complicates surgical therapy. Localized colon resections may suffice for limited areas of involvement, but total colonic involvement usually requires total colectomy. Involvement of the entire colon and the ileum portends a complicated, often recurrent form of the disease. Under these conditions conservative treatment must be tried as long as possible.

Specific infections
Pseudomembranous colitis

Pseudomembranous colitis is discussed in Chapter 24.

Amebiasis

Amebiasis of the colon is uncommonly seen in our country, with the exception of inmates in mental institutions. Amebic infiltrates have a predilection for the rectum and cecum. They may mimic carcinoma, or a diffuse amebic colitis may be confused with ulcerative colitis. Sigmoidoscopic examination with biopsies and stool cultures usually confirm the diagnosis. Emetine and other antiamebic drugs control most cases. Complications such as perforation necessitate surgical therapy.

Tuberculosis

Tuberculosis of the colon is almost always secondary to pulmonary tuberculosis. A primary form, probably of bovine origin, seldom arises in our country. The typical granulomatous nature of tuberculosis involves, in the large bowel, chiefly the cecum and right colon. Although the diagnosis can be suspected preoperatively, it is seldom confirmed except at operation. When obstruction occurs, resection of the involved portion of the large bowel may be necessary. Antituberculous drugs must be used to control the systemic infection.

Bacillary infections

Bacillary infections may be confused clinically with chronic ulcerative colitis. The sigmoidoscopic findings are also similar, but bacterial culture establishes the diagnosis of bacillary dysentery.

Actinomycosis

Actinomyces bovis is a rare cause of human intestinal disease, although it is a relatively common inhabitant of the gastrointestinal tract. Biopsy, cultures, or hanging-drop preparations usually reveal the diagnosis. Persistent (and confusing) abdominal wall fistulas may occur, sometimes months after an operation. Treatment with new penicillin preparations has been gratifying.

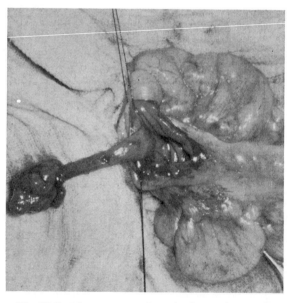

Fig. 25-7. Adenomatous polyp of colon on long stalk.

NEOPLASMS

Adenomatous polyps and adenocarcinoma are the most common tumors of the colerectum. Although polyps may bleed and occasionally cause bowel obstruction, their overwhelming significance resides in the possibility of associated malignancy.

Polyps

Polyps are sessile or pedunculated (Fig. 25-7). About 70% arise within range of the sigmoidoscope and most of the others are visible through the colonoscope. Barium studies, especially air contrast studies, outline most polyps in the upper colon (Fig. 25-8 and Table 25-3). Five chief types of polyps are seen: adenomatous, villous, juvenile, hereditary familial, and those associated with the Peutz-Jeghers syndrome.

Pseudopolyps

Pseudopolyps are discussed in the section on mucosal, or ulcerative, colitis, p. 366.

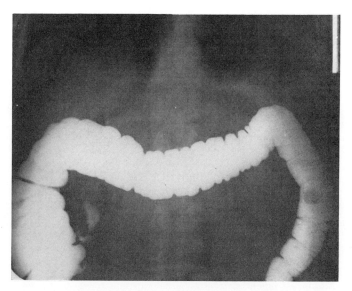

Fig. 25-8. Polyp of colon shows as filling defect on barium enema.

Table 25-3. Comparison of polyps of the large bowel

Type	Frequency	Site	Malignancy	Treatment
Adenomatous	Most common polyp; 10% of all adults; increases with age	Rectosigmoid 70%	Malignant potential is disputed	Endoscopy and biopsy excision; excise larger upper colonic polyps
Villous	Relatively common in the aged	Rectosigmoid 80%	About 25% malignant	Total biopsy; radical operation if malignant
Juvenile	Common in first decade; rare in adults	Chiefly rectum	Never	Excise only for bleeding, intussusception, diagnosis
Hereditary familial	Very rare	Scattered	100%	Total or near-total colectomy
Peutz-Jeghers	Very rare	Chiefly small bowel	Never (?)	Excise for bleeding or obstruction

Adenomatous polyps

Adenomatous polyps (polypoid adenomas, pedunculated polyps) are without question the most common polyps.

Age. Adenomatous polyps reach a peak incidence during the eighth decade. Below the age of 20 years they are nonexistent (except for genetically induced multiple polyposis). Adenomatous polyps are more common in males than females.

Site. About 70% of adenomatous polyps arise in the rectosigmoid area. A similar occurrence for carcinomas suggests, but does not prove, a causal relationship between adenomatous polyps and colorectal carcinoma.

Incidence. The incidence of adenomatous polyps varies with age. Clinical studies suggest that above 40 years, about 10% of patients have rectosigmoid polyps. Autopsy studies suggest a much higher incidence (20 to 50%). Multiple polyps (2 to 10 polyps) occur in about 30% of all patients with polyps.

Malignant potential. The potential for malignancy is the most important factor concerning polyps, and yet the most controversial. Advocates of the malignant potential of polyps cite as corroborative evidence the striking parallelism between polyps and cancer in (1) location, (2) age and sex incidence, (3) frequent association of polyps and cancer, and (4) the absolute 100% incidence of cancer with familial polyposis.

Contrary opinions based on continuing study of patients with untreated polyps, with polyps removed, and with no polyps cite an almost identical incidence of cancer in these three groups as proof that adenomatous polyps are *not* premalignant lesions.

Further study is necessary to clarify this important (adenomatous polyp–cancer) relationship. Until such studies are available, we are left with the conclusion that the concept of malignant *transformation* of adenomatous polyps is as yet *not* verifiable. General agreement exists that wide-based polyps and large (over 2 cm.) polyps are associated with an increased incidence of colorectal cancer. Polyps on stalks are considered to be relatively benign.

Treatment. *Sigmoidoscopic removal* of polyps is usually safely and simply accomplished. Wide-based rectal polyps are removed by transanal excision (after sphincter dilatation) and direct suture closure.

Colonoscopy has added a dramatic new dimension to upper colonic polypectomy (or biopsy). Experienced colonoscopists can reach the cecum in about 90% of all patients and they can successfully visualize (and biopsy or excise) an even larger percentage of polyps within the more distal colon. By preempting laparotomy, colonoscopy has made polypectomy safer for many patients and allowed biopsies of wide-based polyps that help select those lesions that require laparotomy and excision.

Laparotomy and polypectomy. For those patients with polyps that cannot be visualized, the physician must weigh the operative risk against the risk of cancer. Single, pedunculated, nonbleeding polyps (less than 2 cm. in diameter) can be periodically reevaluated, but wide-based, large (greater than 2 cm.) or suspicious polyps demand excision.

The student should realize that repeated diagnostic barium enema studies and endoscopy are time consuming, costly, and uncomfortable. For those patients who accept repeated examinations reluctantly or diffidently, laparotomy may prove to be the most prudent plan.

Villous adenomas

Villous adenomas (villous papilloma, villous tumor, papillary adenoma, and true papilloma) are velvety, broad-based tumors that may grow to encircle the bowel. About 80% reside in the rectum. In contrast to cancer, which they resemble visually, they are usually soft and pliable, so soft, in fact, that they can be missed by digital examination of the rectum.

Malignant potential. Although some surgeons look upon villous adenomas as malignant tumors, only 21% of 112 tumors in our recent experience have been malignant.

Treatment. Most villous adenomas (1) occur in older persons, (2) occur in the rectum, and (3) have broad bases (therefore, small biopsies are inconclusive). Combined abdominoperineal resection, which would be required for most of these rectal lesions, if malignant, carries an imposing mortality in aged patients. Therefore, *total biopsy* of the tumor with frozen section diagnosis of several cross sections of the tumor helps greatly to determine whether radical resection is necessary. If the lesion is benign, nothing more need be done; if malignant, a cancer operation is performed. In some critical risk patients focal cancer has been treated by such local resections alone—or cauterization—in deference to the forbidding mortality of radical operations.

In no instance has malignant recurrence followed total biopsy of benign tumors in our experience. In rare instances severe fluid and electrolyte problems have been caused by the copious diarrhea (mucorrhea) that these patients so frequently exhibit. Potassium loss is especially high. Large tumors can be removed by spreading the sphincters and by direct excision. Coccygectomy and posterior proctotomy help to expose lesions high in the rectum.

Juvenile polyps

Juvenile polyps are hamartomas, not true neoplasms. Grossly they are smooth, round, and cherry red and exude mucus when cut across; microscopically they are characterized by mucoid cystic spaces with a large amount of interstitial fibrous tissue. Generally single, they occur most frequently in the first decade of life, and tend to disappear spontaneously. Because of bleeding they may be a persistent nuisance. They rarely induce intussusception, and *malignancy never occurs* in juvenile polyps. Biopsy excision to control bleeding or to differentiate familial polyposis should be the extent of treatment. Indiscriminant radical colectomy for juvenile polyposis is a surgical tragedy. The polyps in a patient with multiple or scattered polyps will almost invariably share the same histology; thus, if the physician can prove microscopically that one accessible polyp is of the juvenile variety, he need not remove any of the others unless symptomatic.

Familial polyposis

Familial polyps will become malignant in 100% of the cases. A rare inheritable trait, the tendency can be transmitted by either parent. Most cases appear between the ages of 20 to 40 years subsequent to bleeding or diarrhea. In some cases the polyps number in the thousands and the diagnosis is obvious (Fig. 25-9). If less than 12 polyps are found, the diagnosis is highly questionable. Histologically these polyps are *adenomatous,* with a great variation in gross size.

Treatment. Either total removal of the rectum and colon (and ileostomy) or total colectomy with preservation of the rectum (and ileoproctostomy) must be done. The inexorable carcinomatous transformations in familial polyposis allow no other options. If the surgeon spares the rectal stump, he must reexamine every patient periodically and destroy all recurrent polyps.

After he diagnoses familial polyposis, the physician's responsibility includes surveillance of all other members of the family who might carry the inheritable trait.

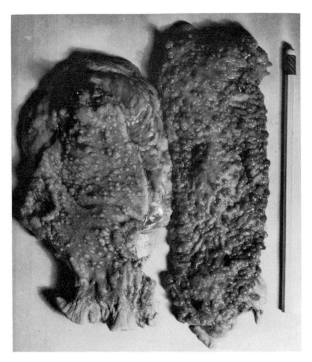

Fig. 25-9. Multiple polyposis of colon.

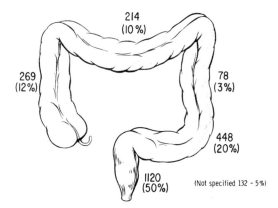

Fig. 25-10. Sites of 2,261 colorectal cancers at University of Iowa Hospitals, 1940 to 1960.

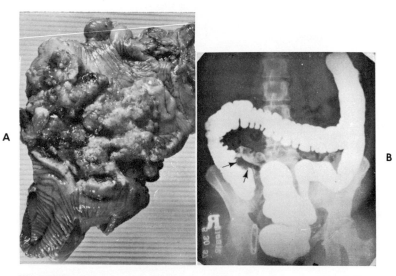

Fig. 25-11. A, Polypoid, ulcerating carcinoma of cecum. Distal ileum at left. **B,** Barium enema with arrows marking the filling defect of cecal carcinoma.

Peutz-Jeghers syndrome

Peutz-Jeghers syndrome is discussed in Chapter 24.

ADENOCARCINOMA

Adenocarcinoma of the colon and rectum runs slightly ahead of lung cancer as the most common killing cancer in humans. About 60% of these tumors lie within range of the sigmoidoscope; now that the colonoscope can reach the remaining 40%, diagnostic efficiency should improve (Fig. 25-10).

Epidemiology. Mortality rates for colorectal cancer are high in North America, western Europe, and Australia and in patients with ulcerative colitis or familial polyposis. Burkitt theorizes that low-fiber, high-sugar diets induce colon and rectal cancers.

Age. The relative incidence of colorectal cancer increases with age; 90% appear in patients past 40 years of age. Under 30 years of age, familial polyposis or ulcerative colitis often coexist. The prognosis in youthful cases (mostly mucoid carcinoma) is depressingly poor.

Symptoms. Alteration in bowel habits, blood in or with the stools, obstruction, and anemia keynote the symptoms. *Anemia* is most common with right colon lesions because the tumors are characteristically polypoid, and the ileal contents that bathe these tumors are caustic (Fig. 25-11, *A*). *Obstruction* predominates in left colon lesions because of a narrower lumen, firmer feces, and the characteristic annular and infiltrating lesions (Fig. 25-12, *A*).

Diagnosis. *Physical signs* are often scant. Masses are sometimes palpable, most often by rectal examination, and stools usually show blood, sometimes grossly, most often in the occult form. Endoscopy greatly aids early diagnosis.

Barium enema examination and *colonoscopy* help detect colonic cancers above the reach of the sigmoidoscope (Figs. 25-11, *B,* and 25-12, *B*).

Differential diagnosis. Since large polyps that resemble carcinomas should be removed (Fig. 25-13), they present few diagnostic problems. Distinguishing diverticulitis from cancer, usually in the sigmoid colon, is the major diagnostic problem. Even at laparotomy some cases defy diagnosis until the specimen is opened. (Cancers always involve mucosa; diverticulitis causes mucosal edema.) Since diverticulosis and cancer of the colon may coexist, preoperative barium studies seldom exclude carcinoma absolutely.

Tuberculosis and other infections and benign tumors (lipoma, fibroma, mucocele of the appendix, endometriosis) are, on rare occasions, mistaken for carcinoma of the colorectum. In all such cases, biopsy diagnosis must exclude colorectal cancer.

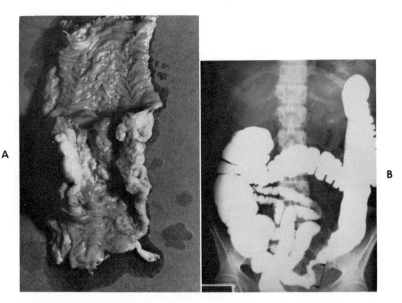

Fig. 25-12. A, Annular, constricting carcinoma of sigmoid colon. **B,** Barium enema outlining "apple core" defect of sigmoid carcinoma shown in **A.**

Metastases. Metastases from large bowel cancers spread in 6 ways: (1) intramural, (2) lymphatic, (3) venous, (4) implantation within the bowel lumen, (5) direct extension, and (6) transperitoneal. Most of these tumors are slow growing and metastasize late; thus *staging* of the disease is important in determining treatment and prognosis.

Duke's staging helps the surgeon to predict prognosis.

Duke's classification	*Extent of disease*	*5-yr. survival (%)*
A	Confined to bowel wall	80–90
B	Extension into pericolic tissues; nodes—negative	50
C	Involving adjacent structures; nodes—positive	20

Distant spread. With distant spread the cancer is incurable, but palliative resection often provides temporary symptomatic relief.

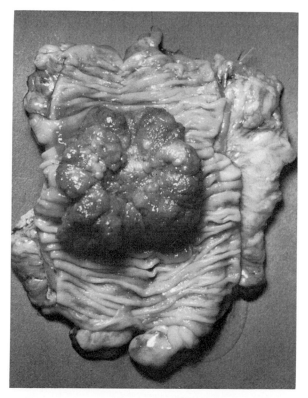

Fig. 25-13. Large polypoid carcinoma of the colon.

Significance of nodes. When regional nodes are negative for contained tumor, the 5-year survival rate is almost double the rate when nodes are involved.

Treatment. The aims of treatment of colorectal lesions are to remove the cancer, the areas of lymphatic spread, and areas of local extension (when such contiguous spread is limited). During these procedures early ligation of venous return and ligation of the bowel above and below the tumor help to prevent operative dissemination of cancer cells.

Operations are designed to remove the lymph-bearing tissue, yet

Table 25-4. Operations for colorectal carcinoma

Tumor site	Operation	Anastomosis or colostomy
1. Cecum Ascending colon	Right colectomy	Ileum to midtransverse colon
2. Hepatic flexure	Right and transverse colectomy	Ileum to midtransverse or left transverse colon
3. Transverse colon	Right, transverse, and upper left colectomy	Ileum to upper descending colon
4. Splenic flexure	Right, transverse, and upper left colectomy	Terminal ileum to descending colon
5. Descending colon Sigmoid colon	Left colectomy	Left transverse colon to rectosigmoid
6. Rectum	Left lower colectomy with low anastomosis or anal anastomosis; abdominoperineal resection	Descending colon to rectal stump; terminal sigmoid colostomy

permit sufficient vascularity of the remaining bowel to sustain the anastomosis.

Procedures are preceded by thorough cleansing of the bowel by (1) clear liquid diet, (2) laxatives, and (3) enemas. Some surgeons use preoperative antibiotics to sterilize the gut; others do not. All agree that thorough cleansing is the most important factor in preoperative preparation of the colon.

Operations for colorectal cancer vary according to the site of the cancer. With some individual differences the operations listed in Table 25-4 are commonly employed.

Prognosis. Results vary with age, extent of tumor, pathological type of tumor, location of tumor, the presence or absence of involved nodes, associated diseases (ulcerative colitis or familial polyposis), and the operation performed. A summation of the prognostic importance of these factors follows, highlighted (as in many other cancers) by the presence or absence of involved lymph nodes:

1. Without positive lymph nodes, the 5-year survival is about 60 to 65%; with positive lymph nodes, the 5-year survival is about 30%. In *all* cases the 5-year survival is about 40%.
2. Right colon cancers have a better prognosis than left colon cancers.
3. Women show a slightly better prognosis in all age groups.

4. Large bowel cancers in young people (below 40 years) have a poor prognosis.
5. Rectal cancers that originate *above* the peritoneal reflection have a better prognosis than those that originate *below* the peritoneal reflection.
6. Obstructing cancers of the colon have a more dismal prognosis than nonobstructing cancers.
7. If the colon is not removed in *familial polyposis,* almost all patients will develop cancer by 50 years of age.
8. Cancer associated with chronic mucosal colitis is especially vicious.

TRAUMA

Trauma to the large bowel may be *penetrating* or *blunt. Penetrating* wounds may occur from *outside* (knife wounds, missile wounds) or *inside* from objects inserted into the rectum (thermometers, sigmoidoscopes, enemas) or swallowed (safety pins, toothpicks, fish bones). *Blunt trauma* is most common from automobile accidents in civilian life and from blast injuries in combat military personnel. Improperly worn seat belts (which ride too high) can themselves induce intra-abdominal injury.

Diagnosis. The extent of *penetrating* wounds from the outside is usually indeterminant from examination of the wound. Probing small abdominal wall wounds is misleading, since contraction of the musculofascial layers overrides and obscures the original tract. Most penetrating abdominal injuries demand immediate laparotomy.

In all instances of abdominal trauma two serious threats arise: (1) *bleeding* and (2) *perforation.* If sufficient blood is lost (1,000 to 1,500 ml.), shock occurs. The bleeding vessel must be ligated. With losses of lesser amounts of blood, the findings are more subtle. In these instances, paracentesis or peritoneal lavage (500 to 1,000 cc. of balanced salt solution through a peritoneal dialysis catheter, then evacuated by placing the bottle on the floor) gives the most accurate information. Blood (above 100,000 RBC/cu. mm.), bile bacteria, or amylase indicates intraperitoneal disease.

Perforation is suggested by abdominal pain and tenderness (the "hot abdomen," discussed in Chapter 20). The diagnosis of perforation of a hollow viscus is not always easy, since trauma to the abdominal wall may induce both pain and tenderness within the wall itself.

Plain and upright films of the abdomen are helpful, since free peritoneal air is diagnostic of perforation of a hollow viscus. Negative films for free air, however, do *not* rule out perforation since small amounts of free air may be overlooked. Thus frequent, repetitive examinations, abdominal films, and peritoneal lavage form the core of successful management of the patient with possible intraperitoneal damage.

Treatment. When intraperitoneal hemorrhage or perforation is diagnosed, operative treatment must be immediate. In perforation, the elapsed time since the injury determines treatment. When the patient arrives soon (within 4 to 6 hours) after the wound, and peritoneal soilage is limited, simple closure of the wound may suffice. When the patient arrives late and peritoneal soilage is extensive, exteriorization of the damaged bowel segment (when possible), or a bypass colostomy with drainage of the contaminated area, is the preferred, and often the only possible, treatment. In penetrating wounds of the abdominal wall, when uncertainty exists concerning intraperitoneal damage, watchful waiting and diagnostic laparotomy are the two main therapeutic options. Laparotomy is, of course, the most certain plan, but under battlefield conditions or with multiple person injuries in civilian practice, the physician must sort out the patients who demand operation from those he can watch. In battle wounds, high-velocity missiles may damage a wide area about the wound because of shock waves. Wide debridement of the bowel wall before closure is necessary to prevent necrosis.

CHAPTER 26

The anorectum

SAMUEL D. PORTER
RICHARD D. LIECHTY

In terms of physical agony (from painful anorectal disorders) or mental anguish (from concern with bowel function or cancer) the anorectum assumes an importance that belies its insignificant anatomic status; e.g., hemorrhoids are one of the commonest of all human ailments. The pain from one small, thrombosed, external hemorrhoid can completely overwhelm an otherwise healthy person.

In our cancer-conscious generation, fresh blood on the toilet paper or a lump appearing at the anus sends patients trembling to their physicians, even though both signs often result from simple hemorrhoids.

The anorectum, the gatekeeper of defecation and the site of a variety of disorders (both simple and complex), is an area of understandable patient concern.

ANATOMY

Pertinent anatomic points are shown in Figs. 26-1 and 26-2:
1. The anatomic *key* to the anorectum is the *pectinate line*.
2. *Above it* pain sensation is absent, blood drains to the portal system and vena cava, and lymph drains along the superior rectal vessels or lateral to the obturator or iliac nodes.
3. *Below* the pectinate line pain is notably present, blood drains to the inferior vena cava, and lymph drains to the inguinal nodes.
4. *Anal glands* empty into anal crypts at the pectinate line. When obstructed or infected, these glands become the source of abscesses and fistulas.

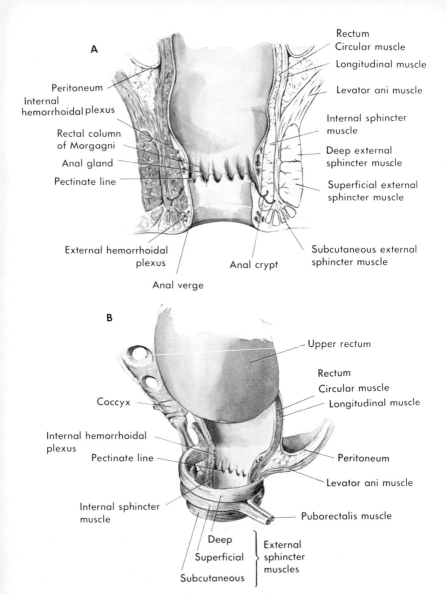

Fig. 26-1. A, Vertical section of anorectum. **B,** Anorectum. Three-dimensional diagram showing relationship of external sphincter to internal sphincter; note that superficial portion of external sphincter inserts into both coccyx and pubis.

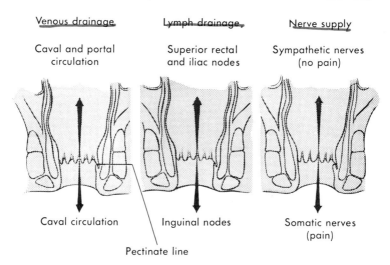

Venous drainage · Lymph drainage · Nerve supply

Caval and portal circulation · Superior rectal and iliac nodes · Sympathetic nerves (no pain)

Caval circulation · Inguinal nodes · Somatic nerves (pain)

Pectinate line

Fig. 26-2. The pectinate line marks important differences in nerve supply, venous drainage, and lymph drainage.

PHYSIOLOGY

When the rectosigmoid colon distends with feces, autonomic nerve impulses stimulate the colon to contract involuntarily, forcing the feces toward the anus. Voluntary relaxation of the tonically contracted puborectalis and external sphincter muscles permits this passage.

Chronic or injudicious use of laxatives thwarts this remarkably efficient mechanism by stimulating the colon when the rectum is *not* distended with feces. This process, repeated many times, results in temporary loss of the natural response. Thus, habitual laxative (or enema) use becomes physiologically disrupting in the vain effort to "regulate" (or coerce) bowel movements.

When laxatives liquefy the stool another disruption occurs. Normal stools (the consistency and shape of bananas) gently compress the anal canal, "milking" the anal glands and crypts. Chronically liquid stools lack this milking effect. Thus, liquid stools bathe the crypts and glands with bacteria; chronic cryptitis and anal gland infection result. The increased frequency of anal disease in patients who practice chronic self-purgation is, we are convinced, more than coincidental.

Regular bowel movements are obtained by a balanced diet, exercise, adequate fluid intake, and heed to nature's demands. Laxatives and

enemas for constipation in an otherwise healthy person should be
condemned for what they are—nostrums.

EXAMINATION

In no other area of the body is physical examination more important than in the anus and rectum. For complete examination, three
important factors are good illumination, proper positioning, and patient cooperation.

Inspection of the perinanal area can yield much information. Ex-
coriations from scratching (in pruritus), fissures, external fistulas,
external hemorrhoids, abscesses, and occasionally tumors can be seen.
Digital examination of the rectum should be an integral part of *all*
physical examinations except when preempted by pain (anal fissure).
In this situation the digital examination is performed with anesthesia
or is deferred until acute inflammation subsides. Sphincter tone, prostatic size, point tenderness, extrinsic or intrinsic rectal masses, pelvic
hernias, or a "rectal shelf" (tumor deposits in the cul-de-sac) is noted.
Remember that *up to 50% of all large bowel malignant tumors can
be palpated by rectal examination.* A specimen of stool from the examining finger is immediately available for testing for occult blood.
Anoscopy is carried out simply and without prior enemas. The
diseases of the anorectum that can be observed or palpated are discussed in the next section. (Sigmoidoscopy is discussed in Chapter 25.)

DISEASES OF THE ANORECTUM
Hemorrhoids

Internal hemorrhoids are dilated veins of the superior and middle
rectal plexuses that occur above the dentate line and underlie mucosa.
External hemorrhoids are dilated inferior rectal veins that lie below
the dentate line and are covered by squamous epithelium. Factors
that increase pressure in these venous systems are theoretically responsible for development of hemorrhoids. The common ones are constipation, straining at stool, hereditary varicose tendencies, pregnancy,
prolonged upright position, abdominal or pelvic tumors, and portal
hypertension. Chronic anal infection from colitis or ileitis, or chronic
laxative usage may also dilate the vein walls by causing chronic
cryptitis and anal vein phlebitis with consequent dilatation.

Bleeding, protrusion, dull *pain,* and *pruritus* (in any combination)
characterize uncomplicated hemorrhoids. Thrombosis or acute prolapse (with edema or ulceration) is exquisitely painful. Toxic symptoms may accompany acute episodes.

The diagnosis is usually obvious from inspection, but diagnostic
efforts must *always* include barium studies and sigmoidoscopy to rule

out other large bowel disease. Many patients with colon cancer have had hemorrhoidectomies *shortly before* the cancer was diagnosed.

Treatment. The three common indications for hemorrhoidectomy are *pain, prolapse,* and *bleeding.* Since most adults eventually develop hemorrhoids, excision is advised only when symptoms warrant the risk and inconvenience.

Treatment of an acutely thrombosed external hemorrhoid is incision and evacuation of the painful clot, followed by warm sitz baths. Small internal hemorrhoids may be injected with a sclerosing solution with good success. This promotes microthrombi formation and ultimate fibrosis of the hemorrhoid. Sodium morrhuate and 5% phenol in oil are commonly used solutions for injection. Rubber band ligation of internal hemorrhoids has also proved to be effective.

Larger external hemorrhoids and internal hemorrhoids, which are symptomatic, are surgically excised. The aims of all the various methods of hemorrhoid removal are the complete removal of the hemorrhoids with preservation of an intact, functional anus.

After hemorrhoidectomy an important problem is control of pain. Pain followed by perianal muscle spasm is responsible for many postoperative complications, such as urinary retention, constipation, fecal impaction, and pulmonary difficulties caused by immobilization. Pain is alleviated by warm, moist packs, adequate analgesia, and maintenance of a soft stool. Gentle daily digital dilatation for several days promotes normal healing and discourages stenosis.

Anal fissure

Anal fissures are slitlike ulcers in the anal mucosa. They are, of course, always infected. Commonest causes are (1) trauma, usually from passage of hard stool, (2) sequelae to cryptitis when the anal crypts become inflamed and subsequently develop a mucosal break that extends distally, and (3) ulceration of mucosa over a thrombosed hemorrhoid. Spasms of the anal sphincters (by decreasing blood flow) help sustain anal fissures.

These fissures occur most frequently in the posterior midline. A "sentinel tag," a small projection of skin, usually lies just below and marks the fissure.

Severe pain with defecation and blood-streaked stools characterize anal fissures. The anus is, of course, markedly sensitive to digital examination.

Anal fissures are treated conservatively by scrupulous anal hygiene, hot sitz baths, and stool softeners. If the fissure does not heal within 3 weeks, *sphincter dilatation* (under anesthesia), *fissurectomy,* and *partial sectioning* of the *internal sphincter* or the *external sphincter* (subcutaneous portion) are the operative options. These procedures used alone or in combination are advocated with varying degrees of enthusiasm. They have in common relaxation of the sphincter mechanism. We prefer excision of the fissure and division of the subcutaneous portion of the external sphincter. With sphincter muscle spasm relieved, stool passage is easier, which aids healing. Complicated fissures occasionally progress to abscesses, fistulas, or anal stenosis.

Anorectal abscesses and fistulas

Since fistulas are the end result of perianal abscesses, these diseases will be discussed together. *Perianal abscesses* almost invariably result from infected anal glands that erode into underlying tissues. Chronic use of purgatives, regional enteritis, and ulcerative colitis have liquid stools in common, as a probable causative factor. Uncommon infections (actinomycosis, tuberculosis, other fungal diseases), pelvic inflammatory disease, prostatitis, and cancer may rarely be associated.

Fig. 26-3 shows the common locations of these abscesses. Opinions vary as to frequency of occurrence in various anatomic sites. In our experience the ischiorectal abscess is the commonest.

Early symptoms of dull rectal aching and mild systemic complaints progress to severe, throbbing perianal pain with fever, chills, and malaise. A fluctuant, "pointing" area is not always apparent because

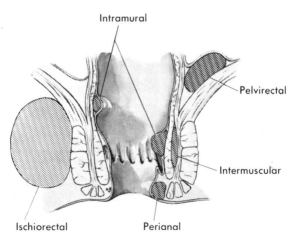

Intramural

Pelvirectal

Intermuscular

Ischiorectal   Perianal

Fig. 26-3. Location of pelvirectal and perirectal abscesses. Infections in anal crypts are the usual source.

of the thick perianal skin. Redness, tenderness, and a generalized bulging are the usual findings. Prompt incision and drainage *without* waiting for fluctuation (as in other subcutaneous infections) can prevent serious extensions. We have seen mutilating extensions that involved thighs, scrotum, and even the abdominal wall. Because of severe pain, general or regional anesthesia is preferable, but some surgeons drain perirectal abscesses under local anesthesia.

Supralevator abscesses. Supralevator abscesses are uncommon. Anal gland infections and pelvic or intraperitoneal infections engender these abscesses.

Intramural abscesses. Intramural abscesses cause little discomfort since the bowel wall has no pain sensation. They are drained through a sigmoidoscope. Pelvirectal abscesses are drained through the skin. Drains are always brought out through *external* incisions.

Perirectal fistulas. Probably three out of four perirectal abscesses, after drainage, eventually heal with no sequelae. But those that fail to heal primarily evolve into fistulas. The external opening may close temporarily only to recur when pus accumulates in the tract and eventually the tract becomes lined with epithelium. Multiple openings ("pepper pot anus") may occur in complicated cases. Extensions to the urinary tract, perineal area, thighs, or bone may occasionally occur.

Usually the fistulous tract follows a variable course, but a few general rules are available for simplification:

1. The primary or internal opening is usually found in one of the anal crypts.
2. Most lie at one side or the other of the posterior midline.
3. If the cutaneous opening is anterior to a *transverse* line drawn through the anus, the internal opening is on a radial directly into the anorectum. If the cutaneous opening is posterior to the line, the internal opening will probably be in the posterior midline (Fig. 26-4, *A*).

Symptoms are usually confined to intermittent swelling, drainage, pruritus, and varying discomfort. The history of an abscess is of obvious help in the diagnosis.

The cutaneous opening is characteristically a slightly raised, gray-pink papule of granulation tissue. In time scarring along the tract becomes palpable. A probe can sometimes be passed through the fistula and observed at the pectinate line. This is ordinarily not painful. Common courses of anal fistulas are shown in Fig. 26-4, *B*.

Simple, early fistulas are incised with saucerization (excision of the overhanging margins) of the tract. In severely scarred fistulas, excision of the tract, leaving the skin open, is the best method of removal. In either case the internal opening must be obliterated or the fistula

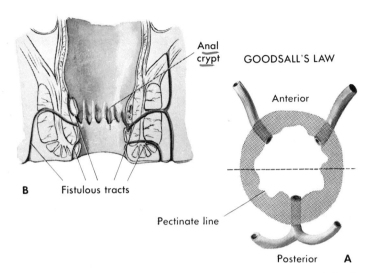

Fig. 26-4. A, Anorectal fistulas. The location of the external fistulous opening is a key to the position of the internal opening. **B,** Common courses of anorectal fistulous tracts. Internal (primary) opening is almost always in a crypt; fistulas are usually single and involve only portions of the sphincter muscles; multiple fistulas or fistulas that involve all the external sphincter muscles are less common.

will recur. If the fistula follows a course that necessitates cutting of the sphincter, the incision must traverse the muscle fibers perpendicularly and *at only one level;* none of the muscle should be removed.

If the fistula is the result of carcinoma, tuberculosis, Crohn's disease, or mucosal colitis, the primary disease must, of course receive treatment priority. Most surgeons are extremely reluctant to perform anorectal operations on patients with mucosal colitis or Crohn's disease because of local recurrence with failure of wound healing.

Pruritus ani

Pruritus ani, intense itching of the perianal area, is a symptom, not a disease. Common and frequently debilitating, it offers a constant therapeutic challenge. A busy general paractitioner will see numerous patients every month with this complaint.

A classification of etiological factors is listed below:

Surgical: Hemorrhoids, fissures, fistulas, prolapse, cryptitis, neoplasm

Nonsurgical:

> *Local:* Dermatitis, bacterial, fungal, contact; pinworms, antibiotic irritation
>
> *Systemic:* Jaundice, diabetes, psoriasis, syphilis, seborrheic dermatitis, leukemia
>
> *Idiopathic:* Including psychophysiological

With such a broad spectrum of causes, the necessity for cultures and other pertinent laboratory tests is obvious.

Treatment. Underlying anatomic factors are treated surgically (fissures, fistulas, hemorrhoids, or neoplasm). Similarly, in systemic conditions, like diabetes or jaundice or with local irritants and infestations, such as antibiotics or pinworms, the offending cause is specifically treated. "Smothering" symptoms with local treatments (for specific disorders) is as foolish as treating a brain tumor headache with aspirin.

Even after extensive search a cause of pruritus ani often cannot be found. *Idiopathic pruritus* accounts for approximately half of the patients seen. The single common denominator in all patients with this complaint is feces being excreted through the anus and thus, perianal fecal irritation. Immaculate perianal hygiene is therefore imperative for effective relief of the itching. The perianal area should be washed with water and dried with cotton or a soft cotton cloth. Cornstarch applications help to keep the area dry. Hydrocortisone ointment, 1%, is nonspecific, but usually helpful. Anxiety states are associated in many patients.

Subcutaneous alcohol injections, radiation therapy, and presacral neurectomy are heroic treatments reserved for a very few, truly intractable patients with pruritus ani.

Prolapse of the rectum

The three types of rectal prolapse (Fig. 26-5) are: (1) mucosal prolapse, (2) rectal intussusception, and (3) true prolapse.

Mucosal prolapse (Fig. 26-5, *B*) occurs with an intact sphincter and involves extrusion through the anus of *rectal mucosa* only. The remainder of the wall is not involved. It becomes symptomatic because of irritation and, occasionally, ulceration of the prolapsed tissue. Soiling results from mucosal secretions. This condition is common in infancy (theoretically because of the lack of sacral curvature) and in the aged. Infant prolapse almost invariably disappears by 5 years of age. In the adult, radial incisions, similar to hemorrhoidectomy incisions, result in scarring, which holds redundant mucosa in place.

Rectal intussusception (Fig. 26-5, *C*) involves protrusion of the entire rectal wall, without a peritoneal sac. It starts above the pec-

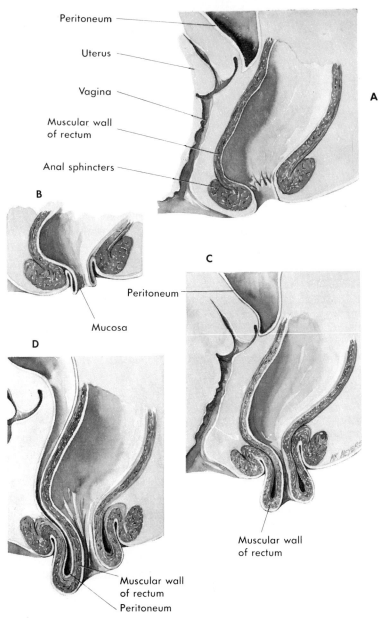

Peritoneum

Uterus

Vagina

Muscular wall
of rectum

Anal sphincters

B

Mucosa

C

Peritoneum

D

Muscular wall
of rectum

Peritoneum

Muscular wall
of rectum

A

Fig. 26-5. For legend see opposite page.

Table 26-1. Venereal diseases *that affect anorectal region :*

Type	Cause	Diagnosis	Treatment
1. Lymphopathia venereum	Virus	Frei test; biopsy	Noneffective
2. Condyloma acuminatum	Virus	Biopsy; multiple warts	Podophyllin (25%)
3. Syphilis	Spirochetes	Biopsy; dark-field examination	Penicillin
4. Gonorrhea	Bacteria	Smear; intracellular diplococci	Penicillin

tinate line. The palpable full-thickness wall in the prolapsed portion and concentric folds distinguish it from mucosal prolapse. A sulcus can be palpated along the periphery of the prolapsed part of the anal ring that is *not* present in true prolapse.

True prolapse (Fig. 26-5, *D*) occurs by herniation of the pelvic peritoneum through the pelvic diaphragm, the anterior rectal wall, and the anus. The anal sphincter tone is poor. This type occurs mainly in infants, men in their twenties or thirties, and women at any age. In men it probably represents a congenital weakness because the prostate and seminal vesicles lend adequate support anteriorly to prevent this.

Several operations have been devised for correction of intussusception and true prolapse, and, as is usually the case when several operations are used for a particular condition, all leave something to be desired. The operations that give the best results utilize: obliteration of the peritoneal sac, shortening and fixation of the rectosigmoid colon, and approximating the levator ani muscles.

Specific infections

Specific infections of the anorectum are uncommon, yet must be remembered when sinus tracts, ulcers, or tumors appear that defy the usual categorization or treatment. The venereal diseases listed in Table 26-1 may be the offenders in such instances.

Fig. 26-5. Rectal prolapse. **A,** Normal. **B,** Mucosal prolapse most common type of prolapse; mucosa shows radial folds. **C,** Rectal intussusception; all layers of rectal wall prolapse—peritoneum does not. **D,** True prolapse; all layers of rectal wall prolapse; peritoneum descends as a hernial sac anteriorly. Both **C** and **D** show concentric folds from accordionlike effect of mucosa that has not been depicted.

Anorectal tumors

Basal cell carcinomas and *melanoma* of the anus are curiosities treated by wide excision (as in other parts of the body) with or without preoperative irradiation.

Epidermoid carcinoma of the anus occurs in the elderly, is associated with chronic infection (an excellent reason for biopsy of chronic lesions), and metastasizes to pelvic and inguinal nodes. (Inguinal nodes are also involved with anal infections.) Radical abdominoperineal resection with resection of involved inguinal lymph nodes (or, in low, early lesions, conservative resection) appears to offer about the same 5-year survivals as rectal adenocarcinoma.

Pilonidal sinus   *in ♂ more*

Although not arising from the anorectum, pilonidal disease often enters the differential diagnosis of anorectal diseases; it can mimic anorectal abscesses or fistulas.

As the name suggests, a nidus of hair is almost invariably found within these sinus tracts. Almost all of the hairs enter the sinus *root end first*. Hair scales pointing away from the root end (like feathers on an arrow) apparently are driven inward by a rolling action between the buttocks. Hair *follicles* or other skin appendages are *never* found within the sinus walls. These lesions occur in the intergluteal region of young hirsute males, and less commonly in females. Pilonidal disease is common in young military personnel. It almost never occurs in persons 45 years of age or older. An analogous pilonidal sinus occasionally afflicts the hands of barbers by indriven hairs.

Infection with rupture through the skin (which forms sinuses), chronicity, and recurrence keynote the problem. Simple incision and drainage of infected cysts and excision with open healing of chronic sinuses have evolved, since World War II, as the most prudent treatment. Excision with primary closure is preferred by some surgeons.

CHAPTER 27

Abdominal hernia

ROBERT T. SOPER

A *hernia* is an abnormal protrusion of an organ or tissue through an aperture, or opening. Thus the brain may herniate through the foramen magnum, or the lung through a thoracotomy incision. Usually, however, the word is restricted to describe an abdominal hernia, i.e., an abnormal opening in the abdominal wall through which protrusion of intra-abdominal viscera occurs.

Hernial apertures, or openings, generally represent defects in the musculofascial tissues surrounding and supporting the abdominal cavity. These defects may be congenital or acquired. A pouch of peritoneum (the hernial sac) pushes through the fascial defect (the hernial ring) and then, because of continuity with the intra-abdominal cavity, abdominal contents enter this sac. The neck of the hernia sac is that portion protruding through the musculofascial defect and defining its narrowest dimension. The omentum, small bowel, large bowel, stomach, and urinary bladder are the most common organs that herniate into hernia sacs in roughly descending frequency.

The anatomic location of a hernia is a convenient method of identification or classification. The following is a list of the more common hernias according to *location:*

Inguinal (indirect or direct)	Femoral
Umbilical (infantile or adult)	Epigastric
Incisional (postoperative, ventral)	Pelvic
Diaphragmatic (congenital or hiatal)	Lumbar

The status of the contents of the hernial sac is of extreme clinical importance and is defined by the following descriptive adjectives:

1. A *reducible hernia* is one in which the organs contained within the hernia sac can be returned to the abdominal cavity.

397

2. In an *irreducible hernia* the hernia sac contents cannot be returned to the abdominal cavity without operative reduction.
3. The term *incarcerated hernia* (Fig. 27-1, *B*) is used synonymously with irreducible. Neither of these terms implies intestinal obstruction or vascular interference.
4. A *strangulated hernia* is one in which the blood supply to the herniated viscus is occluded. Infarction of the viscus occurs if surgical reduction is not promptly carried out. If intestine is involved, obstruction is generally present. A strangulated hernia is generally irreducible or incarcerated, but an irreducible hernia is generally *not* strangulated.

Further definitions might clarify for the student certain points about hernias:

A *ventral* hernia is one that occurs through the ventral abdominal wall and generally includes umbilical, epigastric, and incisional hernias.

An *incisional* hernia is one that occurs through an incisional wound that fails to heal completely. Thus, an incisional hernia is also a ventral hernia only if the incision is made through the ventral abdominal wall.

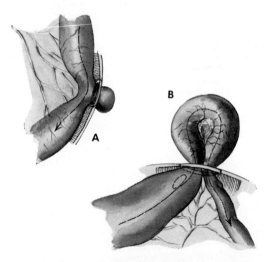

Fig. 27-1. A, Richter's hernia. Only a portion of bowel passes through hernial ring; arrow indicates that bowel need not be obstructed mechanically even with strangulation. **B,** Incarcerated hernia. Distended bowel in hernia cannot return to abdomen through narrow fascial defect.

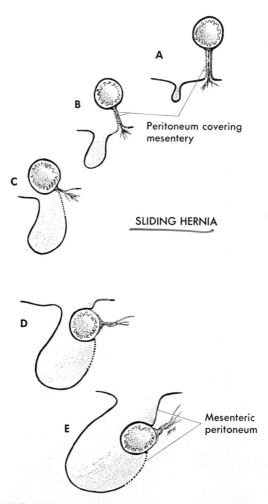

A

B

Peritoneum covering
mesentery

C

SLIDING HERNIA

D

E

Mesenteric
peritoneum

Fig. 27-2. Sliding hernia. Simple hernia evolves in **A** and **B**. It begins to
"slide" with one mesenteric leaf in **C** and the bowel itself in **D**. In its
final evolution in step **E,** the bowel and both mesenteric leaves are part
of the hernial sac.

Richter's hernia (Fig. 27-1, *A*) is herniation of only a part of the circumference of bowel through a fascial defect; it is especially dangerous because strangulation can occur *without* complete mechanical intestinal obstruction. It is most commonly found in femoral hernias because of the small size and sharp and relatively inflexible nature of the fascial ring in this area.

Littre's hernia appears to be similar to Richter's hernia, but it should be restricted to the herniation of Meckel's diverticulum through a fascial ring.

A *sliding* hernia (Fig. 27-2) is one in which a portion of the sac of a hernia is made up of the herniating viscus itself. Its importance lies in the fact that attempts at surgical removal of the entire sac will, of course, remove or injure the viscus which is "sliding." The most common sliding hernias involve the bladder in direct inguinal hernias, the sigmoid colon in left indirect inguinal hernias, and the cecum in right indirect inguinal hernias.

INGUINAL HERNIA

The surgical treatment of inguinal hernia is the most common major operation performed in the United States (Table 27-1). In-

Table 27-1. Inguinofemoral hernias

	Femoral	*Indirect inguinal*	*Direct inguinal*
Age at onset	Young to middle-aged adult	Infant, child, young adult	Middle to old age
Sex	Female > male	Male 20:1	Almost always male
Cause	? congenital	Congenital (*indir*)	Wear and tear (*direct*)
Incidence	Uncommon	Most common	Second most common
Origin	Femoral canal	Internal inguinal ring	Hesselbach's triangle
Neck size	Small, rigid	Small to medium	Large
Course of sac	Variable	Oblique to scrotum	Local protrusion
Incarceration	Common	15 to 20%	Rare
Strangulation	Common	5 to 10%	Hardly ever
Sliding	Rare	Common if long-standing; right-cecum, left-sigmoid	Common (bladder)
Treatment	Always surgical	Always surgical	Surgical if symptomatic

guinal hernias are 20 times as common in males as in females because of the defect in the abdominal wall occasioned by descent of the testis into the scrotum in the male and also perhaps because of the protection to the inside of the lower ventral abdominal wall afforded by the uterus in females.

Inguinal hernias are of two types: indirect and direct. The fascial defect in an indirect inguinal hernia (Fig. 27-3) lies lateral to the inferior deep epigastric artery, and the defect in the direct hernia (Fig. 27-4) lies medial to this structure. Usually the indirect type has a preformed or congenital sac, occurs in the infant to young adult male, and is more symptomatic and more prone to develop complications; in contrast, the direct inguinal hernia is much less common, is seen in the elderly male as part of the "wear and tear" process of aging, almost never becomes complicated by strangulation, is generally less symptomatic, and is almost unheard of in the female. The distinction between the two is perhaps academic in the good-risk patient, since both should be corrected surgically at an elective time. However, in the poor-risk elderly patient the distinction between the two becomes important in selecting the appropriate treatment; a low-risk direct hernia in a high-risk patient might better be treated by a well-fitted truss or other conservative methods.

Etiology. Most indirect inguinal hernias arise because of retention or imperfect obliteration of the embryological outpocketing of perito-

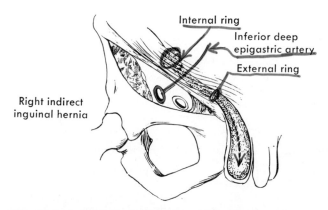

Fig. 27-3. Right indirect inguinal hernia. Hernial sac begins at the internal inguinal ring lateral to the inferior deep epigastric artery, and exits from the inguinal canal at the external ring to descend into the scrotum. The sac lies anteromedial to the cord structures.

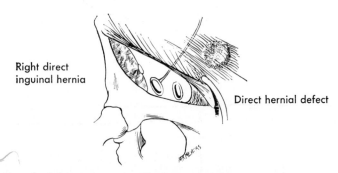

Right direct
inguinal hernia

Direct hernial defect

Fig. 27-4. Right direct inguinal hernia. Hernial sac arises in Hesselbach's triangle medial to the inferior deep epigastric artery and just above the pubic tubercle. It does not descend into the scrotum.

neum accompanying testicular descent into the scrotum known as the *processus vaginalis.* The testis originates along the urogenital ridge in the retroperitoneum and migrates caudad during the second trimester of pregnancy to arrive at the internal inguinal (abdominal) ring at about the sixth month of intrauterine life. During the last trimester it proceeds through the abdominal wall via the inguinal canal and descends into the scrotum, the right slightly later than the left. The processus vaginalis then normally obliterates postnatally except for that portion surrounding and serving as a covering for the testicle (tunica vaginalis). Failure of this obliterative process results in an indirect inguinal hernia at birth or during the first few months or years of life (coincident with the highest age peak of incidence of this hernia). The incidence then diminishes to rise again in young adult males. Herniation at this latter age probably results from the stress of muscular activity and the increase in intra-abdominal pressure forcing open a previously imperfectly obliterated processus vaginalis. Indirect inguinal hernias seldom arise after the age of 40, to underscore the importance of this congenital, or preformed, sac in its genesis.

A hydrocele is an unobliterated processus vaginalis in which the communication with the peritoneal cavity is large enough to allow peritoneal fluid to enter but not large enough to admit bowel. About 15% of inguinal hernias in infants and children are preceded by a hydrocele, but the vast majority of hydroceles in the very young disappear spontaneously as the continuing obliterative process closes off the peritoneal connection. Hydroceles do not require treatment unless they persist into childhood; surgical treatment involves simply division and ligation of the communicating tract.

Diagnosis. Early complaints of indirect inguinal hernia include a bulge or swelling in the groin that appears only when the patient strains, cries, or assumes an upright position and that disappears when reclining. Commonly the budge is associated with a nagging, dull discomfort locally. Occasionally forceful straining or lifting precipitates an acute hernia, heralded by sudden groin discomfort and a bulge in the area. With time, the groin bulge increases in size and pursues an oblique course from the internal inguinal ring downward and medially along the course of the inguinal canal, and when it descends to the bottom of the scrotum it becomes a *complete* hernia.

Physical examination is the key to diagnosis. Demonstration of an oblong swelling in the groin that appears with pressure and extends downward and medially into the scrotum, disappearing in a reverse direction upon assuming the supine position, is the classic finding. Inversion of scrotal skin by the examining index finger confirms that the external (subcutaneous) inguinal ring has been dilated by the hernia. Asking the patient to cough or strain (cough impulse) will bring down the bowel or the end of the sac against the end of the examining finger. After an indirect inguinal hernia has been completely reduced, finger pressure over the internal (abdominal) inguinal ring (located 1 cm. superior to the midpoint of a line drawn from the anterosuperior iliac spine to the pubic tubercle) prevents recurrence unless a direct hernia coexists (so-called *pantaloon* hernia).

Treatment. Indirect inguinal hernias should be repaired surgically unless specific contraindications exist because of the discomfort that they evoke, certainty that once established they will persist and even become larger with time, and the constant threat of complications of the hernia developing. In the infant and young child, adequate surgical treatment (Fig. 27-5) consists of simple division of the sac with high ligation of the sac neck. There is usually no need for fascial reconstruction since the basic defect is retention of the sac itself rather than a deficiency of the supporting musculoaponeurotic structures. The distal sac can be left in situ as normal cord and testicular coverings.

In the older child or young adult, division and closure of the neck of the sac are caried out after reduction of the herniated viscera. In addition, the abdominal ring (aperture in the transversalis fascia) is snugged up closely around the carefully identified (and undamaged) cord structures over the top of the ligated sac. In those hernias that, through neglect, have grown to enormous proportions, destroying a good part of the supporting transversalis fascia and displacing the inferior deep epigastric vessels medially, a more extensive fascial repair

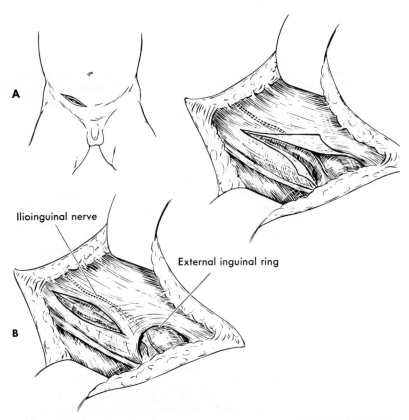

Fig. 27-5. Repair of right indirect inguinal hernia in infant. **A,** Groin-crease skin incision. **B,** Incision in external oblique aponeurosis exposes hernia and cord structures; ilioinguinal nerve should be protected. **C,** Hernial sac has been separated from cord structures and divided, and the contents have been reduced; suture-ligature is closing neck of the sac.

is necessitated after the sac has been ligated. Reattachment of the fresh superior edge of transversalis fascia to Cooper's ligament and the prefemoral fascia (McVay operation) is one of the more popular operations designed to restore the integrity of the musculoaponeurotic support. Recurrence of the hernia is seen in only 1 to 2% of the smaller hernias of infancy and childhood and in up to 5% of the very large hernias of adulthood.

Complications. Acute incarceration of a previously reducible hernia is associated with local pain and, if not reduced promptly, may produce edema and increased pressure at the narrowed sac neck with strangulation of the herniated viscera. Acute incarceration sometimes heralds the onset of the inguinal hernia, especially in the infant and young child. Nonoperative reduction may be attempted, provided that the irreducibility is only a few hours in duration and there is no localized tenderness, redness, or signs of intestinal obstruction to suggest early strangulation. To accomplish mechanical reduction, the patient should be placed in the supine position with the hips flexed and the foot of the bed elevated; a sedative or analgesic agent will help produce relaxation, after which gentle pressure over the hernia is applied.

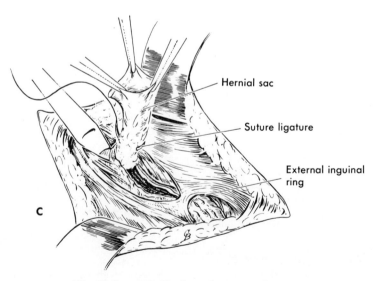

Fig. 27-5, cont'd. For legend see opposite page.

If gentle attempts at manual reduction are unsuccessful, or if there is any suggestion of early strangulation, surgical correction of the hernia must be carried out as an emergency. The techniques of repair are the same, namely: opening of the sac, careful inspection of the herniated viscera to assure their viability, following which they are reduced into the intraperitoneal cavity, high ligation and division of the sac neck, and fascial repair if indicated.

A long-standing hernia often becomes less completely reducible and ultimately may be completely irreducible or incarcerated. A chronically incarcerated hernia is not likely to be symptomatic, nor does it carry the threat of immediate strangulation. It often indicates that the hernia is really a sliding hernia (Fig. 27-2) rather than the more common nonsliding type. Surgical repair of a sliding hernia is more complicated in that complete sac dissection and division and closure of the sac neck are impossible because a portion of the sac wall itself is composed of the sliding viscus. Only that portion of the sac not made up of viscus can be excised, and the entire remaining sac and its sliding viscus must then be reduced en masse; repair of the musculoaponeurotic supporting tissue can then be made superficial to the sac to prevent its recurrence. The morbidity, mortality, and recurrence rates after surgical repair of a sliding hernia are all higher than with a nonsliding hernia, and justify early hernia repair before the sliding hernia has time to develop.

Strangulated hernia

A hernia is more likely to strangulate if it has a capacious sac with a rather narrow sac neck surrounded by a rigid and unyielding fascial ring. Pressure at the ring first slows venous return, producing stasis and edema, thereby ensuring irreducibility. An inflammatory response adds to the vicious cycle and culminates with impedance of arterial inflow to the strangulated viscus with necrosis and gangrene. Small intestine is the most commonly strangulated viscus and is, of course, associated with mechanical intestinal obstruction at this point. Delay of surgical repair by attempts at forceful reduction will further traumatize the friable viscus, often resulting in perforation and spreading peritonitis. Surgical treatment should be undertaken promptly with resection of the strangulated organ, followed by anatomic repair of the hernia. The morbidity, mortality, and recurrence rates after strangulated hernias are understandably higher than for nonstrangulated types.

Direct inguinal hernia

Direct inguinal hernia (Fig. 27-4) is only about one-fifth as common as the indirect counterpart, originates after the age of 40, and is (almost) never seen in the female. The bulge is medial to the inguinal canal just above the pubic tubercle and is likely to be circular and diffuse, rather than distinct and elongated as is the bulge in the indirect variety. The fascial edges are indistinct in keeping with its origin as a gradual and diffuse weakening of the fascia transversalis in Hesselbach's triangle, associated with aging and increasing intra-abdominal pressure from coughing (asthma), straining to micturate (prostatism), obesity, constipation, and nutritional defects. This very fact, however, is the reason direct inguinal hernias, although uncomfortable, rarely become complicated by incarceration. As they get larger, the bladder commonly "slides" into the medial edge of the direct hernia sac, a factor that must be remembered at the time of surgical repair.

On physical examination the distinction between the indirect and direct hernias is not difficult. When the examining finger is placed through the external (subcutaneous) ring and then directed posteriorly, the weakness in the fascia transversalis forming the floor of the inguinal canal is the most distinctive finding. After reduction, finger pressure over the internal (abdominal) ring does not prevent a direct hernia from appearing immediately when the patient strains or stands. Direct hernia sacs have no direct relationship to the testicular cord structures, nor do they commonly descend into the scrotum. In view of the low complication rate, a direct inguinal hernia may be conservatively treated in the high-risk, debilitated patient. A well-fitted truss, although cumbersome, can relieve the symptoms.

The more expedient treatment consists of surgical repair. Direct inguinal hernia sacs are simply reduced and the defect in the floor of the inguinal canal repaired by bringing down the strong superior margin of fascia transversalis and reattaching it by suture to Cooper's ligament medially and to the prefemoral fascia laterally (McVay repair). Recurrence rates are twice as high as with indirect hernias.

FEMORAL HERNIA

A femoral hernia (Fig. 27-6) is one that occurs through an enlarged femoral ring, the medialmost compartment of the femoral canal. The femoral canal lies below the inguinal (Poupart's) ligament and above the pubic bone and is bounded medially by the rather unyielding lacunar ligament. The contents of the femoral canal from lateral to medial spell out the word *nave* (standing for femoral *n*erve, *a*rtery, *v*ein, *e*mpty space). It is through this empty space that a femoral hernia occurs.

Femoral hernias occur more commonly in women than in men and are probably acquired rather than congenital. The narrowness of the

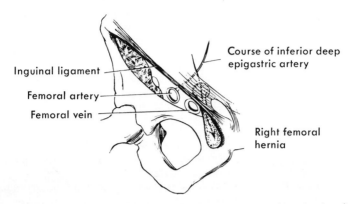

Inguinal ligament

Femoral artery

Femoral vein

Course of inferior deep epigastric artery

Right femoral hernia

Fig. 27-6. Right femoral hernia. Hernial sac arises below the inguinal ligament and medial to the femoral vein.

sac neck and the rigidity of its boundaries predispose to the high incidence of irreducibility, strangulation (up to 20%), and Richter's type of strangulated hernia (Fig. 27-1, *A*). It is understandable why symptoms occur earlier and why prompt surgical treatment should be carried out more urgently than with inguinal hernia.

Initially the bulge of a femoral hernia lies below the inguinal (Poupart's) ligament medial to the femoral arterial pulse. However, as the sac enlarges with time, it is likely to turn upward anterior to the inguinal (Poupart's) ligament and then present as an inguinal swelling difficult to distinguish from an indirect inguinal hernia. Careful inspection will often reveal that its neck is located low and that reduction occurs in a different direction from the indirect inguinal hernia.

Surgical repair is the only recommended treatment for femoral hernia, preferably undertaken before complications occur. The surgical approach is through the same skin incision (inguinal crease) as that used for the two more common types of inguinal hernias, and the essentials of repair are the same, namely, opening of the sac, reduction of the herniated contents, ligation and high closure of the sac neck, and reattachment of the fascia transversalis to Cooper's ligament to close off completely the empty space in the femoral canal without compromising the femoral vein.

Table 27-1 compares and contrasts the three varieties of inguino-femoral hernias.

Differential diagnosis of inguinofemoral masses

The three types of inguinofemoral hernias (direct inguinal, indirect inguinal, and femoral) can often be distinguished from among themselves on careful physical examination, and they *must* be distinguished carefully from other disorders that produce swelling in the same general area. A few of the more common considerations in differential diagnosis of inguinofemoral masses are discussed briefly:

1. *Hydrocele* of the cord and/or testis (pp. 402 and 470) is distinguished from indirect inguinal hernia by the fact that it cannot be quickly reduced, is not attended by discomfort, transilluminates brilliantly, and often is associated with a thickening of the cord structures above the hydrocele.

2. *Undescended testis:* Careful palpation of the scrotal sac should make the diagnosis of cryptorchidism clear. When the testicle is within the inguinal canal, it is palpated as a firm mass that cannot be brought down by traction to within the scrotum; this distinguishes it from simply a high-riding or retractile testicle that, with gentleness, persistence, and often exposure to warm water, can be brought down into the scrotum and is not truly undescended. Cryptorchidism is almost invariably associated with an indirect inguinal hernia that, in itself, commonly justifies early surgical treatment of the hernia and concomitant replacement of the testicle within the scrotum.

3. *Inguinal lymphadenitis:* Enlarged inguinofemoral lymph nodes generally are multiple rather than solitary and are sometimes tender. The site of infection within the extremity resulting in the inguinal node enlargement should be apparent on examination. The nodes do not reduce nor transmit a cough impulse.

4. *Varix of upper greater saphenous vein:* A localized varix or thin-walled enlargement of the proximal portion of the greater saphenous vein presents as a soft swelling below the inguinal ligament that is commonly confused with femoral hernia. It is generally associated with varicosities of the rest of the saphenous system. It transmits a cough impulse that is felt in the remainder of the dilated vein, and percussion of the veins transmits a percussion thrill to the varix to distinguish this clearly from femoral hernia. The varix swelling promptly disappears when the patient is recumbent.

5. *Lipoma of the cord:* A lipoma surrounding the cord structures is difficult to distinguish from indirect inguinal hernia. It occasionally is associated with a hernia and constitutes part of the inguinal canal swelling. Lipoma of the cord is not reducible, is not painful, and does not transmit a cough impulse.

UMBILICAL HERNIA

There are three general types of umbilical hernia that differ markedly in causation, prognosis, and treatment: omphalocele, infantile hernia, and adult hernia (Table 27-2).

An *omphalocele* is not a true hernia because its covering is made up of amniotic sac, it has no true inner peritoneal lining or skin covering its outer surface; it really represents a failure of the extra-coelomic midgut to return to the peritoneal cavity after the tenth to twelfth week of intrauterine existence (p. 442). The prognosis of an omphalocele is grave because of its propensity to rupture, a high incidence of associated congenital anomalies elsewhere, and extreme difficulty in reducing the herniated viscera even at operation. Surgical treatment is aimed at excising the sac and closing the abdominal wall in layers, when the contents can be reduced without tension and the defect in the abdominal wall is not large. If these two features are absent, the sac is simply covered by surgically undermined skin of the abdominal wall; this maneuver converts an omphalocele into a large infantile umbilical hernia, and more definitive surgical reduction and repair can then be carried out at a later date. Recently, a sheet of Dacron-reinforced Silastic has been sutured to the edges of the defect to temporarily cover the exposed viscera, allowing staged reduction of the viscera and skin closure.

Infantile umbilical hernia is very common, occurring in upwards of 5% of Caucasian infants and 20% of Negro infants. The incidence is higher among premature than among term infants. It represents protrusion of a hernia sac through an aperture created when the um-

Table 27-2. Umbilical hernias

	Omphalocele	*Infantile*	*Adult*
Age at onset	Newborn (premature)	Newborn (premature)	Middle to elderly
Sex	Equal	Female > male	Female > male
Race	None	Negro > Caucasian	None
Incidence	Rare	Very common	Common
Cause	Congenital	Congenital	Wear and tear
Skin cover	None	Intact	Intact
Other anomalies	Frequent	Average	Average
Neck size	Large	Small to large	Often small
Incarceration	Rare	Rare	Frequent
Strangulation	Rare	Rare	Frequent
Treatment	Surgical	Observe	Surgical

bilical vessels thrombose and rapidly involute at the time of delivery. Because the infantile type of umbilical hernia never becomes complicated by incarceration or strangulation, and almost always disappears spontaneously by the seventh year of life, the indications for surgical repair are few. Trusses do not speed up the involution of an umbilical hernia and may even entrap and irritate herniated intestine; their use is therefore discouraged. In the occasional case that is symptomatic, or so large as to predispose to external trauma, surgical repair is indicated.

The *adult type of umbilical hernia* occurs more commonly in the obese and multiparous female. It originates through a dilated and weakened umbilical ring or through a weak spot in the linea alba just above the umbilicus. Adult hernias in this region are dangerous because, like the femoral hernias, the neck remains small and unyielding in spite of often a very capacious hernia sac. This results in a high incidence of incarceration and strangulation, a feature that demands early surgical repair.

The surgical treatment of umbilical hernias is carried out through a curving infraumbilical incision; the sac is opened, the contents reduced, and the neck of the sac closed flush with the entrance into the abdominal cavity. The fascia surrounding the resultant defect is then brought together and often overlapped (imbricated) for a 2-layer repair.

EPIGASTRIC HERNIA

Epigastric hernias occur in the linea alba between the xiphoid process and the umbilicus. These hernias are probably initiated by the protrusion of properitoneal fat through apertures created by perforating vessels, which then gradually enlarge with continuing stress (a rise in intra-abdominal pressure) to allow a peritoneal sac to protrude. They cause local pain and tenderness, even though small in size, and are generally seen in middle-aged men doing manual labor. The pain can mimic other types of intra-abdominal surgical disease that must be ruled out before elective hernia repair is undertaken. The repair consists of excision and closure of the sac and repair of the defect in the fascia.

INCISIONAL HERNIA

An incisional hernia is one that occurs through an old operative incision in the abdominal wall that has partially dehisced. Incisional hernias develop more commonly in vertical than in transverse incisions and in patients with poor wound healing, *postoperative wound infections,* or with conditions causing increased intra-abdominal pressure.

Poor wound healing may occur because of faulty surgical technique (placement of sutures too close to the edges being apposed, use of too small or too large suture material, knots tied so tightly as to necrose abdominal wall layers, knots becoming untied, or interruption of a running suture that then unravels for the length of the incision). Hematomas and infections of the wound produce delayed and imperfect healing; foreign bodies brought through the wound (drains, catheters) prevent sound approximation of wound edges and are associated with a high incidence of herniation. Postoperative cough, distension, and hiccups all markedly elevate intra-abdominal pressure and place undue strain upon the sutures, which may then give way to initiate an incisional hernia.

The symptoms are those of a variable-sized swelling in an old incision line, generally attended by only mild symptoms of local discomfort. Incarceration is fairly common, but strangulation is rare because of the large size of the sac neck.

Treatment is generally surgical, although satisfactory control of the moderate-sized hernias can be afforded by girdles or trusses for the poor-risk patient. Small and symptomatic hernias should be repaired surgically because of danger of strangulation, and the large and diffuse ones should be repaired because of failure of control by binders or girdles. In the large hernias with attenuated fascia, fascial grafts and prosthetic replacement to bridge gaps in the fascia are commonly necessary.

INTERNAL HERNIA

Internal hernia is the name given to the herniation of intestine through an aperture (natural or acquired) within the abdominal cavity. Thus, small bowel herniation through the foramen of Winslow into the lesser sac would be termed an internal hernia. There are recesses in the paraduodenal and paracecal areas in which internal hernias may occur. Postoperative adhesions may form an aperture through which an internal hernia occurs.

Internal hernias are dangerous because they may remain undiagnosed until complications of intestinal obstruction or strangulation occur that necessitate emergency surgical exploration. Treatment is directed at relieving the obstruction or strangulation by appropriate means and then closing the aperture through which the herniation occurred.

RARE EXTERNAL HERNIAS
Lumbar hernia

Most lumbar hernias are really incisional hernias occurring in old nephrectomy incisions. However, occasionally they occur spontaneously either just above the iliac crest posteriorly or just below the twelfth rib. The hernias generally remain reducible, do not tend to strangulate, and can usually be controlled by a corset or belt.

Obturator hernia

A hernia may accompany the obturator vessels and nerve into the thigh via the obturator foramen. Obturator hernias are uncommon at any age but more often occur in elderly women. Obturator hernias an be diagnosed by a swelling in the upper and medial aspect of the thigh associated with pain radiating to the medial aspect of the knee, aggravated by sudden increases in intra-abdominal pressure but not by hip or knee movements. Hypesthesia in the area of pain radiation indicates irritation of the sensory component of the obturator nerve. The neck of the sac is often palpable on vaginal or rectal pelvic examination. Strangulation and incarceration are common, and the morbidity-mortality rate remains high because of delay in diagnosis. Treatment is reduction of the viscera at the time of exploratory laparotomy with closure of the peritoneum over the aperture.

Sciatic hernia

Sciatic hernias can occur either through the greater or the lesser sciatic notches to present as bulges inferior to the gluteus maximus muscle. They become symptomatic either by producing intestinal obstruction or by pain that has a sciatic nerve distribution.

Spigelian hernia

A spigelian hernia sac, by definition, originates at the junction of the semilunar and semicircular lines just lateral to the rectus muscle in its lower one quarter. As the hernia sac enlarges, it may track from this location interstitially in almost any direction to present a most puzzling clinical picture. Strangulation may occur.

Respiratory diaphragm hernias

The respiratory diaphragm separates the thoracic from the abdominal cavity and is breached by the esophagus, the aorta, and the major veins of the caval and portal systems. It is an extremely important muscular organ that assists in respiratory efforts and can remarkably affect pressures within the thoracic and abdominal cavities and vessels. It is formed embryologically by peripheral muscularization and the septum transversum. Hernias occur either through apertures resulting from imperfect development (congenital) or are acquired by increases in intra-abdominal pressure, rupturing weakened points, or enlarging the preexistent apertures.

Congenital diaphragmatic hernia is one of the true surgical emergencies of the newborn period of life; 70% occur through the left posterolateral foramen of Bochdalek, and 20% occur through a similar defect on the right side—presumably the tamponade effect of the liver on the right side accounts for this difference in incidence. Most Bochdalek hernias have no sac. Since the aperture in the diaphragm occurs early during intrauterine life, before rotation of the midgut has occurred, it is commonly associated with malrotation; for the same reason, the involved lung is frequently immature and incapable of immediate normal expansion after surgical correction.

Rapid respiratory decompensation demands urgency in diagnosis and treatment of congenital diaphragmatic hernia. The sequential pathophysiology is as follows: the intestine rapidly fills with swallowed

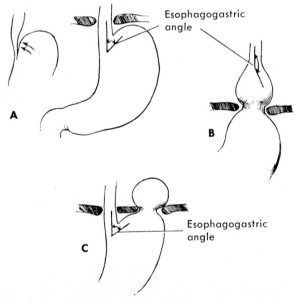

Fig. 27-7. A, Normal relationship of stomach and esophagus to diaphragm; acute esophagogastric angle helps prevent reflux from stomach into esophagus (inset). **B,** "Sliding" type of esophageal hiatus hernia; esophagogastric junction above diaphragm; obtuse esophagogastric angle favors reflux. **C,** Paraesophageal hiatus hernia; esophagogastric angle is normal, and no reflux into esophagus occurs.

air postnatally, which expands the size of the herniated viscera in the chest, producing progressive mediastinal shift to the contralateral side with interference in respiratory exchange in the normal lung and impedance of venous return to the heart. The diagnosis is established by a plain upright radiograph demonstrating gas-filled loops of bowel in the chest with a contralateral mediastinal shift. Emergency endotracheal intubation and assisted respiration temporarily stabilize the child. Nasogastric suction halts the lethal ingress of swallowed air prior to early surgical reduction of the abdominal viscera from the chest and suture approximation of the edges of the defect in the diaphragm.

Acquired diaphragmatic hernias (Fig. 27-7) generally involve the stomach, herniating either through an enlarged esophageal hiatus (the sliding type of esophageal hiatal hernia) or through a defect in the diaphragm just lateral to the diaphragmatic crura encircling the esophagus (paraesophageal or parahiatal type). The sliding hiatal hernia is many times more common than the paraesophageal; since it increases the acute esophagogastric angle, there is free reflux of stomach contents into the esophagus to produce the outstanding symptoms of esophagitis: regurgitation, heartburn, mild bleeding, and later scarring with stricture formation and dysphagia. Hiatal hernias are

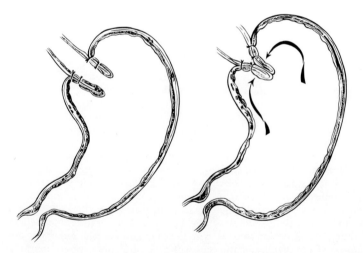

Fig. 27-8. Fundoplication. Left: gastric fundus is wrapped around lower esophagus. Right: when stomach fills, pressure closes the gastroesophageal junction, preventing reflux.

seen either in infants or in middle-aged to elderly patients with obesity and increased intra-abdominal pressure for one reason or another. The symptoms are aggravated by lying down and improved by sitting up. Often an acid-peptic diathesis is associated.

Treatment is tailored to the severity of symptoms and the patient's general operative risk status. Hiatus hernias that are small and only mildly symptomatic or that occur in very poor-risk patients can be satisfactorily managed by restricting the patient to an upright position postprandially, elevating the head of the bed while sleeping and introducing an antacid medical regimen. Reduction of body weight and other factors that reduce intra-abdominal pressure also assist in the treatment program. Hiatus hernias that are large, progressively more symptomatic, or associated with complications of ulceration, bleeding, or stenosis should be treated surgically: the stomach is pulled down below the diaphragm, and usually the hiatal aperture is closed around the esophagus. Usually some sort of antireflux operation is then performed (Fig. 27-8) to further discourage gastroesophageal reflux. If acid-peptic diathesis is present or if the patient has an actual peptic ulcer, vagotomy and an appropriate emptying procedure are commonly added. The poor-risk patient who must be treated surgically because of complications can be improved by simple suture fixation of the reduced stomach to the anterior abdominal wall.

The less common parahiatal diaphragmatic hernias produce symptoms of vague epigastric and lower anterior chest pain aggravated by increases in intra-abdominal pressure and recumbency. Since the esophagogastric junction is undisturbed, none of the symptoms of esophagitis are present. Complications include ulceration and bleeding within the herniated stomach, incarceration and strangulation, and progressive enlargement until most of the stomach is intrathoracic (giving an "upside down" radiographic appearance to the stomach).

Treatment principles are similar to those of the sliding type of hiatal hernia: surgical reduction and repair of the aperture in the diaphragm.

Indirect or direct trauma to the diaphragm may produce tears or weaknesses through which hernias develop. These are almost always on the left side because of the protection afforded by the liver to the right side of the diaphragm. Respiratory and gastrointestinal symptoms coexist, and the diagnosis is confirmed by plain films of the chest as well as barium studies of the upper and lower intestine demonstrating loops of intestine within the thorax. Surgical reduction and closure of the diaphragmatic rent will prevent complications (intestinal obstruction, strangulation, atelectasis).

CHAPTER 28

Pediatric surgery

ROBERT T. SOPER

Twenty-five years ago, medical (infectious) disorders accounted for most hospitalizations and deaths of children in this country. However, today 60% of hospitalized children have diseases with surgical overtones and, of all surgical patients, one-fourth are children. Since there are approximately 70 million people under 14 years of age in the United States, these figures have staggering logistic and professional implications. Surgical disease in children is becoming more important for two reasons: (1) antibiotics, immunizations, and good medical care have dramatically decreased the infectious diseases that were responsible for most hospitalizations and deaths of children a quarter-century ago, and (2) new drugs, instruments, and better training now allow routine correction of abnormalities hitherto considered inoperable, with open heart surgery being a prime example.

Ill infants and children cannot be treated as small adults. There are enough differences in the etiology, course, and pathophysiology of disease in the very young to adequately justify special consideration and training. The obvious problems imposed by the small size of the patient, his different maintenance requirements, inability to give a history, and the magnitude of certain corrective operations all add to the need for a chapter devoted to the very young surgical patient.

THE NEONATAL SURGICAL PATIENT

The newborn infant epitomizes the profound differences that exist between the adult and the very young surgical patient. These differences become less striking and important as the patient grows into adolescence. About 0.5% of live born babies require emergency neonatal surgery, generally on account of congenital anomalies obstructing flow through one of the vital body conduits (food through the G.I. tract, air through the trachea, CSF through the central nervous system, blood through the heart or major vessels).

In the following ways newborns tolerate operations surprisingly well:

1. The body systems that have developed correctly function remarkably well, despite measurable anatomic and physiological evidence of immaturity. The cardiovascular system is perhaps the outstanding example: the heart muscle is hypertrophied at birth because during gestation it pumps 20 to 30% more blood (through the placental circuit) than the postnatal circulatory volume. The heart therefore possesses relatively more functional reserve at birth than it will have later.

2. The newborn infant enjoys a higher relative circulating blood volume than he will have subsequently because of (a) return of extra blood to the fetus from the placenta at the time of delivery and (b) relative to size, the newborn has 50% more extracellular fluid, part of which is blood, than does the adult.

3. The newborn's blood has a higher oxygen-carrying capacity than it will have later, with hemoglobin and hematocrit levels often 50% higher than those in adults. A relative hypoxemia in the fetus (from inefficient transport of oxygen across the placental barrier) stimulates fetal blood production. Increased tolerance to hypoxemia is carried over into the neonatal period.

A strong heart pump, hypervolemia, and a high oxygen-carrying capacity of the blood combine to make the newborn a relatively good operative risk.

Fluid therapy. The newborn contains 10 to 15% more total body water relative to weight than does the older child or adult. This excess fluid is soon lost as urine. It dictates the low maintenance fluid requirement of 50 ml./kg. for the first day, which progressively rises to 100 ml./kg./day by the end of the first week of life. Thus the daily maintenance fluid of the week-old infant is three to four times that of the adult when calculated per unit of body weight. These requirements must be computed carefully on the basis of body weight, surface area, or calories expended.

One of the simpler methods for calculating daily maintenance fluid requirements for children is as follows: about 100 ml./day is needed for each of the first 10 kg. of body weight, about 50 ml./day for each of the second 10 kg. (from 10 to 20 kg. body weight), and about 20 ml./day for each kg. above 20 kg. body weight. The average adult requires about 30 ml./kg./day.

Another method of calculating daily maintenance fluid is on the basis of body surface area. Surface area is expressed in square meters ($M.^2$) and is calculated from a nomogram using the patient's body length (height) in centimeters and body weight in kilograms. Daily fluid for maintenance normally is 1,500 ml./$M.^2$ of body surface area, a figure that does not vary with age. Representative body surface areas for babies of given body weights are as follows:

Body weight (kg.)	Body surface area ($M.^2$)
1.8	0.15
2.7	0.2
4	0.25
5	0.29
8	0.4
10	0.5
20	0.8
30	1

The fluid that I prefer for maintenance purposes when parenteral feedings are required is N/5 saline in 5% dextrose solution. This solution contains 30 mEq. of NaCl per liter. To this is added KCl, 20 mEq./L. after adequate urinary output is assured.

Parenteral (intravenous method is preferred) fluids must be calculated precisely for volume and content and should be given at a rather steady rate over the entire 24-hour period. Unusual body fluid loss such as vomiting, diarrhea, nasogastric suction, and sequestered body fluids must be measured or estimated accurately and added to maintenance requirements. Hyperthermia or exposure to a dry environment increases fluid requirements. Oral feedings are self-regulated.

A newborn infant weighing 3 kg. has a total circulating blood volume of roughly 250 ml. Blood loss in the relatively modest amount of 25 ml. (less than 1 ounce) constitutes a significant hemorrhage that proportionately in the adult would approach 600 ml.

Environment. The newborn infant is much more sensitive to environmental temperature and humidity than is the adult because (1) he has almost three times the amount of skin exposed to the environment in relation to weight and (2) he has a meager insulating blanket of subcutaneous fat. The neonatal surgical patient must be nursed in an incubator. Advantages gained from the incubator include:

1. Humidification of the air to nearly 100% to reduce insensible fluid loss.
2. Oxygenation of air breathed to 30 to 35% concentration to facilitate adequate oxygenation of tissue.
3. Control of air temperature at about 85° F. that will allow easy maintenance of normal body temperature; lower air tempera-

ture will induce body heat loss and require expenditure of energy to generate more body heat (by shivering).

The lack of subcutaneous fat in the neonate (in contrast to the adult) is significant for one other reason: fat provides calories when oral caloric intake is insufficient. Thus, correction of factors preventing oral intake of food in the newborn is vital, since adequate calories cannot be supplied by conventional parenteral fluids.

Respiration. Four factors, unique to the newborn, influence respiration:

1. Air exchange in the lungs and blood flow through the pulmonary circuit have just been initiated, and commonly a few days elapse before lung function becomes optimal.
2. The right upper lung lobe is predisposed to atelectasis for anatomic reasons (a dependent position of its bronchus).
3. The newborn depends entirely on diaphragmatic descent for lung expansion, because the ribs are horizontal and cannot "lift" on inspiration as in the adult. Anything impeding free motion of the diaphragm jeopardizes respiration: congenital diaphragmatic hernia, faulty innervation of the diaphragm muscles, and an increase in intra-abdominal pressure (intestinal obstruction).
4. The newborn breathes by preference through his nose rather than mouth, and anything narrowing or occluding the nasal passages (choanal atresia, mucous plugs, nasogastric tubes) impairs respiratory exchange.

These factors of (1) inefficient early lung function, (2) atelectasis, (3) inhibition of diaphragmatic motion, and (4) obstruction of nasal passages must all be diagnosed and managed promptly to assure normal respiratory function.

Types of operations (newborn versus adults). Congenital anomalies are the most frequent indication for operations on the newborn, in distinction to infection, trauma, and degenerative and neoplastic diseases in the adult. Thus, neonatal intestinal obstruction is generally caused by webs, bands, membranes, faulty innervation, or other abnormalities of development. On the other hand, intestinal obstruction in the adult is generally caused by hernias, postoperative adhesions, and neoplasms.

Surgical disease—rapid progression. The speed at which surgical disease progresses is often dramatically accelerated in the newborn patient and may result in death in just a few hours. Small actual volume of body fluids, low energy and nutritional reserves, and poor defenses against infection contribute to this rapid progression. Furthermore, the newborn must communicate his illness by indirect and often subtle signs such as changes in color and rates of pulse and respiration, inability to feed, irritability, and lethargy. The good pediatric nurse or physician must be an astute observer, for the baby is a poor historian. Time is truly of the essence in the newborn surgical patient.

THE NEWBORN AND THE OPERATING ROOM

Temperature. Body temperature must be monitored continuously. Body heat of the infant is conserved by warming the operating room air, shortening the time periods out of the incubator before and after operation, avoiding large volumes of rapidly evaporating fluids to prepare the skin, and using a heat exchange blanket on top of the operating table mattress. Infrared lights also may be used to deliver heat to the baby during operation.

During operation, body heat is lost rapidly when major body cavities such as the thorax or abdomen are opened, and this loss must be countered by lavages of normal saline heated to just above body temperature. Clear plastic adhesive drapes (such as Vi-Drape) reduce convection loss of heat, provide a sterile barrier impervious to water, allow better visualization of the entire patient by the operating room team, and are therefore highly recommended.

Technique. Placement of a plastic catheter in a vein via "cutdown" must precede all major operations performed upon infants, as a dependable route for blood transfusion. Good surgical principles are never more important than in the neonate: precision (magnification is sometimes helpful), gentleness, protection of exposed viscera, miniaturized instruments, and fine suture material are essential. Gastrostomy tubes are preferable to irritating nasogastric tubes if lengthy suction or tube feeding is anticipated. Subcuticular closure of the skin incision will avoid the need for later suture removal, and clear plastic sprayed on the wound obviates the use of restricting conventional dressings that prevent observation and easy examination of the area. Above all, the *proper* operation must be performed *correctly*. The margin for error in neonatal surgery is narrow.

Postoperative care. Postoperative convalescence of the newborn surgical patient is generally gratifyingly rapid. Sedative and analgesic drugs are seldom required because of an apparently high pain threshold. The infant should be checked frequently visually through the transparent incubator, but all manipulations should be held to a minimum, e.g., at regular 2-hour intervals.

Postoperative complications in the newborn patient are mainly those of the operation itself plus infection and aspiration of vomitus. The postoperative complications common in the adult patient (paralytic ileus, pneumonia, urinary retention, deep vein thrombophlebitis) are almost unheard of in the newborn surgical patient. Aspiration of vomitus, anastomotic leaks, adhesive postoperative intestinal obstruction, and wound infections are poorly tolerated by the infant; they are best prevented, or diagnosed and treated rapidly.

The results of surgical treatment are very gratifying when the anomaly is completely corrected, no other anomalies are present, and no complications ensue. Multiple anomalies, incomplete surgical correction, prematurity, and postoperative complications are discouraging features that favor morbidity and mortality. There is no greater satisfaction to the surgeon or nurse than a newborn patient who has been given a normal life expectancy, surgically cured of an otherwise lethal anomaly.

CONGENITAL ANOMALIES

Congenital anomalies are simply abnormalities of development that are present at birth. Location, magnitude, and mode of origin differ. They constitute the most important single type of surgical problem in the newborn.

Cause. Congenital anomalies are the result of three basic causes:
1. Abnormal genes or chromosomes of the sperm or egg.
2. Abnormalities that develop in previously normal genes or chromosomes (mutations) often because of noxious environmental influences.
3. Unfavorable environment that alters normal development of the fetus without any detectable chromosome or gene alteration.

Abnormal genes or chromosomes. Some congenital disorders are caused by gross chromosomal abnormalities that can now be verified microscopically (mongolism, Turner's syndrome, Klinefelter's syndrome, and intersex problems). These are characterized by multiple widespread and often severe changes in the developing fetus.

Other congenital anomalies are thought to result from an abnormality of a single autosomal gene (congenital cataract, achondroplasia, and syndactylism). Some of these are *dominant* (polydactylism, familial polyposis coli) and are expressed in the patient regardless of the fact that the other gene for this trait is normal. If the gene abnormalities are *recessive,* both members of the genic pair must be abnormal (albinism, cystic fibrosis) before it is expressed in the offspring. Some of the genetically determined abnormalities are sex-linked (such as hemophilia), are exhibited only in the male offspring, and are merely carried or transmitted without expression in the female.

Environment. Far more common than these are congenital abnormalities induced by exposure of the developing fetus to harmful stimuli, usually in early gestation. Vulnerability is directly proportional to the rapidity with which the body systems are developing;

therefore, the first trimester of pregnancy is the time when these harmful stimuli have their greatest effect. Some of the noxious environmental stimuli that have been identified are the following:

1. *Chemical:* Thalidomide, female hormones, nitrogen mustard, cortisone, lead, mercury, alcohol, nicotine.
2. *Nutritional deficiencies:* Riboflavin, pantothenic acid, vitamins A and D, copper, iodine.
3. *Infection:* Viruses, rickettsia, bacteria, especially cytomegalic disease, toxoplasmosis, and rubella.
4. *Irradiation:* X-ray, radium, natural background irradiation.
5. *Mechanical:* Malposition of the fetus (extended knees, ankylosis), mechanical pressure (atrophic single extremity), hydraulic pressure (all four extremities atrophic).
6. *Defective fertilization and implantation:* Tubal pregnancy.
7. *Parental age:* Mongolism, more frequent when parents are older.
8. *Anoxia:* May be ultimate pathway in many of the conditions mentioned.

Incidence. Over 25% of stillborn babies have congenital anomalies that caused the stillbirth; 3% of live babies will be found to have congenital anomalies on immediate careful examination, although an additional 4% harbor occult abnormalities. Fortunately, most of these are minor and do not significantly affect growth, development, or life expectancy; 75% are single, but 25% are multiple—thus, when one congenital anomaly is discovered in a baby, others must be anticipated. Anomalies are about 15% higher in the male than in the female sex. The incidence is 2.5 times higher in multiple than in single births. When one anomalous child is born into a family, there is a 25 times greater chance that subsequent children will have anomalies than if previous siblings were normally developed. In two malformed siblings in a family, there is about a 50% chance that the anomalies will be similar in location and severity. The central nervous system, cardiovascular, skeletal, and intestinal systems appear to be most commonly involved in abnormal development.

History. The history is most important in diagnosing congenital anomalies, keeping the preceding causes in mind. Questions should be directed to anomalies in previous generations and the maternal health and habits during the pregnancy. Maternal hydramnios (excessive amount of amniotic fluid) is associated with a 50% incidence of fetal anomalies and should be investigated carefully. Normally, the fetus continually swallows amniotic fluid, which is absorbed from the proximal small intestine to circulate as tissue fluid, plasma, and cerebrospinal fluid before being excreted via the kidneys back into the amniotic sac. Interruption of this cyclic flow at any point in the

Text continued on p. 432.

Table 28-1. Important aspects of the more common congenital anomalies

Type	Anatomic deformity	Clinical characteristics	Treatment, age	Prognosis
A. Central nervous system				
Myelomeningocele	Defect in bony and soft tissue coverings of neural canal, generally lumbar level	Protrusion of cord coverings in back; paralysis and no sensation in lower extremities, anus, and bladder; about 75% will later develop hydrocephalus; meningitis a constant threat	Cover exposed nerve elements with tissue and skin in infancy	No improvement in nerve function
Hydrocephalus	Obstruction to flow or absorption of C.S.F. with increasing pressure of fluid	Enlarging head, deterioration of cerebral function, tense fontanelles	Shunt C.S.F. from brain to bloodstream or body cavity via plastic tubing and valve system; done in infancy	Malfunction of shunt in majority requires revisions
Craniosynostosis	Premature closure of skull sutures (growth lines)	Small head, progressive cerebral deterioration	Osteotomy of suture lines to prevent closure; done in infancy	Good; repeat operations may be necessary
B. Cardiovascular system				
Interatrial septal defect	Hole in wall between left and right atrium	Systolic precordial murmur, some decrease in growth and exercise tolerance	Closure by suture or patch during heart-lung bypass; done in childhood; some close spontaneously	Excellent

Ventricular septal defect	Hole in wall between left and right ventricle	Systolic precordial murmur; if neglected, cyanosis and serious lung complications	Closure by suture or patch during heart-lung bypass; done in infancy or childhood	Excellent if repaired early
Tetralogy of Fallot	Interventricular septal defect, stenosis of pulmonary outflow tract, and takeoff of aorta from both ventricles	Cyanosis and breathlessness with exercise, stunted growth, systolic precordial murmur	Closure of septum to right of aorta, enlargement of pulmonary valve during heart-lung bypass; done in childhood	Higher risk operation, results good if complete correction can be achieved early
Malformation of heart valves	Stenosis or imperfect valves that allow regurgitation of blood	Systolic and/or diastolic murmur; dilatation, hypertrophy, and failure of heart with edema and breathlessness	Enlargement of stenotic valve, suture correction or replacement of deformed valve during heart-lung bypass; done in childhood	Good if complete correction can be achieved, guarded if not
Coarctation of aorta	Narrowing of descending aorta	Headache, heart enlargement, hypertension in upper body, hypotension in lower body, absent femoral pulses	Excision under hypothermia or during heart-lung bypass; done in childhood	Excellent
Patent ductus arteriosus	Retention of fetal vessel joining pulmonary artery to aorta (to bypass lungs in utero)	"Machinery" type of continuous murmur heard in chest and back	Suture closure; in infancy or childhood	Excellent

Continued.

Table 28-1. Important aspects of the more common congenital anomalies—cont'd

Type	Anatomic deformity	Clinical characteristics	Treatment, age	Prognosis
C. Otolaryngological system				
Cleft lip and/or palate	Cleft, or opening, in lip or palate; often seen together	Obvious cosmetic defects, difficulty in feeding, speech, and dentition	Plastic surgical closure of lip in infancy, palate in young childhood	Good; generally requires large team of surgeons, dentists, speech and hearing experts for complete rehabilitation
Branchial cleft abnormalities	Retention of part, or all, of the embryonic branchial structure	Cysts, sinus, or fistula of lateral neck	Complete excision at time of election	Excellent
Thyroglossal abnormalities	Retention of embryonic thyroid tract from base of tongue to low anterior neck	Cyst or tract in anterior midline neck	Complete excision at time of election	Excellent
D. Gastrointestinal system				
Atresia: complete closure of intestinal lumen; rare in stomach and colon	1. Esophagus: generally has blind proximal pouch, plus fistula connecting bronchus to distal esophagus	Blind pouch: saliva and feedings vomited Fistula: air distending bowel, stomach; HCl bathing lungs to cause pneumonia	Division and closure of fistula, anastomosis of ends of esophagus in neonatal period	Good; often some scarring and narrowing of anastomosis
	2. Anorectal: no anal opening, closed rectum; 70% have narrow fistula con-	Abdominal distension, bilious vomiting; either no meconium passed, or—females:	Division and closure fistula, "pull-through" of end of rectum to perineum	Good early results; ultimate fecal control is variable

...necting rectum to vagina and perineum in females, or to bladder, urethra, and perineum in males	meconium per vagina or perineum; males: meconium in urine or perineum	through anal muscles; may need preliminary colostomy in neonatal period	Excellent
3. Ileum, jejunum: complete closure of lumen by membrane, or with loss of continuity of bowel	Abdominal distension, bilious vomiting, scanty meconium per rectum	Excision and end-to-end anastomosis; in neonatal period	Excellent
4. Duodenum: complete closure by membrane beyond ampulla of Vater (where bile and pancreatic juice enter); about one-fourth are mongoloid	Little abdominal distension, copious bilious vomiting, scanty meconium per rectum	Surgical bypass of membrane by side-to-side anastomosis of duodenum above the block to (a) jejunum or (b) duodenum, below the block; done in neonatal period	Excellent
Stenosis: narrowing of intestinal lumen; rare in esophagus, stomach, or colon			
1. Duodenum: partial obstruction by membrane with a hole in it; one-fourth are mongoloid	No distension, bilious vomiting of feedings, some diminution in stools	Surgical bypass of membrane by side-to-side anastomosis when discovered	Excellent
2. Jejunum, ileum: partial obstruction by membrane with a hole in it	Moderate abdominal distension, bilious vomiting of feedings, some diminution in stools	Excision and end-to-end anastomosis when discovered	Excellent

Continued.

Table 28-1. Important aspects of the more common congenital anomalies—cont'd

Type	Anatomic deformity	Clinical characteristics	Treatment, age	Prognosis
Malrotation of midgut	Abnormal embryological rotation of gut with extrinsic band across duodenum, small bowel in right side abdomen and colon in left; 50% have volvulus, or twisting, of gut around vessels	Bilious vomiting when duodenum obstructed by band; symptoms may be vague, intermittent or absent; volvulus produces pain, strangulation, and shock	Lysis of extrinsic duodenal band; derotation of volvulus, resection if bowel dead; operate whenever discovered or symptomatic	Excellent if no volvulus
Meckel's diverticulum	Outpocketing on the surface of distal ileum, vestige of embryonic tract, seen in 2% of people; 15% contain stomach mucosa, secrete HCl acid, and produce symptoms of ulceration, inflammation, or bleeding	Many are asymptomatic; intermittent abdominal pain, distension, vomiting, and melena are characteristic symptoms	Excision and closure when diagnosed or symptomatic	Excellent
Hirschsprung's disease (congenital megacolon, or aganglionosis)	Absent autonomic nerve cells in wall of distal colon causing obstruction at this point because peristaltic waves not propagated	Abdominal distension, constipation since birth	Excision or bypass of involved colon; may require preliminary colostomy	Good

Meconium ileus	Seen in 8% of babies with mucoviscidosis (fibrocystic disease of pancreas); undigested meconium obstructing small bowel	Abdominal distension, bilious vomiting, scanty meconium passed	Irrigation or bypass of obstructing meconium block; administration of pancreatic digestive enzymes; done in neonatal period	Poor because of generalized mucoviscidosis and pneumonia
E. Genitourinary system Congenital obstruction	1. Ureteropelvic junction (at kidney outlet): due to extrinsic band or vessel, or intrinsic narrowing; may be unilateral or bilateral; results in hydronephrosis and often infection	Flank pain or mass, fever, pus in urine, uremia if bilateral	Plastic revision to relieve obstruction if kidney good; done whenever diagnosed	Good
	2. Ureterocystic junction (where ureter joins bladder): intrinsic or extrinsic narrowing, poor peristalsis; unilateral or bilateral; produces hydroureter, hydronephrosis, and often infection	Flank pain or mass, fever, pus in urine; uremia if bilateral	Excision of obstructed area, reimplantation of ureter into bladder; done whenever diagnosed	Good

Continued.

Table 28-1. Important aspects of the more common congenital anomalies—cont'd

Type	Anatomic deformity	Clinical characteristics	Treatment, age	Prognosis
3.	Bladder neck (outlet): intrinsic valve or membrane; produces enlarged bladder and often bilateral reflux and infection to both kidneys	Lower abdominal mass, flank pain, fever, pus in urine, uremia if neglected	Resection of valve or membrane, plastic widening of stenosis	Good
Undescended testes	One or both testes in or above inguinal canal, often associated with hernia	Empty scrotal sac one or both sides with groin swelling	Surgical placement in scrotum; in childhood	Good
F. *Lymphatic and vascular systems*				
Cutaneous capillary hemangioma "strawberry"	Pink-red, slightly raised skin lesion	Cosmetic deformity mainly; occasionally ulcerates and bleeds	None; 95% thrombose and disappear in early childhood after growth spurt in infancy	Excellent
Cavernous hemangioma	Large venous channels with abnormal lymphatic and arterial connections	Enlarged, bulky, blue-red lesions with discomfort or dysfunction if extremity involved; occasionally ulcerates, bleeds, or becomes infected; gigantism may occur	Injection of sclerosing agents, partial excision with skin grafts or, rarely, amputation as symptoms necessitate	Poor; recurrence and progression common

Cystic hygroma	Enlarged lymphatic spaces that cannot empty watery tissue fluid	Cystic, soft, indentable mass of neck or axilla that transilluminates; rarely produces tracheal deviation and airway obstruction	Conservative excision or breaking down of loculations at age of election	Excellent
G. *Skeletal system* Congenital dislocation of hip	Dislocation of femoral head out of shallow hip joint	Asymmetry of fat folds of leg and buttock; inability to abduct and externally rotate hip	Reduction by manipulation, plaster cast in neonatal period	Excellent
Clubfoot	Foot points downward and is twisted inward	Inability to elevate foot	Manipulation and plaster casts in increasing degrees of dorsiflexion in neonatal period	Excellent if begun early
H. *Abdominal wall* Umbilical hernia	Enlarged umbilical fascial ring with protrusion of intestines into sac covered by skin	Umbilical swelling, larger with straining; asymptomatic	None; almost all will spontaneously disappear by the age of 7 years	Excellent
Omphalocele	Enlarged umbilical fascial ring with protrusion of intestines into thin opaque amniotic sac not covered by skin	Grayish sac bulging around base of umbilical cord at birth filled with viscera	If small, immediate excision and repair of abdominal wall; if large, cover sac with abdominal wall skin	Good

fetus (proximal small bowel: atresia; central nervous system: anencephaly, hydrocephaly, myelomeningocele; urinary tract: atresia, renal aplasia) may upset the delicate balance of amniotic fluid to produce volume abnormalities (oligohydramnios or polyhydramnios).

Physical examination. Physical examination must be meticulous and detailed. It should include inspection of the freshly cut umbilical cord to see if one of the umbilical arteries is missing; this often is a clue to the presence of a hidden anomaly in the body. Small catheters passed into both ends of the gastrointestinal tract can rapidly diagnose obstruction. Special tests are listed under specific congenital anomalies.

Treatment. The treatment of congenital anomalies must be individualized. No treatment is possible if the anomaly is so serious as to be immediately lethal or incorrectable, and none is necessary if the anomaly is so minor as to produce no significant change in function. Important aspects of the more common congenital anomalies are summarized in Table 28-1.

TRAUMA

The individual is probably subjected to more trauma during childhood than at any later period of life. Some is self-occasioned by poor judgment, imperfect muscular and nervous coordination during the toddler years, and some by poor parental supervision. Thanks to the resiliency of young tissue, most of the trauma is well tolerated, and few of the scars are carried into adulthood.

However, accidents are still the most common cause of death in the United States during the first half of life, and an estimated 15 million children incur significant accidents yearly. The general heading of accidents includes (roughly in decreasing frequency) lacerations, contusions and abrasions, fractures, ingestion of poisons, drugs, and foreign bodies, bites, sprains, head injuries, puncture wounds, eye trauma and burns.

Roughly two-thirds of accidents occur in or near the home and can be prevented by intelligent parental supervision and removal of the more common hazards. Safer playthings, supervised playgrounds, less accessible and tasty medications, and the manufacture of nonflammable clothing are public health measures that can diminish this toll. Automobile and bicycle accidents injure or kill thousands of children. Improved automobile safety engineering (seat belts, accident-proof door locks) and education of the adult driver and the child pedestrian or bicycle rider are worthwhile efforts to lower the number of children injured in this manner.

Battered child

Battered child is a term recently coined for the child deliberately injured by physical beatings administered by parents or guardians. The battered child is generally under 3 years of age (too young to communicate the cause of his injury) and often comes from a family that is deprived socially, economically, and emotionally. Multiplicity of injuries is the rule: many fractures in different phases of healing and many ecchymoses and hematomas in various stages of resolution. Occasionally fatalities occur. Almost all states in this country have now enacted legislation to remove the threat of litigation (for false accusation) for the attending physician who reports a suspected case of a battered child to the proper authorities. In many states the physician who fails to report a suspected case of child battering may be prosecuted.

Surgical treatment of all of the traumatic wounds mentioned is varied according to the type and location of the trauma.

CANCER

During the past 25 years cancer has risen from twelfth to second place among the causes of death in young children in the United States. There is little to indicate an actual increase in the frequency of childhood malignancies, but rather a decline in other causes of death as described in the introduction to this chapter.

Comparison of adult and childhood cancer

Many basic differences distinguish adult from childhood cancer. Cancer in the adult generally arises from epithelial tissue lining glands, external surfaces, or hollow organs of the body. In contrast, childhood cancer emerges from mesenchymal tissue or cells of very primitive embryological origin. The organ systems involved are different; the adult has a high incidence of cancer arising from skin, breast, lung, prostate, and intestinal epithelium. Cancer of these structures is almost unheard of in the child. About half the malignancies of children arise from lymphoid tissue in the form of leukemias and lymphomas. Another 15 to 20% are located within the central nervous system, and 10% arise from the adrenal glands and 10% from the kidneys.

Causes of cancer

A few tumors of childhood seem to have hereditary implications, including retinoblastoma, familial polyposis, and Hodgkin's disease. The incidence of cancer within the first decade of life exceeds that of the second decade, suggesting that some of the malignancies are congenital. Leukemia in the mother has been transmitted across the placenta to her fetus; cancers of the adrenal glands and kidney occur in newborns. Irradiation delivered to children for other causes has been incriminated in later development of some cancers, particularly of the thyroid gland and lymphoma family.

Treatment of cancer

Generally the results of treatment of childhood malignancies are discouraging, partly because of their rapid growth rate, early spread, and a delay in diagnosis occasioned by either absence of symptoms or the inability of the child to communicate such symptoms. However, there is no room for a "defeatist" attitude in the treatment of childhood malignancy. The resiliency of the young and the occasional spectacular response to therapy in the face of seemingly hopeless odds justify an aggressive, confident approach to treatment.

All of the treatment modalities employed in adult cancer are used in children; the field of chemotherapy shows particular promise in this age group. Combinations of therapy are the rule rather than the exception. A 2-year salvage rate in the child with cancer is considered equivalent to 5-year survival in the adult patient.

Specific types of childhood cancer
Lymphoma-leukemia family

Leukemia is the single most common malignant neoplasm seen in children. About 90% are of the acute lymphogenous type, with the peak incidence at about 4 years of age. Prognosis is poor, although radiation and antitumor drugs are achieving increasing numbers of cures. Chemotherapy is the treatment of choice at the present; the surgeon is restricted to an occasional diagnostic node or bone marrow biopsy.

Neuroblastoma

Neuroblastoma is a malignancy arising in primitive elements of the sympathetic nervous system. Two-thirds originate in or near the adrenal gland, about 20% in the posterior mediastinum, and about 5% each from the neck and pelvic areas. The average age at diagnosis is 18 months, and the growth rate is typically rapid.

Symptoms of neuroblastoma are nonspecific; bone pain and fever frequently herald the presence of bone marrow metastases. Diarrhea, weight loss, anemia, and irritability are often seen. About 80% of patients have an abdominal mass that often extends across the midline, occasionally associated with metastases palpable within the liver. Diagnosis is confirmed by plain radiographs showing the mass (which often contains calcium stippling) displacing hollow viscera, and intravenous pyelograms that show kidney displacement. Roentgen-ray examination reveals metastases to bone in about 30% and to the lungs in 10%.

The most diagnostic test of neuroblastoma is the presence of specific hormones (vanilmandelic acid and homovanillic acid) in the urine or blood, representing metabolic end products of tumor origin. Treatment consists of surgical removal of as much tumor as possible, generally followed by low-dosage irradiation. Chemotherapy in the form of vincristine and cyclophosphamid combinations effectively palliate neuroblastoma.

Onset within the first year of life, or tumors primary in the neck, pelvis, or mediastinum command a favorable prognosis. Curiously, about 5% of neuroblastomas spontaneously transform into benign ganglioneuromas. Tumor antibodies have been demonstrated in some cured patients.

Wilms' tumor

Wilms' tumor, or nephroblastoma, is a cancer arising in embryonal kidney cells that grows rapidly to destroy the normal kidney tissue. Again, the symptoms are nonspecific and include vague abdominal discomfort, fever, and occasionally hematuria. Early spread to perirenal tissues is the rule, with metastases to lung and liver in one-third of the patients by the time a diagnosis is established; 90% of patients have a mass in the abdomen on physical examination, and intravenous pyelograms will differentiate from neuroblastoma. About 5% of patients regrettably develop Wilms' tumors of both kidneys. Treatment is combined surgical removal, roentgen-ray therapy, and chemotherapy with actinomycin D and vincristine. Recent reports indicate the salvage of over half of these patients for a 2-year period.

Central nervous system tumors

Most central nervous system tumors arise below the membrane, or tentorium, which separates the cerebrum from the lower centers. Most of these cancers stem from supporting tissues within the brain and produce symptoms by disturbing balance and motor activity, or by blocking the flow of cerebrospinal fluid to increase intracranial pressure. Surgical excision is the most effective treatment at this time. In keeping with central nervous system tumors of all ages, no distant metastases are seen.

Bone cancers

Bone cancers have a peak incidence later in childhood, probably because of increasing bone growth rates at this time of life. Striated muscle cancers *(rhabdomyosarcoma)* in infancy are most commonly located in the bladder or genital tracts; in older children they are chiefly seen in the head and neck, but they may occur in any striated muscle. Surgical excision, roentgen-ray therapy, and a number of therapeutic drugs are used in combination for treatment of these less common childhood malignancies. Prognosis is poor, with salvage of the patient in less than one-fourth of all cases.

NEONATAL GASTROINTESTINAL OBSTRUCTION

Obstruction of the gastrointestinal tract in the newborn is both serious and unique enough to justify special consideration. Obstruction may occur anywhere from esophagus to anus, having a curious numerical predilection for both ends of the tract. All neonatal gastrointestinal obstructions are secondary to congenital anomalies that, however, arise from a host of different influences. Together they constitute by far the most common surgical emergency of the neonatal period of life.

Neonatal gastrointestinal obstructions are no exception to the rule that anomalies are often multiple. Two causes for intestinal obstruction may coexist at different levels, as exemplified by the association of esophageal atresia with duodenal atresia or anorectal atresia—or the associated anomaly may involve a totally different system, such as the major congenital heart defects that accompany esophageal or anorectal atresia. The intestine may be obstructed simultaneously by two different mechanisms at the same level (extrinsic duodenal obstruction resulting from malrotation, and intrinsic obstruction from duodenal membrane) or at different levels by the same mechanism (about 15% of patients with intestinal atresia have additional atretic areas downstream from the most proximal one). About one-fourth of babies with neonatal gastrointestinal obstruction have other anomalies, which must be diagnosed and managed along with the primary obstructing lesion.

Prematurity (birth weight below 2,500 Gm.) is associated in about one-third of babies with congenital gastrointestinal obstruction. Both prematurity and serious associated congenital anomalies markedly worsen prognosis. The mortality for full-term newborns with obstruction who have no other major anomalies is about 10%, contrasting unfavorably with an 80 to 90% mortality expected in the obstructed premature baby with other major anomalies. If the obstruction is complicated by peritonitis, the mortality is 50%. If the intestine must be opened to relieve the obstruction, the mortality (40%) is much higher than it is when the obstruction is extrinsic (5%). Overall, the salvage rate for neonatal gastrointestinal obstruction is about 75%.

Family and maternal pregnancy history. Some causes for neonatal gastrointestinal obstruction are familial or inheritable, and therefore a carefully taken history of the genealogy is helpful. Fibrocystic disease of the pancreas (with meconium ileus), congenital aganglionosis of the colon (Hirschsprung's disease), and hypertrophic pyloric stenosis are all examples of this tendency. Mongolism has a familial tendency, as well as a predilection for duodenal atresia (about 2 to 3%).

The maternal pregnancy history is important in terms of illnesses, ingestion of drugs, and exposure to irradiation or other of the noxious environmental influences associated with congenital anomalies. Polyhydramnios, the presence of excessive amounts of maternal amniotic fluid, has a high association with obstructions to the proximal gastrointestinal tract, as explained on p. 423.

Patient history. Bile vomiting, abdominal distension, and obstipation are the three cardinal signs of obstruction of the gastrointestinal tract at any age. However, exceptions to this rule occur frequently enough in the obstructed newborn baby to justify special attention. Thus, esophageal atresia with tracheoesophageal fistula produces regurgitation of feedings and saliva unstained with bile; the abdominal distension is profound but is associated with free passage of meconium. The newborn with duodenal obstruction will indeed have copious bile vomiting but only mild epigastric distension and may pass one or two normal meconium stools. Paradoxically, the functional (nonmechanical) type of colonic obstruction produced by congenital aganglionosis (Hirschsprung's disease) is sometimes associated with diarrhea and only late and infrequent vomiting, although abdominal distension is marked. Notwithstanding these exceptions, any newborn baby who (1) fails to pass meconium per rectum within 24 hours after birth, or (2) vomits bile, or (3) exhibits abdominal distension should have a plain radiograph of the abdomen taken in the erect position as a minimal initial step to investigate intestinal obstruction.

Relative incidence. Atresias of the esophagus and anorectal area are numerically the most common causes for neonatal gastrointestinal tract obstruction, each comprising roughly 25% of cases. An additional 20% is caused by atresia and stenosis of the small intestine, and another 25% will be about equally divided among midgut malrotation, meconium ileus, and congenital aganglionosis; 5% of cases are comprised of a miscellaneous group of very diverse causes.

Diagnosis. The diagnosis of gastrointestinal obstruction may often be made in the newborn baby before symptoms occur, by gentle passage of a small, soft, plastic catheter into both ends of the gastrointestinal tract. If the tube passes into the stomach, esophageal and choanal atresia can be ruled out; if 10 ml. or less of clear fluid is aspirated from the stomach, congenital obstruction of the small bowel is extremely unlikely. However, if more than 20 ml. of bile-stained material is present in the stomach, the diagnosis of obstruction should be entertained seriously, and an upright radiograph of the abdomen should be taken. Passage of the catheter through the anus and into the rectum rules out anorectal atresia.

Plain radiographs of the abdomen and chest in the supine and upright positions are the first step in diagnosis. Abnormal distribution or amounts of intestinal gas often allow a specific enough diagnosis to be made that no additional radiographic procedures are necessary. Occasionally barium enema is indicated, especially for showing the size and position of the colon. Upper gastrointestinal contrast studies are rarely needed—they are sometimes dangerous from the standpoint of barium aspiration or conversion of a partial to a complete obstruction by inspissation of barium at the point of narrowing.

Differential diagnosis. There are many nonsurgical conditions that can simulate intestinal obstruction in the newborn baby. Some are very serious diseases in their own right, and it is tragic to compound an already grave medical problem by laparotomy undertaken with a mistaken diagnosis of intestinal obstruction. Examples of these nonsurgical conditions follow:

1. *Feeding problems:* Underfeeding, overfeeding, or improperly administered feedings are probably the most common cause for neonatal vomiting. Generally the material vomited consists simply of the feeding itself, or nonbile-stained material. Observation of a feeding or a carefully taken history of the feeding program should allow a proper diagnosis to be made.

2. *Infections:* Septicemia in the newborn can produce vomiting and abdominal distension, whether the infection is primary within the gastrointestinal tract or elsewhere. Cultures of the blood, pharynx, and stool plus detection of a source for the infection establish the correct diagnosis.

3. *Increased C.S.F. pressure:* Cerebral edema, hemorrhage caused by birth trauma, or hydrocephalus often cause vomiting in the newborn. Evaluation of fontanelle pressure and careful neurological examination should rule out these causes for neonatal vomiting.

4. *Obstructive uropathy:* Congenital obstruction of the urinary tract producing azotemia is associated with vomiting and difficult feeding of the baby. Observation of the urinary output, serum BUN determinations, and intravenous pyelography are helpful clues in diagnosis.

5. *Endocrine and metabolic:* Adrenal failure (adrenogenital syndrome), abnormalities of glucose metabolism (hypoglycemia,

galactosemia, glycogenosis), and tetany from hypocalcemia can be associated with vomiting and/or abdominal distension in the newborn. Appropriate studies of the serum and urine electrolyte and glucose levels establish the appropriate diagnosis.

6. *Chalasia:* Chalasia, or congenital incompetence of the esophago-gastric sphincter, allows easy regurgitation of gastric contents and feedings and is occasionally confused with surgical causes for vomiting. The nonbile-stained character of the regurgitated material and its relationship to the supine position are clues to the diagnosis, which is confirmed by upper gastrointestinal tract barium studies. Competence of the sphincter develops within a few days or weeks, and interim treatment consists of positioning the baby in the upright position in an appropriately constructed seat and offering thick feedings.

Embryology of the gastrointestinal tract

Misadventures that occur to the fetus resulting in abnormal development of the gastrointestinal tract are the most frequent cause for neonatal obstruction. This section reviews briefly the major stages of gastrointestinal tract development and some of the more common anomalies that occur.

For convenience and better understanding of its embryological development, the gastrointestinal tract is divided into three subdivisions: (1) the foregut, which embraces the esophagus, stomach, and proximal duodenum (including the bile ducts, liver, and pancreas), vascularized largely by the celiac axis, (2) the midgut, running from the ampulla of Vater in the second portion of the duodenum to the splenic flexure of the colon and supplied with blood by the superior mesenteric artery, and (3) the hindgut, extending from the splenic flexure of the colon to the rectum and having as its major blood vessel the inferior mesenteric artery. The venous return from all three embryological gut subdivisions is largely through the portal system to the liver.

In the early embryo, the gastrointestinal tract is a straight tube running in the midline from the oral cavity to the anus, suspended by both a dorsal and a ventral mesentery. The ventral mesentery is lost early, but the dorsal mesentery is retained with the blood supply to the developing gastrointestinal tract. By the fourth gestational week the lung anlage separates from the proximal end of the foregut; incompleteness of this splitting mechanism results in the various forms of esophageal atresia and tracheoesophageal fistula.

Beginning at the fifth week of intrauterine life, the stomach sacculates and the midgut begins to proliferate, enlarge, and elongate in a very accelerated manner. Epithelial proliferation tends to narrow

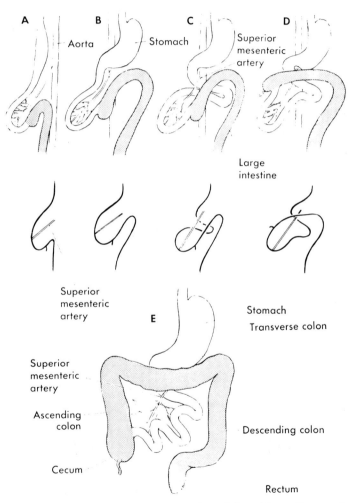

Fig. 28-1. Normal embryological rotation of the midgut. (See text.)

the intestinal lumen; in lower animals the proliferation continues until the lumen is obliterated to form the so-called *solid cord stage*. In the human embryo the solid cord stage develops rarely, and only in the duodenum; vacuolization and coalescence of vacuoles rapidly reestablish the internal lumen of the tract.

Linear growth of the midgut rapidly outstrips the volume of the peritoneal cavity, resulting in elongation of the mesentery and herniation of the entire midgut into the base of the umbilical cord. The resulting *extracoelomic phase* (Fig. 28-1) of midgut development occurs from the sixth to the tenth weeks of intrauterine life.

As one views the fetus from the front, the midgut rotates 270° in a counterclockwise direction around its vascular axis (the superior mesenteric artery) (Fig. 28-1, *A* to *C*) during this extracoelomic phase of development, after which an orderly return of the midgut to the enlarged peritoneal cavity occurs during the tenth to twelfth weeks of intrauterine life. Return of the midgut occurs in an aboral manner from proximal to distal, the duodenum returning to the right upper abdominal quadrant after the first 90° of rotation (Fig. 28-1, *B*), where it is fixed retroperitoneally. This forces the stomach to rotate 90°, so that its original left side is now anterior and its right side the definitive posterior wall. This is correlated with elongation of its dorsal mesenteric surface into what we refer to as the greater curvature of the stomach.

As the proximal jejunum returns, the 270° counterclockwise rotation is completed (Fig. 28-1, *C* and *D*) so as to carry the distal portion of the duodenum inferior (caudad) to the superior mesenteric artery and across the midline, where the duodenojejunal junction is fixed in a nearly retroperitoneal manner by the ligament of Treitz. The hindgut is pushed to the left by the returning small bowel (Fig. 28-1, *C*), and the cecum and the right colon are directed above (cephalad) the superior mesenteric artery with the cecum ending in the right upper abdominal quadrant (Fig. 28-1, *D*). The embryological changes in the midgut are completed leisurely during the succeeding months of gestation and on into the first few weeks of postnatal life by the gradual descent of the cecum to the right lower abdominal quadrant (Fig. 28-1, *E*), where it becomes attached to the right posterior parietes in the normal adult position.

Two pathological states involving the midgut are attributable to misadventures occurring during these critical fifth to twelfth weeks of gestational life. *Omphalocele* (exomphalos) (Fig. 28-2) may be thought of as a retention of the extracolonic phase of midgut development, with failure of both normal rotation and return of the midgut. It complicates about 1:4,000 live births. The midgut is contained extra-

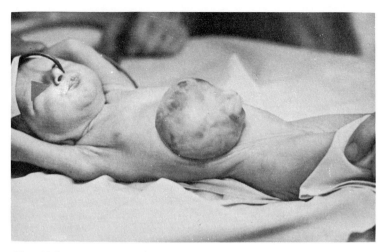

Fig. 28-2. Omphalocele—note the lusterless, semiopaque sac that contains herniated midgut.

peritoneally at the umbilicus in a sac composed of amniotic membranes devoid of skin. It is characterized by abnormalities of intestinal rotation and invariably is associated with a small peritoneal cavity, which has not been stimulated to enlarge by a normal return of the midgut viscera.

The omphalocele sac is friable and poorly vascularized; 10% rupture during intrauterine life to provoke a chronic peritonitis reaction of the bowel, which is bathed in amniotic fluid (foreshortening, matting of loops, lusterless serosal exudate). The sac ruptures in an additional 25% during or shortly after labor and delivery. In either event, the exposed viscera must be covered immediately.

Treatment of omphalocele is individualized:

1. *Sac ruptured:* Emergent surgical protection of exposed bowel by either (a) total repair of the abdominal wall defect (if < 4 cm. in diameter) or (b) coverage of viscera by synthetic sheets or abdominal wall skin (defect > 4 cm. in diameter).
2. *Sac intact:*
    a. *Nonsurgical* (generally restricted to poor-risk babies). Daily painting of sac with an astringent (1% Mercurochrome) to thicken and toughen it as the abdominal wall skin gradually overgrows and replaces the sac during the ensuing weeks.
    b. *Surgical.* Total repair or coverage of exposed viscera in line with the principles just mentioned.

A principle vital to the surgical treatment of all omphaloceles is to avoid an excessively high intra-abdominal pressure when returning bowel to the abnormally small peritoneal cavity. Elevated intra-abdominal pressure is tolerated poorly by the newborn because of (1) reduced respiratory exchange from restricted motion of the diaphragm, and (2) impedance of venous return to the heart from the lower compartment by compression of the inferior vena cava. Gastrostomy decompression of the G.I. tract and intraoperative manual stretching of the abdominal wall help avoid this disaster. Recently, synthetic sheets, which house the bowel extracoelomically for 2 or 3 weeks, have been sutured to the edges of the abdominal wall defect and allow slow, progressive reduction of bowel back into the gradually enlarging abdominal cavity. Total parenteral feeding avoids early postoperative oral feedings, which are poorly tolerated in the crowded abdominal cavity, especially by bowel that is temporarily aperistaltic by having been bathed in amniotic fluid throughout gestation.

Gastroschisis is an anomaly clinically identical to the antenatally ruptured omphalocele, in that midgut protrudes through a small paraumbilical aperture in the abdominal wall, generally on the right side, throughout gestation. The bowel suffers the same chronic, aseptic, chemical peritonitis that characterizes the antenatally ruptured omphalocele, and treatment principles are the same. Embryologically, gastroschisis probably arises from simple failure of a paraumbilical segment of abdominal wall to develop.

Malrotation of the midgut is the second major problem resulting from faulty embryological development of the midgut. It is characterized by various degrees of incompleteness of the rotation mechanism. Most commonly, rotation occurs only through the first 90° arc (Fig. 28-1, *B*) with a normal position of the stomach and the proximal duodenum. The duodenojejunum descends to the right of the superior mesenteric artery, and in general the entire small intestine lies in the right hemiabdomen while the large bowel occupies the left hemiabdomen. The base or root of the midgut mesentery is invariably narrow.

With normal midgut rotation (Fig. 28-1, *E*), the base or root of the mesentery in the adult measures about 20 cm. in length and extends from the ligament of Treitz (to the left of the second lumbar vertebra) obliquely downward to the ileocecal area in the right lower abdominal quadrant. With failure of normal midgut rotation, the mesenteric root or base is very narrow, measuring only the width of the superior mesenteric artery and vein (Fig. 28-1, *B*). The combination of a narrow mesenteric vascular root and a very lengthy fan-shaped periphery (along which the midgut itself courses) provides the setting for the most significant and lethal complication of midgut malrotation, namely, twisting or *volvulus of the midgut*. Volvulus occurs in about 50% of patients with midgut malrotation. It involves a clockwise twist of the midgut around the very narrow vascular base or root to produce varying degrees of occlusion of the lymphatic, venous, and arterial vessels of the mesentery. The volvulus always occurs in a clockwise direction for an unknown reason (perhaps because the liver developing in the right upper quadrant prevents an initial counterclockwise thrust) and may involve twisting through three or four complete turns.

Two potentially lethal conditions occur, then, with volvulus of the midgut: the twist (1) closes off the midgut on both ends to produce *"closed loop intestinal obstruction"* and (2) results in varying degrees of mesenteric vascular stagnation as venous outflow and later arterial inflow are occluded. These two features set the stage for midgut perforation and infarction, either of which can be fatal.

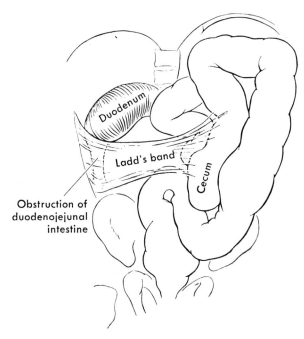

Fig. 28-3. Malrotation of the midgut—entire colon in left hemiabdomen and Ladd's band running from cecum to right posterior parietes to cross and obstruct the duodenojejunal intestine.

Midgut malrotation without volvulus is generally symptomatic because of some degree of duodenal obstruction. Extrinsic duodenal obstruction occurs from peritoneal bands *(Ladd's bands)* (Fig. 28-3) stretching from the right posterior parietes across the duodenum to the cecum and ascending colon in the left upper abdominal quadrant; they can be thought of as bands that would have fixed the cecum and ascending colon in the right gutter had normal rotation occurred. Approximately 15% of patients with extrinsic duodenal obstruction on this basis also have an intrinsic obstruction caused by a duodenal membrane. The duodenal obstruction is generally intermittent and partial, reflected by bouts of bile-stained vomiting associated with epigastric distension. If volvulus ensues, the morbidity is sharply increased by trapping fluid within the closed midgut loop, thereby producing more abdominal distension and obstipation, and perhaps less vomiting. Strangulation will precipitate signs of peritoneal irritation progressing to shock and a critically ill patient within a matter of hours.

The diagnosis of midgut malrotation often must be made in the operating room, since it is difficult to distinguish duodenal obstruction occurring in young patients on this basis from other causes, such as duodenal stenosis, atresia, and annular pancreas. Plain abdominal radiographs and barium studies of the upper gastrointestinal tract will show a dilated stomach and duodenum without clear differentiation as to cause. A barium enema is helpful if it clearly shows the colon lying entirely within the left hemiabdomen and the cecum at or near the epigastric midline. When the signs of intestinal strangulation are associated with duodenal obstruction in an infant or child, malrotation with midgut volvulus becomes the most likely cause and demands early laparotomy.

Surgical treatment of uncomplicated midgut malrotation involves (1) complete division of Ladd's bands, thereby allowing the cecum to lie freely within the left upper abdominal quadrant with the duodenum and jejunum proceeding down the right posterior parietes in an unobstructed manner, (2) prophylactic appendectomy so that left upper quadrant appendicitis will not later be a confusing clinical entity to diagnose, and (3) proof of intrinsic patency of the duodenum. If volvulus has occurred, the twist must be derotated completely in a counterclockwise direction, and necrotic bowel must be resected. Recurrent volvulus virtually never occurs, probably because intestinal fixation from adhesions generated during the operation.

Early in embryonic development, the hindgut and allantois are joined as the cloaca. Division into a urogenital sinus anteriorly and rectum posteriorly occurs during the sixth to eighth weeks of gestation

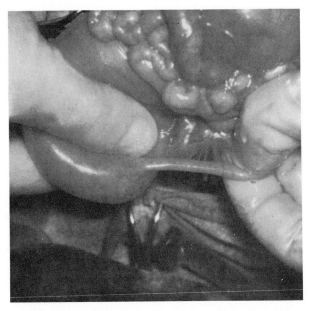

Fig. 28-4. Intestinal atresia with intrinsic membrane occluding lumen. Dilated and obstructed small intestine to the left, and unused but patent "wormlike" bowel distal to the membrane to the right.

by descent of the urorectal septum. Shortly thereafter, rupture of the cloacal membrane in the proctoderm produces separate genital and intestinal orifices. Defects in these mechanisms produce the many anatomic variations that characterize rectal atresia and imperforate anus.

Origin of intestinal atresia and stenosis

Gastrointestinal atresia implies total closure of the bowel lumen. It may be composed simply of a membrane or diaphragm stretched across the lumen (Fig. 28-4), or it may be extensive with total loss of continuity and may even be multiple (Fig. 28-5). Stenosis results in a narrowing of the lumen without complete obstruction, often represented by a diaphragm or membrane with a small aperture; it never involves loss of continuity of the intestine or complete obstruction.

Some dispute exists as to the embryogenesis of atresias and stenoses

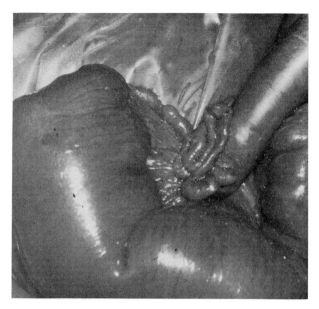

Fig. 28-5. Intestinal atresia with loss of intestinal continuity. Dilated and obstructed proximal bowel to the left and below, and unused distal bowel to the right.

of the gastrointestinal tract. The traditional concept is that they represent a failure of canalization (vacuolization and coalescence of vacuoles) after the so-called solid core stage at about the fifth week of embryonic life, wherein the lumen of the developing intestine is occluded by hyperplasia of the mucosal epithelial cells. The basis for this solid core theory stems largely from embryological studies done on lower animal forms. More sophisticated and recent studies of the human embryo demonstrate a somewhat abortive epithelial cell hyperplasia that produces total obliteration of the lumen (only rarely) in the duodenum. Therefore this mechanism is a logical explanation for congenital atresia and stenosis of the human duodenum only. The solid core theory does not explain many of the features of jejunal and ileal atresia: loss of bowel continuity, defects in the adjacent mesentery and visible remnants of volvulus, intussusception, and meconium peritonitis.

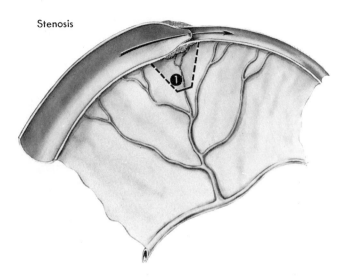

Fig. 28-6. Diagram of thrombosis of small mesenteric "end artery" of developing fetal intestine, producing a sterile infarction of a short segment of bowel nourished by this vessel. The resulting phagocytosis and repair reaction produce an intrinsic diaphragm, which in the diagram has a small aperture through which some of the intestinal content may pass.

A more recent and attractive explanation for congenital stenosis and atresia of the jejunum and ileum implicates a thrombosis of the mesenteric vessels arising some time during gestation, which provokes a sterile infarction of that segment of developing intestine supplied by the vessels. Thrombosis of a small terminal artery (Fig. 28-6) would infarct only a short segment of gut, with the resulting granulation and scar tissue forming a membrane characteristic of stenosis or the minor forms of atresia. Occlusion of major vessels (Figs. 28-7 and 28-8) nourishing longer segments of developing intestine would better explain the more gross and extensive degrees of atresia. Spontaneous thrombosis, or strangulating misadventures such as intussusception or volvulus, might be the basic origin of the mesenteric vascular occlusion.

Deliberate experimental production of mesenteric vascular occlusion in unborn animal fetuses has successfully reproduced all degrees of stenosis and atresia of the intestine, lending experimental credence to this thesis of origin. Because of the short dorsal mesentery nourishing

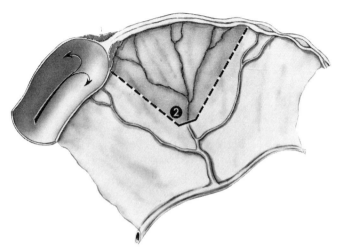

Fig. 28-7. Thrombosis of larger mesenteric artery of developing fetal intestine, producing a sterile infarction of a longer segment of bowel. External continuity of the bowel is retained, but the intrinsic membrane totally obstructs the lumen. (See Fig. 28-4.)

the esophagus and duodenum and the nonmesenteric collateral circulation to the developing rectum, this seems to be a less attractive and plausible explanation for the embryogenesis of atresia of the esophagus, duodenum, and rectum.

Esophageal atresia with tracheoesophageal fistula

There are many anatomic variations of congenital esophageal stenosis and atresia, but approximately 90% have a blind proximal esophageal pouch extending to the low cervical or upper thoracic level, with the distal esophagus connected to the tracheobronchial tree near the carina (Fig. 28-9). Because of its frequency, this is the only type that will be discussed.

A glance at Fig. 28-9 allows the student to predict the symptoms produced by this anatomic arrangement. The blind proximal esophagus fills with saliva, which is then regurgitated back into the mouth, producing a seemingly "mucusy" baby who is salivating excessively. The first feeding provokes gagging and immediate regurgitation, with explosive coughing and cyanosis if any spills over into the trachea. The fistula between the trachea and the stomach via the distal esophagus

Atresia without continuity

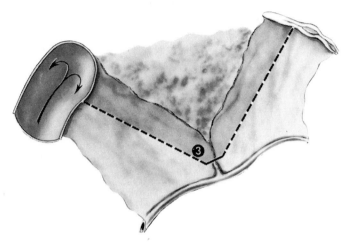

Fig. 28-8. Thrombosis of major mesenteric artery of fetal intestine, infarcting a long segment of bowel and mesentery; the sterile phagocytic reaction that this provokes causes loss of bowel and mesenteric continuity and total intestinal obstruction. (See Fig. 28-5.)

is a "two-way" street. Some of the inspired air is diverted into the stomach and on downstream to produce unusual degrees of abdominal distension and tympany. When the infant is recumbent, hydrochloric acid from the stomach flows up into the lungs via the distal esophagus to produce the most serious complication of this variety of esophageal atresia, namely, a severe chemical pneumonitis.

Diagnosis is quickly made by passing a soft, small, plastic catheter through the nose and finding that it meets an obstruction within 10 cm. A single upright radiograph taken after 1 to 2 ml. of a radiopaque material has been injected into the tube outlines the blind proximal pouch and reveals pneumonitis and the unusually large accumulation of intestinal gas characteristic of this disorder. Until further treatment can be carried out, the infant should be positioned upright, and continuous suction should be applied to the nasoesophageal tube to retrieve saliva.

Definitive treatment of esophageal atresia must be individualized according to the degree of pneumonitis, the weight of the baby, and the precise anatomic form of the anomaly. In good-risk babies, primary

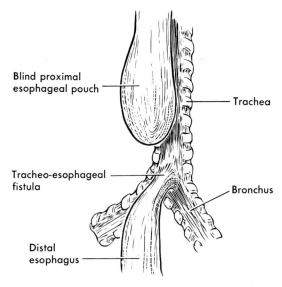

Fig. 28-9. Esophageal atresia with tracheoesophageal fistula.

repair may be carried out either transthoracically or retropleurally, with ligation and division of the fistula and end-to-end anastomosis of the two esophageal ends. If the infant is premature and has other major anomalies or a severe pneumonitis, preliminary gastrostomy is carried out under local anesthesia to remove the threat of further chemical pneumonitis; the baby is then nourished parenterally until repair can be safely undertaken. If the proximal pouch is short, it may be elongated by daily dilatations during this waiting period to facilitate primary anastomosis later.

Neonatal duodenal obstruction

Most neonatal obstructions of the duodenum occur distal to the ampulla of Vater, with bilious vomiting the outstanding clinical feature. If the obstruction is complete, plain radiographs of the abdomen taken in the upright position show the classical "double bubble" sign (Fig. 28-10), which results from air-fluid levels in the stomach and proximal duodenum.

Duodenal atresia is the most common cause for complete duodenal

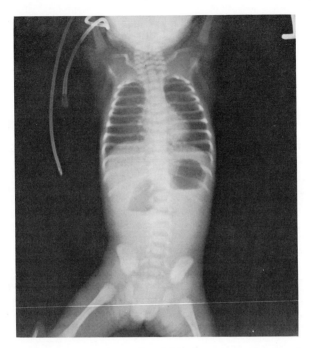

Fig. 28-10. "Double bubble" radiographic sign of complete duodenal obstruction in the newborn. The air-fluid level in the left upper quadrant is in the dilated stomach, that to the right of the midline is in the dilated and obstructed duodenum.

obstruction, about one fourth of the babies also being mongoloid. Malrotation of the midgut with or without volvulus can cause total neonatal duodenal obstruction but also is capable of producing intermittent obstruction at various times during infancy and young childhood. Duodenal stenosis is the most common cause for partial obstruction, and the most rare cause of all is annular pancreas. Diagnosis of partial or intermittent duodenal obstruction often requires an upper gastrointestinal tract barium series.

Duodenal atresia, stenosis, and annular pancreas are treated by surgical bypass; a side-to-side anastomosis is created between the duodenum proximal to the obstruction and either the distal duodenum or the first portion of the jejunum. The treatment of malrotation with duodenal obstruction is discussed in detail on p. 445.

Jejunal and ileal obstruction

Neonatal obstruction of the jejunum and ileum is generally caused by congenital atresia or stenosis and less commonly by meconium ileus. Clinically the obstruction is manifested by bilious vomiting with abdominal distension proportionate to the level of the obstruction, its degree of completeness, and the time elapsed since delivery. Plain radiographs of the abdomen taken in the upright position will diagnose the level and completeness of the obstruction but will not label the cause precisely.

Atresia is a much more common cause of complete ileal or jejunal obstruction than meconium ileus, with stenosis the most likely cause of partial obstruction. Resection and anastomosis is the preferred treatment of atresia and stenosis.

Meconium ileus complicates about 8% of children with generalized mucoviscidosis, or fibrocystic disease of the pancreas. The obstruction is caused by extremely inspissated and tenacious meconium occluding the lumen because of insufficient digestive enzymes of pancreatic origin. A specific diagnosis is suggested by a family history of cystic fibrosis of the pancreas and palpation of cordlike masses of meconium within the abdomen. Plain abdominal radiographs show variable-sized small bowel loops plus a "soap bubble" appearance of gas dispersed within tenacious meconium.

Surgical treatment consists of disimpaction of the undigested meconium by irrigation with mucolytic agents if only a short segment of bowel is involved. Surgical bypass, or temporary ileostomy to allow direct instillation of proteolytic enzymes into the distal small bowel, is necessary if a lengthy segment of ileum is filled with undigested meconium.

Recently a nonsurgical method of relieving the obstruction has been reported, successful in about two-thirds of the cases. Radiopaque, water-soluble material (Gastrografin) is introduced per rectum into the well-hydrated newborn (the hypertonicity of Gastrografin may quickly dehydrate the baby). Under direct vision (by means of cinefluoroscopy) the Gastrografin flows retrogradely through the colon and the obstructed ileum, liquefying and breaking up the tenacious meconium enough to allow its expulsion per rectum. If unsuccessful, prompt surgical intervention must follow.

The prognosis is poor from the intestinal obstruction itself and is compounded by tenacious bronchial mucus predisposing the patient to atelectasis, pneumonia, and bronchiectasis.

NEONATAL OBSTRUCTION OF THE COLON

The most common cause for congenital obstruction of the colon is the various forms of *anorectal atresia;* additional causes are the *me-*

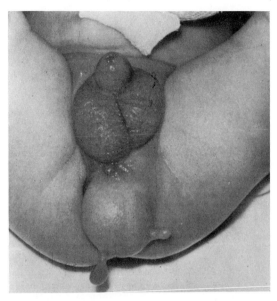

Fig. 28-11. Anorectal atresia, with an abortive attempt at formation of a perineal fistula marked by the bluish, meconium-filled tract in the scrotal raphe. A large lipoma occupies the intergluteal cleft.

conium plug syndrome, congenital aganglionosis (Hirschsprung's disease), and *congenital atresia* of the colon, in descending order of frequency.

There are many anatomical variations of *imperforate anus* and *rectal atresia,* but the most common type consists of an absent anus with a dilated and obstructed rectum terminating somewhere in the pelvis. In *high rectal atresia* the rectum ends above the levator sling (the muscular pelvic diaphragm through which the rectum normally courses and which contributes most to fecal control), and in *low rectal atresia* the rectum passes through the sling (anterior to the puborectalis muscle) before terminating. Seventy to 80% will have a fistula that, in the male, connects the rectum to the bladder neck, urethra, or perineal skin. In the female the fistula opens into the vagina or perineum.

Obstipation with progressive abdominal distention and late bilious vomiting characterize the disorder clinically. Diagnosis can generally

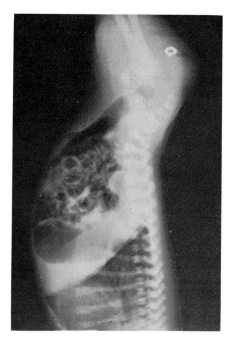

Fig. 28-12. Lateral radiograph taken after baby was inverted for several minutes, showing the distance from the perineum (radiopaque marker) to the end of the atretic, air-filled rectum.

be made by inspection alone (Fig. 28-11). A plain radiograph of the abdomen taken after the infant has been inverted for several minutes (Fig. 28-12) gives a clue as to the distance between the end of the rectum and the perineum. Much more precise documentation of the abnormality is afforded by transperineal needle injection of radio-contrast material into the atretic rectum. Probes are helpful in locating perineal and vaginal fistulas, and meconium or air in urine is diagnostic of a rectourethral or rectovesicle fistula in male infants.

Relief of the colonic obstruction is the first aim of treatment and can occasionally be satisfied by dilating the larger perineal and vaginal fistulous tracts. In good-risk patients primary perineal anoplasty (Fig. 28-13) is carried out as definitive treatment of the low-lying rectal atresia. Colostomy is necessary with the higher rectal atresias or in poor-risk newborns to allow temporary relief of the obstruction. Later,

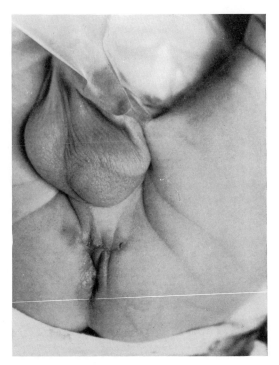

Fig. 28-13. Photograph taken 2 weeks after anoplasty repair of anorectal atresia in baby shown preoperatively in Fig. 28-11.

the rectum is "pulled through" to the perineum by a posterior (trans-sacral) and/or a transabdominal approach. The most crucial aim of the operation is to draw the rectum in front of the puborectalis muscle so that the sling's anterior pull will provide effective fecal continence.

Congenital aganglionosis of the colon (Hirschsprung's disease) may produce an acute obstruction in the neonatal period of life. It is characterized by abdominal distension with the passage of little or no meconium per rectum and late bilious vomiting. Occasionally, paradoxical diarrhea may occur to confuse the diagnosis of obstruction. Diagnosis is suggested by rectal digital examination that reveals a narrow rectal ampulla and often provokes explosive passage of gas and meconium upon withdrawal of the finger. Barium enema reveals a narrow rectum that enlarges at some point proximally, with poor evacuation of barium. Absolute confirmation rests with biopsy demonstration of absent ganglia in the autonomic nerve plexuses in the submucosal and intermuscular planes on rectal wall biopsy.

Initial treatment consist of relieving the intestinal obstruction. Occasionally, saline enemas and frequent rectal dilatations are sufficient, but commonly colostomy (within ganglionated bowel) is necessary. Definitive corrective operation can be carried out primarily on a good-risk baby; it is best delayed in small or otherwise compromised babies until later in infancy or young childhood.

The *meconium plug syndrome* consists of obstruction generally of the transverse, descending, or sigmoid colon by a long, pale, and stringy plug of inspissated meconium. Delayed passage of meconium per rectum, gross and progressive abdominal distension, and late bilious vomiting are the clinical signs and symptoms. Plain radiographs show nonspecific dilatation of multiple bowel loops with air and fluid.

Both diagnosis and treatment rest upon barium enema examination, which reveals a long *filling defect* of the plug of meconium, proximal to which the colon is dilated and obstructed; dissection of the barium around the plug commonly dislodges and allows passage of the obstructing bolus of meconium. Clinical signs of obstruction are relieved promptly. A few of these babies later are found to have Hirschsprung's disease or cystic fibrosis. The cause of the inspissated meconium is unknown.

Besides the stomach, the colon is the least likely site for atresia or stenosis of the gastrointestinal tract to occur. It will produce complete (atresia) or partial (stenosis) obstruction at the site of the membrane, which must be distinguished from other causes of colonic obstruction by barium enema examination. Excision and anastomosis constitute proper surgical treatment.

NECK MASSES IN INFANTS AND CHILDREN

Cervical masses in infants and children are extremely common; a careful examiner is able to find neck nodules in virtually every youngster from 2 to 10 years of age. Fortunately, most of these are innocent lymph nodes that are simply residua of previous upper respiratory infections.

Lymph nodes

Acute cervical lymphadenitis arises from a primary infection (usually in the pharynx) and in itself justifies no specific therapy other than that directed to the inciting primary inflammation. Less commonly, acute lymphadenitis becomes suppurative, manifested as a fluctuant, tender neck mass; specific treatment in the form of warm soaks followed by surgical incision and drainage should be undertaken at this point, and cultures usually show *Staphylococcus* as the guilty organism. The use of antibiotics depends on the organism, the status and site of the primary infection, and the general condition of the patient.

Chronic cervical lymphadenitis is less common than acute or sub-acute forms. In this country chronic cervical adenitis is rarely attributed to tuberculosis and is generally caused by atypical *Mycobacterium,* cat-scratch disease, or fungal infections.

Neoplasm

Cervical adenopathy in children can also herald a malignancy, generally primary and belonging to the lymphoma family and less commonly cervical neuroblastoma or rhabdomyosarcoma. Metastatic carcinoma to cervical lymph nodes is much less common in the child than in the adult and is most likely to originate from a primary thyroid neoplasm.

The surgeon is frequently asked to perform a biopsy on a persistently enlarged cervical lymph node for histological confirmation of diagnosis. Neck dissection for therapy of cervical malignancy is limited to localized cervical neuroblastoma or rhabdomyosarcoma and for the surgical treatment of thyroid carcinoma, commonly adjunctive to roentgen-ray therapy and chemotherapy.

Branchial remnants

Embryological *remnants* of the *branchial arch system* produce *sinuses, cysts,* and *fistulas* that occur from the external pinna to the clavicular insertion of the sternocleidomastoid muscle in infants and children. Only the first two branchial arch systems are usually involved in these vestigial remnants.

Preauricular sinuses and skin tabs constitute about one-third of branchial remnants, representing residuals of the *first branchial arch.* They usually produce only cosmetic defects, but the sinuses can become infected. Either of these conditions represents a valid indication for surgical excision. However, excision must be carried out in the operating room with proper anesthesia, exposure, and light because the sinuses must be removed in their entirety to avoid recurrences and injury to the facial nerve.

Second branchial arch remnants present as cysts, sinuses, or fistulas in the anterior triangle of the neck. The cysts generally arise later in childhood as fluctuant swellings just anterior to the upper half of the sternocleidomastoid muscle; they represent approximately 10% of all branchial abnormalities. The cysts are prone to recurrent bouts of infection, thus justifying prophylactic complete excision.

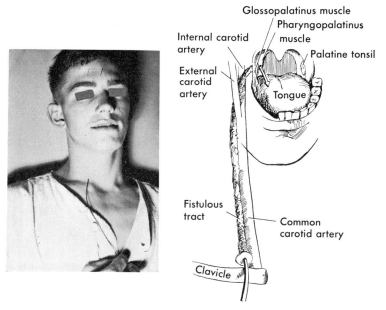

Fig. 28-14. Branchial fistula. Ureteral catheter passes from the external ostium on up the tract to the tonsillar fossa.

Cervical fistulas and sinuses constitute the bulk of branchial remnants and in about 15% of patients are bilateral. The external ostia always open on the skin along the anterior border of the sternocleidomastoid muscle, usually in its lower one third (Fig. 28-14). The sinuses extend cephalad for varying distances to terminate blindly. The fistulas extend completely cephalad to empty into the pharynx at the tonsillar fossa; the tract invariably passes behind the posterior belly of the digastric muscle and between the branches of the carotid artery (in keeping with its second branchial arch derivation). Both cysts and fistulas are lined by epithelium and are prone to become infected. Prophylactic total excision is the treatment of choice; long fistulas often require two parallel neck crease incisions (stepladder incisions) to allow the exposure necessary for their safe and total removal. Recurrences are certain with incomplete excision.

Cystic hygroma

Cystic hygroma (cavernous lymphangioma) is the classical developmental abnormality of the lymphatic system. It consists of multiloculated cysts filled with watery tissue fluid that may appear as relatively asymptomatic masses anywhere on the body; however, 85% are confined to the lateral neck and face area (Fig. 28-15) (the left is slightly more common than the right side); 2 to 3% of the cervical cystic hygromas have extensions into the mediastinum. The axilla is the second most common location of cystic hygroma.

Cystic hygromas are generally present at birth and commonly enlarge rapidly during infancy. They tend to invade or displace surrounding structures, thereby producing their only serious symptoms: interference with deglutition and the airway. Pathologically, they are

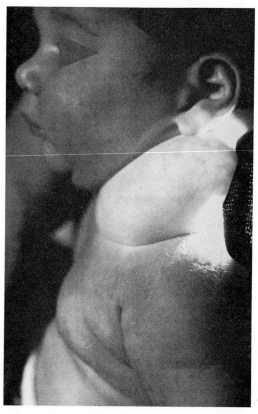

Fig. 28-15. Cystic hygroma of neck. Note how brilliantly it transilluminates

considered hamartomas rather than neoplasms. Cystic hygromas seem to represent lymphatic spaces that receive tissue fluid via afferent channels but that do not establish the proper efferent connections to the venous system, resulting in accumulation of lymph. Correct diagnosis is made by palpation of a soft, cystic mass that does not change the color of the overlying skin, which is nontender and transilluminates brilliantly (Fig. 28-15).

Treatment by aspiration of cystic hygromas has largely been abandoned: (1) the needle cannot penetrate into all the multiple cysts, and (2) it carries the risk of introducing infection, which can be acute and progressive. The rare solitary cyst, or cysts that recur after surgical treatment, may be aspirated and hypertonic glucose injected to favor sclerosis and obliteration. The most commonly accepted treatment of cystic hygroma is excision of as much of the lesion as possible without damaging vital neurovascular structures. Excision is carried

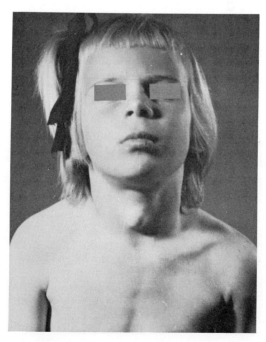

Fig. 28-16. Thyroglossal duct remnant.

out at an elective age, except in the rare instance when the airway is threatened by displacement or involvement.

Thyroglossal duct remnants

Thyroglossal duct remnants (Fig. 28-16) produce masses in the anterior midline of the neck, generally at about the level of the hyoid bone. They represent cystic dilatation of remnants of the thyroglossal duct, the embryological anlage of the thyroid gland that normally involutes and disappears. The thyroglossal tract arises as a midline diverticulum from the back of the tongue *(foramen cecum)* and moves caudally through the midportion of the hyoid bone before splitting into the two definitive lateral thyroid lobes in their normal position low in the anterior cervical area.

Thyroglossal cysts may appear anywhere along this tract but are most common in and around the hyoid bone. They must be differentiated from other midline neck masses in children:

1. *Submental lymph nodes* are generally multiple, movable in a lateral plane, and not cystic in consistency.
2. *Dermoid cysts* are generally lower in the anterior midline of the neck than thyroglossal duct cysts, are more superficial, sometimes actually attaching to the skin, and are not elevated by protruding the tongue.
3. *Ectopic thyroid tissue* can arise anywhere along the thyroglossal tract, is solid rather than cystic, and concentrates iodine on diagnostic radioactive iodine uptake studies. Ectopic thyroid tissue should *not* be removed if it is the *only* thyroid tissue that the patient possesses.

Thyroglossal duct cysts are fairly deep-seated, are cystic in consistency, are not tender unless secondarily infected, and move cephalad upon protrusion of the tongue. Treatment is surgical excision of the cyst plus the remnant of the thyroglossal tract that connects the cyst to the foramen cecum of the tongue; this makes obligatory the removal of a 1 cm. block of midline hyoid bone and the entire tract up to the base of the tongue.

VASCULAR ANOMALIES
Hemangiomas

The *capillary hemangioma (strawberry mark, raspberry mark)* is the most common peripheral vascular abnormality in infants and children. It is generally present at birth but can appear after a few weeks or even months of life. Histologically it is composed of numerous tiny vascular channels. Grossly the capillary hemangioma is a bright red mass that may be small and flat or quite elevated and nodular, but that retains the characteristics of blanching with compression, best observed by pressing a glass slide firmly over the lesion. About 70% of the lesions are confined to the upper torso, head, and neck.

Although initially small, capillary hemangiomas almost uniformly display a growth spurt for the first 6 to 12 months of life, often at an alarming rate, with a slowing of growth during young childhood. Well over 90% begin to regress spontaneously during the middle childhood years, with progressive diminution in size by thrombosis of the vascular channels. The thrombosis typically begins centrally as whitish areas that appear within the pink-red lesion; these whitish areas then coalesce and spread peripherally to encompass the entire lesion.

Because of their tendency to regress spontaneously, active treatment of capillary hemangiomas is not recommended unless they compromise a vital function by virtue of their location, or if their growth rate is continuous and entirely out of proportion to body growth rate. Surgical excision, injection of sclerosing agents, radiation therapy, or local cryotherapy are accepted methods of active therapy, which often are more disfiguring than the ultimate result of the untreated lesion.

Cavernous hemangioma (Fig. 28-17) is numerically only about one-tenth as common as its capillary counterpart. It consists principally of

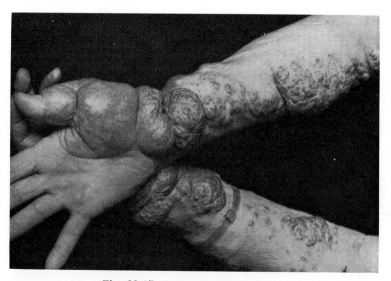

Fig. 28-17. Cavernous hemangiomas.

larger-sized vascular channels that often contain some lymphatic elements, as well as abnormal connections with the arterial vascular tree. Cavernous hemanigomas most commonly involve the dermis and subcutaneous tissues of the extremities to produce an irregular, soft mass that imparts a red to blue discoloration to the overlying skin. They may diminish in size upon compression, reverting quickly to their former size upon release of pressure and enlarging during periods of increased venous pressure (Valsalva effect, crying, or straining).

Cavernous hemangiomas are much more serious than the capillary type because (1) they infrequently involute, (2) they are cosmetically more disfiguring, and (3) local gigantism results when the member is extensively involved, probably because of the increase in blood flow to the tissue. Treatment is generally unsatisfactory, whether by injection of sclerosing agents, excision and skin grafting, or irradiation. Complete surgical excision is performed safely only on small cavernous hemangiomas. Extensive lesions must be approached cautiously and conservatively, with therapy individually tailored to forestall or treat ulceration, infection, and hemorrhage, and to ablate gigantism.

OTHER COMMON PEDIATRIC SURGICAL DISEASES
Tonsils and adenoids

Tonsils and adenoids are structures that are part of the lymphatic system of the body. The tonsils are paired clumps of lymphoid tissue lying on each side of the pharynx at the base of the tongue, and the adenoid tissue is in the nasopharynx behind and above the uvula. As with lymphoid tissue elsewhere in the body, they enlarge with infections as mechanisms of defense. Because of the frequency of upper respiratory tract infections in children they are commonly enlarged at this age.

Tonsils are not removed because of their size alone. Untreated tonsillitis can result in peritonsillar abscesses or bloodstream infections. Enlargement of the adenoids blocks nasal respiration and obstructs drainage of the eustachian tube connecting the middle ear with the pharynx to produce recurrent bouts of otitis media. Chronic adenoid enlargement encourages a mouth-breathing habit, poor humidification of inspired air, and resultant episodes of bronchitis and cough.

Tonsillectomy and adenoidectomy are performed if tonsil and adenoid enlargement are associated with repeated middle ear infections, recurrent bouts of bronchitis or pneumonia, or a chronic habit of breathing through the mouth. Introduction of antibiotics has reduced the number of tonsillectomies and adenoidectomies performed in recent years.

Appendicitis

Appendicitis is the most common cause for emergency abdominal operation in the child, although its actual incidence appears to be declining. Extremely rare in the infant and unusual under the age of 5 years, its incidence increases rapidly thereafter with the peak incidence at about 11 years of age.

Obstruction of the lumen initiates appendicitis (Fig. 28-18). This occurs either from enlargement of the lymphoid tissue underneath the lining mucosa of the appendix (generally in the younger child) or by a concretion of feces and undigested vegetable matter called a fecalith (Fig. 28-19) (generally in the older child or adult). The obstruction traps the mucoid secretions of the appendiceal cells to progressively build up intraluminal pressure; intestinal organisms cause infection and abscess. Occasionally the obstruction relents and the attack of appendicitis is aborted; if it persists, the appendix becomes turgid, swollen, edematous, and inflamed, which then progresses by vascular thrombosis to gangrene and perforation. Perforation results in peritoneal contamination with rapid development of peritonitis with generalized abdominal pain, high fever, paralytic ileus, and abdominal rigidity (an acute surgical abdomen).

The speed of progression from obstruction to perforation is rapid in the very young since defense mechanisms are limited and the symp-

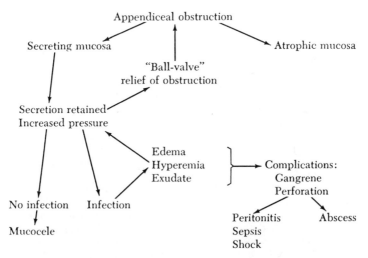

Fig. 28-18. Pathophysiology of appendicitis.

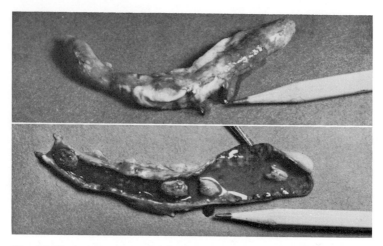

Fig. 28-19. Acute suppurative appendicitis. Note in the top photograph the distended, injected, and edematous appendix. The opened specimen shows the obstructing fecalith to the left and other fecaliths, pus, and debris filling the lumen.

toms difficult to communicate. The complication rate of appendicitis in children under the age of 5 years is understandably high, approximately 80% by the time operation is undertaken. The older the child, the slower the progression, the more accurate the history, the lower the complication rate.

Symptoms begin with epigastric pain that gradually migrates to the umbilical area and then localizes to the right lower abdominal quadrant as the parietal peritoneum in this area becomes involved in the inflammatory process. Anorexia, nausea and vomiting, low-grade fever, leukocytosis to a range of 9,000 to 14,000 cells/cu. mm., and malaise are common findings. Diagnosis can be difficult because of early nonspecificity of symptoms and findings. Localized tenderness in the right lower abdomen is the most accurate sign. Occasionally plain abdominal roentgen rays show an opacified obstructing fecalith.

Many nonsurgical illnesses mimic appendicitis: right lower lobe pneumonia, mesenteric lymphadenitis, and enterocolitis to mention but a few. Because of the very serious potential complications of appendicitis, exploration is indicated whenever the possibility of appendicitis exists. The surgeon is wrong in about 20% of cases, but he accepts this in order not to miss the "difficult-to-diagnose" case that, if un-

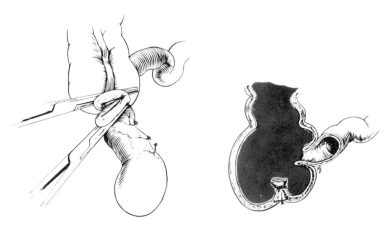

Fig. 28-20. Removal of inflamed appendix.

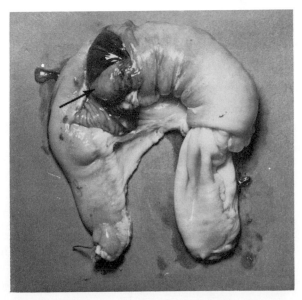

Fig. 28-21. Intussusception of the small bowel. Note the telescoping of bowel toward the left side of the specimen, which has been opened in its midportion to disclose a polyp *(arrow)* causing the intussusception.

treated, would become complicated by perforation and peritonitis. Surgical treatment involves removal of the inflamed appendix, closure of the base of the appendix leading into the cecum, and drainage of localized pus (Fig. 28-20).

Intussusception

Intussusception is an invagination or telescoping of one segment of bowel into another (Fig. 28-21); its cause is not known. Intussusception results in intestinal obstruction with the threat of strangulation of the involved bowel as the blood supply becomes shut off. The majority involves the distal ileum telescoping into the cecum with propagation on or around the colon to varying levels. Intussusception is characteristically seen in the 6-month-old to 18-month-old well-nourished child. Abdominal pain occurs every 5 to 10 minutes (intestinal colic), during which the child cries and doubles up, followed by a period of disarming quiet. Vomiting of bile and the passage of bloody stools resembling currant jelly are classic features. The intussuscepted bowel can often be palpated as a tubular mass across the upper abdomen when the child relaxes between episodes of intestinal colic.

Barium enema (Fig. 28-22) confirms diagnosis and also can be used to reduce the intussusception safely (in about two-thirds of the patients). This reduction is observed by fluoroscopy; the barium column is elevated no higher than 30 to 36 inches above the table to avoid perforation of the bowel or reduction of strangulated bowel. Surgical reduction and sometimes bowel resection are required when barium reduction is ineffective or when strangulation is suspected.

Hypertrophic pyloric stenosis

Hypertrophic pyloric stenosis is the most common cause for intestinal obstruction in the baby 2 to 6 weeks of age (occurring once in 200 births). Forceful vomiting of gastric content not discolored by bile is the outstanding feature of the history. Prominent waves travel from left to right across the epigastrium; these represent forceful peristaltic contractions of the stomach attempting to squeeze gastric material through the narrowed pyloric channel. The pylorus, the muscle surrounding the outlet of the stomach, becomes thickened (Fig. 28-23, *A*). Its lumen (the pyloric channel) narrows, obstructing the outflow of material from the stomach. The basic cause for this hypertrophy is unknown.

The diagnosis is confirmed in about 80% of the patients by palpation of the thickened muscle, the "olive" mass, in the right upper abdominal quadrant. If the age, history, or findings are atypical, an upper G.I. series establishes the diagnosis by outlining the narrow pyloric

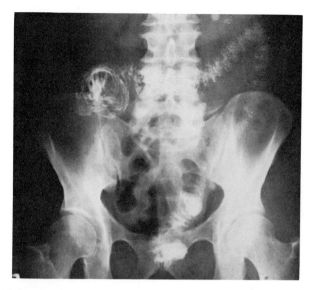

Fig. 28-22. Barium enema showing the diagnostic "coil-spring" appearance of ileocolic intussusception at about the hepatic flexure of the colon in the patient's right upper abdomen.

channel. Acute pyelonephritis and the adrenogenital syndrome occasionally mimic the symptoms of pyloric stenosis.

Operative treatment is simple; the thickened pyloric muscle is incised and spread apart (Fig. 28-23, *B* and *C*), thereby enlarging the channel and relieving the obstruction. Pyloromyotomy (Ramstedt procedure) has perhaps the highest success rate and the lowest morbidity and mortality of any common operative procedure.

Inguinal hernia, hydrocele

Inguinal hernia in the male child results from retention of an embryological outpocketing of peritoneum known as the *processus vaginalis,* which accompanies testicular descent into the scrotum. The walls of this structure normally adhere to obliterate the sac (Fig. 28-24, *A*), but if obliteration fails, the sac will remain and allow bowel to enter as a hernia (Fig. 28-24, *B* and *C*).

Surgical correction is carried out when the diagnosis is made because of possible complications of incarceration or strangulation of the

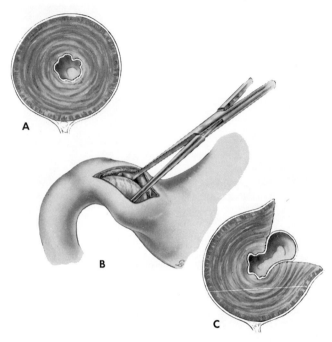

Fig. 28-23. Hypertrophic pyloric stenosis. **A,** Cross section of thickened pyloric muscle and narrow channel. **B,** Ramstedt pyloromyotomy showing instrument spreading the muscle apart after it has been incised longitudinally, allowing the intact mucosa to bulge outward as in **C** to greatly enlarge the lumen of the pyloric channel and relieve the obstruction of the stomach.

herniated bowel; this occurs in 5 to 15% of babies with a hernia. Hernia repair requires division and closure of the neck of the sac to remove the connection with the peritoneal cavity.

A hydrocele is embryologically related to the hernia (Fig. 28-24, *D* and *E*), the difference resting in the size of the connection of the patent *processus vaginalis* with the peritoneal cavity. In a hydrocele, the connection is large enough to allow fluid to gravitate into the unobliterated sac, but not large enough to allow bowel to enter. The majority of hydroceles spontaneously disappear when the small peritoneal connection becomes obliterated, allowing no further peritoneal fluid to enter. Only rarely is surgical closure of this connection neces-

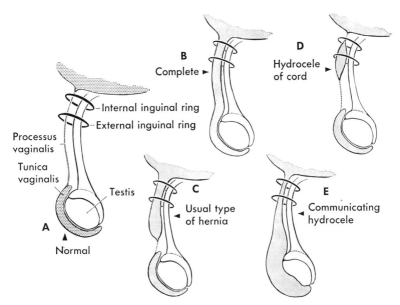

Fig. 28-24. A, Normally obliterated processus vaginalis. **B,** Complete failure of obliteration of processus vaginalis, with large opening into peritoneal cavity allowing bowel to enter as a complete, or scrotal, hernia. **C,** Proximal part of processus vaginalis does not obliterate, allowing bowel to enter as the usual type of indirect inguinal hernia. **D,** Hydrocele of cord. **E,** Communicating hydrocele; connection with peritoneal cavity is large enough to allow peritoneal fluid to enter the sac, but not large enough for bowel to enter.

sary. About 15% of hernias are preceded by a hydrocele, the peritoneal connection having enlarged sufficiently to allow bowel to enter the sac.

Hirschsprung's disease of the older child (congenital aganglionosis of the colon, congenital megacolon)

Hirschsprung's disease is the most common functional congenital obstruction of the colon. The colonic obstruction is caused by absence of peristalsis within that segment of colon in which the autonomic ganglion cells (both intermuscular and submucosal) are congenitally absent. Proximal to the aganglionic segment, the colon dilates and

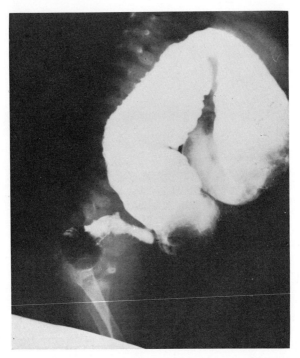

Fig. 28-25. Congenital aganglionosis (Hirschsprung's disease). Barium enema shows narrow, spastic rectum and rectosigmoid (aganglionic) flaring into megacolon (ganglionated bowel) at sigmoid colon.

hypertrophies to warrant the descriptive term "megacolon." The obstruction may be acute and relatively complete immediately after birth (discussed in section on neonatal obstruction of the colon, p. 437). Bouts of distension, vomiting, and paradoxical diarrhea interspersed with constipation characterize the disease during the first year of life. As the child grows older, chronic constipation emerges as the dominant complaint. Life-threatening complications of bowel perforation, enterocolitis, and sepsis accordingly bear an inverse relationship to age.

In about 80% of children, aganglionosis is limited to the rectum and rectosigmoid but occasionally extends higher in the colon and in nearly 5% of cases involves the entire colon. There are reported cases of aganglionosis of the entire gastrointestinal tract. Regardless of its proximal point of origin, the aganglionosis invariably extends from that point on down to include the internal anal sphincter, therefore allowing completely reliable diagnosis by the simple expedient of rectal wall biopsy carried out transanally. Abdominal distension and evidence of poor nutrition parallel the degree of obstruction. Children with Hirschsprung's disease are predisposed to acute necrotizing enterocolitis (Chapter 24), a complication that carries approximately a 50% mortality.

The history given by children with congenital aganglionosis may be extremely varied, although abnormal bowel function of some degree is present from the day of birth. There often is a delay of 24 to 48 hours in the passage of meconium per rectum after delivery, with varying degrees of constipation and/or explosive diarrhea thereafter. Abdominal distension, vomiting of feedings, and poor weight gain are common complaints. Invariably changes in formula and the use of laxatives, enemas, and suppositories have all been attempted for symptomatic control.

Physical examination reveals a somewhat pale and malnourished infant or child with soft abdominal distension. Loops of colon are often palpable, distended by gas and hard feces. Rectal digital examination reveals a small rectal ampulla. If the aganglionosis extends only to the rectosigmoid, the examining finger may reach the dilated and stool-filled sigmoid colon and provoke an explosive escape of liquid stool and gas upon withdrawal of the finger.

Barium enema is helpful in diagnosis, characteristically showing a narrow or normal-sized rectum that flares into a megacolon above the point of obstruction (Fig. 28-25); only small amounts of barium should be used, with no effort made to fill the entire colon, since tardy expulsion of the barium is a second feature of the radiographic diagnosis. Confirmation of diagnosis rests upon rectal wall biopsy.

The treatment of Hirschsprung's disease is surgical, except in rare instances of a very short aganglionic segment that can be easily controlled by conservative methods (stool softeners and enemas). Initial efforts are directed toward relief of the intestinal obstruction, generally by performing a colostomy; the proximal extent of aganglionosis is histologically determined by seromuscular biopsy of the colon obtained at appropriate levels. The colostomy must be placed within an area of normal ganglion cells.

Definitive treatment consists of resection of the aganglionic colon to within 1 to 3 cm. of the anus. Anastomosis of the ganglionated colon to the rectal pouch is achieved by one of a variety of abdominoperineal techniques. Prognosis is good.

CHAPTER 29

Geriatric surgery

SIDNEY E. ZIFFREN

According to mortality statistics, about two out of three Caucasian males born today in the United States will reach the age of 65 years. At 20 years of age, their chances of living to 65 years of age are about 70%. The survival likelihood for a Caucasian female is slightly more favorable. These figures have increased about 10% during the past 25 years. If this favorable survival trend continues to the year 2000, there will be over 32 million people in this country over 65 years of age.

Using Table 29-1, one may calculate the years of life expectancy among people in this country, once they have achieved Senior Citizen status. The "weaker" female sex enjoys greater longevity at all age levels.

Table 29-2 contrasts causes of death among Caucasian United States males in the first two decades with the eighth decade of life. Cardiovascular-renal diseases and cancer account for only 5% of deaths in the young, but over 80% of deaths in the aged. These figures do not support the contention, however, that if medical science could effectively reduce deaths from cardiovascular-renal disease and cancer, longevity would greatly increase. On the contrary, if mortality from malignancy at age 70 were decreased by 10%, it would add only approximately 0.1 year to life expectancy; reduction of 20% would add 0.2 year, and decrease of cancer deaths by 30% would add only approximately 0.4 year to life expectancy.

From time to time the suggestion is made that in A.D. 2000 man may expect to live to be 100 years old. Of the Caucasian offspring born at the present time in the United States, only about 15% of the males and 23.5% of the females will live to 90 years of age. The average life expectancy beyond 90 years has remained virtually un-

Table 29-1. Average years of life expectancy among Caucasian American males and females*

Age	Caucasian males	Caucasian females
65	13.0	16.0
70	10.3	12.5
75	8.0	9.4
80	6.2	7.0

*Calculated for the different ages that have already been achieved in the left-hand column; females are expected to live longer than males at all ages.

Table 29-2. Comparison of causes of death in Caucasian American males up to 20 years of age with those of men in the eighth decade of life*

Cause of death	Ages 0-19 (%)	Ages 70-79 (%)
Cardiovascular-renal disease	1.7	65.9
Cancer	3.7	16.3
Accidents	16.9	2.7
Pneumonia and influenza	6.2	2.5
Tuberculosis	0.2	0.8
Diabetes mellitus	0.1	1.5
All other causes	71.2	10.3

*Accidental death is most prominent in the young, whereas death from cancer and degenerative disease causes the majority of deaths in the aged.

changed since 1840. It is expected to improve only slightly in the future. Even if we were to assume that sometime in the future all deaths could be prevented before the age of 90, which is very unlikely, the expectation of life at birth would still be less than 95 years. The time is still unforeseeable when a man can expect to live for 100 years.

CHARACTERISTIC DISEASES OF THE AGED

Certain conditions are far more common in the elderly than in the young, the prime example being *degenerative diseases,* such as arterio-sclerosis. Degenerative disorders are manifested in many different forms and systems, such as cardiac failure or myocardial infarction, peripheral vascular insufficiency, aortic aneurysm, or cerebrovascular accidents from hemorrhage or thrombosis.

Other diseases, including fractures and probably cancer, are dependent on degenerative processes. These diseases, common in the aged, are discussed in more detail in relevant chapters. The proximal femur is the bone most commonly *fractured* in the aged, both the neck and intertrochanteric regions being especially vulnerable. Forearm fractures are rarely encountered in the elderly patient, whereas fracture of the neck of the humerus is not uncommon. Vertebral fractures are common among elderly females because of the frequency of osteoporosis. *Colon diverticula* progressively increase with age, and their complications of inflammation, perforation, and bleeding are serious problems. The elderly male is plagued with *hyperplasia* of the *prostate* leading to urinary tract obstruction and infection, and emphysema is the most common respiratory tract problem in the aged. The incidence of *cancer* rises steadily with each decade of life. Between 20 and 60 years of age, the frequency of cancer of the breast and female reproductive system leads to a higher malignancy incidence in women than in men. Above the seventh decade of life, however, this figure is reversed and males develop cancer more than females. The incidence and mortality of all cancers increase with age to reach a maximum in the eighth decade of life and then decline because of the fewer survivors exposed to this risk.

PREOPERATIVE PROBLEMS OF THE AGED
Blood volume

The most common and difficult problem in the aged surgical patient is a *diminished total blood volume.* Old people tolerate fluctuations in blood pressure poorly because of homeostatic mechanisms that are not as flexible as those of a younger person, and a small blood loss in the elderly patient may precipitate irreversible shock, myocardial infarction, or a cerebrovascular accident. A diminished blood volume must therefore be diagnosed and treated prior to any operation in the elderly. Experience has shown that hypovolemia of some degree can be anticipated in the aged patient with *cancer, infection,* or *intestinal obstruction.* The physician must recognize and correct this diminished volume before operation is undertaken; otherwise a tragic result may occur on the operating table or during the postoperative period.

Many sophisticated instruments and techniques are available in hospitals for measuring total circulating blood volume. However, hypovolemia can and should be recognized clinically. Clinical criteria that should arouse suspicion of hypovolemia are recent weight loss, an emaciated, chronically ill appearance, and poor skin turgor. The blood pressure tends to fall when a patient with diminished blood volume stands up, and the pulse accelerates slightly. Hemoglobin and hematocrit levels are often deceptively normal, but one must remember that these measure only the *concentration* of red cells in the blood, and do *not* indicate *total blood volume*. The patient with chronic hypovolemia has become adjusted to a lower blood volume, and his vascular space contracts to compensate for the volume deficit. If he were to suffer an acute blood loss, the vascular compartment could not compensate by further contraction and shock would quickly ensue.

Occasionally, total blood volume is preserved in the aged patient who has slowly developing anemia (chronic blood loss, iron deficiency) by an increase in the plasma volume, giving hematocrit and hemoglobin levels that accurately reflect the red blood cell deficit. Attempts to correct this type of anemia hastily by transfusions of whole blood may produce hypervolemia with pulmonary edema; packed red blood cell transfusions are preferable to whole blood.

A handy clinical guide to total blood volume in the aged is the response of hemoglobin and hematocrit levels to transfusions. A 500 ml. whole blood transfusion raises the hemoglobin level approximately 1.5 Gm./100 ml. when plasma volume is normal, and the hematocrit rises approximately 3 to 6 vol.%. If a blood transfusion produces less of a rise than this, the patient is quite likely hypovolemic. The plasma volume gradually adjusts to these increments of transfusions by renal excretion of excess fluid, and slow daily transfusions may safely be given until a hemoglobin of 12.5 to 13 Gm./100 ml. is reached and the expected incremental rises of hemoglobin and hematocrit are achieved.

Nutrition

Ideally, every aged patient should be brought to a healthy nutritional state preoperatively, with ample body stores of glycogen and protein. However, this ideal is impossible to achieve for a number of reasons. Preoperative priming of the elderly surgical candidate with intravenous amino acids, fats, alcohol, albumin, or plasma is costly in time and money and must be given through a large vein (subclavian). Many patients cannot take enough food by mouth because of the nature of their disease (intestinal obstruction, paralytic ileus), or the urgency of treating their disease (cancer) precludes the time required for nutritional repletion by oral means. Tube feedings of rich formulas often provoke diarrhea, and nasogastric tubes are poorly tolerated by the elderly patient. Consequently, no long-term attempts are usually made to correct nutritional deficiencies completely before operation.

In contrast, vitamin deficiencies require short-term attempts at replacement. Many elderly surgical patients are in borderline vitamin deficiency because of the reduction in both vitamin requirements and intake imposed by the semistarved state associated with many surgical disorders. Under these conditions, if caloric intake is suddenly increased, the depleted vitamin stores are rapidly used up, resulting in an acute vitamin deficiency. Consequently, some multivitamin preparation is given for several days preoperatively to exclude this possibility.

Cardiopulmonary status

Heart and lungs require especially careful evaluation in the elderly preoperative patient. Complex pulmonary tests are ordinarily not done, since no simple method is as yet available. However, if serious lung disease is suspected on the basis of history, physical examination, or radiographic examination of the chest, then more detailed studies of pulmonary function are indicated, especially if a thoracotomy is anticipated. (See Chapter 30.) Arrhythmia, tachycardia, rales, heart murmurs, elevated venous pressure, and dependent edema are simple clinical signs that justify further cardiac evaluation and consultation.

Renal function

Renal function must be assessed carefully, especially in the elderly male so prone to bladder neck obstruction from prostatic enlargement. The history of urinary tract difficulties or evidence of urinary infection or bladder distension on the routine work-up justifies additional investigation. Measurement of residual urine, determination of blood urea, and intravenous pyelography and cystography are simple and helpful tests to document urinary tract disorders that might well take priority over the patient's surgical disease, or influence the surgeon's method, choice, or time of operation.

Hydration

Acute surgical disease that requires emergency operation often imposes an additional requirement on the physician: evaluation of the patient's state of hydration and electrolyte balance. Commonly the aged patient has low cardiac reserve and impaired renal function that demand especially judicious replacement of fluid and electrolyte deficiencies before operation may be undertaken safely.

OPERATIVE PROBLEMS IN THE AGED

What can we expect in terms of operative mortality in the aged? In Table 29-3 are listed some of the standard operations and their mortalities in patients below the age of 60 in contrast to later decades of life. In general, low mortalities are found in operations that (1)

Table 29-3. Mortality percentages of standard operations performed at the University of Iowa during a recent 10-year period, broken down according to different age groups

Operation	Under 60	60-69	70-79	80 and over
Thyroidectomy	0.0	0.0	0.0	0.0
Radical neck dissection	0.0	2.8	5.9	13.6
Simple mastectomy	0.0	0.0	1.1	0.0
Radical mastectomy	0.0	0.0	2.8	8.5
Below-knee amputation	1.7	1.8	6.3	3.3
Above-knee amputation	3.7	7.1	17.1	16.5
Inguinal hernioplasty	0.1	0.2	1.6	3.3
Partial colectomy	6.4	6.8	5.4	9.0
Cholecystectomy	0.8	2.8	5.5	5.4
Partial gastrectomy for ulcer, cancer, and massive hemorrhage	3.9	5.0	11.2	19.8
Transurethral prostatectomy	0.4	2.2	2.3	5.0

are of short duration, (2) involve little blood loss, and (3) have low rates of postoperative infection. The opposite qualities characterize high-mortality operations. It is clear that operative procedures done as emergencies carry a much higher operative mortality than when the same operations are performed electively; e.g., elective chole-cystectomy is much safer in uncomplicated gallbladder disease than emergency operative procedures for acute cholecystitis, gallbladder perforation or gangrene, or obstructive jaundice. This is perhaps the most compelling justification for prophylactic surgical treatment of potentially serious problems such as hernias, "silent" gallstones, colonic polyps, and enlarging aortic aneurysms, even when they are not espe-cially symptomatic in the elderly patient who at the time is a good operative risk.

POSTOPERATIVE PROBLEMS IN THE AGED

In the postoperative period the aged patient is vulnerable to many of the same complications that occur in younger persons, plus many that are unique to the aged. However, his responses to these complica-tions may be much different from those seen in younger age groups; e.g., it is common for the elderly patient with infection to show no fever or leukocytosis. Such nonspecific complaints as apathy and de-lirium may herald the onset of a postoperative complication in the aged patient that might be more explicitly manifested in the young. Constant observation and alertness on the part of the surgeon are needed to interpret these vague complaints correctly and to detect the development of a complication.

The incidence of postoperative pulmonary complications is much higher in the aged than in the young. Inefficient coughing and deep breathing lead to retained secretions, atelectasis, poor alveolar exchange, and pneumonia. Generalized weakness and immobility, apathy, depression by analgesic drugs, or respiratory splinting because of operative pain initiate what develops into a vicious cycle. Immobility and weakness favor development of venous thrombosis, with the constant threat of embolization and pulmonary infarction. In general, one complication in an aged patient seems to promote another and yet another, in almost arithmetic progression. Prophylaxis, early detection, and early treatment of complications are the key to successful postoperative management of the elderly surgical patient.

It is easy to overload the aged patient in the immediate postoperative period with fluids and electrolytes, forgetting that his renal mechanisms are below par and that edema develops more easily in this group than in the younger group. Unfortunately, the edema does not remain confined to the dependent portions of the body but involves all of the organs, including the lungs.

The aged patient can be brought through most surgical procedures quite easily. However, in no other branch of surgery is more care required of the surgeon in the technical delicacy, speed, and precision of the operative procedure, and in the manner in which he handles the postoperative period. The experienced surgeon recognizes all these fine nuances, and the pitfalls that are likely. He is constantly engaged in preventing complications from occurring because he anticipates them. Surgery in the elderly is a great but rewarding challenge.

CHAPTER 30

Thoracic and pulmonary surgery

NICHOLAS P. ROSSI
DONALD B. DOTY

Thoracic surgery deals primarily with dynamic structures, mainly the heart and lungs; their integrated function is vital to life. To this end, the thoracic surgeon operates on these structures to correct abnormalities of development, relieve obstruction, drain and contain infections, and extirpate tumors. Adequate function of the heart and lungs must be maintained during operation, which often requires highly sophisticated techniques and instruments.

Diseases of the heart and lungs are among the most common and important in man. Most of them have become amenable to surgery within this century, mute testimony to great advances in understanding the pathophysiology of the thoracic viscera. This chapter summarizes the most important surgical diseases of the thorax and lungs.

SPECIAL PROCEDURES

Certain procedures are commonly used for diagnosis and treatment of patients with thoracic and pulmonary disorders that every student should understand. Since they will be referred to often on the succeeding pages of this section, their principles are discussed here.

Thoracentesis

Thoracentesis is simply needle aspiration of the pleural cavity. It is performed both for diagnosis and for treatment of disorders causing abnormal accumulations of gas or fluid within the pleural space. The accumulations may consist of air (pneumothorax), blood (hemothorax), serum (pleural effusion), chyle (chylothorax), pus (empyema), or varying combinations thereof (hemopneumothorax, pyopneumothorax).

Normally, the pleural cavity is simply a *potential* space that is under negative pressure (−5 to −10 cm. H_2O) during inspiration (expansion of the rib cage and depression of the diaphragm) and under positive pressure (up to +5 cm. H_2O) during expiration. The space is bounded by *parietal pleura* lining the inside of the chest wall and *visceral pleura* covering the surface of the lungs. Normally, the pleural cavity contains only a few milliliters of lubricating serum to allow frictionless gliding of the apposed pleural surfaces during respiratory excursion.

Since the chest wall is relatively unyielding, accumulations within the pleural space first collapse the ipsilateral lung to impair its expansion and aeration, proportionate to the volume accumulated. Progressively greater volumes shift the mobile mediastinal structures to the other side, impairing expansion of the contralateral lung and diminishing the return of venous blood to the heart. Cardiopulmonary dysfunction results that is proportionate to the volume and speed with which the gas or fluid accumulates within the pleural space.

The technical details of thoracentesis are sketched in Fig. 30-1. Thoracentesis is performed aseptically after shaving, scrubbing, and painting the skin with an antiseptic solution. The operator is gloved and often wears a mask and gown. The needle is introduced just *above* an appropriate rib, to avoid the intercostal vessels that travel along the *inferior* rib surface. The patient with pneumothorax is supine and the needle is introduced parasternally in the second or third intercostal space, since air gravitates upward. When fluid is to be removed, the needle is introduced into the seventh or eighth intercostal space in the midaxillary line while the patient is in an upright position, since fluid gravitates inferiorly (Fig. 30-1, *C*). If the fluid is loculated or localized, radiographic examination of the chest or fluoroscopy should guide placement of the needle.

Diagnostic thoracentesis is performed when physical examination and radiographic examination of the chest disclose pleural collections (generally fluid) of an unknown type. Generally, only a few milliliters of the fluid are aspirated, with no attempt being made to tap the pleural space dry. The aspirate can be inspected, cultured, stained, examined cytologically, and tested for clotting properties, specific gravity, pH, and chemical constituents. Definitive treatment is facilitated by knowing the precise nature of the pleural effusion.

An attempt is made to evacuate the pleural fluid or air totally in a thoracentesis performed for *therapeutic* purposes. The visceral and

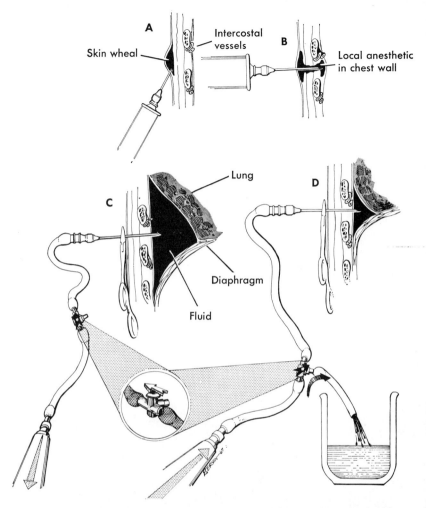

Fig. 30-1. Thoracentesis for removal of pleural fluid. **A,** Skin wheal with local anesthetic agent. **B,** Infiltration of chest wall with local anesthetic agent. **C,** Thoracentesis needle introduced above the superior surface of the appropriate rib so that its tip just enters the pleural space; needle clamped by hemostat at skin level to prevent further advancement; fluid aspirated into syringe. **D,** Stopcock changed to allow delivery of fluid from the syringe into the side arm and container; the system is not disconnected until the needle is withdrawn, to avoid air entering the pleural space.

parietal pleural surfaces are thereby apposed to one another and help seal off the source of leakage of air or blood. Removal of large amounts of pus aids in the supportive treatment of empyema and thins the fibrous "peel" that subsequently forms. Occasionally, drugs are injected into the pleural space (fibrinolytic enzymes, antibiotics) before withdrawing the needle. Diagnostic and therapeutic thoracenteses are often combined.

Complications of thoracentesis are few: (1) bacteria may be introduced if the needle is dirty, if the skin is inadequately prepped, or if the needle is inserted through a contaminated area of the chest wall, (2) air is sucked into the pleural space if the needle, tubing, or syringe becomes disconnected, because of the negative intrapleural pressure, and (3) the lung may be punctured by the needle tip, provoking a pneumothorax or hemothorax. These complications are minimized by careful attention to the technique illustrated in Fig. 30-1.

Pleural space drainage

Underwater-seal drainage is the standard technique of *closed tube drainage* of the pleural space to remove pleural space air or fluid aseptically and encourage lung expansion. It is selected in preference to thoracentesis when the leakage is expected to continue for some time (hours or days), with rapid reaccumulation likely after simple needle aspiration.

In keeping with the principles outlined for thoracentesis, the chest tubes are introduced aseptically high anteriorly for the removal of air, and low and laterally when fluid is removed. They may be inserted through a trochar under local anesthesia, but more commonly are left indwelling at the conclusion of thoracotomy operations in which functioning lung tissue remains in that hemithorax. Tube drainage is *not* used after total pneumonectomy because the risk of postoperative air leak or infection is low, and the serum that fills the empty hemithorax obliterates dead space to prevent dislocation of mediastinal structures, and the other lung, to the operated side.

Fig. 30-2 diagrams the principles of underwater-seal drainage. The fluid or blood enters the bottle under the surface of the water, with the length of glass tubing immersed determining the positive-pressure that must be exerted by the patient before drainage occurs. Air bubbles off through the vent in the top of the bottle, while fluid accumulates in the bottle. The fluid cannot backtrack up the tubing to reenter the pleural space. If the tubes are not plugged, one can tell that an air leak has sealed when bubbling ceases and that pleural fluid has disappeared when the fluid level in the bottle stabilizes. The tubes are generally removed at this time.

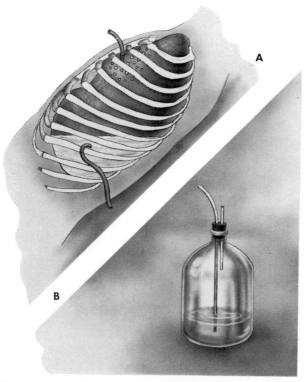

Fig. 30-2. Intercostal chest tubes with underwater-seal drainage. **A,** The tube to remove air from the pleural space is introduced through the second intercostal space at the midclavicular line; the tube to remove liquid (blood, pus, and postoperative fluid collection) is introduced through the eighth intercostal space at the anterior axillary line. **B,** The tubing is connected to the glass rod on the bottle that is covered with sterile water; the pleural air bubbles into the bottle and escapes to the outside, while the fluid collects in the bottle.

Open tube drainage of the pleural space simply communicates the pleural space directly to the outside, generally via one or two hard rubber tubes. The tubes are introduced through an appropriate intercostal space, or (preferably) through the bed of a short segment of resected rib. Open tube drainage is simpler and quicker than closed tube (underwater-seal) drainage, but it can be used only under the following circumstances: (1) when contamination is already present (empyema), (2) when the negative intrapleural pressure has been lost, and (3) when the lungs and mediastinal structures are fairly fixed, or stabilized, so that they cannot be dislocated. With these limitations, the open tube method is usually restricted to the drainage of chronic empyema.

Tracheobronchial toilet

Good tracheobronchial toilet is essential at all times and is automatically carried out by all of us as we periodically change position, sigh, breathe deeply, clear our throat, or cough. Maintenance of a clear airway is especially important in patients with lung disease or patients who are recently postoperative. It is accomplished best by the patient himself with frequent changes in position, periodic deep breathing, and vigorous coughing. When the patient cannot or will not carry out tracheobronchial toilet himself, it must be supplied by the nurses and physicians responsible for his care.

Endotracheal suction is one of the techniques to facilitate tracheobronchial toilet, as outlined in Fig. 30-3. The irritation that the tube provokes in the trachea generally itself induces uncontrollably vigorous coughing, raising sputum and dislodging mucous plugs that are then sucked out. Saline and mucolytic agents can be injected through the tube to liquefy secretions and improve cleansing of the respiratory tree. A "trap" in the tubing allows collection of the aspirate for examination and culture. The apparatus must be sterilized before using.

Periodic assisted ventilation and *tracheostomy* are more extreme measures in tracheobronchial toilet that are used without delay if simpler methods fail. Ventilation can be assisted by bag and mask but is administered more effectively by passing an endotracheal tube and ventilating with a bag. Irrigation and aspiration can be performed through the tube, and poorly aerated or atelectatic areas of lung are expanded to improve respiratory exchange.

Tracheostomy allows irrigation, aspiration, and assisted ventilation to be performed by a nurse or technician and, in addition, reduces respiratory "dead space." However, it is accomplished at the expense of increased nursing care, desiccation of inspired air, loss of phonation, and occasionally misadventures such as erosion of the trachea and bleeding.

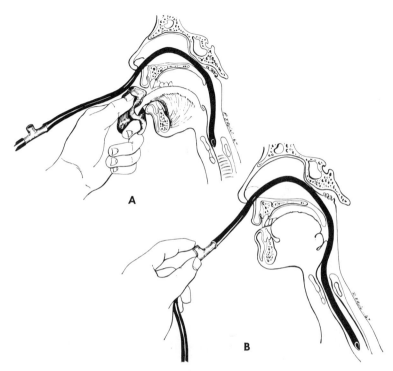

Fig. 30-3. Endotracheal suction. **A,** Patient in sitting position, tongue grasped and retracted forward to enlarge hypopharynx; suction catheter introduced through nose curves around posterior pharynx to enter larynx and upper trachea. **B,** Suction applied to remove secretions brought to catheter tip by violent coughing that the catheter provokes; the suction is intermittently broken by removing finger from the adapter, to prevent mucosa from being sucked into catheter tip, and to minimize arterial hypoxemia that accompanies aspiration of gas from the airway. Administration of oxygen before, during, and after endotracheal suction reduces hypoxic complications.

Bronchoscopy

Bronchoscopy allows visualization of the interior of the trachea and main stem bronchi through an illuminated, rigid, tubelike instrument. The bronchoscope is introduced with topical anesthesia in the cooperative and sedated adult but requires general anesthesia in children and uncooperative adults. Mucosal ulceration, inflammation, or tumors can be seen at bronchoscopy, as well as deviation, distortion, and narrowing of the trachea and bronchi. Secretions can be aspirated, foreign bodies removed, and suspicious mucosal lesions biopsied through the bronchoscope. The rigid bronchoscope complemented by use of telescope lens systems allows visualization of the airway to segmental bronchi and is therefore of greatest use in centrally located proximal lesions.

Direct examination of subsegmental bronchi is possible by means of the flexible bronchofiberscope, which utilizes the fiberoptic principle allowing the visual image to be transmitted along a curved pathway. Because of this unique property and a relatively small diameter, the device can be manipulated into subsegmental bronchi, thereby expanding direct airway visualization. In addition, the instrument provides access to distal bronchi for the passage of brush catheters and small biopsy forceps. These devices can be guided under fluoroscopic control into peripheral lung lesions, allowing diagnosis in 80% of cases.

Bronchography

Bronchography allows radiographic visualization of the smaller ramifications of the tracheobronchial tree. Radiographs are taken in different projections after a rather viscid radiopaque material has been injected endobronchially via a nasotracheal catheter. The patient is positioned appropriately to allow filling of any or all of the lung segments. Bronchography outlines filling defects caused by tumors or foreign bodies, localizes endobronchial obstruction, and diagnoses bronchiectasis and abnormalities of position of the various lung segments.

Prescalene lymph node biopsy

Occasionally a diagnosis of known pulmonary disease cannot be made by radiographic examination of the chest, bronchoscopy, bronchography, sputum analyses, and other routine measures. In such patients, biopsy of the prescalene lymph nodes is sometimes helpful in diagnosis. The procedure is done under local anesthesia for all but children and uncooperative adults, a supraclavicular transverse incision being preferred. The incision is made on the side of palpable nodes, and a diagnosis is nearly always secured. If the nodes are not palpable, a diagnosis is provided in only 10 to 15% of cases, and lymph node pathological changes are nonspecific in the remainder. With nonpalpable nodes, the left pescalene nodes are biopsied if the pulmonary disease involves the left upper lobe (which drains to this side), but the right prescalene nodes are biopsied if the disease predominantly involves the right lung or the left lower lobe. This choice of sides is made to avoid the thoracic duct, which is on the left side at the junction of the jugular and subclavian veins, and also because of the known crossover of the lymphatic drainage of the left lower lung to the right prescalene lymph node chain.

Prescalene lymph node biopsy is especially helpful in the diagnosis of Boeck's sarcoid, obscure lung carcinoma, hilar masses, and diffuse bilateral pulmonary infiltrates, but there is a low yield in tuberculosis, pulmonary mycoses, solitary peripheral lung lesions, bronchopneumonia, and pleurisy.

Mediastinoscopy and anterior mediastinotomy

Biopsy of mediastinal lymph nodes is more likely to yield a diagnosis in patients with pulmonary disease than biopsy of more distant regional lymph nodes. These procedures require general anesthesia. Mediastinoscopy is performed by inserting a lighted scope through a small cervical incision in the suprasternal notch. The instrument is passed along the anterior surface of the trachea deep to the pretracheal fascia to the level of the bifurcation of the trachea. Lymph nodes adjacent to the trachea, proximal right and left bronchi, and subcarinal area are visualized and biopsied. Anterior mediastinotomy is an extrapleural mediastinal exploration through the bed of the second or third costal cartilages. These procedures are nearly always diagnostic in sarcoidosis or lymphoma with hilar adenopathy and are of great value in assessing mediastinal spread of bronchogenic carcinoma.

Lung biopsy

For diffuse disease of the pulmonary parenchyma it may be necessary to obtain a specimen of the lung for analysis. A trephine air drill or cutting needle may be used percutaneously to biopsy the lung but carries the hazard of pneumohemothorax. Open biopsy of lung through small anterior thoracotomy is usually the best means of obtaining adequate, representative tissue.

LUNGS
Pulmonary function tests

Pulmonary function tests are as much a part of medicine as are tests for hepatic, renal, or cardiac function. They are valuable in de-

Table 30-1. Pulmonary function tests*

Test	Definition	Normal value	Explanation and remarks
Vital capacity (VC)†	The volume of gas exhaled by maximum voluntary effort after maximum inspiration	Depends on age, weight, sex, nutrition, height	The VC alone is of very limited value; it is useless in evaluating obstructive disease and correlates poorly with dyspnea; it is reduced in the restrictive lung diseases
Timed vital capacity (TVC)†	The amount of the vital capacity exhaled in a given time interval: 1, 2, or 3 seconds; in 1 second it is called the forced expiratory volume or FEV 1	About 85% of VC is normally exhaled in 1 second	This test relates much better to the overall evaluation of ventilatory function and to dyspnea than does the VC; the shortest 1-second volume correlates best with symptoms
Air-velocity index	$\dfrac{\% \text{ predicted MBC}}{\% \text{ predicted VC}}$	A value below 0.8 is indicative of airway obstructive disease; a value greater than 1 indicates restrictive airway disease	The actual value of the two components must be considered first
Maximal voluntary ventilation (MVV)	The amount of gas exchanged per unit of time during maximum voluntary hyperventilation; usually done over 10 to 15 seconds, or to 1 minute if possible	Formulas based on age and surface area	Unlike single-breath tests, it reflects the integrity of the respiratory bellows as a whole, including fatigue, muscular strength, blood supply, and air trapping; better correlates with dyspnea
Mean maximal inspiratory flow (MMIF)	The mean maximal flow measured between 200 ml. and 1,200 ml. on the inspiratory spirogram	400 to 600 L./min.	Normally is a straight line throughout

Test	Description	Normal value	Significance
Mean maximal expiratory flow†	The mean maximal expiratory flow rate for that portion of the VC between 200 and 1,200 ml.	From formulas: 400 to 600 L./min., average adult	A reduction indicates that a mechanical problem exists; this is serious because it decreases the patient's ability to cough and remove secretions from his airway because of excessive air trapping
Dyspnea index	The percentage of the MBC required for a standard exercise	8 to 15% walking at 2 m.p.h.	An increase in the dyspnea index is most commonly the result of a decreased ventilatory capacity and rarely the result of increased respiratory requirement
Transfer factor for carbon monoxide (D_{CO})	A test for evaluation of the diffusion capacity of the lungs; several techniques; the simplest is a single breath test in which the amount of CO entering the blood is measured after inspiring a gas mixture of known CO concentration and holding the breath after one preliminary breath	25 ml./min./mm. Hg; frequently reported as a percentage of a predicted value based on known dependent factors	Depends on many factors— position, body size, hematocrit, and alveolar P_{O_2}; normal value indicates normally functioning pulmonary capillary membranes; does not require patient cooperation
Single-breath nitrogen test	Another test to evaluate diffusion capacity	Less than 1.5% N_2	Used to determine uneven distribution of the inspired air; may be normal in obstructive and restrictive lung disease but means serious lung disease when abnormal

*These tests are readily available and require minimal instructions; all are used in screening.
†Part of the routine physical examination.

terming the location or type of process causing respiratory impairment, and in serially documenting changes that occur during therapy. Table 30-1 outlines commonly used pulmonary function tests. For more elaborate tests the student should consult other references.

Blood gases

When the lungs cannot maintain arterial O_2 pressures and saturation at normal levels, pulmonary insufficiency for oxygenation (hypoxemia) results. When they cannot prevent the increase of arterial CO_2 tension, insufficiency exists for CO_2 elimination (hypercapnia or hypercarbia).

Hypercapnia is always caused by alveolar hypoventilation that is secondary to severe impairment of the mechanics of breathing. The trouble may be in the lungs (pneumonitis), the airways (mucous plug), the pleural space (pleural effusion), respiratory muscles (tetanus), or respiratory center (cerebrovascular accident). Impairment of diffusion does *not* cause hypercapnia because the tissue CO_2 solubility quotient is 20 times that of O_2. Arteriovenous shunting also is not an important cause. Hypercapnia is almost always associated with hypoxemia, but hypoxemia can coexist with a normal CO_2 arterial pressure and saturation.

Hypoxemia, unlike hypercapnia, may be caused by several mechanisms and may exist with no measurable impairment of the mechanics of breathing. The most important causes of hypoxemia are venoarterial shunts (as seen with congenital intracardiac shunts, or in areas of lung atelectasis), underventilation, poor diffusion (thickened alveolar-capillary membrane), and when breathing air of low O_2 content (high altitudes).

Congenital malformations
Congenital lobar emphysema

Congenital lobar emphysema is an important cause of respiratory distress in the newborn, and at times is life threatening. The involved lobe (usually the left upper and right middle lobes) is markedly overdistended because of a ball valve effect of a partially obstructed bronchus; air readily enters the lobe but cannot escape. The lesion may be associated with insufficient blood supply to the involved portion of the lung, or the bronchus may have faulty cartilaginous support, but frequently the cause is obscure. In cases in which carefully pathological study has been carried out, a cause can be found in no more than half. Progressive respiratory distress (tachypnea, dyspnea, cyanosis) is the chief clinical problem. Serial plain chest radiographs show an enlarging, air-filled cyst. Resection of the involved lobe gives excellent results.

Pulmonary intralobar sequestration

Pulmonary sequestration is a bronchovascular anomaly produced when the bronchus supplying a part of the lung (usually the lower lobes) develops abnormally and loses its connection with the tracheobronchial tree and receives its arterial supply from the lower thoracic or abdominal aorta. The involved lung contains many cysts lined by ciliated or mucus-producing columnar epithelium. Recurrent infection is common. The chest radiograph may simulate the changes of bronchiectasis, abscess, localized empyema, and occasionally a tumorlike form. Aortography showing the abnormal vessel may be diagnostic. The lesion is four times more common in males. Excision of the sequestered lesion is the treatment of choice.

Arteriovenous fistulas

Congenital connections between a pulmonary artery and vein occasionally occur. This anomaly, in a diffuse form, may be related to hereditary hemorrhagic telangiectasia. Congenital arteriovenous fistulas are multiple in more than 50% of the cases and vary from miliary proportions to large communications occurring peripherally in all lobes. Symptoms include dyspnea, cyanosis, clubbing, hemoptysis, and easy fatigability. Central nervous system manifestations are related to the associated polycythemia or to intracranial vascular abnormalities. Bruits may be heard on auscultation of the chest. In the localized form, the disorder is very rarely recognized during childhood, but when widespread, it causes severe respiratory disorders in the newborn. In long-standing cases severe complications, such as hemoptysis, stroke, and brain abscess, have occurred.

Single lesions are excised. In the miliary form, surgical therapy has little value. Ligation of the supplying vessels is worthless.

Agenesis, hypoplasia, aplasia of the lungs

The lesions of agenesis, hypoplasia, and aplasia of the lungs are rare. They may be bilateral or unilateral and may involve a lobe or an entire lung. Bilateral pulmonary agenesis is the rarest and severest form, is associated with cardiac defects, and, of course, is incompatible with life. Unilateral agenesis of the lung also causes a high toll in infant mortality but is in itself compatible with life. There is usually a history of some respiratory difficulties, and the chest film shows a homogeneous density. An incorrect diagnosis of massive atelectasis may be made, as with foreign body inhalation.

In hypoplasia the lung is underdeveloped, as are the corresponding artery and bronchus, and this is sometimes associated with congenital diaphragmatic hernia. In aplasia no aerated lung tissue is present in the involved segment, and the bronchus is rudimentary. Recurrent infection is common. Surgical excision is the usual therapy of both hypoplastic and aplastic lung segments.

Congenital bronchogenic cysts

Congenital bronchogenic cysts are usually found in the mid-mediastinum near (but not communicating with) the tracheal bifurcation and main stem bronchus. They are usually single but may be multilocular. They are lined by respiratory epithelium, and the walls often contain smooth muscle and cartilage. Infection may destroy the epithelium to make specific histological identification difficult. Symptoms depend on the size, location, and the presence of infection: wheezing, pain, cough, atelectasis, and nonspecific symptoms of infection are all possible. Excision should be performed.

Acquired disease
Chylothorax

Chylothorax, an uncommon clinical entity, is associated with tumor, trauma, or tuberculosis. By far the most common is trauma (about half the cases). It also occurs after operations, especially after dissections around the subclavian artery for patent ductus, coarctation of the aorta, Blalock shunts, and esophagogastrectomy. It may follow some abdominal operations, such as vagotomy and gastric resections. It may be the presenting sign of an unrecognized lymphoma.

Spontaneous chylothorax occurs in the newborn and causes symptoms of tachypnea, cyanosis and chest wall retractions. In older children, chylothorax with symptoms of respiratory difficulty, cough, or recurrent pneumonia suggests an intrathoracic anomaly.

Aspiration alone is effective therapy in children. It will usually be successful in benign cases but is frequently ineffective for chylothorax caused by tumors. The cause should always be sought.

Inflammatory bronchiectasis

Inflammatory bronchiectasis is a chronic suppurative disease of lung segments resulting from pulmonary infections, asthma, and bronchial obstruction (i.e., aspirated foreign body). In the group derived from infections, bronchiectasis begins in the first 5 years of life. The pathogenesis is now generally believed to be a necrotizing infection around the branches of segmental bronchi. The smaller bronchi become obliterated, and the larger proximal bronchi undergo dilatation and widening during the healing, fibrotic phase of the inflammatory process. Sinusitis and allergy are common.

Bronchiectasis is described according to anatomic type: cylindric, saccular, fusiform, or cystic. Mild cylindric bronchiectasis is reversible, but otherwise anatomic classification is not clinically significant. In children, bronchiectasis is commonly associated with aspiration of foreign bodies, chronic upper and lower respiratory tract infections, and cystic fibrosis of the pancreas. Bronchiectasis is a disease of the lower lobes, except when found in conjunction with tuberculosis.

The symptoms are those of recurrent pulmonary infection: fever, morning cough, production of foul-smelling sputum, hemoptysis, chest pain, and retarded physical development. Socioeconomic problems are common. Bronchography is the most important diagnostic examination, also documenting the extent and location of the disease. Bronchoscopy rules out tumor or foreign body. Complications of the disease are hemorrhage, empyema, and metastatic spread of the infection (brain abscess).

Treatment of bronchiectasis consists of rest, adequate nutrition, antibiotics, and postural drainage. Operative removal of the involved segments is carried out during a quiescent phase in selected patients with adequate pulmonary function, and with appropriate antibiotic coverage. In bilateral cases the operations are staged, the more advanced areas in one lung being resected first.

Empyema

Empyema, or infection of the pleural space, is a complication of lung disease and not a primary disease in itself. The diagnosis is sus-

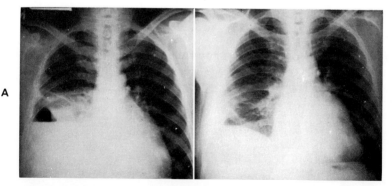

Fig. 30-4. Empyema. **A,** Air-fluid level in right pleural space in patient with pneumonia; indeterminate nature of fluid (blood, pus, serum) by radiograph, but thoracentesis yielded pus. **B,** Same patient after 2 weeks of closed pleural drainage via intercostal tube; pus virtually gone and lung expanded.

pected by signs of fluid within the pleural cavity on physical examination (absence of breath sounds, dullness to percussion, tracheal deviation to the other side) and radiographic examination of the chest (Fig. 30-4) and is confirmed by diagnostic thoracentesis with smear and culture of the purulent fluid. The physician's first duty is to rule out underlying obstructive lung disease by bronchoscopy. Then he must consider if the infection is coming from the lung (lobar pneumonia), from the esophagus or the mediastinum, or from below the diaphragm.

The aim of treatment is the restoration of normal respiratory function. This demands full expansion of the lungs with obliteration of the empyema space, as well as restoration of normal mobility of the lungs, diaphragm, and chest wall. In the acute phase, when the pus is thin and no organizing exudate has formed over the lungs, one or more thoracenteses may accomplish these ends. In the chronic phase, closed tube drainage of the pleural space may suffice; the most common mistake is premature removal of the tube, which should remain in place with periodic shortening until the lung has fully expanded. Decortication is necessary in chronic forms when a fibrous peel encases the collapsed lung (captive lung), the operation consisting of excision of the peel to allow reexpansion of lung.

Lung abscess

Lung abscess is a destructive, suppurative process in the lung caused by microorganisms (Fig. 30-5). The infection is usually polymicrobic. Unlike bronchiectasis, which follows an anatomic segment of the lung, the destructive process of lung abscess crosses segmental lines. Several underlying causes must be considered:

1. *Aspiration of vomitus:* Probably the most common cause of lung abscess, it happens especially in alcoholics, epileptics, patients with central nervous system diseases, and patients who have been unconscious for long periods of time.
2. *Bronchial obstruction with infection distal to the point of obstruction:* Carcinoma, bronchial adenoma, and foreign body are causes.
3. *Pneumonia:* The type of organism determines the pattern of resulting lung abscess. The pneumococcus (type III) and *Klebsiella* produce multilocular cavities, usually in the upper lobes. *Staphylococcus,* the most common cause of lung abscess in infants and children, produces a necrotizing bronchopneumonia leading to multiple abscesses, which can become huge from bronchial obstruction and air trapping.
4. *Abscess from infected cysts or from breakdown of a bronchial*

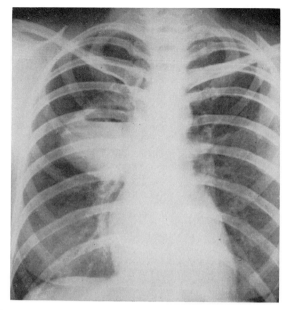

Fig. 30-5. Lung abscess. Underlying cause was carcinoma of the lung; the air-fluid level indicates connection with a bronchus.

carcinoma: Infection destroys the lining of a cyst, making it very difficult to determine its true nature. The "carcinomatous abscess" is one of the many faces of lung carcinoma (Fig. 30-5).

5. *Abscess caused by trauma:* Infection of a hematoma or imbedded foreign material.

6. *Extension from abdominal infection:* Subdiaphragmatic abscess and amebic infection of the liver are the usual precursors.

7. *Metastatic septic abscess:* Seeding of the bloodstream from a distant focus (prostate, soft tissue, liver, etc.) is the method of spread of the infected material to the lungs. The abscesses are usually small and multiple.

Complications of lung abscess include brain abscess, empyema, septicemia, and endotoxic shock.

Clinical signs of lung abscess are fever, cough, production of purulent sputum, anemia, and clubbing of the fingers. Radiographic examination of the chest generally confirms the diagnosis of lung abscess, but bronchoscopy and bronchography are often helpful.

The treatment of acute lung abscess is conservative: postural drainage, bronchoscopic aspiration, bed rest, high caloric diet, blood, and antibiotics. Resection of involved lung is indicated when stenosis of the bronchus is present, empyema is associated, localized lung damage is extensive, and conservative therapy has failed.

Middle lobe syndrome

Middle lobe syndrome refers to intermittent or chronic collapse of the middle lobe of the right lung (Fig. 30-6). Etiology is obscure and variously ascribed to pressure from lymph nodes surrounding the middle lobe bronchus or to its acute angle of entry into the stem bronchus. Tuberculosis is one of the known causes for lymph node enlargement leading to this syndrome, but often no specific infection is found.

The three predominant symptoms are recurrent pneumonia, hemoptysis, and dull chest pain aggravated by breathing. Cystic bronchiectasis is commonly present in the atelectatic lobe. Bronchoscopy and bronchograms rule out carcinoma, tuberculosis, and foreign body. Resected specimens may reveal congenital bronchial stenosis, cysts, specific infections (coccidioidomycosis or histoplasmosis), chronic nonspecific pneumonia, or granuloma.

Characteristically, radiographic examination of the chest shows a triangular density best seen on the lateral projection (Fig. 30-6).

Some cases can be treated conservatively by postural drainage and

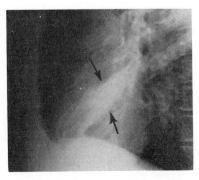

Fig. 30-6. Middle lobe syndrome. Triangular density of the collapsed middle lobe is best seen between arrows on lateral chest radiograph.

specific antibiotic therapy. If this is not successful, the middle lobe should be resected.

Pulmonary tuberculosis

Pulmonary tuberculosis has long been a scourge of mankind, but with epidemiological methods and modern drug therapy it can be controlled, if not eradicated. Despite this control, the incidence of new cases in the United States currently is in the range of 28.7 per 100,000 population, with a death rate of about 5 per 100,000. These figures indicate that tuberculosis is still a health problem of major proportion.

The surgical treatment of pulmonary tuberculosis has changed radically since the introduction of streptomycin and para-aminosalicylic acid in the late 1940s, isoniazid in 1952, and rifampin in the late 1960s. Those who lived through this era recall the "old days" with the same terror invoked by other infectious diseases. Their records show that 70% of patients who had a persistent tuberculous cavity died within 5 years. Total cure was impossible, and methods of treatment, such as induced pneumothorax, often produced more harm than good. Sanitariums were crowded to overflowing, since each patient required an average of 2 years' confinement. All of this has changed for the better, and now the indications for surgical treatment or institutional care are few.

Pathogenesis. Clinically, an initial primary or "childhood" type of tuberculous infection occurs in the lungs that requires about 2 years to develop into the adult type of disease, in those few whose disease progresses. In children pulmonary tuberculosis is frequently accompanied by pleural effusion and by mediastinal and cervical adenopathy. A conservative approach of combined drug therapy is most rewarding in this group. The adult disease is caused by reinfection from a previous tuberculous focus, or a new infection from without. Reactivation is seen more commonly in untreated patients, or in those who were inadequately treated with drugs.

Types of pulmonary tuberculosis. Types of pulmonary tuberculosis are tuberculoma, cavities, bronchitis and bronchostenosis, empyema, bronchiectasis, tuberculous lymphadenitis, and pericarditis.

Tuberculoma. Tuberculoma is a somewhat confusing term, since it has been applied to a first infection focus in the lung. It should be restricted to describe a focus of reinfection, or to a cavity filled with caseous material. Without treatment, about 25% of tuberculomas break into a bronchus and cause endobronchial spread.

Cavities. Tuberculous cavities are lung abscesses that cross segmental barriers between lobes. The cavities may attain a large size, sometimes because the tension produced by air trapped within them. Some become inspissated with caseous material to form tuberculomas. Sometimes they are small and multiple, and as healing progresses with increasing fibrous tissue reaction, a honeycomb or bronchiectatic appearance is produced.

Bronchitis and bronchostenosis. Tubercles in bronchi produce bronchitis. The resultant scarring may so narrow the bronchus as to cause bronchostenosis, which may lead to tension cavities, tuberculomas, persistent cavities, or heavy scar formation in the involved segment or segments.

Empyema. Tuberculous empyema results from tuberculous pleurisy or may follow induced pneumothorax, spontaneous pneumothorax, or resection. Pyogenic organisms may also be present, usually after bronchopleural fistulization.

Bronchiectasis. Bronchiectasis results from bronchostenosis caused by healing endobronchial disease, or by compression of the bronchus by tuberculous lymph nodes. Fistulous connection between the bronchiectatic sacs differentiates it from nontuberculous bronchiectasis. Differentiation, however, may be difficult.

Tuberculous lymphadenitis. Tuberculous lymphadenitis may have serious sequelae: bronchostenosis, erosion into a bronchus with endobronchial spread, or spread to the esophagus, pleura, or pericardium. Many of these problems are seen in children with untreated disease.

Pericarditis. In the past, constrictive pericarditis was most often caused by tuberculosis. Recently, viral and other forms of pericarditis have become more important clinically.

Diagnosis. The protean clinical manifestations of pulmonary tuberculosis suggest that the diagnosis is difficult to establish. Ordinarily this is not so. The vast majority of cases are diagnosed correctly by skin tests, radiographic examination of the chest (Fig. 30-7), and multiple examinations of sputum or gastric washings (swallowed sputum) for acid-fast organisms on smears, culture, and guinea pig inoculations. Thoracentesis, bronchoscopy, bronchography, and prescalene lymph node biopsies are occasionally necessary for diagnostic confirmation. A few obscure cases defy diagnosis by all conventional methods.

Surgical treatment of pulmonary tuberculosis. The aim of treatment in pulmonary tuberculosis is to inactivate the disease permanently (sputum negative for tubercle bacilli). The disease can be prevented by chemoprophylaxis in persons known to be high risks: people (especially children) who are exposed to patients with active pulmonary infection, patients with inactive tuberculosis who have

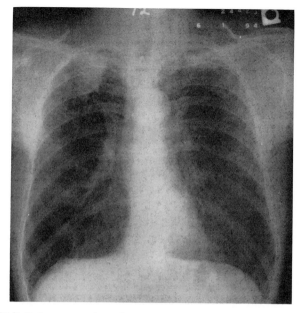

Fig. 30-7. Pulmonary tuberculosis. Bilateral apical fibronodular densities, upward retraction of both lung hila, and compensatory emphysema of both lower lobes.

never been treated with drugs, especially if they are diabetics, receiving steroids, or have had gastrectomy.

Operations used in the surgical treatment of pulmonary tuberculosis fall into two groups:

1. *Relaxant procedures* designed to collapse the involved lung to promote healing.
2. *Resectional therapy.* The trend in the last two decades has been toward this group, but the need for all operative procedures is decreasing.

The *relaxant procedures* are as follows:

1. Induced pneumothorax and pneumoperitoneum.
2. Creation of an extrapleural space by stripping the parietal pleura from the chest wall.
3. Extraperiosteal plombage, filling the space between the lung and ribs with leucite balls or some other inert material.

Text continued on p. 506.

Table 30-2. Fungus diseases of the lungs

Disease	Agent	Endemic geographic distribution	Transmission	Radiographic findings	Laboratory diagnosis	Symptoms	Treatment
Sporotrichosis	*Sporotrichum schenckii*	Worldwide	Direct inoculation into skin from puncture wound	Pleural effusion and fibrocavitary appearance similar to tuberculosis Variable degree of infiltration, cavitary miliary disease (in the disseminated form)	Fusiform organism on biopsy or from sputum or exudate	Involves all organs	KI Amphotericin Hydroxystilbamidine
Aspergillosis	*Aspergillus*	Worldwide	May be normal saprophyte in sputum; usually found in sick patients with lymphoma, carcinoma, tuberculosis	Pneumonic abscess, intracavitary fungus ball	Only dependably established by tissue biopsy	Bronchitis, acute or chronic pneumonia, allergic form Hemorrhage a serious threat	KI value limited Amphotericin B Resection

Monilia-sis	*Candida albicans*	Worldwide	Invasion under conditions of reduced resistance, prolonged antibiotic or steroid therapy	Pneumonia or miliary spread	Only when organism is found in blood or seen in tissue	Those of a severe bronchopneumonia	Amphotericin B
Actino-mycosis	*Actinomyces bovis*	Worldwide	Aspiration from mouth to lower respiratory tract; not a contagious disease	Dense, progressive infiltrates; abscess	Organism seen as sulfur granules in pus or sputum; gram-positive, anaerobic; skin or serology tests no good	Seldom acute cough, purulent sputum, weight loss, low-grade fever; occasionally constrictive pericarditis	Sulfa drugs, penicillin, drainage of abscesses or empyema
Nocar-diosis	*Nocardia aster-oides*	Worldwide	Saprophytes in soil also found in respiratory tract associated with tuberculosis, lupus erythematosus, leukemia, pulmonary alveolar proteinosis	Dense infiltrates; abscess or cavity formation common	Acid-fast gram-positive, cultured early from pus, sputum	Acute or chronic cough, hemoptysis, night sweats, weight loss, pleural involvement, brain abscess and meningitis, mycetoma on foot (madura foot)	Sulfadiazine, drainage of pus and abscess; pulmonary resection only occasionally

Continued.

Table 30-2. Fungus diseases of the lungs—cont'd

Disease	Agent	Endemic geographic distribution	Transmission	Radiographic findings	Laboratory diagnosis	Symptoms	Treatment
Histo-plasmo-sis (Fig. 30-8)	*Histo-plasma capsu-latum*	Most common in Mississippi River basin	From soil contaminated by excreta of birds, bats, and rodents	Variable pneumonia: dense infiltrates, miliary pattern, coin lesion, Ghon type of complex, sclerosing mediastinitis	Demonstration of organism in sputum or lung tissue; complement fixation test 1:8 is regarded as significant	Primary infection is transient; heavy infiltration results in acute pneumonia, protean symptoms in the disseminated form	Amphotericin B; resection of localized disease, otherwise biopsy and drug therapy
Coccidioidomycosis	*Coccidioides immitis*	Southwestern United States	Airborne, highly infectious but not contagious; can be passed on by fomites	Variable: thin-walled cavity, solitary lesion, infiltrates; pneumonitis, pleural effusion, adenopathy	PAS stain of biopsy material; organisms grow readily on Sabouraud's; any complement fixation titer significant	Primary infection, "flu-like," erythema nodosum (20% in females); 1:1,000 clinically ill; small number hematogenous spread with meningitis	Amphotericin B, but not for most cases that are self-limited; surgery for persistent cavities

Cryptococcosis	*Cryptococcus neoformans*	Worldwide; soil especially contaminated by pigeon excreta	Common in leukemia, Hodgkin's disease, diabetes, sarcoid, prolonged steroid therapy; lung principal portal of entry	Solitary or multiple nodules, pneumonitis, mediastinal adenopathy; cavitation rare	Organisms in tissue, C.S.F., or sputum; no skin or complement fixation test available	Human infection usually subclinical; meningitis common; diagnosis made in only half of patients before operation	Amphotericin B is only agent of value; localized pulmonary disease; resection and drug coverage
North American blastomycosis	*Blastomyces dermatitidis*	United States and Canada	Inhalation of spores, not contagious, common in persons in contact with soil	Variable, usually dense pneumonitis or infiltration; may resemble bronchogenic carcinoma	Budding yeast found in sputum, pus, gastric juice, prostatic secretion; treated with potassium hydroxide without staining; skin test not reliable	Similar to those of tuberculosis; suspect with lesions in skin, bone, and lung	Amphotericin B; pulmonary resection rarely indicated

4. Thoracoplasty, removal of the ribs and section of bands of deep cervical fascia attached to the apex of the lung (apicolysis); extensive thoracoplasty is used to close bronchopleural fistulas.

Resectional therapy is indicated for the following:

1. Tuberculosis bronchiectasis
2. Destroyed lung
3. Thick-walled cavity unsuitable for collapse
4. Tuberculoma
5. Giant cavity
6. After a thoracoplasty that has not rendered the patient sputum-negative
7. Suspicion of carcinoma—the incidence of carcinoma of the lung is three times as great in tuberculous patients as in the general population; any patient receiving adequate antituberculous drug therapy whose disease has been stable but who shows a change in his roentgenograms becomes highly suspicious for carcinoma

Pulmonary infections caused by atypical mycobacteria

In recent years atypical mycobacteria (*M. Kansasii* and *M. intracellulare*—the Battey bacillus) have caused pulmonary lesions that are amenable to treatment. In properly selected patients the chance of obtaining negative status has been three to four times greater in surgically treated patients than in medically treated ones.

Fungus diseases

Table 30-2 includes the agent, endemic geographic distribution, transmission, radiographic examination, laboratory diagnosis, symptoms, and treatment of fungus diseases of the lungs.

Pulmonary neoplasms
Bronchial carcinoma

Fifty years ago lung cancer was an infrequent disease. Today it kills more men than any other type of cancer, and its incidence is still rising (Chapter 11). Several environmental materials are known to be related causally: asbestos, arsenic, nickel, chromium, and uranium. Average male smokers of cigarettes are ten times more likely to develop lung cancer than are nonsmokers, and for heavy smokers the risk is twenty times greater. Carcinomas arise from surface epithelium of the bronchus, progressing from squamous metaplasia to carcinoma in situ and on to invasive cancer.

Histologically, lung carcinoma is classified as squamous (epidermoid) cell carcinoma, adenocarcinoma, alveolar carcinoma, and undifferentiated carcinoma.

Squamous (epidermoid) cell carcinoma is slow-growing, involves lymph nodes by direct extension, and tends to be central (toward the hilum) in origin.

Adenocarcinoma is more common in young women than in men, but in women is still less common than epidermoid carcinoma. It tends to be peripheral in location and spreads rapidly by vascular and lymph node involvement.

Alveolar carcinoma (bronchial carcinoma, pulmonary adenomatosis, bronchoalveolar carcinoma) occurs diffusely or as an area of consolidation. It spreads endobronchially through the lung. A multicentric origin is suspected but not definitely established. Histologically the picture is one of well-differentiated, full columnar mucosa. It is usually asymptomatic until it becomes diffuse.

Undifferentiated carcinoma consists of small cells (oat cells, polygonal cells) or large cells. Oat cell carcinoma begins in the main bronchi but rapidly involves the hilar lymph nodes to form a collar

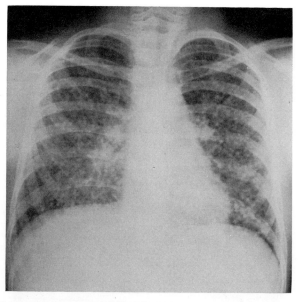

Fig. 30-8. Histoplasmosis. Innumerable tiny calcific nodules scattered diffusely throughout both lungs.

of neoplastic tissue around the bronchus. Early metastasis is common, and the prognosis is poor.

Symptoms. The symptoms of bronchial carcinoma are cough, weight loss, recurrent or unresolving pneumonia, hemoptysis, chest pain, weakness, fever, and wheezing. Extrapulmonary manifestations are clubbing (usually seen in epidermoid carcinoma), Cushing's syndrome (undifferentiated neoplasm), hypercalcemia, carcinomatous neuropathy, phlebitis, osteoarthropathy, and connective tissue disorders.

Diagnosis. Lung carcinoma presents many faces radiographically: hilar mass (Fig. 30-9), atelectasis, single nodule (Fig. 30-10), abscess (Fig. 30-5), pleural effusion, and parenchymal infiltrate.

The big three in the diagnosis are chest radiographs, bronchoscopy and biopsy (positive in only 20 to 30% of cases), and sputum cytology. Prescaline lymph node biopsy is helpful if the nodes are enlarged. Additional diagnostic measures that are useful in selected cases are mediastinoscopy, mediastinal biopsy, intraosseous azygography, pul-

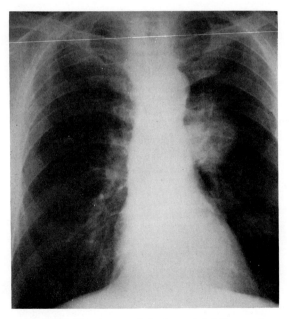

Fig. 30-9. Carcinoma of the lung; left hilar mass.

monary angiography, needle biopsy, thoracentesis, and bronchography. The biggest advance in diagnosis in recent years has been the bronchial brush biopsy. In this technique, undiagnosed peripheral lesions can be identified histologically in a much greater number of patients. We have been able to make the diagnosis by the brushing method in 70% of those patients in whom the standard methods have failed.

The treatment is surgical extirpation (segmental resection, lobectomy, or pneumonectomy). Preoperative irradiation is helpful in treating apical thoracic tumors (Pancoast's disease), but its place in the treatment of cancer elsewhere in the lung has not been clearly established. Prognosis is poor, with those who survive 5 years ranging from 5 to 20%.

Sarcoma

Lymphosarcoma may originate in the lung without involvement of lymph nodes in other areas of the body. Primary thoracic lymphosarcoma is rare but has a slow rate of growth, making it a suitable

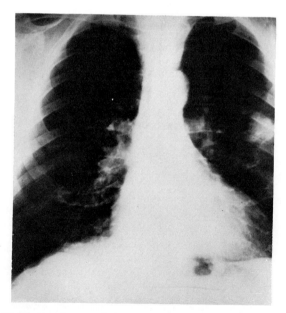

Fig. 30-10. Carcinoma of the lung; nodule in left midlung field.

lesion for surgical excision. Roentgen-ray therapy is also frequently employed. Radiographic examination of the chest reveals an area of consolidation around a patent bronchus, giving an air-bronchogram effect.

Primary sarcomas arising in the lung parenchyma are rare. They present in young patients as solitary lesions, large masses, or atelectasis. A radiolucent meniscus is sometimes seen over the mass on the chest film. Few symptoms occur unless atelectasis is produced by bronchial obstruction. Leiomyosarcoma has the best prognosis, rhabdomyosarcoma has the worst, and angiosarcomas with spindle cell sarcoma are intermediate.

Bronchial adenoma

Two types of bronchial adenoma occur, the carcinoid and the cylindromatous. They account for about 5% of all pulmonary neoplasms. These two types are morphologically and histologically different but are usually separated from carcinoma (Table 30-3).

Table 30-3. Types of bronchial adenoma

	Carcinoid	*Cylindroma*
Location	Proximal bronchus	Primary bronchi and trachea
Comparative incidence	85%	15%
Histological features	Squamous metaplasia, small uniform cell with acidophilic neoplasm; mitosis and argentaffin granules rare	Cells less uniform, smaller, occasionally oncocytic
Lymph node metastasis	Uncommon	Twice as common (30%), also distant metastases more common
Bronchoscopic appearance	Smooth, rounded protrusion into lumen, mucosa intact, bleeds freely	Extends along the bronchus wall; paler and firmer
Invasiveness	Local iceberg effect common: small intraluminal component with rather large endobronchial or extrabronchial component	Recurrence rate 7 times that of carcinoid
Symptoms	Obstruction, infection, bleeding, wheezing	Same

Bronchoscopy is diagnostic in 90% of patients with bronchial adenoma, but bronchoscopic removal should never be attempted. Bronchotomy with local excision may be used in some of the smaller lesions, but if any doubt remains as to the completeness of removal, appropriate excision (lobectomy, pneumonectomy) is required.

Hamartoma

Hamartoma is a developmental error that produces an abnormal arrangement and mixture of normal tissue and is the most common benign tumor of the lung. It must be considered in the differential diagnosis of solitary lesions in the lung. Generally this is not difficult because of the extreme peripheral location of the hamartoma, increased radiodensity, and characteristic eccentric, lobular, or "popcorn" type of calcification. Hamartomas of the lung contain cartilage, fibrous connective tissue, cubical or columnar epithelium, fat, and smooth muscle. They are not encapsulated, but readily shell out. If their characteristic pattern of calcification is not present (which is quite often), they must be distinguished from other peripheral lesions by thoracotomy.

Other benign tumors of the lung are mesothelioma, pseudotumors, lipoma, leiomyoma, hemangioma, mixed tumors, intrapulmonary teratomas, and thymomas.

Tumors of the trachea are rare. The most common is the squamous cell carcinoma of the distal trachea. Cylindromas are next most common but usually occur in the upper third. Reconstruction of the trachea after partial excision is generally unsatisfactory, and direct suture approximation must be done. The prognosis for carcinoma of the trachea is very poor but is very good for cylindroma.

Metastatic lung cancers

After the liver, the lungs are the most common site of visceral metastases of cancer. All the circulating blood must pass through the pulmonary capillary bed on each circuit, as does lymph after it enters the venous system at the jugular-subclavian confluence in the root of the neck. Thus, tumor emboli from neoplasms that spread either via the venous or lymphatic systems ultimately pass into the rich lung capillary bed. If conditions (which we do not understand) are right, the tumor emboli filter out and begin growing as pulmonary metastases. Undoubtedly, many more tumor emboli die or remain dormant in, or pass on through the pulmonary capillary system, then lodge there, and grow as metastases.

Usually, lung metastases produce multiple, rounded, discrete nodules in the periphery of both lungs, which gradually enlarge in size.

Plain chest radiographs are generally diagnostic. Carcinomas can secondarily metastasize to hilar lymph nodes, but sarcomas do not. Pulmonary complaints are often nonspecific and include vague chest discomfort, cough, breathlessness, and pulmonary osteoarthropathy, tending to mimic symptoms of primary lung cancer. Rarely, biopsy is necessary to distinguish metastatic from primary cancer of the lung.

Treatment of metastatic lung cancer is generally palliative (chemotherapy, roentgen-ray therapy) if the patient's general condition is good enough to justify any treatment at all. Surgical resection of cancer that is metastatic to lung is restricted to the occasional patient who has (1) no recurrence of the primary cancer, (2) no metastases elsewhere, and (3) lung metastases confined to one area, making surgical resection of that area possible. The slower the doubling time of the tumor, the better the prognosis.

Pulmonary embolism

Pulmonary embolic disease is a major problem. Intriguing new methods of diagnosis and treatment have been developed, but the clinical diagnosis is often difficult to make, and the efficacy of treatment is difficult to judge.

The true incidence of this disease is unknown. Pulmonary emboli are much more commonly found at autopsy than are diagnosed clinically. This dichotomy exists because of the subtle and variable clinical manifestations of pulmonary emboli. This variability occurs because of the following:

1. *Size of the occluding thrombus:* Small emboli that do not involve the visceral pleura frequently produce no symptoms because of the enormous reserve of the pulmonary vascular bed and because of natural mechanisms of clot lysis that are present in the lungs.

2. *Extent of the occlusion:* A single massive embolus produces the catastrophic picture characteristic of pulmonary embolism, but repeated small emboli produce a picture of respiratory insufficiency of obscure cause.

3. *Infarction:* Pulmonary emboli need not produce infarction of the lung. Infarction depends on other factors, such as collateral bronchial artery supply, infection, and the degree of ventilation of the involved segment.

4. *Condition of the lung:* Other diseases can influence the symptoms greatly—if congestive heart failure exists, or if the pulmonary vascular bed has been reduced by previous emboli, a small embolus may produce severe effects.

Predisposing factors. Pulmonary emboli most commonly arise as thrombi within veins of the legs and pelvis that become detached and travel through the vena cava and right side of the heart to become lodged in the narrow pulmonary artery branches. Many patients with pulmonary emboli have no history of previous venous disease, or evidence of thrombophlebitis on examination. Certain patients are predisposed to peripheral vein thrombosis: patients *immobilized* for long periods of time, the *elderly,* the *obese,* those with *malignancies, congestive heart failure,* previous emboli, and other serious medical disease (the incidence is three times higher in medical than in surgical patients). Prevention of peripheral thrombophlebitis and phlebothrombosis will obviate the problem of pulmonary emboli. (See Chapter 33.)

Diagnosis. Massive pulmonary emboli produce a catastrophic picture of collapse, shock, cyanosis, extreme dyspnea, restlessness, and chest pain followed by cough and blood-tinged sputum. The time from onset to death may be minutes to days. Small emboli produce only minimal symptoms of pleuritis, pain, and hemoptysis, and in many instances no symptoms at all. Nonspecific effects are low-grade fever, leukocytosis, and elevation in the serum lactic dehydrogenase. Signs of lower extremity thrombophlebitis are helpful, but inconstant.

Dyspnea and *tachypnea* are seen with pulmonary emboli, and the lungs demonstrate a *loss of compliance.* The second cardiac sound is exaggerated, and the *electrocardiogram* shows signs of right ventricular strain or bundle branch block. Radiographic examination of the chest often shows a prominent *pulmonary artery shadow.* Hypoxemia is mild in minor episodes of embolization but is increased with activity. Major emboli produce *cyanosis* and *pulmonary edema.* In either case, oxygen does not alleviate the hypoxemia. *Arterial CO_2 tensions* are higher than expected because increased hypercarbia from the poorly perfused lung (dead space) offsets the hypocarbic effect of tachypnea.

Lung scanning and pulmonary angiography are sophisticated studies that have been developed recently to aid in diagnosing pulmonary embolus. The lungs are scanned after infusion of macromolecular particles of ^{131}I-tagged serum albumin; poor uptake of ^{131}I is seen in areas of the lung that are perfused by vessels plugged with emboli. This method is still in developmental stages. Pulmonary angiography allows radiographic visualization of the pulmonary artery tree, outlining clearly which branches are occluded by clot, and is the most reliable diagnostic test of pulmonary embolism.

Treatment. Treatment of pulmonary emboli consists of rest, oxygen, allaying of anxiety, and anticoagulation. Vena caval ligation is required with repeated episodes of embolization. When to perform pulmonary embolectomy is an agonizing decision, since the operative mortality is 50 to 60%. Complicating the problem is the fact that even massive emboli may resolve spontaneously. In several instances patients have been operated on only to find that the diagnosis was incorrect. The procedure should be used when all else fails in a deteriorating patient in whom the diagnosis has been definitely established.

Intravenous heparin is the most reliable anticoagulant drug for treating pulmonary embolus. It possesses the distinct advantage of rapid onset, short period of activity (6 to 8 hours) to allow good control, with anti-inflammatory and some fibrinolytic activity, and has a specific antidote (protamine sulfate). Initial dosage is 10,000 units every 8 hours, with subsequent size and frequency of administration depending on the response to treatment as reflected by coagulation times, which should be two to three times the patient's control levels. Fibrinolytic drugs (streptokinase and urokinase), which effectively lyse clot already present, currently are being evaluated and may well be added to treatment in the near future.

Fat pulmonary embolism

Fat embolism is a most common and important cause of complication and death after fracture. It affects many organs, the most important being the lung, brain, and kidneys, but the lung is such a good filter that in 75% of autopsied cases fat embolism can only be found there. The heart is secondarily involved when the fat emboli elevate pulmonary resistance to produce cardiac dilatation, tachycardia, hypotension, and increased central venous pressure. The physician may ascribe shock entirely to the injury, forgetting that fat embolism may be the basic cause. When shock coexists, a smaller fat pulmonary embolus produces serious consequences earlier, with a higher death rate.

The patient develops tachypnea, dyspnea, and cyanosis. There may be a lag of 24 to 48 hours between injury and the clinical appearance of symptoms, with this "latent" period representing the time taken for the lung to filter out enough fat to be symptomatic. Confusion, disorientation, acute psychosis progressing to coma, and stupor may exist. Their significance must be evaluated in light of whether the patient has suffered a head injury or was intoxicated.

Other variable clinical signs are bubbling rales; white, fluffy, patchy retinal exudates; and petechial hemorrhages on the neck, shoulders, chest, soft palate, and conjunctiva but rarely over the abdomen.

The chest roentgenogram shows diffuse, small, nodular infiltrates, enlarged pulmonary arteries, and perhaps cardiomegaly. In the absence of bleeding, a sharp drop in the hemoglobin is also suggestive.

In the first few days after injury fat droplets appear in the urine. Sputum examination for fat is of no value. Later an elevated serum lipase is of diagnostic and prognostic (the higher, the better) value.

Treatment. Treatment consists of respiratory support, immobilization of the fracture, heparin (increases lipase activity) dextran, and steroids.

Spontaneous pneumothorax

Acute collapse of the lung caused by the sudden escape of air from the lung into the pleural space is known as spontaneous pneumothorax (Fig. 30-11). It occurs typically in young robust males about three times more frequently than in females and is caused by rupture of a subpleural bleb (Fig. 30-12). The pneumothorax occasionally coincides with a period of physical exertion, but generally it develops when the patient is engaged in routine activities. Pain, commonly referred to the shoulder, can be excruciating and is associated with

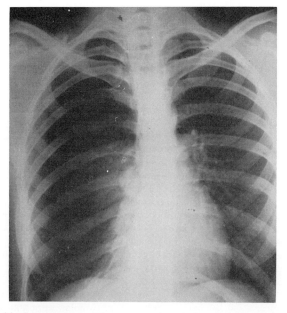

Fig. 30-11. Spontaneous right pneumothorax; lung about 60% collapsed by the pleural air.

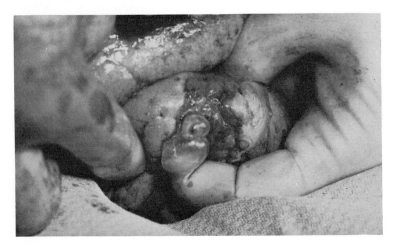

Fig. 30-12. Subpleural bleb, rupture of which produces spontaneous pneumothorax.

some degree of dyspnea. Other conditions occasionally associated with spontaneous pneumothorax are tuberculosis, emphysema, chronic bronchitis, giant bullae, and obstructive emphysema.

In infants and children, tension pneumothorax is caused more often by staphylococcal pneumonia than by rupture of true congenital blebs. Sometimes no predisposing lung disease is identified. Spontaneous pneumothorax occurs often in the newborn period; 15% of newborns have asymptomatic pneumothorax. In symptomatic neonates pneumothorax is frequently accompanied by pneumomediastinum and is usually related to the aspiration of blood, meconium, or squamous debris during delivery, with resulting obstruction in the bronchial tree. The pneumothorax occurs after the increased respiratory effort of these patients and the frequent resuscitative measures they receive. The condition may be missed if only an anteroposterior chest roentgenogram is taken, but there is almost 100% accuracy of diagnosis with a cross-table lateral radiograph. Persistence or recurrence of pneumothorax in infants and children suggests another abnormality (e.g., cystic fibrosis or multiple lung cysts).

Physical examination reveals decreased vocal and tactile fremitus, tympany to percussion, tracheal shift to the opposite side, and perhaps cyanosis. Occasionally tearing of a vascular adhesion leads to serious intrapleural bleeding. Radiographic examination of the chest is diagnostic.

Treatment

Bed rest and *anterior thoracentesis* is usually tried in lesser degrees of collapse during the first or perhaps second episode.

Intercostal drainage with a chest tube (Fig. 30-2) inserted in the second intercostal space parasternally is the preferred treatment. The tube is connected to underwater-seal drainage, allowing the egress of air and encouraging reexpansion of the lung by restoration of negative intrapleural pressure. Pleural adhesions seal the leak.

Thoracotomy is employed after multiple recurrences, when blebs or bullae are seen on the chest film, and for chronic states of collapse. The blebs are oversewed or excised, and the parietal pleura is abraded to stimulate the formation of adhesions between the parietal and visceral pleura. Parietal pleurectomy accomplishes a similar end. Chemical irritants are seldom employed to produce pleural abrasion.

MEDIASTINUM

Inflammation

Mediastinitis is uncommon. Once uniformly fatal, it can now (in most cases) be treated successfully (Table 30-4).

Mediastinal neoplasms

Mediastinal tumors arise from (1) the mediastinum proper, (2) adjacent structures, and (3) outside the thoracic cavity. In general, they produce symptoms by compression or interference with function of mediastinal organs, or by the development of infection or malignant change in the tumor itself.

Extraneous lesions *simulating* primary mediastinal neoplasms are the following:

1. *Thyroid.* Extension of a cervical goiter through the thoracic inlet, or truly aberrant thyroid tissue (very rare).
2. *Chest wall neoplasms.* They may have no palpable external component: chondroma, chondrosarcoma, chordoma, Ewing's sarcoma.
3. Congenital or acquired *herniations* through the *diaphragm.*
4. *Aneurysms* of the great vessels.
5. Mediastinal *meningoceles.* 70% have stigmas of neurofibromatosis.
6. *Achalasia* of the esophagus.

Neurogenic tumors make up about 30% of all mediastinal tumors, teratomas about 15%, cysts 15%, thymomas 10%, goiter 10%, and all others 20%; about 15% are malignant. Each of the different types of mediastinal tumor tends to occur in a characteristic part of the mediastinum, making an important clue to diagnosis (Fig. 30-13).

Table 30-4. Mediastinitis

	Method of contamination	Symptoms and signs	Etiology	Radiographic findings	Treatment
Acute	1. Direct penetrating trauma 2. Hematogenous, or spread from thoracic viscera (heart, lungs, esophagus, or from chest wall) 3. From the neck along fascial planes 4. Direct extension from the lungs or pleura	High fever, pain under the sternum; highly toxic state; dysphagia; hacking cough; mediastinal and subcutaneous emphysema; edema of chest wall; prominence of veins on chest wall	1. 60% due to ruptured esophagus (carcinoma, from endoscopy) 2. Spread by blood or lymphatic drainage from thoracic viscera 3. Spread from neck along the visceral fascial planes from infection in neck 4. Extension from empyema or lung abscess	Widening of mediastinum, displacement of trachea; interstitial emphysema; fluid level of abscess; extravasation of swallowed contrast material	Drainage is most important; antibiotics are only a helpful adjunct

| Chronic | Same as acute | Usually insidious in onset: Weakness Weight loss Chronic cough Anemia Chest pain Low-grade fever Symptoms of superior vena caval obstruction Swelling of face and neck Esophageal obstruction Occasionally esophagobronchial fistula with lithoptysis | A granulomatous infection, often not specifically identified; histoplasmosis is the most common cause, tuberculosis only occasionally in the United States | Paratracheal mass, subcarinal or paraesophageal; 50% not calcified, one-third heavily calcified | Largely nonsurgical; treatment for specific infection if found (tuberculosis, actinomycosis, histoplasmosis); mediastinal granulomas should be removed if heavily calcified |

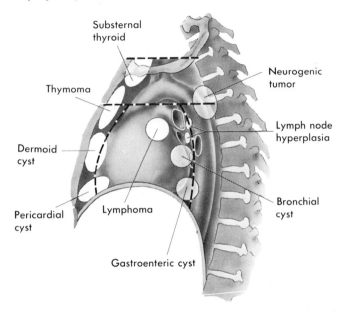

Fig. 30-13. Diagram of mediastinum, indicating typical location of the different mediastinal tumors.

Anterior mediastinum

Intrathoracic goiters are almost always extensions of cervical goiters. The trachea is displaced and the neck veins are prominent because of compression, which accounts for symptoms of dyspnea, stridor, dysphagia, and facial swelling. Plain radiographs show a lobulated shadow high in the anterior mediastinum with displacement of the trachea, and barium swallow proves the mass moves with deglutition; failure of the mass to move with deglutition suggests either that the goiter is malignant or that some other diagnosis must be entertained. Removal is recommended, generally with cervical thyroidectomy.

Thymomas are composed of the normal cellular elements of the thymus, except usually lacking Hassall's corpuscles. Initially encapsulated, they later invade locally as low-grade malignancies, especially when accompanied by *myasthenia gravis*. The degree of malignancy depends on its behavior (i.e., gross findings) and not on histological appearance. Calcification is sometimes seen, but this is not a sign of benignity. They are slow growing, with as long as 10 years elapsing with little enlargement seen. Thymomas often are totally asymptomatic, but when large, they produce pain, venous obstruction, stridor, cough, and dyspnea. Surgical excision is recommended, with postoperative irradiation if the thymoma is malignant clinically.

The relationship of the thymus to myasthenia gravis has long been recognized: about 85% of patients with myasthenia have a normal thymus, and about 50% of thymomas are associated with myasthenia. The role of thymectomy for myasthenia gravis is still unsettled because results are variable. In most instances, anticipated benefits outweigh the operative risk. The best results of thymectomy for myasthenia are obtained in women with symptoms of short duration. Thymomas have been reported to occur with red blood cell aplasia, Cushing's syndrome, megaesophagus, and hypogammaglobulinemia. Steroids may be helpful in patients who are not benefited by thymectomy or anticholinesterase drugs.

Dermoids (benign teratomas) histologically contain only tissue of ectodermal origin. They are usually large and unilocular and are found in middle-aged patients.

True *teratomas* contain elements of all three germ layers, commonly with hemorrhagic or polycystic areas; 70% ultimately become malignant. The usual symptoms of mediastinal teratoma are cough, pain, and dyspnea, but they may rupture into the pleura, pericardium, and blood vessels. Expectoration of hair is pathognomonic; hemorrhage may be severe. Radiographic examination is diagnostic if cartilage, bone, or teeth are seen in a tumor high in the anterior mediastinum. The preferred treatment is surgical removal.

Pericardial cysts are fairly common, arising from a pinched-off portion of the pleuroperitoneal membrane, which occurs during the formation of the diaphragm. They are always anterior (usually on the right side) and close to the cardiophrenic angle. They contain fluid similar to pericardial fluid, prompting the descriptive term "springwater" cysts. They sometimes have a pedicle attached to the pericardium. Pericardial cysts are always benign and usually are asymptomatic.

Posterior mediastinum

Neurogenic tumors comprise over 90% of posterior mediastinal tumors. The main histological types are the ganglioneuroma, neurofibroma, neurilemoma, and the highly malignant neuroblastoma. Neurofibromas and neurilemomas are frequently associated with intercostal nerves, ganglioneuromas with the sympathetic chain. Neurofibromas are least common, and ganglioneuromas are quite common. Immature elements indicate a potentially malignant ganglioneuroma. In some instances, the syndromes of diarrhea and abdominal distension or of hypertension, flushing, and sweating occur with ganglioneuroma. Urinary levels of vanillylmandelic acid may also be elevated.

Neurogenic mediastinal tumors are often asymptomatic, discovered on incidental radiographic examination of the chest as a "cannonball" lesion; spreading of the involved intercostal space and rib erosion are highly suggestive of neurogenic tumor. Occasionally a tumor will proceed dumbbell fashion through an intervertebral foramen to cause paraplegia. Mediastinal neurofibromas are associated with general neurofibromatosis. Neuroblastomas occur in children high in the posterior mediastinum and are highly malignant; calcific stippling characteristically is seen on radiographic examination. Treatment is surgical removal followed by irradiation.

In general, treatment for mediastinal tumors of neurogenic origin is thoracotomy and excision. Those tumors with intraspinal projections require preliminary laminectomy.

Enterogenous cysts are generally seen lying along the right side of the esophagus in infants and young children, probably because of displacement by the aorta. They often are associated with abnormally formed vertebral bodies, to which they may attach, and occasionally extend through the diaphragm juxtaposed to stomach or intestine. Enterogenous cysts have walls of smooth muscle with an inner lining of mucosa. If the mucosa actively secretes, evpansion and perforation may occur, but these cysts are asymptomatic if the lining is inactive. Large cysts cause obstructive symptoms (cough, dyspnea). Total surgical removal is the recommended treatment.

Middle mediastinum

The *lymphoma* family of mediastinal tumors include leukemia, Hodgkin's disease, and lymphosarcoma, the latter accounting for 60% of the total. The disease occurs characteristically in males in the fourth and fifth decades of life. Hepatosplenomegaly, lymphadenopathy, and fever are well-known systemic manifestations of lymphoma. Lymphosarcoma and Hodgkin's disease occasionally are localized to the mediastinum and may then be cured by excision, irradiation, or a combination of the two.

Bronchogenic cysts sometimes occur in the midmediastinum; they have been discussed in the section on congenital malformations of the lungs.

CHEST WALL
Congenital malformations of the chest wall
Pectus excavatum

The most common anterior chest wall deformity is pectus excavatum (Fig. 30-14). Though opinions differ as to etiology, it is most

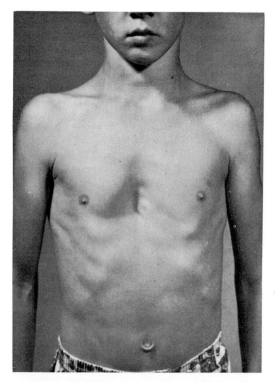

Fig. 30-14. Pectus excavatum, preoperative.

likely caused by a congenitally foreshortened central tendon of the diaphragm, sometimes associated with anomalous attachments to the lower ribs anteriorly. Mechanical factors are mainly responsible for the progression of the deformity during growth of the thoracic cage. The point of fixation at the lower end of the sternum prevents proper respiratory excursion by maintaining the thoracic cage in a position of semiexpiration. As the lower portion of the rib cage and cartilages becomes fixed, the rib cage is forced to expand in a lateral direction. The mediastinal structures are usually displaced to the left as the midline anteroposterior dimension of the thorax foreshortens. Though initially symmetric, growth produces asymmetry during the childhood years. It occurs three times oftener in males than in females.

Mild, nonprogressive deformities require no treatment. Operative correction is indicated for cosmetic and psychological reasons, or if

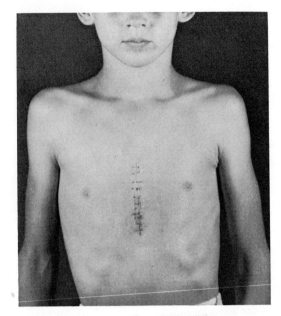

Fig. 30-15. Pectus excavatum, postoperative.

the deformity progresses in early childhood (Fig. 30-15). In adolescents and adults, physiological changes (detected by pulmonary function studies and cardiac catheterization) are occasionally cogent indications for repair.

Pectus carinatum

The rare deformity pectus carinatum produces anterior displacement and bulging of the sternum. It seems to be a counterpart of pectus excavatum, with a fixation point at the lower end of the anteriorly tilted sternum and secondary changes in the rib cartilages.

Neoplasms of the chest wall
Chondroma

Chondromas occur as painless swellings anteriorly near the costochondral junction, or in the sternum. They are benign and cause no symptoms. Radiographic examination reveals bony expansion without bony destruction, and occasionally calcification.

Chondrosarcoma

Chondrosarcomas, on the contrary, occur in the posterior portion of the bony thorax and may involve vertebra and transverse processes. With inward growth they resemble mediastinal tumors on chest roentgenograms. They are usually hard, locally painful external swellings that enlarge slowly and progressively invade surrounding structures. Chondrosarcomas have a great propensity to recur locally after excision, and metastases appear after several recurrences. The differential diagnosis includes osteomyelitis of the ribs, bony tuberculosis, and ununited rib fracture. Total early excision is curative.

Myeloma

Solitary myelomas occur in thoracic vertebrae. They tend to take a benign course, although their osteolytic appearance on radiographic examination always produces concern. The chief symptom is pain.

The ribs are the most common site of solitary *fibrous dysplasia* of bone. They are multilocular and sometimes cystic. A typical "soap bubble" pattern is seen on the roentgenogram. If several ribs are involved, biopsy is required to distinguish fibrous dysplasia from neoplasm.

Eosinophilic granuloma

Eosinophilic granuloma is another benign destructive process of the ribs, most common in children and young adults. The typical history is the acute onset of a painful rib swelling. Fever, fracture, and a history of trauma may confuse the picture. The radiographic appearance is that of a rounded osteolytic lesion. Biopsy is generally needed to rule out malignancy.

Sarcoma

Sarcomas of the chest wall require wide excision and reconstruction of the chest wall with a prosthetic material, such as Marlex mesh.

Chest wall and lung injuries
Chest trauma

Next to cardiovascular disease and cancer, trauma is the most common cause of death in the United States. Urban violence and automobile accidents are in large measure responsible for this. Trauma to the chest is the chief cause of 25% of deaths from auto accidents, and another 50% of patients who die have significant chest trauma.

Multiple rib fractures, often seen after steering wheel injuries (Fig. 30-16), produce an unstable segment of the chest wall that on inspiration moves paradoxically inward and on expiration balloons outward

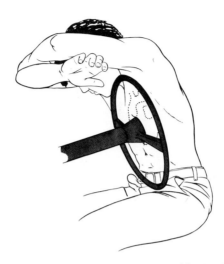

Fig. 30-16. Chest trauma. Chest wall impact with steering wheel may fracture multiple ribs and the sternum, resulting in paradoxical motion of the chest wall (flail chest). Contusion of underlying heart and lung causes reduced cardiac output and arterial hypoxemia.

(flail chest). The inspiratory concavity in the chest wall compresses the underlying lung, shifts the mediastinum to the opposite side, impairs venous return to the heart, and limits expansion of the good lung. Tachypnea increases the movement of the chest wall (mediastinal flutter) to aggravate these changes. Contusion of the underlying lung (traumatic wet lung), however, is the most important factor because of associated severe arterial hypoxia. Interstitial and intra-alveolar hemorrhage accompanying contusive injury to the lung results in marked ventilation/perfusion abnormalities such that deoxygenated blood passes through the lung without proper gas exchange (physiological shunt). Admixture of desaturated blood to pulmonary venous return produces arterial hypoxemia. In addition, blood and debris entering the airway from the area of injury may be aspirated to uninvolved areas of the lung to compound the problem. Splinting of the cough mechanism from pain and chest wall instability prevents adequate clearing of the airway.

Traumatic asphyxia is the term applied to a striking syndrome of petechiae and edema of the face, neck, and upper extremities that occurs after sudden, severe compression of the chest. It is caused by

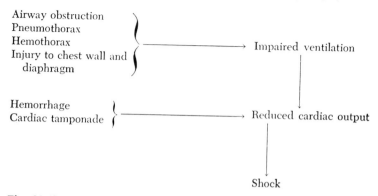

Fig. 30-17. Physiological effects of penetrating thoracic trauma. (After Creech, O., and Pearce, C. W.: Amer. J. Surg. **105:**496, 1963.)

forceful retrograde pulsion into the superior vena cava of blood in the heart reservoir on the right side, producing disruption of small blood vessels and extravasation of blood into the tissues drained by this system.

The physiological derangements accompanying traumatic wet lung and flail chest are best treated by clearing and maintaining an open airway and positive pressure ventilation with a mechanical respirator. The respirator assures adequate alveolar ventilation and also stabilizes the chest wall.

Wounds of the chest caused by penetration of a sharp object or missile may cause pneumothorax or hemothorax. Blood or air entering the pleural space causes collapse of the lung because of compression. If the air or blood accumulates rapidly, the mediastinum is shifted toward the uninvolved side so that the opposite lung is compressed (tension pneumo- or hemothorax). The combined effects of these changes are decreased ventilation, increased pulmonary vascular resistance, and reduced venous return to the heart; cardiac output falls, and circulatory shock results.

When there is loss of continuity of the chest wall, there is a similar chain of events as just described except that outside air enters the pleural space via the "sucking wound."

The physiological effects of penetrating thoracic trauma are summarized in Fig. 30-17. Each of these factors must be evaluated and corrected, with maintenance of the airway and restoration of blood volume taking first and second priority.

Pneumothorax of 20% or less of the volume of the pleural space is often treated expectantly, but if larger than this or if under tension, it requires tube thoracostomy in the second interspace anteriorly and underwater-seal drainage (Fig. 30-2). If blood is present in the pleural space, it is removed by repeated thoracenteses (Fig. 30-1), or by closed chest tube drainage instituted low in the chest (Fig. 30-2). The patient is kept in a semiupright position to facilitate drainage. Persistent bleeding demands thoracostomy to stop the bleeding, expand the lung, and obliterate the pleural space. Failure to remove blood may necessitate decortication later on.

Rupture of a major airway (trachea, larynx, or bronchus)

Most of these injuries are produced by blunt trauma that tears the large airway structures, producing severe air leaks. Dyspnea, cough, hemoptysis, tension pneumothorax, and subcutaneous emphysema are promptly produced, which immediately place the patient in grave jeopardy. Bronchoscopy often confirms the diagnosis. Early thoracostomy and repair are most desirable, since bronchial stenosis, infection, and a destroyed lung may otherwise result. Late repair occasionally improves lung function but does not restore the respiratory tree to normal. Occasionally the esophagus will also be injured; an esophagobronchial fistula may result.

Cardiac trauma

Cardiac trauma may be classified into penetrating and nonpenetrating injuries. The penetrating types involve injury to the heart by a sharp object or missile. If the patient survives the immediate penetrating injury to the heart, he often quickly develops cardiac tamponade. A relatively small amount of blood within the closed pericardial space is sufficient to interfere with cardiac filling, thereby reducing cardiac output. The patient is restless and has air hunger. Heart tones are distant, and there may be a pericardial friction rub; blood pressure is reduced, and pulse pressure is narrow. Venous pressure is elevated and neck veins are distended. Chest films show a normal-sized heart, and the electrocardiogram is helpful in diagnosis only when there is coronary artery injury.

Immediate treatment is pericardiocentesis. A needle is passed into the pericardial space (with electrocardiographic monitoring) to remove accumulated blood. A large bore needle is inserted alongside the sternum at the left sternocostal angle and directed cephalad and posteriorly toward the heart at a 45-degree angle to the sternum. As the needle passes through the chest wall to the pericardial sac, the electrocardiogram is similar to lead V-2. If the needle contacts the myocardium, a current of injury similar to multiple premature ventricular contractions will be noted on the electrocardiogram. The needle is then withdrawn slightly, and the contents of the pericardial sac are aspirated. Blood extracted from the pericardium does not clot, because clotting has already occurred within the pericardium; the substance that is removed is serum and cells, and the fibrin clot is left behind. If blood pressure improves and central venous pressure falls after pericardiocentesis, the patient may be safely observed and closely monitored. Should signs of cardiac tamponade return, immediate operation is indicated to remove blood from the pericardial sac and repair the myocardial injury.

Nonpenetrating injury of the myocardium caused by blunt trauma to the chest wall is probably more frequent than clinically recognized. Steering wheel injury in an automobile accident (Fig. 30-16) and other forms of trauma to the anterior chest wall can produce this injury. The physiological consequences of this injury are cardiac arrhythmia and reduced cardiac output, which are directly related to amount of contused myocardium. In spite of these two complications, it is remarkable that patients often survive tremendous trauma to the myocardium. The diagnosis of cardiac contusion is difficult because of low index of suspicion of the injury and nonspecific electrocardiographic and serum enzyme pattern. New radioisotope techniques involving technetium-labelled phosphate complexes are useful in demonstrating injured myocardium. Treatment of this condition is similar to treatment of myocardial infarction and involves rhythm monitoring and aggressive treatment of cardiac arrhythmia, ionotropic agents to support cardiac output, and bedrest while the myocardium heals.

Aortic injuries

Of patients with thoracic aortic injuries, 85% die at the time of the injury. The most common site of rupture is in the proximal descending aorta just beyond the origin of the left subclavian artery, and the next most common is in the ascending aorta just above the aortic valve. The tears are usually transverse and may involve the entire circumference, with the aorta being held together by thin adventitia in those who survive. The diagnosis is frequently missed because it is not considered. Radiographic examination of the chest shows widening of the mediastinum, and angiography confirms the diagnosis. Other suggestive signs are cervical hematoma, tracheal deviation, hemothorax, asymmetry of radial pulses, and a paralyzed left vocal cord. Immediate repair should be carried out. In the ascending aorta, total cardiopulmonary bypass is required for repair, but a left-sided bypass (left atriofemoral bypass) suffices for injuries distal to the brachiocephalic vessels.

Ruptured diaphragm

Blunt trauma and crushing injuries are the usual cause. Diaphragmatic rupture most commonly occurs on the left side adjacent to the esophageal hiatus, but injury to every part of the diaphragm has been described. The symptoms are not specific, and if there is no evidence of external trauma, the diagnosis can be missed. Progressive cardiorespiratory distress is seen as more and more viscera enter the chest to collapse the lung, push the mediastinal structures to the opposite side, and impede venous return to the heart and expansion of the good lung. Suggestive signs of ruptured diaphragm are bowel sounds heard in the chest and difficulty in passing a nasogastric tube. A chest film is extremely valuable in diagnosis, especially the lateral view, showing bowel loops within the chest. Patients in cardiorespiratory distress must be explored either through the chest or abdomen to allow reduction of the viscera and closure of the diaphragm laceration. Some patients with diaphragmatic rupture are asymptomatic, and the rent is repaired electively after other injuries are treated.

Esophageal lacerations and ruptures

Lacerations of the esophagus, usually caused by instrumentation or by penetrating objects, occur most frequently in the upper third. Any cervical wound penetrating the platysma should be explored. Within a few hours after injury, the rent may be repaired; otherwise drainage, prevention of pleural complications, and antibiotic therapy are required. Chemical injury followed by bacterial infection rapidly produces a life-threatening mediastinitis and empyema.

Injuries of the thoracic esophagus from blunt trauma are rare, and the trauma need not be severe to cause disruption. Penetrating esophageal injuries are accompanied frequently by injuries to the heart and great vessels. In all such cases repair of the injury should be carried out immediately, if possible.

Spontaneous rupture of the esophagus (Boerhaave's disease) occurs usually after large meals and strenuous vomiting. Occasionally it is seen after lifting, seizures, and childbirth. On several occasions we have seen it in newborns.

Perforations and lacerations of the esophagus usually cause dysphagia, vomiting, and subcutaneous emphysema. Movement and inspiration aggravate the pain. Air bubbles, an air fluid level, or widening of the mediastinum on radiographic examination suggest esophageal injury. Pleural effusion (which is potentially an empyema) frequently accompanies esophageal trauma.

If recognized early, the rent should be repaired regardless of location except for small cervical perforations, which may be treated by drainage and antibiotic coverage.

Foreign bodies

Foreign bodies in the chest are not in themselves an indication for emergent removal. They are removed when (1) associated with a nearby infection, (2) very large, or (3) adjacent to the heart, aorta, or some other important structure.

ESOPHAGUS
Benign tumors of the esophagus

Benign tumors are uncommon and may arise from any layer of the esophagus. The majority are leiomyomas, originating in the muscle coats. On plain radiographs they appear as lobulated densities in the posterior mediastinum that on fluoroscopy move with swallowing. Esophagoscopy is often negative. These tumors are usually easily enucleated.

Tumors originating in the mucosa or submucosa project into the lumen and are pedunculated from peristaltic activity. Polyps, adenoma, fibroma, and lipoma are examples. They are more likely to produce dysphagia than the leiomyomas and also may ulcerate and bleed. Excision of the lesions without resection of the esophagus can usually be done.

Carcinoma of the esophagus

Carcinoma is the most important disease of the esophagus and represents about 5% of all malignancies of the gastrointestinal tract. About 90% are epidermoid carcinomas, and the remainder, adenocarcinomas. Therapy is usually only palliative because (1) the prime symptom, *dysphagia*, is delayed (at least a year's tumor growth precedes its onset), (2) most are poorly differentiated histologically (Broders' class III and IV), (3) the tumor extends submucosally both upward and downward, (4) absence of a serosal coat in the esophagus permits early mediastinal invasion, and (5) many of the patients are first seen after severe weight loss and debilitation.

Cancer of the esophagus is more common in men than in women (8:1). In men it occurs more commonly (80%) in the middle and lower thirds, and in women it tends to arise proximally. It spreads mainly by lymphatics.

Dysphagia is generally the first symptom, although unfortunately a very late one. On close questioning, a history of progressive difficulty in swallowing is obtained, first with solids, then semisolids, and finally with liquids. Weight loss is often severe. Pain and hoarseness are grave signs.

The diagnosis of esophageal cancer is established by barium swallow (Fig. 30-18), esophagoscopy, and biopsy. The differential diagnosis includes those diseases in which dysphagia is also a prominent

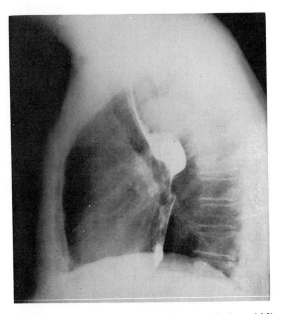

Fig. 30-18. Barium swallow showing carcinoma of the middle third of esophagus producing an abrupt narrowing of the dye column.

symptom: achalasia, peptic esophagitis, foreign body, and diverticulum.

Carcinoma of the esophagus is inoperable if there is also present (1) fistulation into the bronchial tree, (2) vocal cord paralysis, or (3) distant metastasis (liver, lungs, vertebrae, or cervical nodes). Bronchoscopy should always be done to rule out invasion of the bronchial tree.

Curative treatment is total extirpation of the tumor, which is rarely possible. About 50% of patients with cancer of the middle and lower third of the esophagus have metastases to the nodes along the left gastric artery, and removal of these nodes is a necessary part of a curative resection. Palliative treatment is directed at the relief of the esophageal obstruction, if possible. Gastrostomy rarely affords satisfactory palliation. Upper third lesions are usually best treated by irradiation, since the cure rate is extremely low after resection (which usually requires laryngectomy and complicated plastic reconstruction). Middle and lower third lesions are often resected for palliation, with restoration of continuity by esophagogastric anastomosis. Critically ill or debilitated patients are occasionally treated by the insertion of plastic tubes through the tumor and into the stomach, to allow the patient to swallow.

Roentgen-ray treatment provides some palliation of both pain and dysphagia. Adenocarcinomas do not respond well to roentgen-ray therapy and must be resected even for palliation.

Peptic esophagitis

Esophageal mucosa is very susceptible to injury from gastric juice. The source of acid-peptic irritation may be exogenous or endogenous. Endogenous peptic esophagitis is rare; it results from ectopic islands of gastric mucosa in the esophagus, generally toward either end. Esophagitis from reflux of acid gastric juice is far more common and is generally caused by a sliding hiatus hernia (Chapter 27). Rare additional causes of reflux peptic esophagitis are a congenitally short esophagus and operations that destroy the esophagogastric junction or its sphincteric mechanism.

The principal early symptoms of peptic esophagitis from sliding hiatus hernia are "heartburn" and regurgitation of bitter-tasting material, worse when the patient lies down. The regurgitated material may be bloody, and the stools will then contain gross or occult blood. Long-standing, recurrent peptic esophagitis leads to *stricture* by scar formation, at which time dysphagia and weight loss occur. Barium studies of the upper gastrointestinal tract and esophagoscopy are diagnostic.

Treatment should at first be conservative, consisting of rest, antacids, bland diet, abstinence from tobacco, spices, and alcohol, and avoiding the supine position after eating. Dilatation of a stricture by bougienage is helpful unless scar formation is dense. Surgical treatment should return the stomach to the abdominal cavity and restore the obliquity of the esophagogastric angle and markedly ameliorate the symptoms. A number of procedures have been proposed to treat advanced esophageal strictures: esophagogastric resection, cardioplasty, esophagogastrostomy (using the fundus), or resection with intestinal interposition. No uniformly acceptable solution to this problem has been found.

Achalasia

Achalasia is an intrinsic disorder of the esophagus characterized by failure of the lower esophageal sphincter mechanism to relax. The esophagus gradually hypertrophies, dilates, becomes tortuous, and loses effective peristalsis. In the early stages motility is normal or hyper-

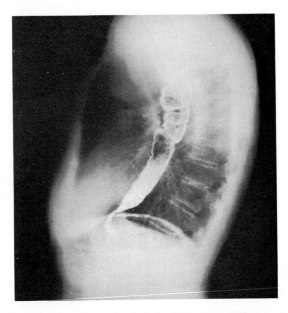

Fig. 30-19. Barium swallow of achalasia. Dilatation and some tortuosity of esophagus, narrowing of esophagogastric junction.

active, but later the esophagus "decompensates" to a saccular, atonic structure. Etiology is unknown; degeneration of Auerbach's plexus is seen on microscopic study of the lower esophagus, but these changes could be secondary; 20% of patients with dysphagia from intrinsic esophageal disease have achalasia, and 10% of patients with achalasia have pulmonary complications.

The classic triad of symptoms of achalasia is dysphagia, regurgitation, and weight loss. The sex distribution is equal. The disease is found at the extremes of age, but the median age at operation is about 55 years. Barium swallow is diagnostic (Fig. 30-19), showing concentric or sigmoid dilatation of the esophagus with abrupt narrowing at its entrance into the stomach. Currently a "modified Heller" procedure is most widely used for both the concentric and the sigmoid types of achalasia, in which the constricting muscle at the esophagogastric junction is divided without opening the mucosa. It gives satisfactory results in 85% of the cases.

Esophageal diverticula

The three most common locations for esophageal diverticula are (1) at the pharyngoesophageal junction (Zenker's diverticulum), (2) in the midthoracic esophagus adjacent to the lung hilum, and (3) in the epiphrenic esophagus just above the diaphragm. They differ enough in origin, symptoms, and treatment to justify individual discussion, although all are diagnosed by barium swallow.

The pharyngoesophageal or Zenker's diverticulum arises in the posterior midline of the esophagus just above the cricopharyngeus muscle, where the pharynx and esophagus join. At this point a triangular area of the inferior pharyngeal constrictor muscle is relatively devoid of muscular support (Killian's triangle), through which the mucosa herniates. Spasm of the cricopharyngeal muscle may be causally related. Collection and stagnation of food occur, elongating the sac generally to the left of the esophagus, large diverticula descending into the mediastinum. Dysphagia, regurgitation, and aspiration are the chief symptoms, and the patient may be aware of a "gurgling" sound in his neck after drinking fluids. These diverticula should be excised if symptomatic or larger than 1.5 cm. Division of the cricopharyngeal muscle also is performed.

Thoracic diverticula are produced by traction on the esophagus by mediastinal tissue, usually inflammatory lymph nodes. The fundus of the diverticulum is higher than the ostium, so that pocketing of food is unlikely and symptoms are rare. Operation is required only in the unlikely instance of fistula formation with the airway.

Epiphrenic diverticula are associated with difficulty in emptying the esophagus at its lower end, with achalasia being the most common predisposing cause. Impaction of food, ulceration, and infection with periesophagitis can result. Excision of the diverticulum and esophagomyotomy are required.

CHAPTER 31

Cardiac surgery

DONALD B. DOTY

Operations on the heart and use of cardiopulmonary bypass techniques have provided increased knowledge of the normal and abnormal function of the circulatory system.

It is the purpose of this chapter to provide a working knowledge of the facts peculiar to surgery of the heart, assuming that the reader will pursue textbooks of cardiology for details of etiology, pathology, diagnosis, and treatment of heart disease.

CARDIAC ANATOMY
Cardiac chambers

The business of the heart is to pump blood. In the heart there are two ventricles (pumping chambers) and two atria (filling chambers). The heart is divided by a septum so that chambers on the right side pump to the lungs and those on the left pump blood to all the rest of the body. The left ventricle, a conical chamber surrounded by a thick-walled muscle (Fig. 31-1), is the focal point of the circulation. As the ventricular muscle mass shortens, blood is compressed and ejected into the aorta and through the arterial system to the cells of the body.

The anatomic relations of the cardiac chambers have been confused by nomenclature and textbook illustrations. The right atrium and ventricle are not only to the right side anatomically, but are also *anterior* to the left atrium and ventricle, which occupy a position to the left and posterior. The dividing septa lie in an oblique plane. The pulmonary artery, which receives blood from the right ventricle, is actually located to the *left* of the aorta because of the complex embryological rotation of the heart.

536

Right Ventricle

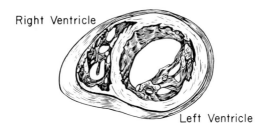

Left Ventricle

Fig. 31-1. Cross section of heart, midportion of ventricles.

Valves

The aortic and pulmonary valves have *semilunar* shaped valve cusps. The cuplike configuration of the sinus of Valsalva allows competence when the valve cusps are approximated during cardiac diastole. The atrioventricular (A-V) valves (mitral and tricuspid) which separate the atria and ventricles are more complex. Valve competence depends on approximation and support of leaflets maintained by the dynamic adjustment of tension on the leaflet by the papillary muscles and chordae tendineae. Hence, abnormal function of ventricular myocardium and papillary muscles may produce malfunction of an otherwise structurally normal valve.

Conduction system

The specialized conduction system of the heart is important because nearly every intracardiac procedure involves manipulating the sinus node, intra-atrial conduction pathways, the atrioventricular node, or the His bundle and its branches. A special surgical landmark is the papillary muscle of the conus, located on the septum below the crista supraventricularis (Fig. 31-2). The bundle of His has divided into bundle branches beyond the base of this muscle in its course through the septum. The first septal branch of the anterior descending coronary artery—which often provides important blood supply to the conduction system—is located in the septum somewhat anterior to the papillary muscle of the conus.

The conus

The crista supraventricularis and its septal and parietal muscle bands separate the body of the right ventricle from the infundibular or conal portion. The conus consists of the crista supraventricularis, the infundibular chamber below the pulmonary valve, the pulmonary

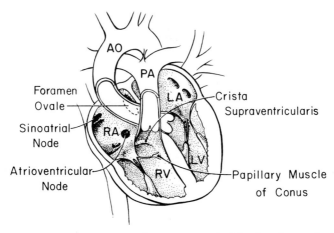

Fig. 31-2. Normal heart. Some important surgical landmarks are demonstrated. *AO*, Aorta; *PA*, pulmonary artery; *RA, LA*, right and left atria; *RV, LV*, right and left ventricles.

annulus, valve, and proximal portions of the pulmonary artery. Abnormalities in the embryological development or rotation of the conus explain many cyanotic congenital cardiac anomalies.

Coronary vessels

The anterior descending and the circumflex branches of the left coronary artery and the right coronary artery are the three vessels that distribute blood to the heart. The coronary artery giving origin to the posterior descending coronary artery supplying the posterior one-third of the intraventricular septum is termed the *dominant* coronary artery because it provides important blood supply to the posterior left ventricle. The nutrient branches of the coronary arteries originate at right angles from the primary coronary arteries and course straight through the myocardium, so that the distant point most vulnerable to ischemia is the endocardial surface. Since these arteries course through contracting muscle, most flow occurs during diastole when the myocardium is relaxed. At the capillary level the vascular channels are sinusoidal and capable of immense dilatation, and they have the remarkable ability to form new flow pathways (collaterals).

CARDIAC PHYSIOLOGY

The heart pumps blood to deliver nutrients to the cells of the body. Oxygen is a critical nutrient, since nearly all metabolic processes

Determinants of Stroke Volume

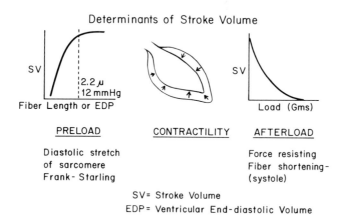

PRELOAD

Diastolic stretch
of sarcomere
Frank- Starling

CONTRACTILITY

AFTERLOAD

Force resisting
Fiber shortening-
(systole)

SV= Stroke Volume
EDP= Ventricular End-diastolic Volume

Fig. 31-3. Factors affecting cardiac output.

require the oxidative pathway. Reduction in oxygen supply to the cell because of reduced blood flow (low cardiac output) or abnormality of oxygen transfer has the same measureable end result: reduced total body oxygen consumption. If this process develops acutely (minutes to hours), usually accompanied by reduced arterial blood pressure, the condition is called *circulatory shock*. When the time course is measured in days to months modified by complex, autoregulatory mechanisms, the condition is called chronic *heart failure*. So, with most cardiac conditions, therapy is directed at improving oxygen consumption and cardiac output.

Determinants of stroke volume

Cardiac output is the product of heart rate and ventricular stroke volume. Heart rate is the major reserve mechanism for increasing cardiac output and is regulated by neurohumoral mechanisms. Stroke volume is determined by three factors:

1. *Preload* (end-diastolic stretch of myocardial sarcomeres, or Frank-Starling mechanism)
2. *Contractility* (contractile state of myocardium)
3. *Afterload* (load resisting shortening of sarcomeres during systole)

The first two factors are related in a positive fashion, while the latter has an inverse relationship (Fig. 31-3). In practice, *preload* in the intact ventricle is taken to mean the end diastolic pressure of the ventricle, provided the A-V valve is normal. *Afterload* is the systolic intraventricular pressure, which is identical to aortic systolic pressure if the aortic valve is normal. Aortic pressure is related to systemic or peripheral vascular resistance, which determines afterload.

Separate performance of the ventricles

There are separate determinants of stroke volume for the right and left ventricles. Obviously, a steady state must be reached in which the output of the systemic and pulmonary ventricles is equal, or all the blood would end up in the lungs or the feet. Inequality of ventricular stroke volume can exist transiently, which explains differences in right and left atrial pressures as they reflect conditions in the ventricle during diastole. As a practical consideration, the highest pressure will be observed in the atrium that fills the ventricle which governs or limits total blood flow. Under normal conditions and in most disease states, this is the left ventricle so that left atrial pressure is greater than right atrial pressure. Great variability can occur, however, so that it is virtually impossible to predict the levels of atrial pressure. It is best to measure pressure simultaneously in both atria. Left atrial pressure may be measured indirectly from the right side as the pulmonary wedge pressure.

MANAGEMENT OF THE CARDIOVASCULAR SYSTEM
General principles

The goal of successful management of the cardiovascular system is to develop *cardiac output* adequate for the metabolic demands of the situation with a *minimum* of pharmacological intervention (because of possible deleterious side effects of drugs). To improve cardiac output, *heart rate, preload, afterload,* and *contractility* may be manipulated. Cardiac output should be measured directly because of inaccuracy of clinical signs used to estimate the cardiac output. Arterial blood pressure, urine flow, cerebral function, appearance of the extremities, and blood gas analysis and pH estimate the *adequacy* of cardiac performance related to perfusion of individual capillary beds.

Monitoring
Arterial pressure

An indwelling Teflon catheter is placed in a systemic artery. In addition to the absolute values for systolic, diastolic, and mean arterial pressure, study of the pulse contour and upstroke relative to time (dP/dT) assists in estimating stroke volume.

Atrial pressure

Small tubes are placed directly in the right and left atria during cardiac surgery. In other patients, a catheter passed from a peripheral vein into the right atrium plus a Swan-Ganz flow-directed balloon catheter placed in the pulmonary wedge position will accomplish the same goal. In the normal heart at rest, mean pressure in right atrium is 4 to 8 mm. Hg and pressure in left atrium is 8 to 12 mm. Hg; these values reflect ventricular end diastolic pressure. Atrial pressure above the normal range generally means diminished ventricular performance and represents the *preload* on the ventricle at that moment.

Electrocardiogram

Continuous monitoring is essential to document cardiac rhythm and rate. Ventricular arrhythmia is important because it not only suggests myocardial ischemia but also may lead to cardiac arrest. Atrial arrhythmia is important because rapid rate may reduce cardiac output. Abnormally slow ventricular rate may also diminish cardiac output. Temporary pacing wires are often placed on the atrium or the ventricle at operation or passed from a peripheral vein to control heart rate and augment cardiac output or suppress arrhythmia.

Cardiac output

Cardiac output may be measured at the bedside by the thermal dilution technique. A thermistor catheter is placed in the pulmonary artery at operation or through a peripheral vein with a Swan-Ganz catheter. This is the sampling site to detect changes in temperature of the blood caused by injection into the right atrium of a bolus of fluid at a predetermined temperature. Though more cumbersome, measurement of oxygen consumption and the content of oxygen in pulmonary and systemic arteries allows calculation of cardiac output by the Fick principle. The result in liters/minute corrected for surface area of the patient is expressed as cardiac index (L./min./M.²).

Practical aspects of management
Normal cardiac output (>3.5 L./min./M.²)

No intervention is necessary. Fluid losses are replaced in addition to maintenance fluids.

Suboptimal cardiac output (2.2 to 3.5 L./min./M.²)

Manipulate *preload*. Blood or other fluid is infused to raise atrial pressure. End diastolic pressure of 12 mm. Hg achieves optimal 2.2 μ stretch of the sarcomere (Fig. 31-3). Atrial pressures above 12 to 14 mm. Hg probably do not increase stroke volume appreciably, but in practice atrial pressure may be taken somewhat higher. Hydrostatic pressure exceeds oncotic pressure at 25 mm. Hg, and a net flux of fluid out of the vascular space (edema) may occur.

Manipulate *afterload*. Occasionally, decreased stroke volume is related to increased peripheral arteriolar resistance. Small doses of chlorpromazine, 2.5 mg./ml., are administered intravenously to reduce afterload. Sodium nitroprusside or trimethaphan (Arfonad) administered as continuous infusion is also useful.

Manipulate *contractility*. Digoxin, 0.9 mg./M.^{2} given intravenously in divided doses should be spaced as determined by urgency. Current evidence suggests that toxicity occurs at half expected doses during the first 24 hours after cardiopulmonary bypass.

Poor cardiac output (<2.2 L./min./M.^{2})

The patient is seriously ill. Manipulation of preload and afterload may help, but usually improvement of myocardial contractility is necessary. Catecholamines are indicated. Epinephrine, 5 to 10 mg./500 ml. 5% DW, is given by continuous intravenous infusion. At low dose levels, the effect of the drug is primarily to increase myocardial contractility, and few peripheral effects are observed. Other pharmacological agents may be equally effective depending upon the clinical situation. Isoproterenol may be used if the heart rate is slow and arterial blood pressure is not too low. If there is oliguria, dopamine may be indicated to increase renal blood flow.

CARDIAC ARREST
Diagnosis

Ventricular *asystole* or *fibrillation* results in cessation of cardiac output. At normal body temperature, loss of consciousness from absence of cerebral blood flow occurs in a matter of seconds, and irreversible brain damage follows in 3 to 4 minutes. Cardiac arrest is diagnosed by absence of pulsation over the carotid or femoral artery, pallor or cyanosis, and loss of consciousness. Gasping agonal respiration or a grand mal seizure is also common. Treatment should be instituted immediately. Precious time should not be wasted listening for heart tones or obtaining an electrocardiogram if circulatory collapse is evident. As treatment is established, however, electrocardiographic diagnosis is a helpful guide to the resuscitative effort.

Treatment
Ventilation

Adequate ventilation of the lungs is the primary step. Initially, this may be established by mouth-to-mouth ventilation. Later, a tight-fitting mask and resuscitation bag may be used. If a laryngoscope and endotracheal tube are available, a tube should be placed accurately and expeditiously in the trachea. Time lost during a difficult intubation or inadvertent, unrecognized intubation of the esophagus can be fatal. Oxygen should be administered to the airway if available.

Cardiac massage

Closed chest cardiac massage should be instituted as soon as possible. With the patient supine on a hard surface (floor or board), the heel of the hand is placed over the lower third of the sternum, and pressure applied so as to depress the sternum 3 to 4 cm. Pressure is applied intermittently at a rate of about 60 compressions per minute. The heart is compressed between the sternum and spine, lateral motion being limited by the pericardium. Effectiveness of massage is measured by restoration of pulsation over the carotid or femoral artery. With effective massage and ventilation, patients have survived cardiac arrest periods of over an hour without irerversible damage to brain or other organs. Fatigability of the person performing the massage is minimized by positioning well above the patient's chest so that pressure may be transferred from the back and shoulders through the arms, locked in full extension at the elbows, to the heel of the hand over the sternum.

Infusion and medications

If no intravenous access is available, a needle-catheter may be readily inserted into the common femoral vein or medications may be injected through a needle penetrating the heart through the chest wall. *Epinephrine* (1 ml. of 1:10,000 solution) may improve quality of fibrillation or restore forceful contraction of the ineffectively beating heart. *Calcium chloride* (5 to 10 ml. of 1% solution) is also helpful as a cardiac stimulant. *Sodium bicarbonate* (44 mEq. every 10 minutes) should be administered to combat metabolic acidosis, which always accompanies cardiac arrest. *Xylocaine* (50 to 100 mg. bolus doses) may stabilize ventricular dysrhythmia. *Propranolol, procaine amide,* and *potassium chloride* are occasionally useful in treating cardiac dysrhythmia.

Electrical defibrillation

Ventricular contraction may be synchronized by applying 20 to 200 watt/seconds of a direct current to the chest wall. A defibrillator unit equipped with special paddle electrodes applies the current through the chest wall between the base and apex of the heart. Vigorous closed chest massage and medications right before the countershock are often helpful. Nearly all fibrillating hearts can be defibrillated, but effective cardiac output may not be established if myocardial contraction produces insufficient stroke volume.

CARDIOPULMONARY BYPASS AND
ASSISTED CIRCULATION

The purpose of cardiopulmonary bypass is to maintain circulation and respiration while the heart is emptied of blood during an operative procedure. Cardiopulmonary bypass involves placing venous cannulae to drain the blood from the body to the pump-oxygenator (heart-lung machine). Gas exchange occurs within the oxygenator, and the blood is pumped through the arterial cannula back to the body, as shown in Fig. 31-4. The driving force for the circulation during cardiopulmonary bypass is the single arterial roller pump. The flow characteristic is essentially nonpulsatile, but depending upon the size of the tubing being compressed and the occlusiveness of the rollers, pulse pressures of approximately 15 to 20 mm. Hg can be developed. As the pump head rotates, blood is forced through the entire circulatory system. Return to the venous side is therefore accomplished by displacement

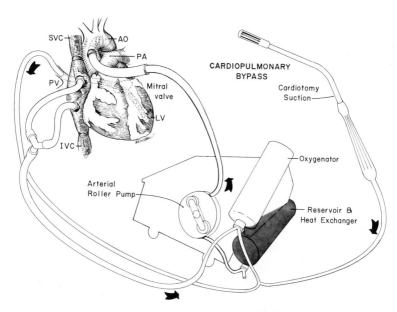

Fig. 31-4. Cardiopulmonary bypass. Blood drains by gravity from the patient to the oxygenator where gas exchange occurs. A single roller pump returns blood to the patient and is the driving force of the circulation.

of the blood, using energy supplied by the arterial pump. Venous return to the oxygenator drains by gravity to the reservoir of the oxygenator.

The principles of this simple system help one understand how the left ventricle functions as the driving force of the entire circulation during normal cardiac action. The left ventricle expels blood through the arterial circulation to the capillaries. Each contraction of the left ventricle displaces blood through the capillaries into the venous system, where it is returned to the heart (again by displacement) for recirculation. The "vis a tergo" (push from behind) is a concept defined by cardiac physiologists. As such, the left ventricle by its own stroke volume becomes a determinant of venous return to the right heart. While this may seem a rather simplistic explanation of venous return, it is reasonable that some source of energy for moving blood through the veins must be supplied. The left ventricle is that energy source for venous return. Trivial sources of energy such as thoracic negative pressure or sucking action of the right ventricle confuse the straightforward nature of the circulation, which can be readily observed during cardiopulmonary bypass when a single pump drives the entire circulation.

Nearly all of the blood is excluded from the heart by diverting venous blood to the pump oxygenator through cannulae placed in the superior and inferior vena cavae. Oxygenated blood which is returned to the aorta does not enter the heart if there is competence of the aortic valve. Blood returning to the cardiac chambers through the coronary circulation may be excluded by occluding the aorta between the aortic perfusion cannula and origin of the coronary arteries. Venous drainage of the bronchial circulation to the pulmonary veins and left atrium is continuous and requires aspiration by vent catheter into the left atrium or left ventricle during operations on the left side of the heart. This source of blood returning to the heart is especially important in the fibrillating heart and in patients with cyanotic congenital cardiac disease who develop marked increase of the bronchial circulation as a collateral pathway for pulmonary circulation.

Oxygenators

Four basic devices are used for exchange of gases during cardiopulmonary bypass.

Screen oxygenator. This type of oxygenator films blood onto a screen in an oxygen-enriched atmosphere.

Disc oxygenator. A series of rotating discs in a reservoir film the blood in an oxygen-enriched atmosphere.

Bubble oxygenator. Microbubbles of oxygen diffuse through a column of blood, and gas exchange occurs on the surface of the bubbles. Microbubbles and foam are removed in a special chamber of the oxygenator system. This oxygenator is available as a disposable device and has the greatest clinical use at the present time.

Membrane oxygenator. A thin membrane of Silastic or Teflon is placed between the blood and the gas. Gas exchange occurs across the membrane, with no direct contact between blood and gas. This system mimics lung and is the least traumatic to the blood elements. Oxygenator size is directly proportional to the size of the patient, as enough membrane surface area must be available for appropriate gas exchange. This system offers the most promise for long-term respiratory support systems.

Hypothermia

The metabolic needs of tissues are directly proportional to the temperature at which metabolism is taking place. At *normothermia* conditions (34 to 37° C.), total body perfusion must exceed 2.5 L./min./M.^{2} to prevent accumulation of products of anaerobic metabolism. As body temperature is lowered, the metabolic requirement is reduced so that many intracardiac procedures are performed under *moderate hypothermia* conditions (28 to 32° C.), at which total body flow rates of 1.8 to 2.2 L./min./M.^{2} are adequate for periods of cardiopulmonary bypass up to 3 hours. As the body temperature is reduced to *deep hypothermia* levels (20 to 24° C.), cardiopulmonary bypass flow rates are reduced proportionally and circulation may be totally arrested for limited periods to either enhance the operating conditions or to reduce the period of cardiopulmonary bypass. This is especially important for intracardiac surgery in infants and small children, in whom deleterious effects of cardiopulmonary bypass are most often observed. Clinical practice has shown that if the body temperature is at 20° C., total circulatory arrest up to 60 minutes is well tolerated in children under the age of 2 years. Adults tolerate circulatory arrest somewhat less well, but limited periods of circulatory arrest at temperatures between 20 and 28° C. have been successfully utilized in adults for various intra- and extracardiac operations.

Consequences of cardiopulmonary bypass and open heart surgery

Cardiopulmonary bypass and intracardiac operation require a large incision, considerable tissue manipulation, and direct trauma to blood elements in the pump oxygenator. Denaturation of protein, abnormalities in platelet function, and destruction of the cellular elements of blood with the liberation of free hemoglobin, aggregates of white cells and platelets, and other microparticles in the blood such as microgas bubbles are consequences of this procedure and will be manifest in the postoperative period as typical physiological response to trauma. Elevation of the body temperature, respiratory insufficiency, mild renal insufficiency, and some observable dysfunction of most other organ systems are also present. Fortunately, the body has good reserve for this type of trauma, and the effects of cardiopulmonary bypass are self-limiting within a few days.

CONGENITAL CARDIAC ANOMALIES
General principles

Abnormalities of embryological development of the heart and great vessels involve about 8 babies out of 1,000 live births. These defects represent a spectrum of disease from simple errors to complex malformations producing gross deformity of the heart or great vessels and severe physiological impairment. As a general principle, complete surgical correction of these abnormalities is the therapeutic goal. Operative mortality and long-term functional results are directly related to the completeness with which the defect is corrected. When total correction of the defect is not possible, temporary or palliative operations are occasionally performed, but the results are not as good as those for total repairs.

Congestive cardiac failure caused by excessive pulmonary blood flow associated with intra- or extracardiac shunt or some obstruction to flow of blood is an indication for surgery. Arterial hypoxemia in patients with cyanotic congenital cardiac disease with increasing polycythemia or loss of consciousness (hypoxic spells) is another common indication for surgery.

Palliative operations
Aortopulmonary shunts

Aortopulmonary shunt is used in patients with defects reducing pulmonary blood flow, such as tetralogy of Fallot or pulmonary atresia with ventricular septal defect, transposition of the great arteries with pulmonary stenosis, and tricuspid atresia.

Three types of aortopulmonary anastomoses are commonly performed to shunt blood between the aortic systemic circulation and the pulmonary circulation (Fig. 31-5).

Blalock-Taussig shunt. The subclavian artery is anastomosed end-to-side to the pulmonary artery. This is the most widely used and perhaps best shunt because the size of the subclavian artery allows optimal controlled increase of pulmonary blood flow.

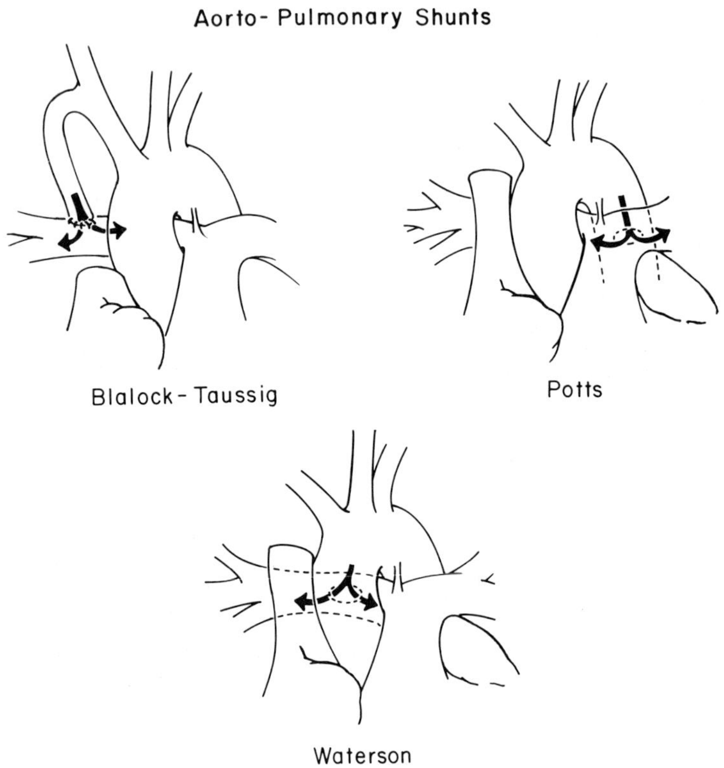

Aorto- Pulmonary Shunts

Blalock - Taussig

Potts

Waterson

Fig. 31-5. Palliative operations. Three common types of procedures to shunt blood from systemic to pulmonary circulation.

Waterston shunt. The ascending aorta is anastomosed side-to-side to the right pulmonary artery. The connection is 3 to 4 mm. in diameter, but occasionally the shunt flow is too great, and pulmonary arteriolar hypertension develops. This anastomosis is used only in tiny babies.

Potts shunt. This is a side-to-side anastomosis of descending thoracic aorta and left pulmonary artery. Size of the shunt is difficult to control and it is the most difficult of the shunt procedures to take down at the time of total repair of the intracardiac defect.

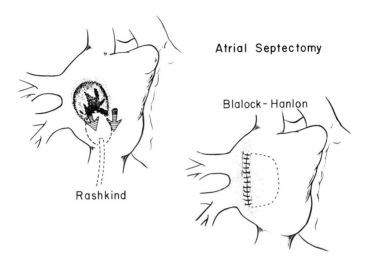

Fig. 31-6. Two methods of producing defects in the atrial septum. Rashkind procedure is rupture of foramen ovale with balloon catheter. Blalock-Hanlon procedure is surgical excision of a portion of atrial septum.

Systemic venous-pulmonary artery shunts

Glenn shunt. This anastomosis of the superior vena cava to the right pulmonary artery is used in older patients with tricuspid atresia. Ordinarily it is a permanent anastomosis, as it is most difficult to revise or take down later.

Atrial septectomy

Rashkind procedure. A defect in the atrial septum is created at cardiac catheterization. A balloon tip catheter is passed via the femoral vein across the foramen ovale into the left atrium. The balloon is inflated and the catheter is forcefully withdrawn, rupturing the membrane of the foramen ovale (Fig. 31-6) to produce a large interatrial communication. This procedure is used in patients with transposition of the great arteries, total anomalous pulmonary venous connection, tricuspid or mitral valve atresia, and hypoplastic right heart syndrome.

Blalock-Hanlon procedure. In this resection of the right lateral portion of the interatrial septum (Fig. 31-6) a side-biting clamp excludes a portion of the right and left atria and septum so that some of the septum can be excised without interrupting blood flow. This procedure is used in patients with transposition of the great arteries who are very young or otherwise not candidates for total intracardiac repair of the defect.

Pulmonary artery banding

Pulmonary artery is narrowed by tightening a band around its external circumference. Blood flow to the lung is reduced by increasing pulmonary outflow resistance. The operation is used in defects such as common ventricle with excessive pulmonary blood flow when there is no means of complete repair.

Total repair—extracardiac anomalies
Patent ductus arteriosus

The ductus arteriosus, which joins the thoracic aorta and the pulmonary artery, closes shortly after birth under the stimulus of air in the lungs and the presence of blood with high oxygen tension in the ductus. If these normal physiological stimuli fail to close the ductus arteriosus, a shunt remains between the aorta and the pulmonary artery that increases pulmonary blood flow (Fig. 31-7). Patent ductus arteriosus is common in premature infants and is associated with idiopathic respiratory distress syndrome. Surgery to close the ductus arteriosus may be lifesaving in these tiny patients. If the shunt is small the patient may be asymptomatic, the diagnosis being made by the presence of a continuous heart murmur. In these patients, the ductus is surgically closed electively because of the threat of congestive cardiac failure developing later in life. The operation consists of either ligation or division of the ductus arteriosus. The risk of operation is small, even in premature infants who require ligation of ductus arteriosus for respiratory distress syndrome.

Coarctation of the thoracic aorta

This anomaly is caused by excessive ductal tissue in the aorta and/or migration of the left subclavian artery during aortic arch resorption so that marked narrowing of the upper portion of the descending thoracic aorta occurs (Fig. 31-7). Circulation to the lower half of the body is maintained by collateral circulation. The diagnosis is made by absence of normal femoral pulsation and hypertension in the upper extremities. Heart failure may occur during infancy, and operative correction has high risk because of associated cardiac anomalies. If the child survives the first year of life, elective operation is performed between 5 and 10 years of age to prevent complications of the anomaly that occur later in life. Operation consists of resecting

Extra - Cardiac Anomalies

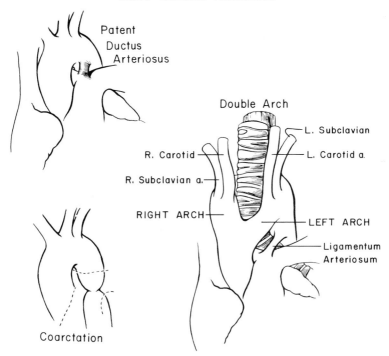

Patent
Ductus
Arteriosus

Double Arch

R. Carotid

R. Subclavian a.

RIGHT ARCH

L. Subclavian

L. Carotid a.

LEFT ARCH

Ligamentum
Arteriosum

Coarctation

Fig. 31-7. Anomalies of great vessels subject to complete repair.

the coarcted segment and end-to-end anastomosis of the aorta. Sometimes bypass graft or enlargement of the aorta by patch angioplasty is performed. The risk of the operation is mostly related to hemorrhage from the enlarged collateral circulation. Complications of intestinal or spinal cord ischemia are rare.

Vascular ring

A number of aortic arch malformations may obstruct the esophagus and/or trachea by compression within a ringlike vascular anomaly. Most commonly the ring is caused by a double aortic arch (Fig. 31-7) or other arch abnormality with compressing ligamentum arteriosus. Symptoms are those of airway obstruction or difficulty in swallowing

552 *Synopsis of surgery*

(dysphagia lusoria). Posterior indentation of the barium-filled esophagus by the vascular ring is seen on roentgen-ray examination. Operation is performed through a left thoracotomy incision with complete dissection of the aortic arch and branch vessels before dividing the ring at an appropriate point. Postoperative complications are related to the loss of airway support because of tracheal malacia at the area of tracheal compression by the vascular ring.

Complete repair—intracardiac anomalies
Anomalies with left-to-right shunts

This group includes atrial and ventricular septal defects, which are the most common forms of congenital intracardiac anomalies, the less common anomalies of the atrioventricular canal, and anomalous pulmonary venous connection (Fig. 31-8). The anatomic abnormality is increased pulmonary blood flow caused by shunting of blood from the left cardiac chambers back to the right heart chambers because of higher pressure on the left side of the heart. Recirculation of the blood through the pulmonary circuit increases cardiac work and leads to congestive cardiac failure if the shunt is large. In addition to dyspnea, heart failure often produces growth failure in children. Late complication of the increased pulmonary blood flow at high pressure is the development of obstructive changes in pulmonary arterioles leading to increased pulmonary vascular resistance. In extreme forms, pulmonary resistance may exceed systemic resistance with reversal of

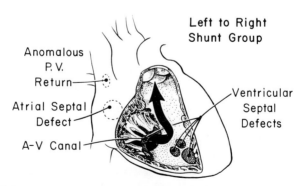

Fig. 31-8. Anomalies producing left to right shunt flow. Increased pulmonary blood flow may cause congestive heart failure and/or increased pulmonary vascular resistance.

shunt flow from right to left (Eisenmenger complex). When the patient reaches this stage, correction of the defect is not possible. With heart failure or increased pulmonary vascular resistance, complete repair is elected regardless of age of the patient. Asymptomatic children are repaired and surgery is performed just prior to school age to avoid heart failure later in life. Defects of the septum are closed by direct suture or by patch material. Pericardium is used to repair atrial septal defects, whereas Dacron cloth is employed to close ventricular septal defects because it is more resistant to the high ventricular pressures. Repair of atrioventricular canal anomalies involves reconstructing the A-V valve as well as closing the septal defect. Anomalous pulmonary venous connection is reconnected to the left atrium by direct anastomosis or by conduit through the atrial septum. In all these repairs, sutures must not be placed in the cardiac conduction system as atrial arrhythmia or complete heart block may occur.

Anomalies with right-to-left shunts

The *tetralogy of Fallot* group of anomalies is associated with pulmonary outflow obstruction, which reduces pulmonary blood flow (Fig. 31-9). There may be severe pulmonary stenosis or total inter-

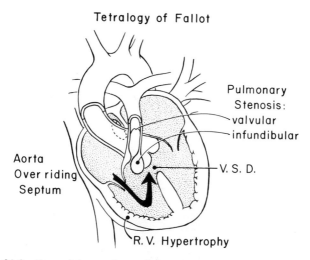

Tetralogy of Fallot

Pulmonary
Stenosis:
valvular
infundibular

Aorta
Over riding
Septum

V. S. D.

R. V. Hypertrophy

Fig. 31-9. Four defects of tetralogy of Fallot. Decreased pulmonary blood flow and direct ejection of right ventricle to aorta (right-to-left shunt) cause arterial hypoxia.

ruption of the connection between the heart and the pulmonary artery (pulmonary atresia) with severe cyanosis. On the other hand, the mildest form will involve little outflow tract obstruction, and the patient will not be cyanotic. There is always a ventricular septal defect and the aorta is positioned to the right, overriding the septum so that the right ventricle ejects deoxygenated blood directly to the aorta. Hypertrophy of the right ventricle is compensatory. The defect results from hypoplasia of the conus portion of the heart with the degree of hypoplasia correlated with severity of the condition. Polycythemia, which follows, is a compensatory response to arterial desaturation. A peculiar manifestation of this condition is the "hypoxic spell." This is related to acute change in right ventricular outflow obstruction resulting from spasm of the hypertrophied obstructing muscle bands of the crista supraventricularis, causing acute reduction of pulmonary blood flow with loss of consciousness. These patients often assume a squatting position as an adaptive mechanism to increase systemic arterial resistance to favor blood flow to the pulmonary circuit by acute angulation of the arteries of the lower extremities.

The diagnosis of tetralogy of Fallot is made by angiography. Contrast media injected into the right ventricle simultaneously fills the aorta and the narrowed outflow tract of the right ventricle. Typically, the outflow tract is obstructed by hypertrophy of the septal and parietal bands of the crista supraventricularis.

Operative repair consists of relieving right ventricular outflow obstruction and closing the ventricular septal defect so that the overriding of the aorta is corrected by placing the patch to the right side of the aorta. When the pulmonary valve annulus is larger than one-third the diameter of the aortic valve annulus, excision of the obstructing septal and parietal bands of the crista supraventricularis and pulmonary valvotomy relieve outflow obstruction. If the pulmonary valve annulus is markedly stenosed, it is widened by placing a Dacron patch extending from the right ventricle across the pulmonary valve annulus into the pulmonary artery. When the pulmonary valve is absent (pulmonary atresia), a new connection is created between the right ventricle and the pulmonary artery by means of an external valved conduit (Rastelli procedure). This procedure is also used in patients with common truncus arteriosus, a condition in which the aorta is the only exit of blood from the heart and the pulmonary arteries originate from the aorta.

The risk of surgical correction of tetralogy of Fallot is directly related to the complexity of the abnormality. When standard repair can be accomplished, the operative mortality is between 5 and 10%. If the anatomy is more complex and the right ventricular outflow tract requires major revision, the operative risk increases. Long-term functional improvement in these patients is remarkable. Patients with a standard tetralogy of Fallot repair enjoy essentially normal exercise tolerance; those who require outflow tract revision may have slight compromise of exercise ability.

Transposition of the great arteries

The attachment of the great vessels to the heart is reversed so that the right ventricle is in continuity with the aorta and the left ventricle empties into the pulmonary artery (Fig. 31-10). Deoxygenated blood returning from the body is recirculated through the systemic circulation without passing through the lungs, and pulmonary venous blood (fully saturated with oxygen) is recirculated through the pulmonary artery (*parallel* circulation). Survival is possible in transposition of the great arteries because of connections that provide mixing between the systemic and the pulmonary circulations, usually at the atrial level through a patent foramen ovale. If a large ventricular septal defect coexists, admixture of the systemic and pulmonary venous blood may bring systemic arterial oxygen saturation to near normal levels.

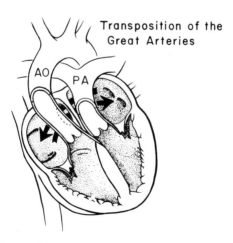

Fig. 31-10. Transposition of the great arteries. Position of great vessels reversed. Defect in atrial or ventricular septum allows mixing of systemic and pulmonary circulation.

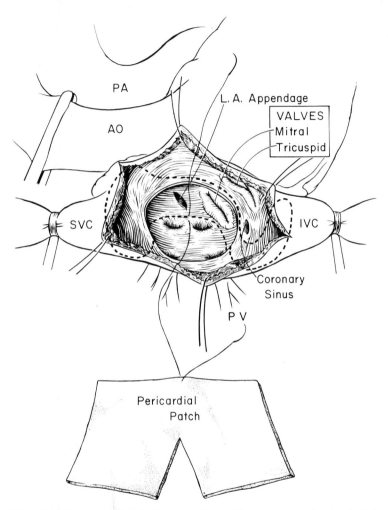

PA

AO

L. A. Appendage

VALVES
Mitral
Tricuspid

SVC

IVC

Coronary
Sinus

P V

Pericardial
Patch

Fig. 31-11. Intra-atrial baffle operation (Mustard procedure). Atrial septum excised. Pericardial patch sewn into atrium along broken line to partition the atrium and redirect venous return. *PA,* Pulmonary artery; *AO,* aorta; *SVC,* superior vena cava; *IVC,* inferior vena cava; *PV,* pulmonary veins.

The diagnosis is made by angiography in a cyanotic infant. Contrast media injected into the right ventricle fills the aorta; when injected into the left ventricle it enters the pulmonary artery. There are a number of variations of this anomaly, and the details of the complex anatomy must be clearly defined by angiography.

A severely cyanotic newborn infant with transposition of the great arteries is treated by Rashkind balloon atrial septostomy. This usually allows adequate oxygenation of blood so that operative intervention may be postponed for several months. If the Rashkind procedure fails to relieve hypoxia, a palliative operation (Blalock-Hanlon procedure) or total repair is performed, but the operative risk is high. If the child is over 4 months of age, intra-atrial baffle operation (Mustard procedure) is usually selected. In this operation, the atrial septum is excised, and a new partition of the atrium is made by means of a pericardial patch (Fig. 31-11). The systemic venous blood returning

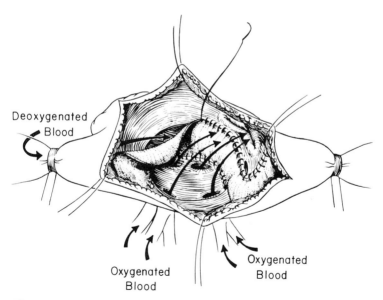

Fig. 31-12. Intra-atrial baffle operation nearly completed. Oxygenated blood returning from pulmonary veins passes through tricuspid valve while deoxygenated systemic blood is redirected behind the patch (to left side) to mitral valve.

through the vena cavae is brought into communication with the mitral valve, left ventricle, and pulmonary artery while pulmonary venous blood is brought into continuity with the tricuspid valve, right ventricle, and aorta (Fig. 31-12). The circulation is then in *series,* physiologically correcting the defect even though it is not a true anatomic correction because the right ventricle remains the systemic pumping chamber. The risk of the operation depends upon a number of complex factors, including age and associated anomalies. Functional results are good, and the right ventricle is capable of supporting systemic circulation in patients followed over 10 years.

Other congenital cardiac anomalies
Valvular lesions

Pulmonary valve stenosis is a common valvular lesion producing outflow obstruction and right ventricular enlargement and hypertrophy. Stenosis of the aortic valve causes obstruction of systemic flow. Children having these valvular lesions are usually asymptomatic but have a loud heart murmur. If the stenosis is severe, however, heart failure may occur within the first few hours or days of life. Severe stenosis of the aortic valve may be associated with scarring of the subendocardial layers of the left ventricle (endocardial fibroelastosis), which impairs left ventricular performance. Operation to relieve valve stenosis consists of incising the valve commissures (valvotomy). Hemodynamics are improved, but blood flow through the abnormal valve may continue to be turbulent so that residual murmur is typical and replacement of the aortic valve is eventually required.

Complex lesions with absence of major intracardiac structure

When atrioventricular valves are stenosed, the stenosis is usually complete (atresia) so there is no communication between the atrium and the ventricle (Fig. 31-13). These complex lesions are associated with hypoplasia of the ventricle and outflow tract distal to the atretic atrioventricular valve. Patients with tricuspid valve atresia and reduced pulmonary blood flow require aortopulmonary shunt or the Glenn procedure. The right atrium may be connected directly to the pulmonary artery by means of a conduit with closure of the septal defect (Fontan procedure). Blood then flows through the lung by left ventricular vis a tergo and a small contribution of right atrial contraction. There is no effective operation for mitral atresia with hypoplastic left heart.

Single ventricle, caused by absence of the ventricular septum or hypoplasia of one ventricle with large ventricular septal defect, may require surgery to alter the amount of pulmonary blood flow. Opera-

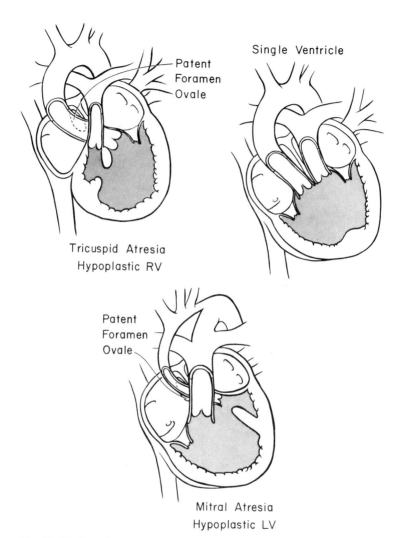

Single Ventricle

Patent
Foramen
Ovale

Tricuspid Atresia
Hypoplastic RV

Patent
Foramen
Ovale

Mitral Atresia
Hypoplastic LV

Fig. 31-13. Complex anomalies with absence of major intracardiac structure. Septal defects and mixing of systemic and pulmonary circulation often allow survival.

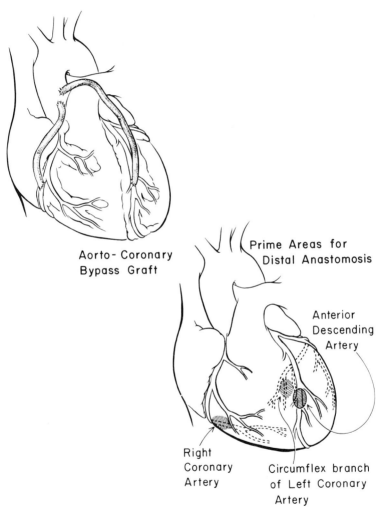

Aorto-Coronary
Bypass Graft

Prime Areas for
Distal Anastomosis

Anterior
Descending
Artery

Right
Coronary
Artery

Circumflex branch
of Left Coronary
Artery

Fig. 31-14. Surgery for coronary artery disease. Segments of saphenous vein used to bypass obstructed portions of coronary arteries. Grafts attached directly to branches of coronary arteries in areas shown on right.

tions for this condition are usually palliative, but some progress has been made toward total correction by creating a ventricular septum with a Dacron partition.

ACQUIRED HEART DISEASE
Coronary artery disease

Coronary atherosclerosis with myocardial ischemia is a significant public health problem. It is estimated that approximately four million people in the United States have coronary artery disease, accounting for 675,000 deaths per year. Surgical treatment of coronary atherosclerosis was made possible by perfection of selective coronary arteriography and the development of surgical procedures that directly revascularize the coronary arteries. About 90% of patients with coronary atherosclerosis will have the major atherosclerotic narrowing confined to the proximal portions of the coronary arteries with the distal portions sufficiently normal to accept revascularization procedures. Using microsurgical techniques, direct vascular anastomosis is possible on vessels as small as 1 mm. in diameter.

The most common operation is the aortocoronary bypass graft utilizing saphenous vein (Fig. 31-14). The saphenous vein is removed from the leg and used to join the ascending aorta and the coronary artery distal to the area of obstruction. The internal mammary artery, freed from its anatomic position along the sternal margin, may also be sutured directly into the left anterior descending cononary artery. Cardiopulmonary bypass quiets the heart while the anastomosis to the coronary artery is made. Usual sites for distal anastomosis to the coronary arteries are shown in Fig. 31-14.

The most common indication for coronary revascularization is in patients with chronic, stable angina pectoris that is intractable to usual forms of medical management. These patients have recurrent attacks of angina pectoris, usually with exercise or emotion, which are not abolished by therapeutic doses of short- and long-acting nitrates and beta adrenergic blocking agents (Propranolol in doses sufficient to reduce resting pulse below 60). When angina pectoris is sufficient to impair quality of life and/or capability of gainful occupation, surgery is recommended. In young patients ($<$ 50 years) or patients with extensive involvement (three-vessel) and/or critical location (left main coronary artery), the indications are liberalized, because it is known that these patients are at highest risk of early death. Similarly, a more aggressive surgical approach is taken in patients who continue to have marked abnormalities in the graded exercise test (treadmill stress test) while receiving optimal medical management. About 75% of patients are relieved of angina pectoris after coronary revascularization, 20% will have continued but less frequent angina, and about 5% will remain the same or worse. There is a general correlation between symptomatic improvement and the graft patency; 66 to 75% of saphenous veins are patent 1 year after the operation, depending on location of the graft. Patency rates approaching 90% have been reported using the internal mammary artery. Mortality rate for aortocoronary bypass graft operations in patients with chronic angina pectoris is about 2%.

Patients with unstable angina pectoris (preinfarction syndrome) require a coronary care facility to monitor cardiac rhythm and intensively treat myocardial ischemia. Enthusiasm for aggressive diagnostic and surgical interventions to prevent myocardial infarction should be tempered by knowledge that infarction in this clinical setting is usually not fatal and that the risk of the operation is higher (10 to 20%) because of the possibility of completed myocardial infarction at the time of surgery. For patients with completed acute myocardial infarction, the place of aortocoronary bypass operations is questionable because of high mortality rate ($> 40\%$) and the short time (60 minutes) after coronary occlusion in which irreversible myocardial damage occurs.

Patients who have congestive cardiac failure resulting from coronary artery disease also are not often helped by aortocoronary bypass operations. Improving myocardial blood flow does not significantly improve ventricular function under these conditions. Congestive heart failure, caused by an infarcted area that subsequently thins out and becomes aneurysmal (ventricular aneurysm), is benefited by excising the aneurysmal portion of the ventricle. This may be complemented by aortocoronary bypass graft. Similarly, patients with heart failure caused by postinfarction ventricular septal defect or mitral valve incompetence secondary to papillary muscle dysfunction respond nicely to surgical intervention, provided the operation is delayed for 30 days after infarction.

Valvular heart disease
Aortic valve

Stenosis or incompetence of the aortic valve results from degenerative changes of a congenitally abnormal valve or from rheumatic pathological changes. Aortic valve stenosis causes muscular hypertrophy of the ventricle, which encroaches on the ventricular cavity, making it effectively smaller. Aortic valve insufficiency, on the other hand, produces diastolic overload and dilation of the ventricle. Unfortunately, symptoms of aortic valve disease do not appear until relatively late in the natural course. Once symptoms of angina pectoris or syncope appear, threat of sudden death is imminent. Heart failure is a late sign and is accompanied by some irreversible changes in left ventricular performance.

Children and teenagers with aortic valve stenosis are treated by aortic valvotomy, but adults and all patients with aortic valve incompetence require valve replacement. Complications of hemorrhage and irreversible tetanic ventricular fibrillation ("stone heart") make operative mortality about 5% for aortic valve replacement. Functional improvement is often dramatic even in patients with poorly functioning left ventricles.

Mitral valve

Stenosis or incompetence of the mitral valve is usually related to rheumatic degenerative changes with fibrosis and thickening of the leaflets and chordae tendineae and ultimate deposition of calcium to produce rigidity of the valve. Pure mitral valve incompetence may result from rupture of chordae tendineae or myxomatous degeneration of the valve. Symptoms of heart failure, especially those related to pulmonary venous hypertension and fluid accumulation, appear gradually. The lengthy course of the disease gives adequate time for diagnostic confirmation and thoughtful timing of surgical intervention. There may be exacerbation of symptoms with change in cardiac rhythm to atrial fibrillation or rupture of chordae tendineae. The decision to operate is usually based on symptoms sufficient to interfere with quality of life that are not adequately controlled medically.

Patients less than 40 years of age with pure mitral valve stenosis having an otherwise pliable, noncalcified valve (good opening snap on auscultation) are treated by closed mitral valvotomy. In this operation, a dilator is passed retrograde through the apex of the left ventricle into the mitral valve. Forceful opening of the dilator opens the fused commissures of the mitral valve. Five to 20 years of symptomatic relief often follow this operation. Older patients and those with calcareous valves or mitral valve incompetence are operated on using cardiopulmonary bypass so that the valve may be visualized. Replacement of the valve with a prosthesis is nearly always required, but in a few patients, especially those with ruptured chordae tendineae, the valve may be reconstructed with appropriately placed plication or annuloplasty sutures. Replacement of the valve with a prosthesis has 5 to 10% mortality and 5 to 10% risk of later thromboembolic complications. Functional improvement is good, but patients with mitral valve disease often require continued medical treatment for fluid retention.

Tricuspid valve

Stenosis of the tricuspid valve caused by rheumatic degeneration is unusual; incompetence with dilated, pulsating neck veins, enlarged pulsatile liver, and immense fluid retention generally follows pulmonary hypertension and right ventricular dilation asociated with severe mitral valve disease. Surgical intervention is based primarily on symptoms similar to the criteria for mitral valve surgery.

Operations on the tricuspid valve are always performed with the cardiopulmonary bypass. A stenosed tricuspid valve must be replaced. When the tricuspid valve is incompetent because of dilation of the annulus, the configuration of the annulus may be restored with a special ring prosthesis (annuloplasty) or the valve replaced with a prosthesis. If mitral valve disease coexists, operative risk is highest of all surgery for valvular heart disease (10 to 20%).

Prosthetic valves

A variety of valve prostheses are used in the surgical treatment of valvular heart disease (Fig. 31-15). The valve most widely used is the ball-in-cage prosthesis of the Starr-Edwards design. This prosthesis has a high cage and the round poppet is bulky, so it occupies a considerable portion of the left ventricular volume when used in the mitral position. In contrast, the disc-in-cage prosthesis offers a low profile, which is more suitable for mitral valve replacement in the

Common Types of Valve Prosthesis

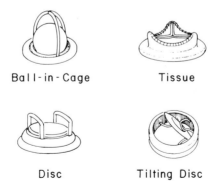

Ball-in-Cage

Tissue

Disc

Tilting Disc

Fig. 31-15. Examples of various devices for replacing damaged heart valves.

small left ventricle. The disc valve, however, creates more turbulent blood flow and sometimes obstructs, impeding blood flow causing pressure gradients. The tilting disc prosthesis has more central flow with favorable hemodynamic properties, especially in replacing valves with a small annulus.

Several tissue prostheses have been devised. The aortic valve taken from cadavers (homograft) is implanted in the aortic position either as a free-hand graft or on a metal stent. Favorable experience with porcine heterograft prostheses is accumulating; the pig aortic valve is mounted on a flexible stent generously covered with Dacron and stabilized in glutaraldehyde. Tissue valves are desirable because of improved hemodynamic properties and low incidence of thrombo-embolic complications even without anticoagulant prophylaxis. Long-term durability of the preserved tissue valve is still unknown.

Bacterial endocarditis

There is a constant threat of infection occurring in any abnormal heart valve or valvular prosthesis. Antibiotics usually control acute or subacute bacterial endocarditis, but irreversible damage with acute valvular insufficiency may accompany the infection. Severely damaged heart valves should be replaced before cardiac decompensation occurs. Risk of operation is increased with associated heart failure and sepsis. A period of 4 to 6 weeks of intravenous antibiotics is recommended, as bacterial infection of a prosthetic valve is very difficult to cure and sometimes progresses to fungal infection, which is nearly always fatal.

Cardiac tumors

Tumors of the myocardium are rare. The most common tumor found within the cardiac chambers is the atrial myxoma. This benign tumor is generally attached to the atrial septum; it is most common on the left side, and the patient presents with either peripheral arterial embolization of the myxomatous tumor or symptoms of mitral valve stenosis from obstruction of the mitral valve orifice by the tumor mass. Operation involves removal of the tumor and the portion of the atrial septum to which it is attached. The only malignant tumor of significance is the rhabdomyosarcoma, which may involve atrium or ventricle and by its anatomic location is often impossible to remove. This highly malignant tumor is generally fatal.

Pericardial disease
Tumors

Benign cyst of the pericardium is a mediastinal mass usually located on the right side of the pericardium. It is filled with yellowish-brown, clear fluid and the term "spring water cyst" aptly describes the contents. The lesion is important in the differential diagnosis of mediastinal masses and is usually removed surgically.

Pericarditis

Inflammation of the pericardium resulting from tuberculosis, viral disease (idiopathic pericarditis), or uremia may produce effusion into the pericardium sufficient to cause cardiac tamponade. Pericardiocentesis relieves the symptoms of cardiac tamponade, after which definitive treatment of the disease process is administered. Rapid fluid reaccumulation requires operative intervention. The operation may excise nearly all of the pericardium (pericardiectomy) or remove a portion of the pericardium on the left side so that pericardial fluid can drain into the left pleural space (pericardial window). This operation is usually both diagnostic and therapeutic.

Some cases of the idiopathic variety may fibrose the pericardium with subsequent scar contraction; this constrictive process in the pericardium also causes symptoms of cardiac tamponade. Operation is indicated to remove the contracted pericardium and involved epicardium.

Heart block and pacemakers

Acquired or congenital disease of the specialized conduction system in the heart may disturb cardiac rhythm. Complete heart block caused by a lesion in the bundle of His produces a slow idioventricular rhythm that may not provide adequate cardiac output, resulting in temporary loss of consciousness (Adams-Stokes syndrome). These patients are initially treated with a temporary electrode catheter passed through a peripheral vein and lodged in the right ventricle under fluoroscopic control. The electrode wire is connected to an external pulse generator which provides electrical stimulation to the myocardium at an appropriate rate. Permanent pacing devices are inserted later.

Electrodes for permanent pacing are placed either transvenously on the endocardium or directly onto the myocardium (Fig. 31-16). The transvenous electrode is passed through a peripheral vein under fluoroscopic control to lodge on the endocardial surface of the right ventricle. Local anesthesia suffices, simplifying the procedure in the high-risk elderly patient, but the electrode is occasionally dislodged in the postoperative period. Dislodgement does not occur when the electrode is attached directly to the myocardium during an open operation in which the heart is directly exposed. Durability of the myocardial electrode is probably enhanced so that this type of electrode is chosen for younger, better risk patients.

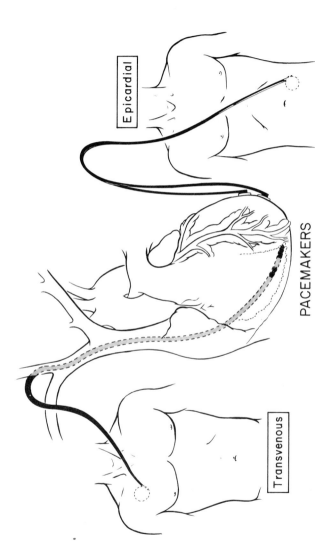

Fig. 31-16. Cardiac pacemakers. Electrodes may be placed through a peripheral vein to contact the endocardial surface of the right ventricle or attached directly to the epicardial surface of the left ventricle. Pulse generator (pacemaker) is attached to electrode and placed in subcutaneous pouch.

The most popular type of pacemaker at the present time is the ventricular inhibited demand type pulse generator, in which electrical stimuli at the rate of approximately 70 per minute are passed through the electrodes. There is a sensing circuit which recognizes spontaneous ventricular depolarization and suppresses the subsequent pacemaker stimulus. Ventricular fibrillation caused by inappropriate stimulus during the refractory period of the heart should not occur with this type of pacing unit.

The pulse generator units rarely fail primarily, but the batteries that provide the energy for the pacemaking stimulus deteriorate with time. It is a simple operation, however, to replace a subcutaneous pulse generator. Most units have a predicted life of approximately 3 to 5 years with standard nickel-cadmium batteries. Pulse generators utilizing lithium energy source, plutonium nuclear energy, or externally rechargeable batteries may offer longer wear, perhaps approaching 20 years.

CARDIAC TRANSPLANTATION, ARTIFICIAL HEARTS, AND ASSISTED CIRCULATION
Cardiac transplantation

Complete removal of the heart with replacement by a cadaver organ has been successfully accomplished for patients with terminal heart failure in many centers throughout the world. The greatest interest in cardiac transplantation came in the late 1960s when these operations were first performed. The operation consists of removal of most of the patient's heart, retaining a portion of the atria to simplify implantation of the donor heart. The donor heart is taken from a patient in whom cerebral death has occurred but myocardial function is normal. The donor organ is placed in the recipient by anastomosing the atria and great vessels. Technically the operation is not difficult, but control of rejection phenomenon is a major problem. Only a few centers have persisted with the clinical experiment of cardiac transplantation, but survival of over one-third of patients for a year or more has been reported.

Another approach utilizes a transplanted auxiliary heart for severe heart failure. In this operation the left atria of the donor and recipient hearts are joined, and the aorta of the donor and recipient vessels are joined such that part of the cardiac output may be taken over by the auxiliary heart to reduce left ventricular load in the patient. Competing heart rates require control by pacemaking. Success of this new concept again depends upon control of the autoimmune mechanism.

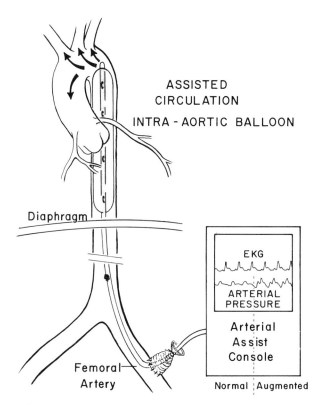

ASSISTED
CIRCULATION
INTRA - AORTIC BALLOON

Fig. 31-17. Assisted circulation. Balloon catheter placed in thoracic aorta via femoral artery is attached to assist device that inflates balloon during diastole and deflates just prior to systole. Displacement of blood produces increased diastolic pressure and better blood flow in coronary and cerebral arteries.

The artificial heart

Implantation of an artificial heart has been successfully accomplished with survival of animals in excess of 30 days. The devices consist of polyurethane ventricles that are compressed by insufflation of air from an external high pressure pulsatile system. The valves utilized in the artificial heart are typically those of the aortic or mitral prosthesis type. Control of attendant pulmonary hemorrhagic disorders, thromboembolism, and inflow obstruction is gradually being solved. On the horizon, of course, is the problem of supplying an energy source that will allow total implantation of the device.

Assisted circulation
Intra-aortic balloon assist

Intra-aortic balloon devices to improve blood flow to critical organs are currently used in patients who have continuing cardiac action but inadequate cardiac output. A balloon catheter is passed into the upper portion of the descending thoracic aorta (Fig. 31-17). The balloon is forcefully inflated and deflated in a pulsatile fashion by an external compressed gas source. Blood pressure and coronary blood flow are enhanced during diastole as the balloon is inflated and blood is displaced from the thoracic aorta. Afterload on the ventricle is decreased as the balloon rapidly deflates just prior to systole. Complex electrical gaiting devices ensure proper timing of inflation and deflation relative to the cardiac cycle. These devices have been used mostly in patients with myocardial infarction and reduced left ventricular performance and in patients after cardiac surgery who have inadequate cardiac output. Indications for using these devices and evaluation of results are under clinical investigation.

CHAPTER 32

Peripheral arteries

WILLIAM H. BAKER

The four basic phenomena (obstruction, erosion, perforation, and a mass) that are so important in other surgical diseases are frequently, and often dramatically, evident in diseases of the arteries. *Obstruction* from arteriosclerosis is one of the most common of all known vascular ailments. Aneurysms may *erode* or appear as pulsating *masses*. *Perforation* of a major artery may dramatically result from degenerative arterial disease or trauma. In addition, there are a variety of rarer but interesting vascular syndromes.

DIAGNOSIS

The most important facet of the vascular evaluation remains the history and physical examination. All of the diagnostic tests have limitations, may at times be misleading, and of necessity must be interpreted with the clinical findings. Calcification in artery walls is often visible on plain roentgenograms (Fig. 32-1). An arteriogram precisely identifies the extent of the pathological process (Table 32-1). Trained technicians can accurately obtain segmental leg pressures using Doppler ultrasound techniques. The pressures are not only of diagnostic value but may also be used to noninvasively follow the progress of the arterial disease. Plethysmography is presently more of a research than a clinical tool.

In patients with chronic arterial disease, there is time for extensive examination. However, in the acute life- or limb-threatening syndromes such as ruptured aneurysms and trauma, time limits diagnostic procedures and exploration may be the first diagnostic procedure.

TYPES OF ARTERIAL DISEASE

Congenital lesions. Congenital arteriovenous fistulas occur as café-au-lait spots, cirsoid aneurysms, or racemose connections between

571

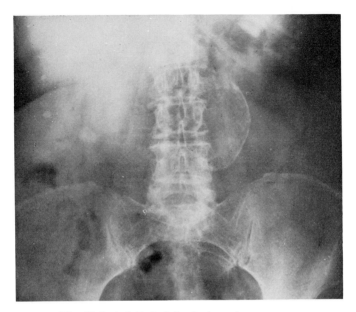

Fig. 32-1. Calcified abdominal aortic aneurysm.

major arteries and veins. Even though the subcutaneous lesions may be disfiguring, nonoperative therapy is usually indicated initially since they may disappear spontaneously or regress in size. Excision or irradiation is indicated if venous lakes or multiple arteriovenous fistulas enlarge or produce changes in cardiovascular dynamics. If localized, excellent palliation may be afforded by the occlusion of major "feeder vessels" surgically or by embolization. However, if there is widespread involvement, amputation is indicated (Fig. 32-2).

Arterial injuries. Three major types of injuries to blood vessels occur: laceration (incision), perforation (ice pick injury, needle injury during arteriography or cardiac catheterization), or contusion (Fig. 32-3). After complete transection of an artery, the ends retract and contract to assist in hemostasis. After partial transection this retraction is impossible and hemorrhage is greater than with complete transection. Contusion of an artery may injure the intima and promote local thrombosis.

These lesions are usually obvious on examination, but, if there is doubt, are confirmed by emergency arteriography. Arterial injury will

Table 32-1. Diagnostic aids in arterial disease

Diagnostic method	Technique	Results
Plain roentgenograms	Usual	Shows calcification in vessel or aneurysm (Fig. 32-1)
Arteriography	Injection of contrast dye in artery	Shows intraluminal contour and abnormalities of flow (Fig. 32-7)
Oscillometry	Pneumatic cuff and aneroid system record pulse amplitudes at various levels in extremity	Locates level of arterial block
Ultrasound velocity detector (Doppler)	Listen over the arterial tree to detect flow characteristics	Locates altered flow characteristics; can be used with a blood pressure cuff to accurately measure the arterial pressure at different levels of the extremity
Ultrasound examination of the abdomen	Noninvasive scan of abdomen	Accurately can measure the size of aneurysms

result in loss of life or limb if not corrected promptly. Concomitantly, hemorrhage is controlled, lost blood is replaced, and the artery is reconstructed. Autogenous tissue (vein grafts, arterial grafts, arterioplasties) is preferred over a prosthetic graft because of the threat of infection. An infected graft produces septic emboli, thrombosis, or disruption of the graft with the threat of false aneurysm or exsanguination.

All too often patients with lower extremity ischemia occurring after injury are treated with the presumptive diagnosis of "arterial spasm." These patients should have either immediate arteriography for diagnosis or exploration for treatment of a suspected arterial injury.

Delayed complications of arterial injury include arterial occlusion with intermittent claudication, rest pain or limb loss, false aneurysms (Fig. 32-4), or traumatic arteriovenous fistulas. These fistulas may become manifest as congestive heart failure (the fistula increasing venous return, dilating the chambers of the heart, and producing cardiac failure), pulsating veins, or typical bruits heard over the involved

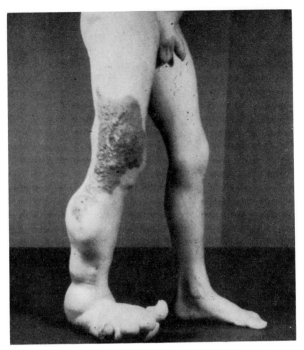

Fig. 32-2. Multiple arteriovenous fistulas in the right leg secondary to hemolymphangioma. Partial amputation was required.

vessels. Resection or ligation of the fistula with reconstruction of the vascular system is the reparative procedure of choice.

Arterial emboli. Arterial emboli usually arise from within the heart. Atrial fibrillation, aortic and mitral valvular disease, recent myocardial infarction with a mural thrombus, or, rarely, myxomas of the heart are antecedent causes. Another source are arteriosclerotic plaques that break off from arterial walls and embolize. The common sites of embolic obstruction are at the bifurcation of the major vessels: femoral, iliac, aorta, and occasionally brachial and carotid arteries.

Peripheral arterial emboli appear as abrupt attacks of ischemia. The classic "five P's" of acute arterial occlusion are: pallor, pain, pulselessness, paresthesias, and paralysis. The latter two findings suggest nonviability and indicate the degree of ischemia is severe enough to

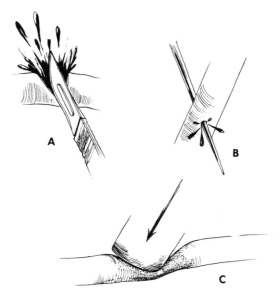

Fig. 32-3. Arterial injuries. **A,** Laceration. **B,** Perforation. **C,** Contusion. *Note:* Partial lacerations usually result in brisk bleeding because the severed ends cannot retract. Complete transections permit the severed ends to retract; spasm and thrombosis often limit bleeding.

cause nerve and/or muscle damage. In spite of prompt, excellent treatment, mortality and morbidity in this group of patients will be increased.

When the diagnosis of an arterial embolus is made, heparin is immediately administered intravenously (usually in the emergency room). This will *not* dissolve the embolus but will prevent propagation of the thrombus in the involved vessels. Embolectomy is performed as soon as possible, preferably within 12 hours. The catheter technique of embolectomy accomplished via a peripheral artery (an aortic saddle embolus is removed through the femoral arteries) can be done under general, regional, or even local anesthesia in poor-risk patients. Although delayed embolectomy (duration of embolus greater than 12 hours) is sometimes successful, it is fraught with increased mortality in patients with nonviable limbs. The source of the emboli is treated to prevent additional embolization (i.e., anticoagulants, valvuloplasty, valve replacement, or cardioversion). Occlusion of arteriosclerotic

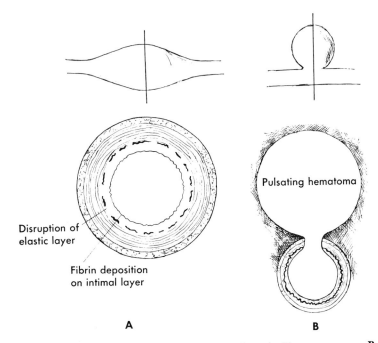

Disruption of
elastic layer

Fibrin deposition
on intimal layer

Pulsating hematoma

A

B

Fig. 32-4. Types of aneurysms in cross section. **A,** True aneurysm. **B,** False aneurysm usually caused by trauma; pulsating hematoma results; intimal layer grows into aneurysm that is covered by clot and later by fibrous tissue.

vessels may indicate combining embolectomy with endarterectomy or bypass grafting.

Aneurysms. Aneurysms are localized dilatations of arteries. They may be true or false (Table 32-2 and Fig. 32-4). Most aneurysms are atherosclerotic in origin; however, a few result from trauma or infection.

The gross pathology of aneurysms includes degenerative dilatation with deposition of fibrin and clot within the lumen. Microscopically the intima is thickened with fatty deposits and the media is disrupted (Fig. 32-4). Many patients (60 to 70%) are unaware of a pulsating mass unless it occurs in a superficial location, such as the extremities.

The diagnosis of aneurysm is usually made by discerning palpation

Table 32-2. Aneurysms

Location	Etiology	Relative incidence	Treatment	Prognosis
Thoracic aorta	Arteriosclerotic, infection, trauma	Occasional	Medical or surgical (depending on anatomic site and patient)	Fair
Abdominal aorta	Arteriosclerotic	Frequent	Resection	Good
Femoral and popliteal	Arteriosclerotic, trauma; infection	Occasional	Resection or exclusion bypass graft	Good
Carotid	Arteriosclerotic	Rare	Resection	Good
Upper extremities	Trauma, arteriosclerotic, infection	Rare	Resection	Good
Splenic	Arteriosclerotic	Occasional	Resection if symptomatic or in females under 40	Good
Renal	Arteriosclerotic	Occasional	Aneurysm resection or nephrectomy, sometimes nonoperative	Good

or by plain roentgenograms that show calcification within the wall of the aneurysm (Fig. 32-1). Abdominal ultrasound scanning accurately measures the aneurysm in two dimensions. Arterial visualization (arteriogram) is unnecessary unless the extent of involvement must be known prior to operation (thoracic aortic aneurysm and aneurysms involving renal arteries), or the distal arterial tree is of questionable quality (popliteal and femoral artery aneurysms). Most aortic aneurysms are asymptomatic, but since their rupture is such a threat to life, the treatment of choice is surgical excision and replacement with a prosthetic graft (Fig. 32-5). All extremity aneurysms should be treated surgically because of the risk of thrombosis and/or distal embolization. Because the thoracic and suprarenal aorta supply organs that do not tolerate prolonged anoxia (spinal cord, kidneys), aneurysms in these areas may require temporary bypass (with the pump oxygenator, atrial femoral bypass, or tube shunts) during repairs.

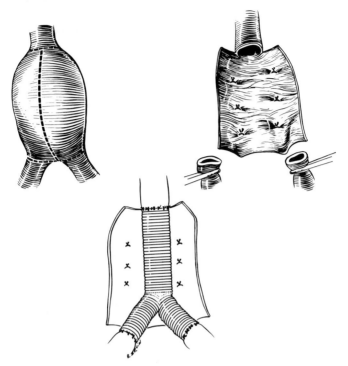

Fig. 32-5. An abdominal aortic aneurysm is incised after obtaining proximal and distal control. Bleeding lumbar arteries are controlled from within the aneurysm. The anterior wall of the aneurysm is resected but the posterior wall is left intact. Vascular integrity is reestablished with a Dacron graft.

Occlusive disease
Lower extremities

Atherosclerosis is the almost universal cause of occlusive disease of the legs. The characteristic pathological features of atherosclerosis (arteriosclerosis) are intimal thickening and degeneration. Lipid deposits on the intima followed by necrosis, fibrosis, and calcification result in progressive obstruction, which may be partial (stenosis) or complete (occlusion).

Clinically, atherosclerosis is characterized by slowly progressive arterial insufficiency. It occurs chiefly in older men but sometimes

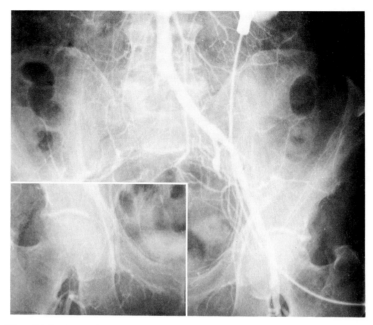

Fig. 32-6. Occlusion of the right common and external iliac artery. Collateral flow from the left internal iliac system supplies the right profunda femoris artery via the obturator and gluteal branches of the right internal iliac artery.

emerges as early as the third decade of life. It is common in diabetics, affecting both the larger, surgically accessible arteries as well as the smaller arteries of the foot and leg.

History. Pain is the most common symptom of arteriosclerosis obliterans. Intermittent claudication, a specific symptom of vascular insufficiency, is a cramping pain in muscles that is relieved promptly by rest after a certain period of continuous exercise. This pain is repetitive with precisely the same amount of exercise. Accumulation of acid waste products from anoxic muscle probably causes the pain. The location of the intermittent claudication (calf, thigh) helps localize the stenotic artery (superficial femoral artery, iliac artery—Fig. 32-6).

Rest pain in the foot occurs from inadequate perfusion in the horizontal position (i.e., sleeping) in the patient with severe occlusive arterial disease. Rest pain is alleviated by placing the foot in a dependent position and must be differentiated from benign leg cramps.

Physical examination. Careful palpation of the pulses is the most important part of examining a patient with peripheral artery disease. The pulse (arterial pressure) is directly related to the inflow of blood and the resistance to flow $(P = F \times R)$. Diminished, absent, or asymmetric pulses often pinpoint the exact site of arterial obstruction. A bruit denotes turbulent flow past a stenotic lesion or through an arteriovenous fistula.

Chronic occlusive disease is characterized by skin coolness, atrophic shiny skin, absent hair, thickened toenails, and sometimes ulcers on the distal extremity. Inadequate blood supply is suggested when the skin blanches with pressure and the color returns slowly after releasing pressure. (In acute obstructions the affected extremity appears suddenly and persistently cadaveric.) Elevation of the ischemic extremity produces pallor, and dependency produces cyanosis. They result from the following chain of events: (1) elevation lowers the perfusion pressure, producing pallor; (2) local anoxia and metabolic acidosis result; (3) capillary dilatation occurs, causing (4) slowing of an already inadequate blood flow, and (5) cyanosis with dependency.

The presence of leg complaints, diminished pulses, and deformed, arthritic joints makes a diagnosis difficult. In other patients typical complaints of intermittent claudication will be combined with satisfactory pulses. It is imperative that the physician exercise the problem patient to produce symptoms and reexamine him at that time. Is the pain really calf pain or joint pain? Are the pulses still present? Are the bruits louder? Is the symptomatic foot paler? Many difficult problems can be solved in the astute clinician's office.

Extracranial cerebrovascular disease

Although arteriosclerosis may involve any neck vessel, typically it causes a localized stenosis at the origin of the internal carotid artery. Symptoms arising from this lesion may result from embolization of atherosclerotic debris or platelet emboli distally, or from low flow past the lesion. In younger female patients, fibromuscular hyperplasia may involve a major portion of the extracranial internal carotid artery. Microscopically the media is alternately thinned (causing aneurysms) and thickened (causing stenosis), producing a "chain of lakes" arteriographically (Fig. 32-7): this is the same picture seen in the renal artery lesion. In addition to standard treatment techniques, arterial dilation is also successful.

Patients with cerebrovascular disease present with at least three neurological syndromes: (1) a transient ischemic attack (TIA) is a

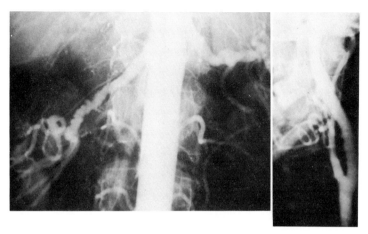

Fig. 32-7. These arteriograms represent fibromuscular hyperplasia. Note the "chain of lakes" present in the right renal artery and the septa present in the carotid artery.

Table 32-3. Classification of cerebrovascular symptoms

Hemispheric:	Unilateral motor and sensory
	Monocular visual
	Dysphasias
Vertebrobasilar:	Vertigo (true)
	Ataxia
	Diplopia
	Bilateral visual aberrations
	Shifting paresis or paresthesias
	Drop attacks
	Dysarthria
	Syncope
Nonspecific:	Dizziness
	Light-headedness
	Decreased mentation
	Headache
	Confusion
	Personality change
	Tinnitis
	Decreased visual acuity
	Seizures

Table 32-4. Chronic occlusive disease

Site	Clinical	Diagnosis	Treatment	Comment
Aortoiliac	Men, fifth to seventh decade, pain, intermittent claudication, impotence	Decreased or absent femoral and distal pulses, bruits over stenotic arteries, aortography shows diseased areas	Thromboendarterectomy, bypass graft, sympathectomy, amputation	Results good if outflow adequate
Femoral	Men, fifth to seventh decade, intermittent claudication, skin changes	Decreased or absent distal pulses, evidence of ischemia in foot or leg	Thromboendarterectomy, patch angioplasty, bypass graft, sympathectomy, amputation	Results good if outflow adequate
Renal	Hypertension, males and females	Bruit over abdomen, renal arteriogram, intravenous pyelogram—small kidney with delayed function, differential renal function, renal vein renin assay	Bypass graft, endarterectomy, patch angioplasty, nephrectomy	Good results if case selection is strict, saves kidney function

Cerebrovascular	Hemispheric, vertebro-basilar, nonspecific	Carotid pulse decrease, bruit over carotid, arteriography shows stenosis or ulceration	Endarterectomy	Good results
Celiomesenteric	Visceral angina: 1. Pain after eating 2. Weight loss 3. Diarrhea (constipation) 4. Abdominal bruit 5. Infarction	Angiography, difficult diagnosis in acute occlusion	Bypass graft, endarterectomy, bowel resection	Good results if done prior to infarction
Upper extremities	Claudication, skin changes, sensory disturbances	Absent pulses, bruit over involved vessel, arteriogram	Endarterectomy, bypass vein graft, resection first rib, cervical sympathectomy, amputation	Fair

neurological deficit that lasts less than 24 hours; (2) a reversible ischemic neurological deficit (RIND) lasts longer than 24 hours but recovery is complete; (3) a permanent neurological deficit (either an acute or chronic stroke) may occur.

The patient's neurological complaints and findings can be further categorized into hemispheric, vertebrobasilar, and nonspecific (see Table 32-3). Diminished carotid or subclavian pulses with overlying bruits may be found. The blood pressure in each arm should be measured. Four-vessel arteriography (both carotids and vertebrals) to include the intracerebral vessels can precisely identify stenotic lesions.

Patients with acute strokes are not operative candidates, in contrast to patients with transient ischemic attacks. Stenosis in the internal carotid artery is typically suited for endarterectomy. The details of the operative procedure (use of an internal shunt, patch angioplasty, hypercarbia or hypocarbia) remain controversial, but the reported results are excellent with a variety of techniques (combined mortality and morbidity of close to 1%).

Visceral arterial stenosis

Atherosclerotic stenosis of any or all of the visceral arteries (celiac artery, superior mesenteric artery, and inferior mesenteric artery) may cause symptoms, as may external compression (by the median arcuate ligament). See Chapters 21 and 24 and Table 32-4 for clinical details.

Renal artery stenosis

Renal artery stenosis is becoming more commonly recognized as a cause of arterial hypertension. In patients in their fifth to seventh decade, atherosclerosis is the most common cause, but in younger women fibromuscular hyperplasia is more common. Rarely, renal artery aneurysms cause hypertension.

On physical examination an abdominal bruit is heard in a hypertensive patient. Intravenous pyelography reveals a small kidney with delayed function. Renal vein renin is elevated on the affected side. Split renal function studies show a diminished urine volume and sodium concentration with an increased urinary creatinine concentration from the involved kidney. The arteriogram reveals the nature and extent of the lesion. Surgical treatment is directed toward correcting or bypassing the responsible lesion.

Treatment of occlusive arterial disease

There are three levels of treatment in vascular disease: (1) maintenance of life, (2) maintenance of limb form, and (3) maintenance or restoration of limb function. The vascular surgeon often resects an aortic abdominal aneurysm in a poor-risk patient since this is a life-threatening lesion. A reconstructive procedure is indicated in less than ideal situations if limb loss is imminent. Operations designed to alleviate intermittent claudication alone must be accomplished by low surgical risk.

Direct reparative arterial surgery is possible for localized segments of occlusive disease in medium to large arteries. When arterial disease is diffuse or involves small arteries, nonoperative therapy, sympathectomy, or amputation are the only treatment options.

Reconstructive arterial surgery. Reconstructive arterial surgery depends on the following fundamentals: (1) an accessible lesion is responsible for the patient's symptoms, or is life or limb threatening; (2) there is adequate inflow and outflow of the proposed reconstructed segment (a superficial femoral artery stenosis is not bypassed with significant aortoiliac obstructive disease); and (3) the choice of operation must be tailored to the patient (a subcutaneous axillofemoral artery bypass is done instead of an intra-abdominal aortofemoral bypass in an extremely poor-risk patient).

There are several methods of arterial revascularization:

1. *Endarterectomy:* The diseased intima is dissected from the media by the open (Fig. 32-8) or closed (loop endarterectomy) method. This is applicable in the aortoiliac system, carotid bifurcation, and visceral arteries, but has met with high recurrence rates in the lower extremities.
2. *Bypass graft:* A graft (either a prosthesis or autogenous tissue) shunts blood around the diseased segment (Fig. 32-9).

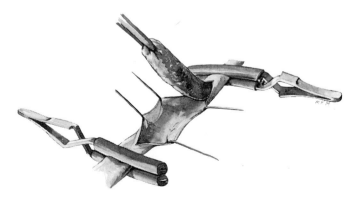

Fig. 32-8. Endarterectomy.

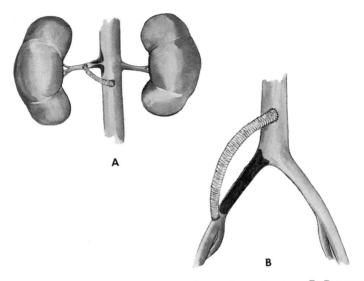

Fig. 32-9. Bypass grafts. **A,** Bypass of stenotic renal artery. **B,** Bypass of occluded iliac artery.

3. *Replacement grafts:* The diseased arterial segment is resected and replaced with a prosthesis or autogenous tissue (usually vein but sometimes another artery).
4. *Patch graft (angioplasty):* Either autogenous tissue or prosthetic material is used to enlarge stenotic arteries (Fig. 32-10).

Nonoperative treatment of ischemic lower extremity. If the arteriosclerosis is diffuse, direct arterial surgical correction is impossible. Nonoperative treatment consists of the following:

1. Avoid pressure by using soft mattresses and adequate-sized shoes.
2. Avoid trauma. Corns and calluses should not be cut.
3. Tobacco is forbidden.
4. The feet are washed carefully and dried daily, followed by bland ointments.
5. We believe vasodilator drugs have little value in generalized arteriosclerosis. (Theoretically, they dilate only pliable arteries.)
6. Ulcers are cleaned by sharp debridement and intermittent saline soaks, and grafted with skin, if possible.
7. Local medications are contraindicated, since the ischemic skin

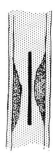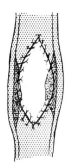

Fig. 32-10. Vein patch graft.

is sensitive to chemical agents; antibiotic ointments are used only against specific organisms resistant to other treatment.

8. Daily exercise to tolerance to optimally develop collateral circulation.

Sympathectomy. Destruction of the sympathetic ganglia in the lumbar chain dilates small and medium-sized arteries. If sufficient collateral arterial supply exists around obstructed arterial segments, sympathectomy may improve a marginal blood supply. Usually at least two ganglia are excised. The first lumbar ganglion is preserved in males to prevent impotence. Plethysmography and skin temperatures before and after sympathetic nerve block may help predict the efficacy of sympathectomy, but a negative test does not rule out a good clinical effect. Sympathectomy is often combined with direct arterial revascularization. Sympathectomy alone will rarely heal large ulcerations or alleviate severe rest pain.

Amputation. Gangrene, advancing infection, recalcitrant ulceration, and unremitting rest pain necessitate amputation. Amputation is a last resort after all nonoperative and direct attempts to treat the ischemia have failed. The level of amputation depends on a blood supply sufficient to heal the incision. Despite an absent popliteal pulse, a below-knee stump can often thrive on collateral circulation. Excellent results have recently been obtained by using plaster dressings. If pedal pulses are both absent, local digital amputations are usually doomed to failure.

The effects of amputation need not be disastrous. With a proper prosthesis the patient may reenter society in a productive role. It is the surgeon's duty to encourage this goal.

Inflammatory and miscellaneous arterial diseases

Buerger's disease

Buerger's disease is an inflammatory disease of unknown cause that involves both arteries and veins. It is included here largely for historic interest for, since the widespread use of arteriography and hence more accurate diagnoses, the incidence of Buerger's disease is rare. It usually occurs in young men (onset at 30 to 35 years) and involves medium-sized arteries (posterior tibial, anterior tibial) in the lower extremities. Besides sex and age, tobacco is the only other important etiological factor.

Pathologically the arteries show an early panarteritis with chronic inflammatory cells and a relatively diffuse scattering of multinucleated giant cells. Fibrosis of the entire artery with small, discontinuous, recanalized channels occurs in late stages.

Clinical examination. Lower extremity pain from inflammation and ischemia with appearance of small segments of migratory, superficial phlebitis, keynote the symptoms. Migrating phlebitis (with no other obvious cause) suggests Buerger's disease.

The course of this disease is variable. In some it smolders for years with minor sequelae. In contrast, we have been forced to amputate a lower extremity in a 19-year-old man after less than 6 months of symptoms.

Treatment. Abstinence from tobacco is probably the most important factor. Bed rest with protection of the extremity is the only other available treatment measure. Antibiotics are used only to treat secondary infections. Sympathectomy may delay or prevent amputation after subsidence of the acute process. Amputation is done only after all other treatment has failed.

Angiospastic diseases

The blood flow to surface areas of the body constantly fluctuates in response to tissue demands, temperature variations, and emotions. Vasomotor control is greatest in the hands and feet, and these areas consequently reflect, most noticeably, abnormalities in vasomotor response. With exaggerated response the skin becomes white (with spasm), cyanotic (from anoxic capillary dilatation), and then intensely red (from reactive hyperemia) before becoming normal.

Raynaud's phenomenon, an intermitent, cold-induced peripheral ischemia, generally involves the upper extremities. It may become chronic, with eventual loss of tissue. The phenomenon is associated with the following numerous conditions, with symptoms fluctuating with progression of the underlying disease.

1. Obliterative arterial disease
   a. Arteriosclerosis
   b. Buerger's disease
   c. Arterial emboli
2. Trauma
   a. After injury or operation
   b. Occupational
      (1) Pneumatic hammer
      (2) Pianists, typists
3. Neurogenic
   a. Thoracic outlet syndromes
   b. Primary neurological diseases
4. Hematological diseases
   a. Cold agglutinins
   b. Cryoglobulins
   c. Hemoglobinopathies (such as sickle cell anemia)
   d. Polycythemia
5. Systemic diseases
   a. Scleroderma
   b. Systemic lupus erythematosus
   c. Polyarteritis nodosa
   d. Rheumatoid arthritis
   e. Malignant disease
6. Drugs
   a. Ergots
   b. Heavy metals

If no underlying conditions causing Raynaud's phenomenon become evident (over a 2-year period), then a diagnosis of Raynaud's disease is made. These patients, usually young females (less than 40 years old), develop numbness and/or a burning pain in the fingers and hands with the typical color changes upon exposure to cold. These changes are bilateral and tissue loss is limited.

A modified Allen's test helps to diagnose vascular disease distal to the wrist. Pressure is maintained over the radial and ulnar arteries by the examiner while the patient clenches his fist to empty blood from the hand. Release of either artery should produce a rapidly spreading erythema of the dependent hand and fingers, thereby demonstrating patency of that artery. Release of an occluded (radial or ulnar) artery will not produce erythema. If a digital or palmar artery is occluded, then the area supplied by that artery will become erythematous later than the rest of the hand..

The diagnosis of Raynaud's disease is made clinically. Arteriography is not indicated unless the physical examination suggests major artery disease. All efforts are made to diagnose an underlying condition. Treatment includes avoiding cold and the wearing of warm clothing. Vasodilators are occasionally beneficial. Sympathectomy is reserved for patients with tissue necrosis but is usually only temporarily helpful.

Erythromelalgia

Erythromelalgia is a rare condition of unknown etiology. Clinically the patient complains of a red, warm, painful area on the lower extremities precipitated by excess heat and dependency. Sympathectomy is contraindicated in these patients.

Thoracic outlet syndrome

The thoracic outlet syndrome is a clinical syndrome of pain in the arm and numbness and coldness of the hand, secondary to compression of the neurovascular bundle as it leaves the chest. The neurovascular bundle is entrapped between a cervical rib and the first rib, the scalenus anticus muscle and the first rib, or the clavicle and the first rib. Clinically, hyperabduction of the shoulders (military position) or tensing the scalenus anticus muscle (Adson maneuver) will diminish the radial pulse in 50% of the patients. Nerve compression, either at the vertebral bodies or distal to the shoulder (i.e., carpal tunnel syndrome) must be differentiated. Treatment is the surgical removal (either transaxillary, transpleural, or transcervical) of the first rib beneath the neurovascular bundle. The surgeon must be aware that a poststenotic dilatation (aneurysm) may harbor thrombus leading to distal embolization. This is repaired to ensure a successful therapeutic effort.

Arteritis

Although Buerger's disease is the most widely discussed inflammation of the arteries, there are numerous other causes of arteritis (Table

Table 32-5. Classification of arteritis

Infective	*Noninfective*
Pyogenic arteritis	Systemic lupus erythematosus
Fungal arteritis	Polyarteritis nodosa
Tuberculous arteritis	Rheumatoid arthritis
Mycotic aneurysm	Pulseless disease
Syphilitic arteritis	Necrotizing arteritis after
	coarctation repair
	Buerger's disease

32-5). Specific infections are caused by direct bacterial invasion (i.e., from the retroperitoneal lymph nodes into the aorta), infection occurring after trauma or surgery, and septic emboli.

The causes of noninfective arteritis are many. Most are manifestations of a "collagen disease." The necrotizing arteritis that occasionally complicates successful repair of an aortic coarctation is allegedly secondary to mechanical stretching of the artery. *Giant cell (temporal) arteritis* causes headaches and visual disturbances. Physical examination discloses a tender, enlarged, superficial temporal artery. *Pulseless disease* (Takayasu's disease, aortic arch syndrome) occurs in young women. Symptoms and findings depend on which arteries of the aortic arch are involved. Pathologically, the artery is thickened with a wrinkled intima, elastic damage, and round cell infiltration in all layers.

Specific arteritis responds to appropriate antibiotics determined by cultures. Surgical therapy is reserved for resistant cases or complications. Autogenous tissue is employed rather than synthetic material. Treatment (usually steroids) of a noninfective arteritis is directed toward the underlying disease. Steroids have also successfully ameliorated pulseless disease and temporal arteritis. Reserpine improves the necrotizing arteritis that sometimes occurs after repair of aortic coarctation.

CHAPTER 33

Peripheral veins

ROBERT T. SOPER
DAVID W. FURNAS

Veins return blood to the heart from the vast capillary system, and, in contrast to their arterial counterparts, flow rates are low, more intermittent, and characterized by progressively lower pressure from peripheral to central areas. Gravity, unidirectional valves, and progressively larger channels with lower pressure determine the direction of flow. The pumping action of the right side of the heart prevents stagnation and a rise in venous pressure. Veins are larger in diameter, thinner walled, and contain much less intramural muscle than do arteries; they are less predictable in location and are closely related anatomically and physiologically to the lymphatics. Obstruction to the flow either of blood within the veins or of tissue fluid within lymphatics elevates interstitial pressure, resulting in stagnation of flow, edema, and poor nutrition of the affected tissues.

ANATOMY

Since the majority of venous surgical diseases involve the lower extremities, the discussion of venous anatomy will be limited to these members. The normal venous drainage of the lower extremity includes (1) a *superficial* network of veins traveling in the subcutaneous areolar tissue above the deep fascia of the leg and (2) the *deep* venous system that lies among the muscle groups in the lower extremity deep to the fascia. These two systems are interconnected segmentally by perforating or communicating channels, with flow normally being from superficial to deep.

The direction of flow in both the superficial and deep venous systems is always from peripheral to central, from higher pressure to

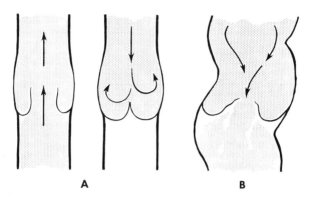

Fig. 33-1. A, Competent vein valve opens to allow forward blood flow but closes snugly to prevent retrograde flow. **B,** Incompetent vein valve cusps cannot close; retrograde flow of blood results.

lower pressure areas. The milking action of the leg muscles is important in generating flow in the deep system in the legs, although gravity does exert some effect. There are several unidirectional valves in both the superficial and deep set of veins, as well as in the communicating (perforating) veins. When competent, the valves prevent retrograde flow with its resultant elevation of tissue pressure distally (Fig. 33-1, *A*).

The *greater* and *lesser saphenous veins* form the superficial set of veins of the lower extremity. The greater saphenous vein arises at the dorsal venous arch of the foot and ascends anterior to the medial malleolus, passing anteromedially up the thigh to empty into the deep venous system (the *femoral vein*) in the groin via a fascial aperture known as the *fossa ovalis*. The greater saphenous system drains blood from the skin and subcutaneous tissues of the entire circumference of the thigh and the medial and anterior aspect of the leg and foot.

The other component of the superficial saphenous system (the lesser saphenous vein) begins behind the external malleolus and ascends posterolaterally in the calf to empty into the deep system (the popliteal vein) in the upper portion of the popliteal space.

VARICOSE VEINS

Numerically, the most common affliction of the veins is varicosities, which are characterized by abnormal *dilatation, elongation,* and *tortuosity.* About 15% of the population eventually develops varicose veins.

Although varicosities can be seen in any of the venous systems in the body (rectum, hemorrhoids; pudendal plexus, varicocele; esophagus, esophageal varices; periumbilicus, caput medusae), the term *varicose veins* is generally reserved for the phenomenon as it so commonly involves the lower extremities.

Veins of the greater saphenous system are most commonly afflicted, only about 10% of patients with varices have significant involvement of the lesser saphenous system. The deep leg veins do not become varicosed because of external support lent by the investing muscle bundles and fascia.

Pathophysiology. Common to all varicose veins is loss of elasticity of the walls and incompetency of the valves. Normally the vein valves are thin, delicate, bicuspid structures that allow blood to pass from peripheral to central areas but close to prevent retrograde flow (Fig. 33-1, *A*). The valves cannot elongate and grow once body growth has been attained; therefore, as the veins lose elasticity and begin to dilate, the valve cusps tend to pull apart and become incompetent (Fig. 33-1, *B*). This allows retrograde blood flow and stagnation. Valves

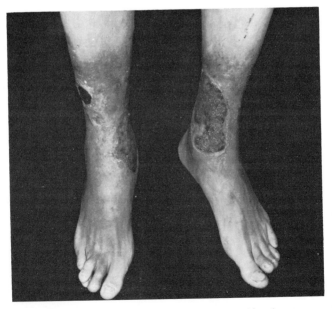

Fig. 33-2. Stasis dermatitis with varicose skin ulcers.

may also be primarily damaged by trauma, infection, congenital factors, and thrombophlebitis.

Regardless of the cause of the initial valve damage, the cycle is self-perpetuating. Each incompetent valve allows retrograde flow of blood that then imposes dilatation of the vein distally to produce incompetence of the next valve downstream. Stagnation and retrograde flow increase venous pressure and favor progressive elongation and tortuosity, to complete the clinical picture of varicose veins.

Sustained increase in venous pressure induces leakage of excessive amounts of protein-rich fluid from the capillary bed into the tissues and reduces the absorption of tissue fluid back into the venules, thereby increasing the volume (edema) and pressure of the fluid within interstitial spaces. Lymph flow is increased, and even intracellular pressure rises. The interstitial edema provokes fibrosis and induration, and cellular nutrition becomes progressively impaired. In time the skin responds by hyperpigmentation, eczematoid changes, and finally ulceration (Fig. 33-2). These are hallmarks of so-called *stasis dermatitis*, the end result of years of varicose veins.

The specific etiology of varicose veins is often difficult to pinpoint. Certainly the upright position of *Homo sapiens* is important, since we do not see varicosities in the upper extremity of man nor at all in quadrupeds. In about 40% of patients with varicosities there is a family history of varicose veins, often with the onset early in adult life (second decade). These perhaps result from a congenital weakness in the elasticity of the vein valves and walls, as well as the supporting tissues of the body generally. Varicose veins have a pronounced female sex incidence (2 or 3:1), presumably related to the smooth muscle-relaxing effect of female sex hormones manifested by cyclic dilatation of veins and increase in tissue fluid premenstrually. Commonly pregnancy is associated with the onset or worsening of varicose veins. Other etiological factors of importance include increase in intra-abdominal pressure from any cause, obesity, increasing age, and occupations that require prolonged inactivity while the legs are dependent. A rare cause of varicose veins is the development of arteriovenous fistulas with the introduction of high arterial pressures within the thin venous channels.

Thrombosis of the deep veins of the lower extremities commonly destroys the valve competency in this system, and even with recanalization the flow in this system henceforth is sluggish. The higher pressure within the deep system produces dilatation of the communicating veins, incompetency of their valves, and reversal of blood flow from deep to superficial veins; in turn, compensatory dilatation of the superficial veins occurs as they become collateral systems draining blood from the deep compartment of the leg.

Clinical features. The most common symptom of varicose veins is a dull, nagging ache or discomfort in the calves and ankles, worsened by prolonged standing. It is often associated with ankle edema and a sensation of heaviness and fullness more pronounced toward the end of the day. Dilatation, tortuosity, and elongation of the superficial veins gradually progress, and the unsightly bluish discoloration that this lends to the legs often brings the female patient in for treatment. Nonpitting edema, eczematoid dermatitis, hyperpigmentation, and superficial skin ulcerations are common late developments, especially in the region of the medial malleolus (Fig. 33-2). Healing of "varicose ulcers" is slow, and often infection and ulceration progress until specific treatment is undertaken.

Rarely, varices rupture and bleed with trauma. In the elderly patient a soft, cystic varix occasionally forms in the groin at the junction of the greater saphenous vein with the deep femoral vein; this mass has a well-marked cough impulse but empties readily upon assuming a recumbent position, to allow easy differentiation from a femoral hernia.

History and physical examination should be complete, looking for etiological factors enumerated earlier. The patient should be examined in the upright position to define clearly the extent and segments of the greater and lesser saphenous veins involved. Skin changes should be noted, especially near the malleoli.

The many tests for varicose veins are designed to answer certain questions about the local cause and extent of the varicosities. The *Schwartz test* is performed with the patient standing and involves sharp compression of the greater saphenous vein at the medial epicondyle of the femur by the fingers of one hand of the examiner, while the fingers of the other hand perceive the percussion fluid wave transmitted up and down the channel. Competent valves dampen the waves, but an intact fluid column in a venous system with incompetent valves transmits the percussion waves into even small tributaries. By moving his hands up and down the vein, the examiner can easily map out the course and extent of the varicosities.

An estimate must be made of the patency and competency of the deep venous system. If the deep veins are obstructed or incompetent, one would be loathe to excise indiscriminately the superficial veins that serve as necessary collateral channels to empty blood from the lower extremity. *Perthes' test* involves placing a tourniquet around the groin tightly enough to occlude flow in the superficial veins—then the patient is walked briskly.

Pain and increasing edema of the extremity indicate obstruction

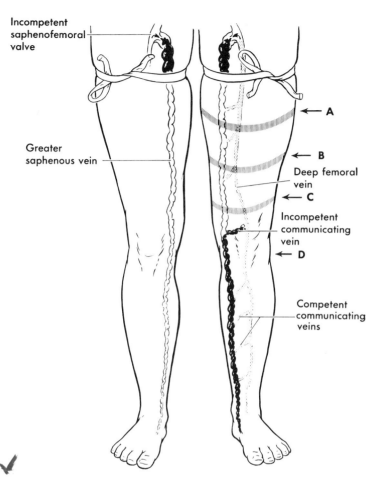

Incompetent
saphenofemoral
valve

← A

Greater
saphenous vein

← B

Deep femoral
vein

← C

Incompetent
communicating
vein

← D

Competent
communicating
veins

Fig. 33-3. Modified Trendelenburg (tourniquet) test for varicose veins. The tourniquet on the patient's *right* leg prevents filling of the varicosed greater saphenous vein distally, proving competency of all the communicating valves and incompetency of the saphenofemoral valve. On the patient's *left* leg, an incompetent communicating vein valve at the knee allows filling of the greater saphenous vein distal to this point, but the tourniquet prevents filling of the vein above the knee. A second tourniquet at points **A, B,** or **C** would not alter the findings. However, had a second tourniquet been placed at point **D,** the greater saphenous vein would have filled only from the knee down to this level.

to the deep veins. An alternative test is to wrap the extremity snugly from toes to groin with an elastic wrap; pain upon ambulation indicates the same phenomenon. Conversely, an improvement in symptoms when the patient walks while the superficial veins are occluded suggests that treatment of the superficial varicosities would be beneficial.

Rarely, *phlebography* is helpful to document more precisely the extent and nature of the disease in the deep venous system. Radiopaque dye is injected into a superficial vein of the foot while an ankle tourniquet is in place, to direct the dye into the deep venous system. Several radiographs of the entire lower extremity are then made, with the patient at rest and after exercise, to note the speed of clearance of the dye as well as size, distribution, and patency of the deep leg veins.

Having determined a normal deep venous system in the extremity, the next question to answer is whether the valve at the saphenofemoral junction is incompetent (by means of the modified *Trendelenburg test,* Fig. 33-3). After the veins have been emptied by recumbency and elevation, a tourniquet is placed at the groin with enough pressure to occlude the superficial veins, after which the patient stands erect. The tourniquet is then released, and observations are made of the speed and direction by which the greater saphenous venous system refills (Fig. 33-4). If the vein fills promptly from above in a retrograde manner, the saphenofemoral valve is incompetent. A similar test can be performed on the valve between the lesser saphenous–popliteal anastomosis in the popliteal fossa, after the vein is emptied and the tourniquet is placed just above the fullness of the calf. If either of these main valves is incompetent, treatment must include ligation and division of these major superficial veins where they empty into the deep venous system.

If the veins fill quickly before tourniquet removal, one must assume that they are filling via incompetent perforators between the superficial and deep system (Fig. 33-3, left leg). One must document the precise number and location of the incompetent perforators so that each can be specifically treated. Often one can palpate the fascial defect through which a dilated and incompetent perforator travels, generally marked as well by especial dilatation of the superficial veins in the immediate area.

The use of two tourniquets simultaneously will locate the incompetent perforators accurately when they cannot be obviously seen and palpated. The veins are emptied, and the high groin tourniquet is reapplied (Fig. 33-3, left leg). The second tourniquet is then applied at midthigh, and the patient stands; if the veins between the two tourniquets do not fill, the perforators in this compartment are compe-

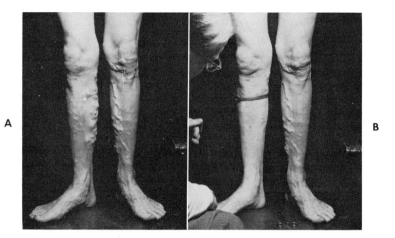

A

B

Fig. 33-4. A, Bilateral greater saphenous varicosities; the veins fill promptly on standing. **B,** The vein does not fill distal to the tourniquet; communicating vein valves are competent below this point.

tent. The test may then be repeated with the second tourniquet placed this time just above the knee. The second tourniquet is moved lower and lower on the leg until a vein promptly fills between the two tourniquets, thus localizing the level at which the incompetent perforating vein lies. When many incompetent perforators are present, application of three or four tourniquets simultaneously at different levels helps to narrow the compartments examined. All perforating veins with incompetent valves must be pinpointed and mapped precisely.

Treatment. The signs and symptoms of mild to moderate varicose veins are generally controlled by conservative measures. These include avoiding constrictive garments (garters) and prolonged periods of inactivity when the legs are dependent, encouraging leg elevation periodically throughout the day, and providing snug external support to the lower extremities. Support is provided by well-fitting elastic hose or by elastic wraps, both applied immediately upon arising and worn until the legs can again be elevated. The foot of the bed should be elevated on blocks 6 to 8 inches high to improve venous drainage while the patient sleeps. Reduction of weight and intra-abdominal pressure should be encouraged.

Injection of sclerosing solution to thrombose the veins is employed in small varicosities, or in those that remain after adequate surgical treatment. Sodium morrhuate and ethanolamine oleate are the most commonly used sclerosing agents. The injections are painful and irritating to tissue, patients can develop sensitivity to the drugs, and the results are variable. Sclerotherapy is most successful in treating the small, cutaneous varices with a radial pattern known as the *"sunburst"* or *"rocket burst"* type, which are seen in menopausal women and which cannot be directly attacked surgically.

✓ Surgical treatment is the most satisfactory method to manage significant varicosities, especially when valvular incompetence exists. If the saphenofemoral or saphenopopliteal valves are incompetent, these veins must be ligated and divided flush with their entrance into the deep venous system. If none of the valves in the perforating veins is incompetent, simple ligation and division (without excision) is adequate therapy.

✓ However, much more commonly the valves of the perforating veins are also incompetent, and their connections to the superficial veins must therefore be interrupted. Since most patients have a series of incompetent perforators emptying into the main channels of the greater and lesser saphenous veins at different levels, this goal is achieved by excising the entire length of the involved main channels. Main channel excision is most easily accomplished by *vein stripping;* a semimalleable instrument is passed down the length of the involved vein, either externally or generally internally, tying the divided vein at its other end to the instrument and pulling out the entire vein upon removal of the instrument. This avulses the main channel from all the perforators, and the latter then thrombose. Perforators that are *away* from the main channel through which the stripper passes have to be individually exposed, ligated, and segmentally excised. Meticulous preoperative mapping of the varicose veins and the incompetent valves allows complete cure of the varicosities to be carried out at one operative sitting, in most cases.

Postoperatively the legs are wrapped with elastic bandages for 6 weeks, after which simply good habits of general leg care are resumed.

If stasis dermatitis or varicose ulcers are already present, adequate surgical treatment of the guilty veins prevents progression of these manifestations of chronic venous insufficiency, provided that the deep venous system is intact. However, if far advanced, direct surgical treatment may indeed be necessary. Excision of the ulcer and the surrounding leathery skin down to muscle fascia, with epithelization via a split-thickness skin graft, is the most expedient method of surgical treatment. Early surgical treatment of the varicosed veins avoids these complications.

THROMBOPHLEBITIS

The term *thrombophlebitis* implies the formation of a clot within a vein associated with acute signs of inflammation (erythema, pain, and tenderness). The acute inflammatory reaction binds the clot firmly enough to the intima of the vessel so that embolization is unlikely. *Phlebothrombosis* designates the asymptomatic formation of a "bland" clot unassociated with heralding signs or symptoms, the clot being soft and loosely attached to the intima and thereby prone to early embolization. Indeed, pulmonary embolus is often the first indication of phlebothrombosis.

The older literature clearly distinguished between thrombophlebitis and phlebothrombosis. However, the distinction between the two forms is not always clear. They are opposite poles of a continuum, any stage of which is potentially dangerous and requires similar methods of prevention and treatment.

Venous thrombosis is favored by varicosities, stagnation of flow, trauma and infection of the soft tissues and vein walls, and certain states of hypercoagulability of the blood. *Thromboangiitis obliterans, polycythemia vera, collagen vascular disease,* and *occult carcinoma* are associated with a higher than normal incidence of spontaneous venous thrombosis. Patients at bed rest are prime candidates for venous thrombosis, especially postoperatively.

Signs and symptoms. Thrombophlebitis of the superficial veins in the lower extremities is generally marked by localized pain, erythema, and a tender induration of the thrombosed vein. It commonly follows trauma and infection to veins that are varicosed and therefore have stagnant flow patterns. The phlebitis is generally self-limited and responds to conservative measures such as elevation, local heat, and rest of the extremity while it is wrapped with elastic bandages. The thrombosis does not commonly extend to involve the deep venous system, nor is embolization likely. Anticoagulants are indicated if the process does not respond quickly to conservative treatment, and rarely the vein must be ligated above the thrombotic process if extension to the saphenofemoral junction appears imminent.

Thrombosis of the deep venous system of the lower extremities may be heralded only by mild ankle edema and superficial vein dilatation detectable only on careful inspection, to be confirmed later by sudden massive pulmonary embolism with chest pain and hemoptysis. About half of people dying from pulmonary emboli of deep vein lower extremity origin have no antecedent signs of thrombosis.

Clinical evidence of deep leg vein thrombosis includes an aching or discomfort in the posterior calf muscles with tenderness to palpation along the course of the involved vein, which may be anywhere

Synopsis of surgery

from the plantar aspect of the foot to the femoral triangle in the groin. *Homan's sign* should be positive (calf pain generated by dorsiflexion of the foot), and there often is edema and subtle dilatation of the superficial veins. Erythema or gross signs of inflammation are rare. Mild pyrexia and leukocytosis are usually present.

Recently, noninvasive techniques using ultrasound have been perfected that evaluate flow patterns within extremity vessels, both arteries and veins. Thrombi and emboli that impede blood flow can be pinpointed quite accurately, often before clinical signs develop. Doppler ultrasound holds much promise for earlier diagnosis of thrombophlebitis. In turn, early treatment should lower the incidence of pulmonary embolus and the postphlebitic syndrome, the dread sequellae of this disease.

Treatment. Specific treatment of deep vein thrombophlebitis initially is bed rest with elevation of the involved extremity and immediate anticoagulation. Heparin is administered intravenously or subcutaneously in dosages of 10,000 units every 8 hours, with serial determination of coagulation times to measure effectiveness of treatment; subsequent dosages are tailored to the response of the individual patient. Three or four days of this therapy will generally relieve the edema, tenderness, and signs of inflammation. When the patient has been asymptomatic for an additional 2 to 3 days, leg exercises are begun and ambulation resumed while the leg is wrapped with elastic bandages.

Heparin is the most effective anticoagulant agent in treating thrombophlebitis because it rapidly prevents propagation of the clot, probably aids in the lysis of clot already present, and possesses a significant anti-inflammatory effect. Furthermore, the effect of heparin is reversed immediately by administering a specific antidote, *protamine sulfate.* Heparin therapy is generally continued for 10 to 14 days until the patient has resumed normal physical activity and remains symptom-free.

The surgical treatment of deep vein thrombophlebitis is directed toward preventing or treating embolic complications. Ligation of the superficial femoral vein proximal to the thrombotic process is effective provided that this is the only source of emboli, which it commonly is not. Too often, the pelvic and contralateral extremity veins are similarly involved. In this case, ligation or placement of a sievelike strainer in the inferior vena cava (inferior vena cava clipping; see Fig. 10-1) arrests emboli from any of the lower torso and extremity veins and prevents further pulmonary embolization.

Occasionally, nonfatal but massive pulmonary emboli are removed surgically with the aid of heart-lung bypass. More commonly, however, prevention of additional emboli from reaching the lungs along with systemic heparinization allow resolution of major pulmonary emboli. Urokinase is being investigated for its embolytic effect in the non-surgical treatment of pulmonary emboli; it may indeed prove superior to heparin.

Phlegmasia alba dolens

The term *phlegmasia alba dolens* ("milk leg") refers to the extreme manifestation of bland phlebothrombosis of the deep veins of the lower extremity. Acute and massive thrombosis of the entire venous system produces an edematous, blanched, painful, and often pulseless leg. A more serious condition is *phlegmasia cerulea dolens* (Fig. 33-5) in which the clot extends to involve the iliac system, with less arterial spasm; this produces an edematous, painful, and plethoric or cyanotic extremity.

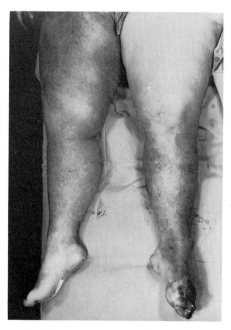

Fig. 33-5. Bilateral phlegmasia cerulea dolens. Note the swelling and mottling of both legs and necrosis of the skin of the left foot.

Pulmonary emboli are uncommon from either of these extreme variations of deep vein thrombosis, because of the intense attachment of the clots to the endothelium of the veins. Treatment early in the course of phlegmasia alba dolens includes surgical extraction of the clot via femoral venotomy. Clot distal to the venotomy is milked up to the venotomy incision via ascending compression of the leg with an Esmarch bandage (rubberized wrap). Extraction of the clot proximal to the venotomy is achieved by suction, or with the help of a catheter. The catheter is introduced cephalad to the clot, a balloon inflated at the tip of the catheter, and the clot and catheter simultaneously removed. The patient is heparinized postoperatively and the leg wrapped with an elastic support to increase the rate and volume of deep vein flow.

If the patient with phlegmasia alba dolens is seen several days after onset, adherence of clot to intima makes physical extraction impossible. Conservative treatment is then necessary, including bed rest, elevation of the wrapped leg, and heparinization to favor gradual resolution of the thrombi and ultimate recanalization.

Postphlebitic syndrome

The postphlebitic syndrome is a late sequela of extensive thrombophlebitis of the deep leg veins. The valves in the deep vein are destroyed or rendered incompetent, and recanalization of the main veins is inadequate. It is actually a state of chronic venous insufficiency with severe stasis dermatitis.

The postphlebitic syndrome is characterized by chronic edema (brawny and nonpitting) associated with hyperpigmentation and poor skin nutrition. The skin is often thin and leathery. Superficial ulceration defies conservative treatment. The superficial veins are dilated, since they serve as collateral networks of venous return; these must be treated surgically with extreme caution lest one worsen the already present venous insufficiency by destroying collateral channels of flow.

The best treatment of the postphlebitic syndrome is its prevention by early and effective management of the original thrombophlebitis process. Lacking this, one is faced with attempts to improve venous drainage conservatively via the measures listed below:

1. Wear elastic bandage or stockings whenever upright. Never stand longer than 30 minutes without elevating the involved extremities at a 45-degree angle; when standing, periodically exercise the calf muscles by standing on tiptoe.
2. Three times a day elevate legs 45 degrees for one-half hour.
3. Elevate foot of bed on blocks 6 to 8 inches so that the legs will be higher than the heart while asleep.

4. Avoid irritation to the skin of the involved leg: trauma, scratches, burns, and infection.

Chronic large skin ulcers must be excised, and "feeding" incompetent perforators in the area are ligated and removed. Skin grafts may then grow if the leg is elevated and immobilized postoperatively.

SPECIFIC LARGE VEIN THROMBOSIS

Acute occlusion or thrombosis of any major vein will produce a syndrome of signs and symptoms specific to the vein, the region drained by it, and the adequacy of collateral venous circulation. Two recognized clinical syndromes are associated with obstruction of the superior vena cava and the axillary (subclavian) vein, respectively.

Acute superior vena caval obstruction occurs with extrinsic compression of the vein by tumor or enlarged lymph nodes or by throm-

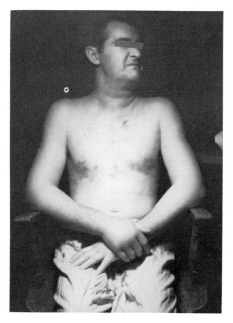

Fig. 33-6. Superior vena caval syndrome—dilated veins on the chest wall, swelling of neck and upper extremities caused by lung cancer obstructing the vena cava.

bosis secondary to direct trauma and infection (Fig. 33-6). Clinically, the *superior vena caval syndrome* consists of a plethora or cyanosis of the skin of the head and neck associated with varying degrees of venous distension and edema of the upper torso and extremities (Fig. 33-6). This is attended by headache, vertigo, tinnitus, epistaxis, and sometimes fainting. Elevated upper extremity venous pressure and delayed arm-to-lung circulation times support the diagnosis; venography confirms the level and length of obstruction. Treatment is directed at the cause of the original obstruction, including surgical resection of the extrinsically compressing tumor or nodes or simply anticoagulation. Rarely the obstruction is bypassed via a vein graft.

Acute axillary (subclavian) vein thrombosis is seen in younger men who strenuously use their upper extremities in sports or occupation, particularly those activities requiring frequent and violent abduction of the arm on the shoulder. Progressive trauma to the vein probably initiates the thrombosis, which then propagates to totally occlude the vessel. Since the venous collaterals are poor at this point, insidious swelling and cyanosis of the upper extremity occur with distension of the superficial veins. Elevated venous pressure, delayed arm-to-lung circulation times, and venography again are useful in diagnosis. Treatment generally is anticoagulation and bed rest with elevation of the affected part, and future avoidance of the activity that provoked the initial thrombosis.

LYMPHEDEMA

The remarkable appearance of lymphedema (excessive lymph in the tissue spaces) caused Caesar's legions to coin the term *elephantiasis* to describe the afflicted lower limbs of their North African opponents, whose lymphatics were obstructed by filariasis.

Primary lymphedema occurs early in life as a result of developmental defects of the lymphatics of a specific site. It may be hereditary or simple (nonhereditary). More frequently the lower limbs and less frequently the upper limbs, the genitals, or facial features are affected. Under the microscope the diseased tissue shows any of three patterns: aplasia, hypoplasia, or dilatation and tortuosity of the lymphatics. Injected vital dyes diffuse randomly through the subcutaneous tissues and are not picked up by the defective lymphatic system. *Congenital (primary) lymphedema* is obvious at birth. (Milroy's disease is congenital lymphedema limited to one or both lower limbs and marked by permanence, steady progress, increasing severity, and absence of constitutional symptoms.) *Lymphedema praecox* has the characteristics of congenital lymphedema except that it becomes obvious only after the patient is 10 to 30 years old (Fig. 33-7). (The rare case of primary lymphedema arising in later years is the *forme tardive*.)

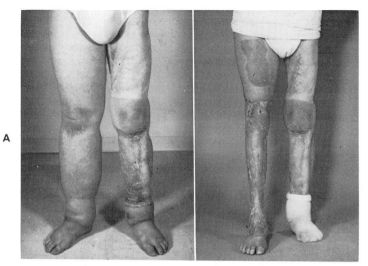

Fig. 33-7. A, Lymphedema precox in a 21-year-old patient; left leg was treated surgically 10 years before; right leg developed recent edema. **B,** Same patient 3 weeks after surgical treatment of right leg.

Secondary lymphedema characteristically occurs later in life and results from obstruction, destruction, or overload of the lymphatics from any of a number of causes, such as (1) repeated lymphangitis or chronic bacterial infections, (2) neoplastic invasion of lymphatics, (3) circulatory changes occurring after thrombophlebitis (postphlebitic syndrome), (4) filariasis (Fig. 33-8), (5) extensive fibrosis and scarring from radiation, burns, or other trauma, and (6) repeated allergic reactions. Lymphedema of the lower limbs beginning after the age of 40 should raise suspicions of intrapelvic carcinoma in women, or carcinoma of the prostate in men, or lymphoma. Lymphedema of the upper limb after radical mastectomy may signal the presence of lymphatic metastases of breast carcinoma, but more frequently it results merely from fibrosis, thrombosis, and localized infections in the postoperative period. A rare malignancy, *lymphangiosarcoma,* appears in a chronically lymphedematous arm (Stewart-Treves syndrome) or leg decades after the onset of the lymphedema.

Treatment. Search out and eliminate the cause if possible. History, genealogy, physical examination, cultures, venograms, and lymphangiograms are helpful. Elimination of infections or parasitic infestations, removal of varicose veins, or excision of neoplasms may be required.

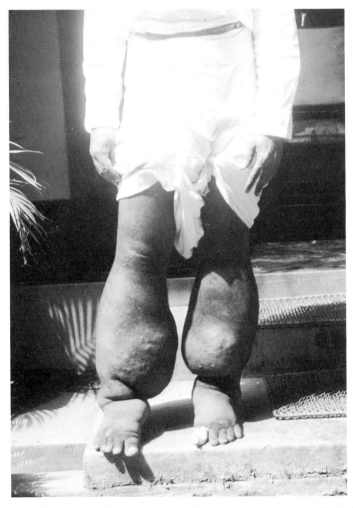

Fig. 33-8. Patient with lower extremity edema secondary to filariasis.

Long-term prophylactic antibiotic treatment is sometimes necessary to prevent repeated episodes of lymphangitis. Well-fitted elastic supportive stockings or garments, intermittent pressure devices, elevation of the affected part, massage, exercises, and protection of areas of vulnerable skin from injury are helpful.

Lymphedema uncontrolled by these measures may be relieved by direct surgical attack (Fig. 33-7, *B*). The defective lymphatics and therefore the lymphedema are chiefly limited to the tissues lying between the superficial one-fiftieth of an inch of skin (epidermis has no lymphatics, uppermost dermis has very few) and the lymphatics superficial to the deep fascia.

In severe, long-standing cases the afflicted skin, often including the investing fascia, is completely excised and split skin grafts are placed directly on the investing fascia or muscles. The grafts may be cut from the excised specimen or from unaffected areas.

A currently popular surgical approach is to supply an escape route for the trapped lymph with a pedicle. One pedicle consists of skin and subcutaneous tissue from the affected leg, which is denuded of its epidermis. The denuded skin is passed through a long incision in the deep fascia and is attached intimately to the underlying muscles, which always have normal lymphatics. The lymph exits from the skin across this bridge to the muscle (Noel Thompson procedure). A novel pedicle consists of omentum tunneled subcutaneously from the abdominal cavity to the limb; lymph is returned from the limb to the abdominal cavity.

CHAPTER 34

Plastic and reconstructive surgery

DAVID W. FURNAS

PLASTIC SURGERY

The word *plastic* stems from the Greek word *plassein,* which means "to form." *Plastic operation* refers to a procedure that "forms" by means of *shifting or transplanting tissues.* Every surgical specialty utilizes plastic operations: the neurosurgeon performs cranioplasties, the thoracic surgeon performs thoracoplasties, the orthopedist performs arthroplasties, etc.

The branch of general surgery that is the specialty of *"plastic surgery"* deals particularly with the facial features (Fig. 34-1), the jaws and oral cavity, the hand, and the body surface in general, including the breasts and the external genitals. The plastic surgeon attempts to *restore a patient to his original state* after injuries, after removal of tumors, or after changes from aging; he attempts to *improve upon the patient's original state* when there are congenital defects, or body features that are thought to fall too short of ideal. The four *C*'s of plastic surgery are Congenital deformities, Calamities, Cancer, and Cosmesis. *Wound care, free grafts,* and *pedicles* are the foundation of the plastic surgeon's art and are fundamental to the craft of surgery in general.

Free grafts

A *free* graft is a piece of living tissue that is detached from one site and transplanted to another site where it survives as living tissue. It is termed an *autograft* (self), *isograft* (identical twin), *homograft* (same species), or *heterograft* (different species), depending on the relationship of the donor to the recipient.

Mechanisms of graft survival or "take"

Skin graft. A skin graft appears white when first placed on a raw defect. It is nourished entirely by the host tissue fluids that bathe its deep surface *(plasmatic circulation).* After a few hours it becomes quite adherent, cemented in place by the formation of a fibrin coagulum. In less than a day the white graft becomes pink by *inosculation* or linking up of the graft capillaries with host capillaries. After 1 to 2 days the graft is *penetrated* by new capillary buds that grow out from the host. As these develop, the graft's original vessels degenerate. The new vessels assume the entire circulatory load and the graft "takes" firmly. Final healing occurs by the same processes seen in other wounds.

Other free grafts. The "take" of grafts of other tissues (dermis, tendon, bone, fascia) is in some ways similar to that of skin; how-

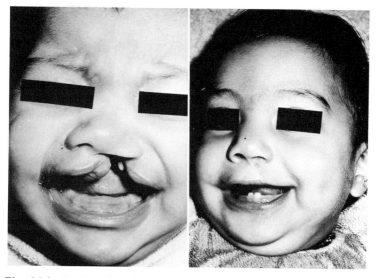

Fig. 34-1. A, Cleft lip. *Left,* Unilateral cleft lip in infant. *Right,* Lip closure several months postoperatively (the scar mimics the left column of the philtrum and will be scarcely noticeable in several years).

Continued.

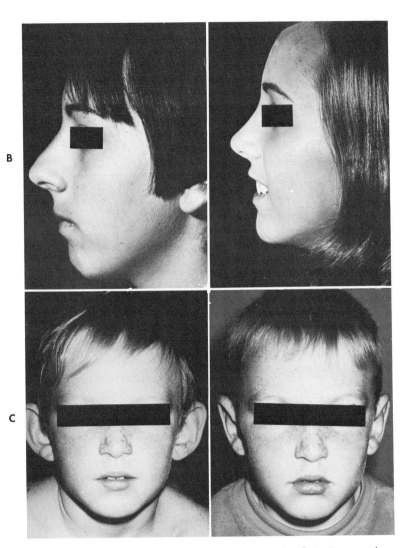

Fig. 34-1, cont'd. B, Nasal hump and receding chin. *Left,* Preoperative. *Right,* Postoperative rhinoplasty and mentoplasty using cartilage and bone from the nasal hump and septum. **C,** Prominent ears. *Left,* Preoperative. *Right,* Postoperative otolasty.

ever, the process is much slower in bone, and fewer of the bone graft's cells remain alive; in cartilage a type of plasmatic circulation is the final form of nutrition. Free muscle grafts will survive: (1) if transplanted as a whole muscle; (2) if denervated 2 weeks before transplant; and (3) if placed in contact with a functioning muscle. Microsurgical techniques have spawned the vascularized free graft. Aided by a microscope, the surgeon performs tiny vessel anastomoses that establish immediate blood flow to the graft. Large blocks of skin from the trunk can be transplanted to the lower limbs or the scalp this way, and toes can be transplanted to replace fingers.

Failure of "take"

The three chief causes of failure of a skin graft to "take" are (1) *bleeding* beneath the graft (Fig. 34-2), (2) *infection,* or (3) *movement* of the graft. If a hematoma forms, the graft is lifted from its bed and dies. *Beta hemolytic streptococci* form exotoxins that lyse the skin graft from its bed and destroy it. *Pseudomonas, Proteus,* and *Staphylococcus aureus* form pus that lifts the graft from the recipient bed. Excessive movement of the graft shears the capillary connections between the graft and host, and the graft dies. Therefore, meticulous

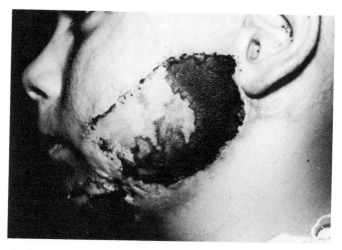

Fig. 34-2. Necrosis of skin graft from hematoma. Bleeding beneath this graft resulted after severe postoperative vomiting. The dark portion of the graft is dead and must be replaced with another skin graft.

Table 34-1. Commonly used free skin grafts

Type	Common donor site	Uses	Comment
Split skin graft (thin, medium, or thick)	Thighs, abdomen, buttocks, back, and elsewhere	To close defects of integument almost anywhere on body	Donor sites epithelialize
Full-thickness skin graft (Wolfe or whole skin graft)	Retroauricular area, supraclavicular area, antecubital fossa	To close skin defects of limited size, particularly on face	Superior appearance and function; donor sites must be closed surgically
Dermis graft (whole graft with a thin graft removed from surface)	Abdomen or elsewhere	To fill out defects in contour or to bolster fascial defects	Buried beneath the skin surface
Dermafat graft (dermis graft with fat attached)	Abdomen, buttocks, or elsewhere	To fill out larger defects in contour	Loses $\frac{1}{4}$ to $\frac{1}{2}$ of bulk after implantation
Hair follicle–bearing skin grafts	Scalp, eyebrow	To repair scalp, eyebrow, or lashes	Usually applied in small patches or strips
Composite skin grafts (whole skin + cartilage; skin + fibrofat or bone)	Helix, anthelix, lobe of external ear / Fingertip (accident)	To repair defects of nose, ear, eyelid / To replace finger part	Only small grafts will survive / Works best for children

Other composite grafts finding occasional use are *nipple-areolar grafts* and *nailbed-nail grafts*

Table 34-2. Commonly used autografts of tissues other than skin

Tissue	Common donor site	Uses	Comment
Fat + dermis	Buttock, abdomen	To fill out defects in contour	Easily reabsorbed; dermafat grafts are much better
Fascia	Fascia lata of thigh and elsewhere	To repair fascia, dura, or tendons; to lash or support other structures	May be used in sheets or strips
Tendon	Palmaris longus, plantaris, extensors of toes	To replace or elongate tendons; to bind other structures	Congenital absence of palmaris longus or plantaris is not infrequent
Bone	Ilium, ribs (especially in children), and sites on long bones	To replace missing bone and correct nonunion of fractures and skeletal contour defects	New ribs regenerate from donor defects in children if periosteum is left
Cartilage	Costal cartilage, nasal septum	To replace missing cartilage or bone; to correct contour defects	Tends to warp if not cut with a symmetrical section
Vessels	Greater saphenous vein	To replace absent or occluded arteries; to patch arterial incisions	Valves must be placed in correct direction
Nerves	Sural, saphenous, greater auricular nerves	To replace absent or damaged nerve segments	The more peripheral the site of injury, the better the results

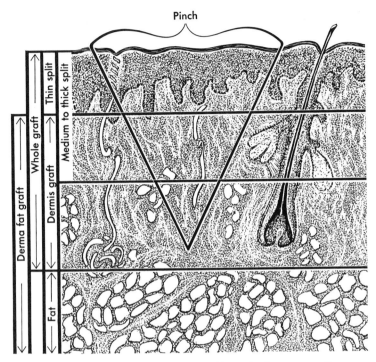

Fig. 34-3. Types of grafts taken from skin and subcutaneous tissue.

hemostasis, aseptic technique, and adequate immobilization of the graft are important for success.

Clinical use of autologous grafts

The factotum among skin grafts is the *split skin graft* (Tables 34-1 and 34-2 and Fig. 34-3). It can furnish viable cover for fresh wounds, granulating wounds, mucosal defects (mouth, vagina, nose), fascia, paratenon, periosteum, even exposed lung, brain, or pericardium. Split skin grafts do poorly if the vascularity of the recipient bed is poor, as in heavily scarred or radiated wounds, or on bare bone, bare cartilage, or bare tendon. Large split skin grafts are cut with special knives or *dermatomes,* small ones with ordinary scalpels. The donor sites heal by *epithelization* in 1 to 4 weeks, depending on the thickness of the graft.

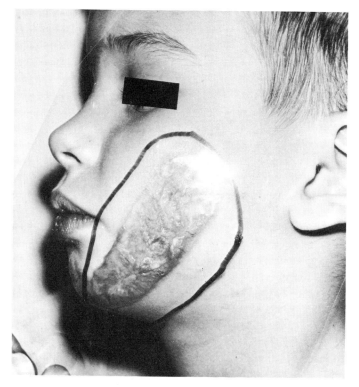

Fig. 34-4. Contraction of thin skin graft. The dark circle represents the original granulating wound that resulted from a full thickness burn. The very thin skin graft was the same size as this inked pattern, but over a period of 3 months it has contracted to half the original size. The graft was later excised and replaced by an advancement flap.

Thin split grafts are more likely to "take" in unfavorable circumstances, but they tend to contract and develop inferior appearance and durability (Fig. 34-4).

Thick split grafts are more likely to perish from excessive movement or from bacterial activity than are thinner grafts, but upon surviving they furnish a more durable surface (Fig. 34-5).

Full thickness grafts furnish a better quality coverage, but "take" is less reliable; the size of the graft is limited by the need to suture or graft (with split thickness skin) the donor site (Fig. 34-6).

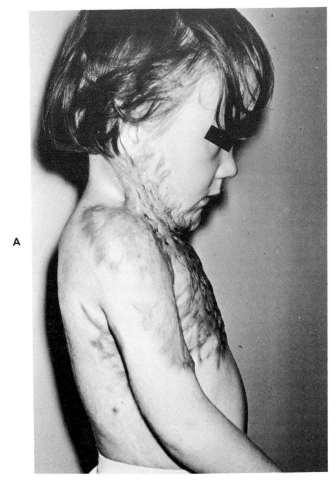

A

Fig. 34-5. Medium thickness split skin graft. **A,** Flaming nightie caused burn scars that have contracted the mandible tightly against the sternum.

Split skin grafts may be cut in sheets, in strips, or in "postage stamps" (small squares). Sheet grafts furnish a superior surface; the smaller grafts are used to expand the area of coverage when donor sites are limited or to improve survival in the presence of infection, movement, or irregular contours.

Composite graft is skin plus other attached tissue. Only small blocks of composite tissue will survive (Fig. 34-7).

Replantation of traumatically amputated limbs, the most complex clinical autograft in current surgical practice, has been performed several times with success, a result of preparedness and teamwork. These grafts, of course, depend on blood flow through major vascular anastomoses for their survival.

Pedicles

Pedicle, flap, pedicled graft, and pedicled flap are synonyms for tissue (usually skin with attached subcutaneous tissue) that is trans-

Text continued on p. 622.

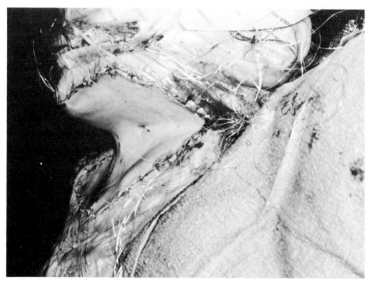

Fig. 34-5, cont'd. B, Raw surface is covered with a single sheet of medium thickness split skin taken from the abdomen.

Continued.

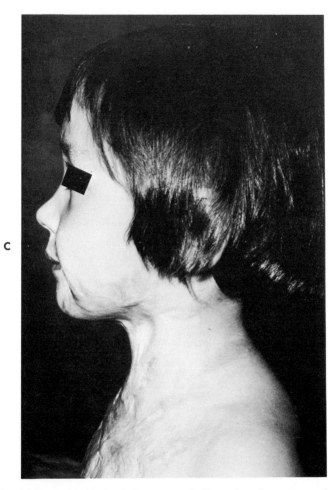

C

Fig. 34-5, cont'd. C, Graft has matured. Even though texture and color are not an exact match, the neck-chin angle has been restored and the potential for deformity of skeletal growth has been greatly reduced.

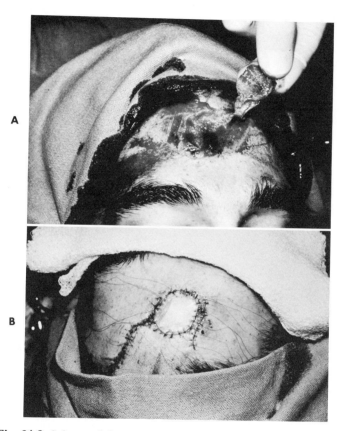

Fig. 34-6. Salvage of doomed flap by conversion into a graft. **A,** Windshield injury to forehead has elevated a flap of skin. The pedicle attachment is too narrow for survival, and the flap is rapidly becoming congested as blood flows in but fails to flow out. **B,** The flap is detached, trimmed, and replaced as a full thickness skin graft.

Continued.

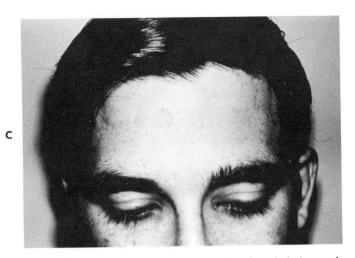

C

Fig. 34-6, cont'd. C, When mature, the replaced graft is inconspicuous and gives a perfect color match.

ferred to a different site *without being entirely detached from its blood supply.* A pedicle is at all times nourished by blood circulating through its own capillaries via a bridge of intact tissue, the *base* of the pedicle. In contrast, a free graft is completely detached from the body and is nourished by suffusion of host tissue fluids. Sometimes the transfer of a pedicle from one site to another leaves a raw defect that must be covered with a free skin graft. Although free grafts are of modern origin (nineteenth century), pedicles have been performed with success since before the time of Christ.

Use of pedicles

Pedicles commonly surpass free grafts as the best procedure in the following instances: (1) where the defect to be treated is *poorly vascularized* (e.g., heavy scar, radiation changes); (2) where *bare tendons, bare cartilage,* or *bare cortical bone* is exposed; (3) where *padding* is needed over the defect (e.g., pressure sores); (4) where *bulk* is required (e.g., replacement of a missing nose, filling out a sunken wound); (5) *where exact match of color, texture, and resilience* is desired (e.g., correction of a cheek defect with a pedicle from neighboring cheek and neck tissue); (6) where a *double facing is*

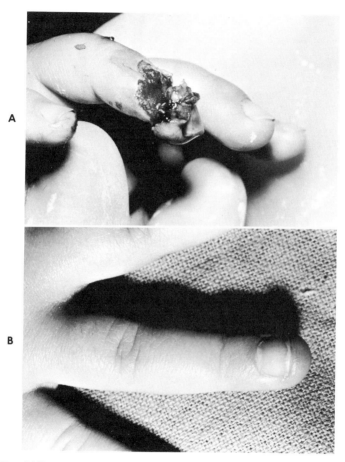

Fig. 34-7. Composite graft. **A,** Tip of ring finger of 3-year-old child was avulsed when caught in car door. It is held in place by tiny dermo-epidermal remnant, but no active circulation is present and thus no congestion occurs. Fingertip was immediately sutured back into place with meticulous care. **B,** Survival of graft is complete. Results of this procedure are generally better in children than in adults.

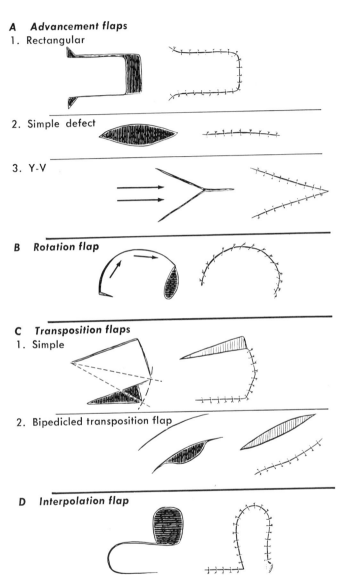

Fig. 34-8. For legend see opposite page.

required (e.g., replacement of full-thickness defect of the cheek or mouth); (7) or where there is likelihood that the new surface will have to be temporarily elevated at a future time to permit further reconstructive surgery (e.g., in anticipation of secondary tendon grafts, tendon transfers, bone grafts, or nerve repairs).

Types of pedicles

Local pedicles. The defect is repaired by the shifting of adjacent tissue by *advancement* (moving tissue margin directly forward into the defect), *rotation* (moving tissue laterally into the defect), *transposition,* or *interpolation* (Figs. 34-8 and 34-10). The original blood-bearing base is usually permanent, and the reconstruction is performed in one stage.

Distant pedicles. Distant pedicles, obtained remote from the defect, may be *direct* as in the case of the repair of a foot defect with a cross-thigh pedicle (Fig. 34-9). They may be *migrated* in stages, as in the case of a facial defect repaired by an abdominal *tube pedicle* by means of a *forearm carrier* (Fig. 34-11). Distant pedicles are always performed in stages to allow growth of a blood supply that will support the pedicle after detachment from the donor site.

"Delay" or vascular reinforcement. "Delay" or vascular reinforcement is a type of preliminary stage in which only part of the required incisions are made initially. The incisions are then completed at one or more later stages. This gives time in the interim for vascular reinforcement to develop: the vessels supplying the pedicle dilate and align their flow in the most favorable direction; also the tissue itself probably develops tolerance to lower blood flow.

Complications of pedicle surgery

Pedicle procedures are subject to the same problems as any other wound (e.g., hematoma, infection, etc.), plus special problems that

---

Fig. 34-8. Types of local pedicles. **A,** *Advancement flap:* (1) stretched directly forward into defect aided by excision of Burow's triangles; (2) advancement of edges of simple defect; (3) **Y-V** advancement flap. **B,** *Rotation flap:* stretched in arc toward defect; donor site closed without skin graft if flap is four to five times bigger than defect; if ratio is smaller, split-skin graft may be required for defect. **C,** *Transposition flap:* (1) moved laterally into adjacent defect; split-skin graft may be required for donor site; (2) bipedicled transposition flap. **D,** *Interpolation flap:* moved over intervening tissue to reach defect, donor site closed with a secondary flap or split-skin graft.

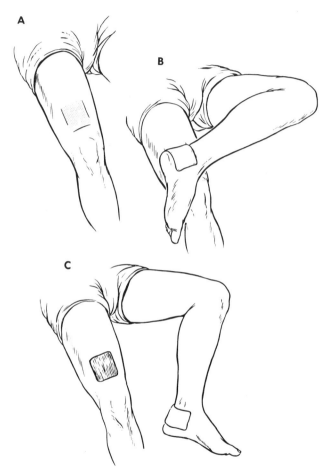

Fig. 34-9. Direct distant flap (cross thigh flap to foot). **A,** Thigh flap, "delayed" by partial incision and undermining. **B,** Incisions completed 3 weeks later, flap elevated and inserted into defect of opposite foot; exposed raw surfaces covered with split-skin grafts. **C,** Flap detached from thigh 3 weeks later, after sufficient blood supply has grown across suture line to support flap.

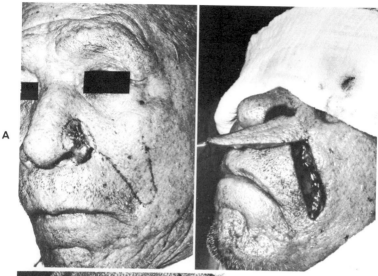

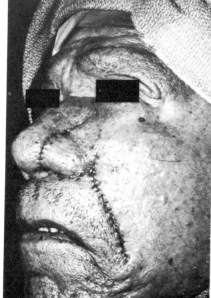

Fig. 34-10. Interpolation flap. **A**, Pigmented basal cell carcinoma of left nasal ala. Excision line and labial interpolation flap have been plotted with ink. **B**, Tumor has been excised. Frozen sections show that margins of specimen are free of tumor, and the flap has been incised, undermined, and moved to nasal defect. **C**, Flap has been trimmed and doubled over to furnish interior lining for the defect. Defect and donor site are closed.

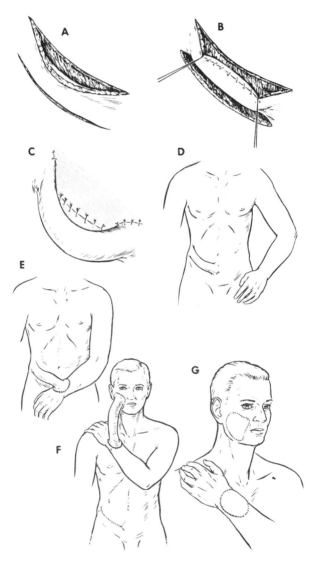

Fig. 34-11. For legend see opposite page.

can threaten the precarious circulation. If a pedicle is too narrow, if it is detached too early, or if the blood flow is obstructed by external pressure (the patient's own weight, tight dressings, heavy bedding), or if it is kinked or twisted, the pedicle may die. If the newly incised free end of a pedicle is placed at a lower level than the base of the pedicle, the pedicle may become congested *(gravitational congestion)* and die from circulatory stasis.

Special pedicles

An axial flap includes a specific artery and vein in its substance, such as the superficial circumflex iliac vessels, or superficial epigastric vessels. These flaps can be made longer and narrower than ordinary *random* flaps.

A *bipedicled* flap consists of two parallel incisions that are connected by undermining; it has two bases. If the two parallel incisions are sutured in apposition, a *tube pedicle* is formed (Fig. 34-11). Either is useful as a "delay," and the tube is convenient for migration.

A *lined* pedicle is surfaced on its raw side with a skin or mucosal graft. Folding a pedicle raw surface to raw surface creates a *double-faced pedicle*. Either furnishes a double surface for reconstruction of full-thickness defects of the mouth, lips, nose, or eyelids.

A complete segment of lower lip can be transferred to the upper lip (or vice versa) via a *lip-switch pedicle*, which is supported by the labial artery.

To form an *island flap*, a complete island of skin is excised and elevated, but its subcutaneous connections with blood vessels are maintained. The artery is dissected free, and the island is burrowed subcutaneously to reach the recipient site with its arterial umbilicus trailing after. An eyebrow may be replaced with a temporal scalp island supported by the superficial temporal artery; or a thumb may be given an area of normal sensation with an island of skin from the

---

Fig. 34-11. Migrated distant flap. Abdominal tube to face via forearm carrier. **A,** Parallel incisions and undermining create a "bipedicled flap." **B,** Incisions are apposed and sutured to form a tube pedicle. **C,** Donor site is closed directly with sutures or with skin graft. **D** and **E,** Lower end of pedicle is detached from abdomen and inserted on forearm 2 to 3 weeks later. **F,** Abdominal end of pedicle is detached after additional 2 to 3 weeks and migrated to facial defect using forearm as carrier. **G,** Flap detached from forearm 2 to 3 weeks later and sutured into facial defect; excess tissue discarded.

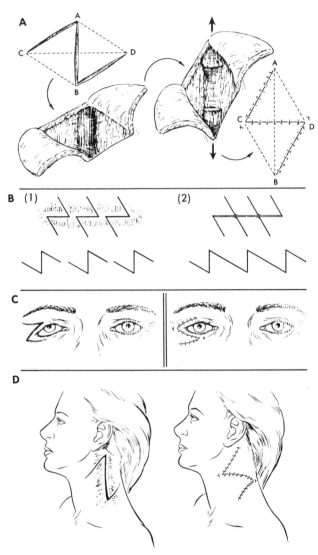

Fig. 34-12. For legend see opposite page.

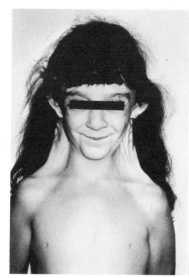
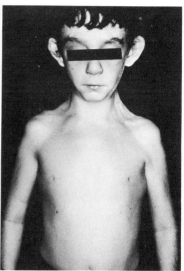

A

B

Fig. 34-13. z-plasty for webbed neck. **A,** Patient with neck webs of Turner's syndrome. **B,** Postoperative obliteration of webs after single z-plasty to each side of neck.

Fig. 34-12. Four functions of z-plasties. **A,** Interpolation of two triangular flaps increases length along path **AB** at the expense of width along path **CD.** (In effect, dimensions are exchanged between **AB** and **CD.**) **B,** Interpolation of series of disconnected (1) or connected (2) series of z's breaks up a straight line (and also gives it increased length). **C,** Shift of topographic landmark. Correction of contracted lateral canthus effected by z-plasty; corner of mouth, eyebrow, or nasal ala may be similarly managed. **D,** Obliteration of a web z-plasty shifts the two planes of a web so that they form the planes of the depression at the base of the neck.

ring finger supported by a digital neurovascular bundle *("sensory island flap")*.

Crossed leg, crossed thigh, crossed finger, and *crossed arm flaps* are direct distant pedicles from one body member to another.

Compound pedicles carry other tissues in addition to skin and fat. A new thumb can be formed from a compound clavicular tube pedicle that carries within it a portion of the clavicle.

Z-plasty

The Z-plasty is a useful surgical technique that may perform any of four basic functions: (1) *increase length along a specific path* (Fig. 34-12, *A*), (2) *break up and reorient a straight line scar* (Fig. 34-12, *B*), (3) *shift topographical landmarks* (Fig. 34-12, *C*), and (4) *deepen webs or obliterate clefts* (Fig. 34-12, *D*).

The Z-plasty is performed by elevating two triangular flaps in the form of a Z and *interpolating* them so that the final figure is a reversed Z. The incisions should be of approximately equal lengths. The angles may be unequal, but the most common form of a Z-plasty has two 60-degree angles. Z-plasties may be single or serial (Fig. 34-13).

CHAPTER 35

Care of the acutely injured patient

CHARLES A. BUERK
RICHARD D. LIECHTY

The most important environmental health problem this nation faces is accidental injuries. Deaths by accident lead all causes of death in the first half of man's life span. In 1973, accidental injuries in the United States killed 117,000 people and disabled 14,028,000 others. The overall cost (including: medical, property loss, insurance claims, working hours lost, etc.) came to a staggering, estimated total of $41.5 billion. Even though the general public accepts this problem almost casually, the medical profession cannot, because accident victims occupy one of every eight beds in a typical general hospital.

This chapter introduces the student to the acutely injured patient and the early, life-saving procedures in the emergency room. Other chapters continue on through the later, specialized care of these patients.

THE EMERGENCY ROOM

Every modern hospital provides accident rooms equipped to receive and treat the injured. Readily accessible to ambulance and automobile, some emergency services feature heliports as well. Probably more important, special centers train paramedics who travel to the accident site and start immediate treatment. A statewide program in Illinois has reaffirmed the worth of these ultramodern, regional emergency centers that initiate treatment on the spot.

Emergency room physicians must become expert at triage—*sorting first things first*. They rapidly scan patients for life-threatening conditions: (1) airway and respiration, (2) heart and circulation, (3) active bleeding, (4) state of consciousness, and (5) obvious threatening injuries (i.e., sucking chest wound, flail chest, sharp bone fragments near major vessels). They know the conditions that threaten life, and they attack these problems rapidly and systematically, the most urgent ones first.

Airway and respiration

The physician can tell at a glance if a patient is breathing adequately. Cyanosis with gasping chest movements means airway obstruction. Knowing that the most common cause in comatose patients is a "swallowed" tongue, the physician should force the jaws open, retrieve the tongue with a finger, and insert an airway for immediate suctioning. If these procedures fail to relieve the obstructed breathing, tracheal intubation (orally or via tracheostomy) will bypass an obstructed larynx and assure an open upper airway. Continuing cyanosis indicates lower respiratory problems; *pneumothorax*, usually resulting from fractured ribs, heads the list. Any fractured rib can puncture a lung, often without gross chest wall deformity. Characterized by a tympanitic hemothorax, absent breath sounds, tracheal displacement (to the opposite side), and subcutaneous emphysema, pneumothorax can become *tension pneumothorax* from a flutter valve defect in the puncture site that forces air into the intrapleural space with each inspiration. As the air builds up, it compresses the opposite lung, sometimes fatally. Aspiration of the entrapped air, by needle or thoracotomy tube, reverses this process.

Crushing chest trauma that fractures several ribs at multiple sites results in *flail chest*. The shattered chest wall, lacking normal rigidity, moves paradoxically (in with inspiration and out with expiration). Although external bracing helps somewhat, tracheostomy and mechanical ventilation continued until the chest wall solidifies (10 to 20 days) have proved most effective. Simple tamponade with an occlusive dressing temporarily repairs open "sucking" wounds of the chest wall.

Acute gastric dilatation (from ileus and swallowed air) may impede diaphragmatic movement and thus hinder ventilation. Nasogastric suction provides instant relief and also helps prevent vomiting and aspiration pneumonitis. Removing gastric juice also decreases stress ulceration.

Circulation

Once assured that the patient has an adequate airway, the physician checks circulation. He should tamponade any serious bleeding site at once, insert a large intravenous catheter, and start crystalloid solutions (after removing a blood sample for typing and matching blood).

Many patients in shock respond to this treatment alone, but if shock (cold clammy skin, weak rapid pulse) persists despite adequate fluid and blood replacement, one of the following causes is likely: cardiac tamponade, tension pneumothorax, internal bleeding (chest, abdomen, or fracture sites), bowel rupture, aortic tear, or, rarely, adrenal failure. At this point, a central venous catheter immensely aids further evaluation.

Cardiac tamponade

In patients with chest trauma, distant, muted heart sounds, low pulse pressure, and a high central venous pressure (CVP) (and often a paradoxic pulse) indicate cardiac tamponade. Echocardiography, if available, can rapidly confirm these clinical signs. Needle aspiration of the pericardial blood, repeated if necessary, will reestablish normal heart action. (See Chapter 31.)

Hemothorax

Because of two factors (collapsible lung tissue and low pulmonary blood pressure), bleeding from lung parenchyma rarely persists. Continued intrapleural bleeding usually comes from severed intercostal or internal mammary vessels. Needle aspiration or insertion of a thoracotomy tube (with suction) removes the blood and allows the lung to expand. Tube drainage provides a constant monitor to assess continued bleeding. (See Chapter 30.)

Hemoperitoneum

The neophyte physician can easily be misled by the relatively normal appearing abdomen that contains 2,000 ml. of blood or more. Thus he should always suspect the abdomen as a likely source of continuing bleeding and persistent shock. Although four-quadrant, intraperitoneal aspiration with an 18-gauge needle serves as a rapid indicator of bleeding, a negative tap means nothing. Peritoneal lavage yields more reliable results. We instill 500 to 1,000 ml. of lactated Ringer's solution through a peritoneal dialysis catheter that enters the abdomen through a tiny skin incision in the lower midline. The bottle, placed on the floor, siphons the fluid from the abdomen. A pink tinge indicates bleeding; bacteria, fecal material, or amylase indicates visceral perforation. Any one of these indicators signals the need for laparotomy. (See Chapter 25.)

Aortic tears

Severe chest trauma may shear the aortic arch, causing dissection along the wall. A widening mediastinum on roentgenography justifies emergency arteriography. (See Chapter 30.)

Adrenal failure

Long-term steroid therapy suppresses normal adrenal response to stress. The physician should suspect adrenal failure in patients who give a history of steroid intake or in comatose patients with stigmata of arthritis, asthma, or chronic dermatoses.

Coma

Head trauma rarely causes shock. In fact, a patient whose skull and brain sustain the shattering impact necessary to produce hemorrhagic shock seldom reaches the emergency room alive. But shock itself produces coma by depriving brain cells of oxygen. Thus our initial efforts to restore airway and circulation aim most urgently at getting more oxygen to brain cells because cerebral cells, unlike other tissues, die rapidly (within minutes) from oxygen lack. These efforts alone often restore consciousness as the brain receives its vital oxygen.

Brain cells suffer hypoxemia from a second major cause after trauma—edema or hemorrhage within the skull depresses local cerebral circulation. Although slowing pulse and respiration, fever, and dilated pupils indicate increased intracranial pressure, the *level of consciousness* remains the most reliable sign. The physician must record his early neurological findings, especially noting state of consciousness, and immediately call for neurosurgical consultation (see Chapter 40). He should also note other possible causes of coma (alcohol, drugs, diabetes, epilepsy).

Other injuries

After he has stabilized the patient's cardiorespiratory function, the physician should systematically review other areas. He should question the patient or those who accompany him for pertinent information concerning the accident and the patient's health (diabetes, cardiac status, renal status, etc.) while surveying the patient for pulses, bony abnormalities, hematuria (after catheterization), and other defects.

The conscious patient can move his digits and respond to pain stimuli from the extremities, but the unconscious patient withdraws from these stimuli. These responses indicate an intact spinal cord. To lessen the chance of vertebral fractures or dislocations injuring the spinal cord, the patient must be moved cautiously and only when necessary.

Treatment priorities

One person, usually a general surgeon or traumatologist, must take charge, coordinate his consultants, and assign immediate priorities throughout this critical period. He arranges priorities as follows: (1) restore cardiorespiratory function (stop bleeding, visible and hidden), (2) repair hollow viscera injuries (intestine, bladder), (3) repair vascular injuries, (4) treat head and spinal injuries, (5) repair open fractures, and (6) treat lacerations and closed fractures. For example, a patient sustains a skull fracture, femoral fracture, colon rupture, lacerations, and shock. The admitting surgeon treats the shock, stops external bleeding by pressure or ligation, and places a simple splint on the fractured femur. As soon as the patient's vital signs stabilize, the surgeon repairs the colonic tear in the operating room and thus interrupts lethal peritonitis at an early, curable stage. Other surgeons meanwhile clean and close the patient's lacerations. Skull films, taken en route to the operating room, show no displaced bone fragments, and echoencephalography reveals no midline shift; thus craniotomy can be deferred. Although the patient is unconscious before and during the operation, his coma does not interdict the life-saving laparotomy.

The team captain must oversee the total care of acutely injured patients. He uses consultants for specialized problems and coordinates their diagnostic and treatment recommendations. Studies have proved that acutely injured patients treated in efficient emergency centers have the best chance of surviving.

SUMMARY

All emergency room personnel must keep clearly in mind the following steps for the care of acutely injured patients:
1. Assure airway and respiratory exchange
2. Assure circulation
   a. Stop bleeding
   b. Treat shock
   c. Prepare to treat cardiac arrest at any moment
3. Determine need for operative control of internal bleeding or bowel rupture
4. Determine need to restore peripheral circulation
5. Determine need for operative decompression of spinal cord or brain
6. Treat open fractures first, then repair lacerations, then treat closed fractures

Because severe injury disrupts many vital functions, critically ill patients require a variety of conduits that connect them to outside supports. Life-sustaining substances flow in through some tubes; displaced bodily fluids (or gases) drain out through others. Some catheters serve mainly as monitors to help us alter, as necessary, this artificial flux. As a rapid reminder of these life-saving priorities, the student should picture a patient with five tubes in place, each serving a necessary function.

Tube	*Reason*
Oral airway or endotracheal tube	Assure adequate ventilation
Intravenous catheter	Restore fluids; treat shock
Central venous catheter	Monitor fluid load, hemopericardium, heart failure
Urinary catheter	Monitor renal perfusion; detect blood from urinary tract
Nasogastric tube	Prevent vomiting and aspiration pneumonia; prevent stress ulcers

Other tubes sometimes indicated

Arterial catheter	Blood gas analyses
Thoracotomy tube	Treat pneumothorax and/or hemothorax

CHAPTER 36

Transplantation

ISRAEL PENN

In 1948, Boston surgeons first successfully transplanted a living human organ, the kidney. Fifteen years later another group of surgeons, at the University of Colorado, pioneered the first unpaired organ transplantation when they replaced a human liver. Five years later, in 1967, a South African surgeon stunned the world by transplanting another unpaired organ—the human heart. Replacement of unpaired organs has added an agonizing new ethical dimension to the many technical problems that face transplanters because the organs must be obtained from cadaver donors.

Since the first primitive efforts of skin grafting, perhaps two thousand years ago, researchers have learned much about immunological responses, delicate vascular anastomoses, and graft rejection. But despite these advances and the encouraging emergence of patients living successfully for years with grafted organs, man's dreams of organ banks and "instant parts" still appear remote.

NOMENCLATURE

The term *autograft* means removal and replacement of an organ or tissue in the same individual, an *isograft* is placement in a geneti-

From the Department of Surgery, University of Colorado School of Medicine, and the Veterans Administration Hospital, Denver, Colorado. This work was supported by research grants from the Veterans Administration, by grants RR-00051 and RR-00069 from the General Clinical Research Centers Program of the Division of Research Resources, National Institutes of Health, and by grants AI-10176-01, AI-AM-08898, AM-07772, and HE-09110 of the United States Public Health Service.

cally identical person, a *homograft* or *allograft* refers to the transfer of an organ to another of the same species, and a *heterograft* or a *xenograft* involves grafting between different species.

An autograft is identified as "self." It never elicits a defensive host reaction and survives indefinitely.

Isografts (transplants between identical twins) are similar to autografts; they remain unrecognized as foreign and have the same life expectancy as the host. Homografts and heterografts are recognized as foreign or "nonself" and are destroyed by an immunological reaction known as *rejection*. The intensity of this response varies with the degree of genetic disparity between donor and recipient. Grafts reject in two phases: first, sensitization of the host; and second, destruction of the graft by sensitized lymphoid cells and humoral antibodies. The first phase begins with the recognition and processing of the foreign antigens by the host, who reacts only against those antigens that he lacks.

TRANSPLANTATION ANTIGENS

Transplantation antigens present mainly on the cell surface, exist in virtually all kinds of cells, though with considerable quantitative differences among the various cell types. The transplantation antigens are produced by *histocompatibility genes* whose positions on the chromosomes are known as *histocompatibility loci*. A series of alternative genes, or alleles, may occur at each locus. The total number of histocompatibility loci varies in different species; rodents, for example, have at least fifteen. The antigens produced by different loci vary in potency. Major and minor loci, with corresponding strong and weak antigens, determine the severity of the rejection. In many species one major locus apparently dominates all others. This locus is known as H-2 in the mouse, AgB in the rat, DLA in the dog, SLA in the pig, B in the chicken, and HL-A in man. (The ABO blood group antigens are also potent transplantation antigens in man.) The antigens at these loci provoke intense rejection reactions.

MEDIATORS OF THE IMMUNE RESPONSE

The immune response has a cellular and a humoral component. In the former, sensitized host lymphoid cells come into direct contact with the foreign organ and destroy it through the release of cytotoxic factors. In the humoral component, stimulated lymphoid cells, mostly plasma cells, produce and release antibodies into the circulating blood and thence the foreign organ. The cells responsible for homograft destruction, whether through cell-mediated immunity or through humoral antibodies, are all ultimately derived from bone marrow stem cells. The thymus gland controls these cytotoxic or *T cells*. Thus neonatal thymectomy greatly depresses cell-mediated reactions but leaves intact humoral antibody formation, at least to certain antigens. In birds a localized structure associated with the hindgut, the bursa of Fabricius, produces humoral antibodies. No such structure exists in mammals, but gut-associated lymphoid tissues or bone marrow may be the functional equivalent of the bursa. Cells of bursal origin (*B cells*), located mainly in the cortical regions of lymph nodes, are arranged in follicles, whereas T cells predominate in the paracortical zones. The T cells, extremely long-lived, constantly recirculate between the blood and the lymphatic system. On stimulation by certain antigens, some of them rapidly transform into large blast cells (immunoblasts) that take up pyronin on histochemical staining. Macrophages, possibly to "process" the antigens, must precede transformation. Activated T cells (*"killer cells"*) play a major role in acute homograft rejection. Other T cells (*"helper cells"*) cooperate with B cells in producing humoral antibodies.

TYPES OF REJECTION

The immunological attack usually proceeds from recipient (host) to donor (graft), i.e., a *host versus graft reaction*.

Acute rejection

Most animal homografts appear initially to be normal. However, between 7 and 10 days after transplantation the graft rapidly deteriorates in a delayed hypersensitivity type of reaction, mediated by sensitized lymphocytes rather than by circulating antibodies. Serial biopsies of untreated renal homografts show this sequence. The first recognizable event, margination of lymphocytes in peritubular capillaries, occurs within 24 hours of transplantation. After 48 hours methyl green pyronin stains indicate rapid RNA synthesis by the marginated cells. At about 72 hours, adjacent cytoplasmic extensions of the endothelial cells withdraw, to leave endothelial defects through which mononuclear cells infiltrate the tubular interstitium. At the same time fibrin and platelets plug the glomeruli, shutting off blood flow. This results in ischemic necrosis of the transplant (if the recipient lives to this stage). The features of untreated cellular rejection appear the same in all organs undergoing acute rejection whether these are liver, kidney, heart, or skin.

Serum antibodies commonly increase in response to homografts, but their role in influencing the outcome of such transplants is poorly understood. Although deposits of gamma globulin accummulate on the vascular endothelium of organs undergoing acute rejection, the evidence weighs heavily in favor of cell-bound immunity destroying the graft.

Although acute homograft rejection can undergo spontaneous remission, most remissions follow immunosuppressive therapy.

Second set rejection

The acute rejection response described above is sometimes referred to as a *first set response* (Fig. 36-1). Homografts placed in recipients that have been sensitized by a previous exposure to donor tissue are usually rejected in an accelerated, or *second set,* fashion (Fig. 36-1). Skin grafts are destroyed in 4 to 7 days instead of the average 10 days. Lymphoid cells mobilize more rapidly than normal because of prior antidonor instruction. Circulating humoral antibodies may also augment the rejection.

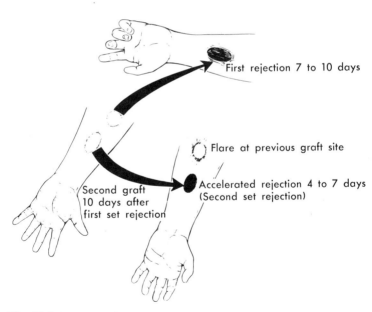

First rejection 7 to 10 days

Flare at previous graft site

Second graft 10 days after first set rejection

Accelerated rejection 4 to 7 days (Second set rejection)

Fig. 36-1. Patterns of homograft rejection. The first graft is rejected by the recipient in 7 to 10 days (first set rejection). The second graft from the same donor to the same recipient undergoes accelerated rejection, indicating prior sensitization of the recipient.

Hyperacute rejection

Humoral antibodies play a much more important role in hyperacute rejection, in which the recipient has previously been repeatedly exposed to donor type antigens. Striking examples of hyperacute rejection have occurred in patients who received renal homografts from ABO blood group–incompatible donors. The ABO blood groups on the red cells also reside in other tissues, including the kidneys. If the kidney of an A, B, or AB donor is placed in a recipient whose serum contains naturally occurring anti-A and/or anti-B isoagglutinins (for example, a patient of O blood type would have both types of isoagglutinins), these antibodies are likely to bind with the renal red cell antigens. This has been confirmed by a fall in systemic isoagglutinin titers when the circulation to a renal homograft is reestablished. Rapid destruction of the homograft follows within minutes or hours of transplantation. Preformed antibodies and antigens of the endothelial cells of the blood vessels of the graft promptly react. The transplanted kidney becomes a trap for antibodies, complement, formed blood elements, and clotting factors with resultant occlusion of the renal vasculature.

The major cause of hyperacute rejection of renal homografts is presensitization of the recipient to transplantation antigens like those of the donor. This may occur from previous exposures through repeated blood transfusions, multiple pregnancies, or retransplantation in patients whose first homografts were rejected and who were presumably immunized to some antigens in the second graft. A variety of antibodies are probably responsible. These may be detected by lymphocytotoxicity, leukoagglutinin, or mixed agglutination tests. However, sometimes hyperacute rejection does occur despite the apparent absence of preformed antibodies. Presumably our currently available techniques lack the sensitivity to detect some antibodies.

Chronic rejection

Humoral antibodies also play an important role in the late rejection of transplanted organs that occurs months or years after the original operation in immunosuppressed recipients. This has been observed following transplantation of the kidney, liver, heart, and lung in man. The outstanding feature of chronic rejection is the development of obliterative vascular lesions. Antibodies specific for donor antigens and complement can be demonstrated in the lesions. The vascular changes probably result from reactions between low concentrations of antibody and antigen. These slow reactions, allowing some repair, eventually lead to narrowing of the vascular lumen with progressive decreasing circulation through the homograft and ultimate organ failure.

Hyperacute xenograft rejection

Organ grafts between animals of different species are rejected with exceptional vigor. The rate of rejection and extent of histological damage depend directly upon the genetic disparity between the species. The relative importance of cellular as opposed to humoral immunity varies with the species combinations. In general, as the combinations become more divergent, the role of humoral antibody increases and that of cellular immunity diminishes. Thus kidney grafts from pigs to dogs violently reject within minutes. Antibodies deposited in the transplanted organ trigger an immunological reaction similar to the hyperacute homograft rejection described above. On the other hand, lungs transplanted from foxes to dogs are tolerated almost as well as canine homografts.

A few attempts have been made to transplant kidneys, livers, or hearts from baboons or chimpanzees to man. In most cases the grafts failed within hours or days, but intensive immunosuppression has permitted some to survive for extended periods (up to 10 months).

Graft versus host reactions

If the donor lacks the recipient's antigens, the graft may mount an immunological reaction against the host when the graft contains immunologically competent lymphoid cells (spleen, thymus, lymph nodes, or bone marrow). Another essential feature is that the host is unable to reject the graft either because of immunological immaturity, as in the fetal or neonatal host, or because the recipient is unable to mount an adequate immunological response as a result of immunosuppressive therapy. The acute form of graft versus host disease is characterized by diarrhea, weakness, dermatitis, alopecia, hepatomegaly, splenomegaly, wasting, and abrupt cessation of growth. Initially, the host's spleen and lymph nodes undergo a striking hyperplasia, followed by atrophy and loss of follicular organization. Atrophy of the thymus and hemolytic anemia develop, and death usually follows. Milder, chronic forms of the disease also occur, and recovery is complete after weeks or months.

MODIFICATION OF THE IMMUNE RESPONSE

A number of methods are available for the prevention or treatment of the rejection reaction: (1) reduction of genetic disparity (tests of histocompatibility), (2) immunosuppression, (3) graft alteration, (4) specific immunological tolerance, and (5) immunological enhancement.

Tests of histocompatibility

Tests of histocompatibility can reduce the genetic disparity between donor and recipient. If we match the donor and recipient so that only minor antigenic differences exist, we can, at least theoretically, attenuate graft rejection. Histocompatibility tests currently in use include serological tests and the mixed lymphocyte culture test (MLC).

Serological tests

The importance of ABO blood group compatibility and of testing donor serum for preformed cytotoxic antibodies has already been emphasized.

In addition, tests for the HL-A antigens employ antisera obtained from persons who had been accidentally or deliberately sensitized to white blood cell antigens. Lymphocytes from several potential donors and from the recipient are tested against these antisera. The HL-A profiles of the donors are then compared with that of the recipient and the combination showing the least disparity is selected for transplantation (Fig. 36-2).

The HL-A system consists of at least two loci on the same chromosome. Each locus has two antigens, and a large number of alternative genes or alleles. In consequence only a remote possibility exists of obtaining a perfect match of all four antigens between randomized members of the nonrelated population. Another disappointing feature of HL-A typing is the lack of correlation between the quality of matching and the clinical outcome after transplantation. The only really significant correlation is in some sibling cases where the donor and the recipient have inherited the same two histocompatibility

	Donor or Recip	Name Last	First	ABO	HLA 1	HLA 2	HLA 3	B 4	HLA 5	HLA 7	HLA 8	B 9	B 11	B 6	B 10	B 12	Cross match
A	R	A	J	A	−	−	−	−	−	−	−	−	−	+	−	+	
	D	W	M, E	A	−	−	−	−	−	−	−	−	−	+	+	+	Neg.
	D	W	J	O	−	−	−	+	−	−	−	−	−	+	−	−	Neg.
	D	W	D	A	−	−	−	−	−	−	−	−	−	+	+	−	Neg.

B	R	R	J, H	O	−	+	+	−	−	−	−	+	−	−	−	−	
	D	R	J, S	O	−	+	+	−	−	−	−	+	−	−	−	−	Neg.

Fig. 36-2. A, Each of the potential donors has a one antigen mismatch with the recipient. **B,** The donor and recipient antigen profiles show complete identity.

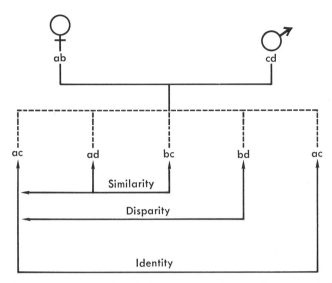

Fig. 36-3. Possible genetic relationships in a family. Since the siblings share one haplotype from each parent there is a 1 in 4 chance of identity, a 2 in 4 chance of similarity, and a 1 in 4 chance of disparity.

haplotypes* and thus have complete identity of the HL-A antigens (Fig. 36-3). Patients with this combination show good clinical results; other donor-recipient combinations have variable outcomes.

Mixed lymphocyte culture (MLC) test

In contrast to serological tests of histocompatibility *typing,* the MLC test attempts to perform histocompatibility *matching.* The aim is to determine the degree of incompatibility between two individuals without defining the responsible antigens.

In the MLC test, lymphocytes from the donor and recipient are placed together in culture medium. As they come into contact, the lymphocytes from each individual are stimulated by foreign histocompatibility antigens of the other. The cells begin to synthesize DNA at an increased rate and undergo mitosis. The degree of stimulation

---

*Haplotype: the group of alleles of linked genes contributed by either parent.

and DNA production can be measured by the uptake of tritiated thymidine by the cells. If donor cells are pretreated with mitomycin-C, a metabolic inhibitor, only the response of the recipient's lymphocytes will be measured. Failure to stimulate implies compatibility at the MLC locus.

The MLC test separates MLC identical siblings from nonidentical ones and helps predict prolonged skin allograft survival. In addition, MLC nonstimulation correlates well with identity for the HL-A leukocyte antigens; that is, siblings whose cells do not stimulate in MLC tests show virtually identical reactions with the serological tests mentioned above. These and other studies suggest that the locus controlling MLC reactivity is part of or closely related to the major histocompatibility locus.

In unrelated individuals who appear to be HL-A identical, MLC tests may show stimulation, suggesting that not all the antigens of HL-A have been defined.

In the selection of sibling donors for bone marrow transplantation, the MLC test helps to minimize potential graft versus host reactions. It is also useful in the selection of donor-recipient combinations for renal transplants between related individuals. However, the MLC test takes 5 to 7 days to complete. This delay negates its usefulness with cadaver donors whose organs must be transplanted within hours.

Immunosuppression

Immunosuppression is the main method to prevent and control rejection. It features a variety of techniques, nonspecific for any particular donor-recipient combination, to suppress the recipient's response. Most procedures either reduce the volume of the host's immunologically competent tissues, or interfere with the functions of the cells that participate in the immune response.

Pharmacological agents

Pharmacological agents constitute the major form of immunosuppressive therapy. These will often suppress the rejection reaction but are toxic agents with potentially dangerous side effects.

Azathioprine has been the basic immunosuppressive drug for almost all clinical transplantation. It interferes with nucleoprotein synthesis, suppresses antibody formation and delayed hypersensitivity reactions, and also has anti-inflammatory properties. The main side effect of azathioprine is bone marrow depression (leukopenia or even agranulocytosis). This drug may also cause liver damage, teratogenic effects, pancreatitis, stomatitis, and temporary baldness.

Cyclophosphamide, a very potent immunosuppressive agent, can substitute for azathioprine, particularly when the latter has caused hepatotoxicity. In large doses, cyclophosphamide may cause bone marrow damage, anorexia, nausea, vomiting, severe cystitis, fibrosis of the urinary bladder, interstitial pulmonary fibrosis, alopecia, and gonadal suppression. These toxic effects have been observed in patients who have received large doses in the treatment of cancer or in bone marrow transplantation. Most of these complications can be avoided with the smaller amounts used in renal, cardiac, or hepatic transplantation.

Prednisone and other adrenal corticosteroids are also basic drugs in clinical transplantation. They appear to exert their beneficial effects through at least two mechanisms—production of lymphopenia and stabilization of lysosomes. Lysosomes, collections of enzymes in the cytoplasm, burst after the cell has sustained a certain degree of injury and destroy it. Unfortunately, the corticosteroids have many serious side effects including obesity, Cushing's syndrome, hypertension, impaired growth in children, osteoporosis with the risk of pathological fractures or aseptic necrosis of bone, diabetes mellitus, peptic ulceration, psychiatric disorders, pancreatitis, and cataracts.

Heterologous antilymphocyte serum (ALS) and its globulin derivative (ALG) are obtained from animals (such as horses, rabbits, goats, sheep, and other species) previously immunized against human lymphoid tissues. The source of the lymphocytes may be the spleen, lymph nodes, thymus, normal peripheral blood, thoracic duct lymph, blood of patients with lymphatic leukemia, or tissue cultures of human lymphoid cells. The antibody response to the injected lymphocytes can be measured by determining the ability of the serum to agglutinate or lyse human white cells in vitro. After intensive immunization, the antiwhite cell titers may rise to levels as high as $1:16,000$. The globulin extract of serum collected from an immunized animal is a powerful immunosuppressive agent. We usually use it in combination with azathioprine (or cyclophosphamide) and prednisone and limit it to a few days before transplantation and the first few postoperative weeks. By using ALG within these guidelines, we can minimize the risks of foreign protein sensitization and anaphylaxis. Other reactions to ALG include fever, local pain, erythema, swelling and tenderness at the site of intramuscular injection, skin eruptions, and thrombocytopenia.

Less frequently used drugs such as actinomycin C, actinomycin D, azaserine, methotrexate, and vinblastine may reverse homograft rejection.

We rarely use one immunosuppressive agent alone. Combinations of drugs yield the most consistent long-term survivals in man. Frequent combinations are azathioprine with prednisone or both of these agents with ALG. Other forms of immunosuppression such as local irradiation of a kidney homograft or a thoracic duct fistula may augment these agents. Our initial dosage of the drugs is high, but as the graft adapts to its hostile new environment, we reduce dosages to maintenance levels and continue them indefinitely.

Irradiation

Total body irradiation has deleterious effects on immunocompetent cells throughout the body. However, this treatment is dangerous because many other cells are sensitive to radiation injury. Death may occur from bone marrow aplasia or from diffuse hemorrhagic gastroenteritis. At present total body irradiation is chiefly limited to use with bone marrow transplantation.

Local irradiation of the graft apparently destroys host lymphocytes that have invaded the transplanted organ. The doses used are too small to alter the antigenicity of the graft. Radiation alone may prolong renal homograft survival in the dog for up to a month. Some transplantation centers routinely combine radiation with drug therapy during the first few days after transplantation. Radiation may help to abort acute rejection episodes.

Lymphoid depletion

Recognition of the major role which lymphocytes play in graft rejection has resulted in attempts to produce generalized lymphoid depletion. Among these are regional lymphadenectomy, splenectomy, intralymphatic infusion of colloidal radioisotopes, extracorporeal irradiation of peripheral whole blood or lymph, removal of lymphocytes through thoracic duct fistulas, and thymectomy. However, regional lymphadenectomy seldom prolongs homograft survival. While the antibody response to many antigens decreases after splenectomy, the value of this procedure in promoting homograft acceptance is unproved. Intralymphatic infusion of colloidal radioisotopes, extracorporeal irradiation of peripheral blood or lymph, and thoracic duct fistulas all exhibit a modest immunosuppressive effect in the laboratory, but not clinically. Neonatally thymectomized animals show profound depletion of lymphocytes in the peripheral blood, lymph nodes, and spleen. Skin grafts placed on these animals enjoy markedly prolonged survival, but thymectomy during adult life has far less impressive results. Thymectomy is rarely used clinically.

Graft alteration

Many of the problems of organ transplantation could be minimized if we could prevent rejection by modifying the homograft rather than the host's immunological response. In certain homografts "passenger leukocytes" and possibly interstitial cells of the transplant may play an important role in the rejection reaction by serving as stimulators of homograft immunity. Elimination of these cells by pretreatment of the donor or of the homograft with immunosuppressive drugs may prolong homograft survival, but these methods have thus far proved to be of little clinical importance.

Specific immunological tolerance

Immunosuppressive therapy is nonspecific; it depresses the recipient's response not only to the homograft but to many other antigens. Consequently infection frequently complicates such therapy. Chronic immunosuppression also increases the incidence of *de novo* malignancies. A form of treatment that is highly specific for a given antigen but leaves the recipient with otherwise normal immune defenses is known as *immunological tolerance*. Tolerance induction depends on pretreatment with donor antigen and results from a poorly understood central failure of the host's immune response. Tolerance requires the continued presence of the specific antigen for its maintenance and decreases if the antigen disappears. It is most easily produced by injection of living lymphohemopoietic cells into embryonic or newborn animals. The recipient not only fails to reject these cells, but also accepts or tolerates subsequent tissue grafts from the same donor. Tolerance can also be induced in adult animals, but less successfully. With minor histocompatibility differences we can usually obtain consistent results. However, with major differences tolerance induction may be extremely difficult. Since tolerance induction depends on the number of cells in the host that can respond to the antigenic stimulus, any means of reducing these cells will augment tolerance. Immunosuppressive therapy with azathioprine, cyclophosphamide, ALS, sublethal irradiation, or thymectomy in conjunction with the antigen will induce tolerance. Unfortunately the graft versus host reaction frequently follows the use of adult donor lymphoid cells. Embryonic donor cells avoid this complication. Alternatively, immunosuppressive agents such as methotrexate given to the host may prevent adult donor cells from reacting vigorously against the host.

Immunological enhancement

Another poorly understood but specific mechanism to prevent homograft rejection involves the development of certain kinds of antigraft antibodies, which either coat the graft antigens and thus prevent the host from recognizing them, or act centrally on the recipient's cellular immune defenses, hampering the development of immunity to graft antigens. Enhancement prolongs the survival of tumor homografts much more than those of normal tissues. Enhancement may be *active,* when it follows treatment of the host with either live or killed tissue syngeneic* with the test graft, or passive, when the host is given previously prepared antigraft antiserum. The administration of both donor antigen and antidonor serum prior to transplantation provides greater suppression of graft rejection than either antigen or antiserum alone.

Unfortunately it is impossible to induce specific tolerance or enhancement consistently with all types of homografts. Some chronically accepted organ homografts in man may reflect tolerance. However, we lack reliable means of consistently producing tolerance in man at the present time. Although a few attempts at producing immunological enhancement in man have recently been reported, we must at present rely on nonspecific immunosuppression to prevent homograft rejection in clinical transplantation.

CURRENT STATUS OF CLINICAL TRANSPLANTATION
Autografts

Certain autografts are commonly performed to reconstruct defects involving skin, fascia, bone, cartilage, tendon, joints, nerve, stomach, and intestines. Autografts of veins and, less commonly, arteries may be used to bypass or replace occluded areas of the vascular system. A patient's own blood may be removed, frozen, and later administered during surgery as an autotransfusion. Occasionally a bone marrow autotransplant may be necessary when a patient receives treatment with an agent which is toxic to the marrow (such as phenylalanine mustard in the treatment of malignant melanoma). Autotransplants of endocrine glands, most commonly the thyroid or parathyroid glands, are sometimes performed when these glands are accidentally or intentionally removed, such as accidental removal of the parathyroid glands during a total thyroidectomy, or removal of all thyroid tissue when a lingual thyroid gland is removed. In the latter instance slices of the removed gland can be reimplanted in the neck. Traumatic amputation of a limb or digit is increasingly being treated by reimplantation of the severed member. Tooth buds and skin containing hair follicles can also be replaced as autografts to correct existing deformities. Autografts of the kidney are becoming more common in the treatment of complicated cases of renovascular hypertension, renal calculi, renal

---

*Syngeneic: having identical genotypes, such as tissues from identical twins or animals of the same inbred strain.

trauma, and renal cancer. The surgeon removes the kidney, corrects the defects, and replaces the organ in the patient.

Homografts and heterografts

Blood. A blood transfusion is the most common type of homograft. Matched red blood cells are apparently nonantigenic, whereas the white blood cells and possibly the platelets are antigenic and may sensitize the patient to transplants of other organs such as kidneys.

Cornea. Corneal grafts have successfully restored vision to patients with corneal opacities. Apparently the fibrous barrier that forms between the host cornea and the graft is almost impervious to blood vessels. In consequence, rejection does not occur. However, should the graft become vascularized it will undergo rejection and become cloudy.

Skin. Skin homografts are useful in the management of burned patients, especially those with extensive skin loss who lack sufficient host skin to use as autografts. The burned patient has some depression of immunity that permits survival of the grafts for longer periods than normal. The homografts are ultimately rejected, but they serve as useful temporary dressings that reduce infection and fluid loss. Recently immunosuppressive therapy has prolonged the survival of skin homografts in a small series of patients. Pig skin heterografts also provide valuable but temporary cover for burned patients.

Bone. Preserved bone homografts and heterografts are nonviable, but provide a temporary support until replaced by host tissue. When autografts are unavailable, surgeons use these foreign bones to treat fractures, to bridge bone defects, to fuse joints, to restore contour, and to replace digits. Transplanted middle ear ossicles have also restored hearing in selected patients with conduction deafness.

Cartilage. Homografts or heterografts have aided facial reconstruction. They resemble corneal grafts in that the donor cells are isolated from contact with host cells while the cartilage matrix itself is avascular and not readily penetrated by the blood vessels of the host.

Tendon. Tendons are composed largely of collagen, which is nonantigenic. Small numbers of tendon homografts have been performed in man with apparent success.

Arteries. Formerly, surgeons replaced arterial defects with arterial homografts, but early degenerative changes leading to thrombosis, rupture, or aneurysm formation have forced them to use synthetic replacement grafts. Enzyme-treated bovine heterografts that consist essentially of tubes of collagen (almost nonantigenic) still have a place in arterial replacement.

Cardiac valves. These consist mostly of collagen and have little antigenicity. Homografts and heterografts can substitute for seriously diseased human heart valves, particularly the aortic valve.

In nearly all the previous examples immunosuppressive therapy is unnecessary because the grafts are nonantigenic, or protected from the host's immune defense, or nonviable and merely serve as temporary struts until the host's tissues replace them. Immunosuppressive therapy, however, plays a critical role in preventing rejection and maintaining adequate homograft function in the following *organ transplants.*

Kidney. Renal transplantation is performed in patients suffering from chronic renal failure. The most common antecedent diseases are subacute or chronic glomerulonephritis. Other predisposing disorders include: pyelonephritis, polycystic kidney disease, familial nephritis, Goodpasture's syndrome, medullary cystic disease, nephrosclerosis, lupus nephritis, diabetic nephropathy, Fabry's syndrome, and renal malignancy.

The patient is prepared for operation by peritoneal dialysis or, more commonly, hemodialysis to correct fluid and electrolyte imbalance, acidosis, hypertension, and pulmonary edema, if present. With hemodialysis, blood is led from a peripheral artery or vein to the hemodialysis machine, where a semipermeable membrane separates the blood from fluid in a bath. Dialyzable wastes from the blood filter through the membrane into the bath and dialyzable electrolytes and other materials inside the bath pass in the reverse direction. The purified blood is then returned to the patient through a peripheral vein.

The surgeon removes the diseased kidneys and places the homograft in a heterotopic* position in the groin (Fig. 36-4).

About 17,000 kidney transplants have been performed throughout the world, and 7,500 of the recipients are still living. The longest survivor, the recipient of a kidney from an identical twin, is doing well 18 years after operation. In our own center, twenty-nine recipients of kidneys obtained from nontwin donors remain alive and well 10 years or more after transplantation. Recipients of consanguineous kidneys have better prospects of survival than those who receive organs from unrelated donors, with a 5-year survival rate of approximately 70 to 80% in the former, compared with 35% in the latter group.

Liver. Patients requiring liver transplantation are in the end state of hepatic disease. Their life expectancy can be measured in days, weeks, or at most a few months. The main indications for the operation include congenital biliary atresia, advanced cirrhosis, chronic

---

*Heterotopic: in an abnormal anatomic location.

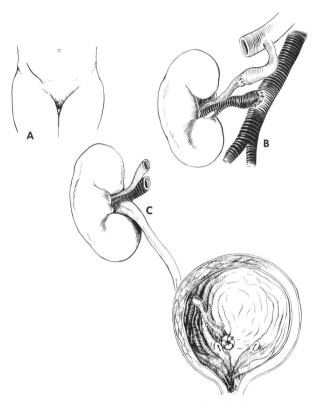

Fig. 36-4. Renal homotransplantation. **A,** The incision is made in the recipient's groin. **B,** The renal artery is anastomosed end-to-end to the hypogastric artery and the renal vein end-to-side to the external iliac vein. **C,** The donor ureter is implanted into the recipient's bladder (ureteroneocystostomy).

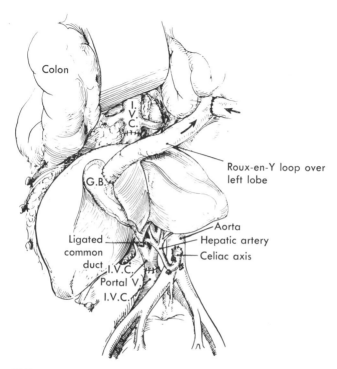

Fig. 36-5. Heterotopic liver transplantation. The patient's own liver is under the retractor at the top of the illustration. The recipient's vena cava was transected below the level of the renal veins and the donor liver was revascularized as follows: The donor portal vein was anastomosed to the recipient's distal inferior vena cava; the donor's suprahepatic vena cava was joined to the recipient's proximal inferior vena cava; the donor celiac axis was anastomosed to the recipient's aorta. The donor's subhepatic vena cava was closed with a suture. The common bile duct was ligated below its junction with the cystic duct and biliary drainage was provided by anastomosis of the gallbladder to a Roux-Y loop of the small bowel. (From Starzl, T. E.: Experience in hepatic transplantation, Philadelphia, 1969, W. B. Saunders Co.)

aggressive hepatitis, and liver-based metabolic disorders such as Wilson's disease. Less common indications are primary hepatic malignancies and acute hepatic failure caused by fulminating viral hepatitis or the ingestion of hepatic toxins.

A liver transplant may be heterotopic, in which case the surgeon leaves the recipient's own diseased liver in situ and places the homograft organ somewhere else in the abdomen (Fig. 36-5). Alternatively, he may remove the host's diseased liver and place the homograft in the normal anatomic position, an orthotopic transplant (Fig. 36-6). Theoretically, the former operation has the advantage that residual function of the host's own liver may help to tide him over a severe rejection crisis involving the homograft. In actual practice the pro-

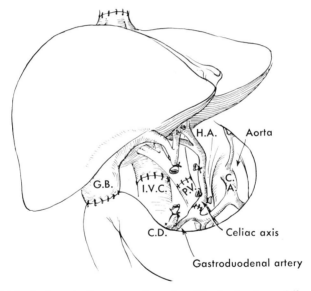

Fig. 36-6. Orthotopic liver transplantation. The host's diseased liver and related segment of inferior vena cava have been removed. The donor liver and the related segment of inferior vena cava have been placed in position with anastomosis of the vena cava above and below the liver, the portal veins, and the hepatic arteries. The donor common bile duct was ligated and biliary drainage provided by anastomosis of the gallbladder to the duodenum. (From Starzl, T. E.: Experience in hepatic transplantation, Philadelphia, 1969, W. B. Saunders Co.)

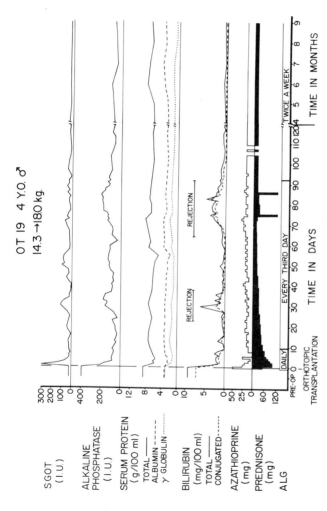

Fig. 36-7. Early postoperative course in a 4-year-old child who underwent orthotopic liver transplantation for congenital biliary atresia. Two rejection episodes were heralded by elevations of the bilirubin and alkaline phosphatase levels. These were successfully reversed and the patient had no further problems with rejection. Standard immunosuppression was with azathioprine, prednisone, and ALG (the last was discontinued after several months). The patient died of severe infection 3½ years after transplantation. (From Starzl, T. E.: Experience in hepatic transplantation, Philadelphia, 1969, W. B. Saunders Co.)

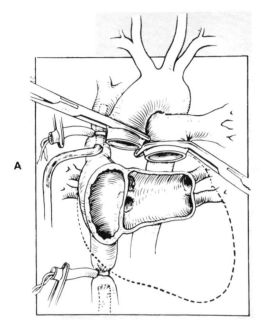

Fig. 36-8. Transplantation of the heart. **A,** Using cardiopulmonary by-pass the recipient's heart has been excised leaving behind the transected posterior portions of both atria, the ascending aorta, and the pulmonary artery. **B,** The entire donor heart has been removed. The superior vena cava has been ligated. The right atrium has been opened by an incision from the inferior vena caval opening extending toward the atrial appendage, taking care to preserve the sinus node and sinoauricular pathways. The left atrium has been opened by an incision joining the orifices of the four pulmonary veins. **C,** The donor heart is sewn into the recipient. The left and then the right atrial anastomoses are completed, followed by anastomosis of the pulmonary artery and the aorta. (From Cooley, D. A.: Transplantation of the human heart; report of four cases, J.A.M.A. **205:**479-486, 1968.)

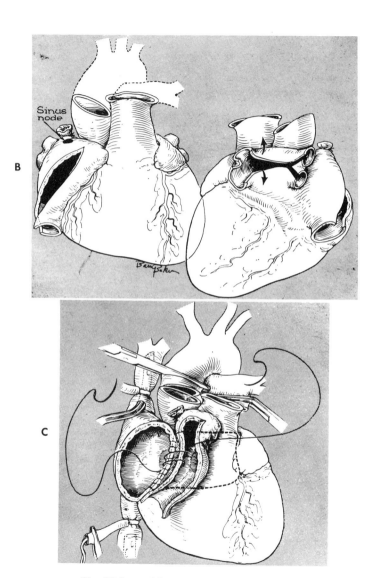

Fig. 36-8, cont'd. For legend see opposite page.

cedure has serious drawbacks. The abdomen lacks space to accommodate a second large organ. Tight closure of the abdomen and upward displacement of the diaphragm cause serious postoperative respiratory problems. Furthermore, the two livers compete functionally, and the organ that receives no blood from the splanchnic area (usually the homograft) atrophies. For these reasons, most surgeons have abandoned heterotopic liver transplantation.

To date, over 200 liver transplants have been performed throughout the world. The early postoperative course of a long-term survivor is shown in Fig. 36-7. At least sixteen recipients are currently alive. The longest survivor is now $5\frac{1}{2}$ years posttransplantation.

Heart. Cardiac transplantation is performed in patients with terminal heart disease not amenable to medical treatment or any other surgical procedure. The most common indication is for heart disease caused by coronary atherosclerosis. Other indications include cardiomyopathy, multivalvular rheumatic disease, and severe congenital anomalies.

The essential features of the operation are shown in Fig. 36-8. Of 240 cardiac transplants performed in 236 patients, 37 recipients are still living. The longest survivor is 6 years post-transplantation.

Pancreaticoduodenal transplants. These have been performed in cases of severe juvenile onset diabetes mellitus complicated by marked retinopathy and nephropathy. Thirty-four such procedures have been performed to date. Two patients are still alive, the longest survivor being 2 years post-transplantation. Because of difficulties with the exocrine secretion of the homograft and rejection of the duodenum, researchers have attempted to isolate and transplant large numbers of viable islets of Langerhans. So far this procedure has been tried successfully only in animals.

Lung. The prime candidates for this procedure are patients who are gravely ill with primary pulmonary hypertension or restrictive lung disease. Other indications include chronic obstructive airway disease and acute respiratory insufficiency caused by toxic pneumonitis or trauma. Lung transplants have been performed in 34 patients. The longest survival was 10 months.

Bone marrow. Bone marrow transplantation may help patients critically ill with the following diseases: accidental whole body irradiation; aplastic anemia; leukemia; immune deficiency diseases including agammaglobulinemia, hypogammaglobulinemia, the Wiscott-Aldrich syndrome, and the DiGeorge syndrome. Several hundred bone marrow transplants have been performed to date. Of the 148 patients transplanted between January, 1968, and April, 1973, reported to the Bone Marrow Transplant Registry, 37 were alive with functioning grafts at the time of their last follow-up report, the longest survivor being 41 months post-transplantation. At the present time the only worthwhile long-term results have been obtained in transplants between ABO and HL-A identical siblings.

Endocrine glands. Because hormonal replacement therapy is so readily available for endocrine (thyroid, adrenal, gonad) glands, little need exists for substitution homografts (and the hazards of immuno-suppression). Severe hypoparathyroidism may represent an exception.

Other organs. Occasional transplants of the spleen, thymus, small intestine, and larynx have been attempted in man, but at present, the complications of immunosuppressive therapy outweigh any advantages of transplanting nonvital organs.

Renal transplantation has yielded many long-term survivals, other organ transplantation relatively few. The reasons for this disparity include greater technical difficulties (liver requires more difficult anastomoses); lack of artificial organs (similar to renal dialysis) to carry patients through periods of acute liver, heart, or pulmonary failure; and problems with the diagnosis of rejection in its early and most reversible phase.

New discoveries in tolerance induction or enhancement, in support systems, and in surgical techniques should extend the benefits of this exciting field of organ transplantation to future generations.

CHAPTER 37

Thermal injuries

CHARLES E. HARTFORD
WILLIAM C. BOYD

Each year in the United States about 80,000 people are hospitalized because of burns; of this number, about 12,000 die. Among the survivors, morbidity is often prolonged because of scarring and disfigurement. In addition, property loss from fire is considerable. The burn problem has become known as the "silent epidemic."

Numerically, most burns occur in and around the home, particularly the kitchen, utility room, garage, and yard. Those at highest risk for burns are the young, the aged, and the mentally and physically infirm. Many of these individuals have neither the physical capability nor the presence of mind to protect themselves from scalding liquids or to extinguish or remove burning clothing. Furthermore, when clothing burns, a lethal injury can easily occur within 1 minute.

Many who treat burns believe the next important advance in this field lies in prevention. In the United States recent federal legislation requires flame retardant material for the manufacture of night wear size 12X and smaller. Although this is an important advance, it is clearly not enough. People in high-risk groups, including the institutionalized and those with seizure disorders, also deserve to be protected with flame-retardant clothing.

PATHOPHYSIOLOGY
The wound

Heat from many sources, including chemicals and electricity, can cause burns. Although pain from heat is perceived at 47.5° C., injury to cells will occur at 45° C. The damage done depends upon the intensity and duration of exposure. Cell death by coagulation of pro-

662

tein begins at 65° C. Instantaneous exposure of the skin to 72° C. produces a blister (a burn of second degree or partial thickness of skin).

The gross appearance of thermally injured tissue ranges from erythema and blisters of more superficial burns to the charred, black, leathery brown or cadaveric white of deep burns. Coagulated veins usually signify full thickness skin injury. Intense and prolonged exposure may cause the skin to split, exposing subcutaneous fat.

The skin is the major organ injured in a burn; an appreciation of its basic anatomy, physiology, and reaction to thermal injury is essential to understand depth of injury and healing. Skin is composed of squamous surface epithelium and epidermal appendages supported by interwoven collagen fibers of the dermis (Fig. 37-1). The epidermal appendages include hair follicles, sebaceous glands (the hair follicle and sebaceous gland together are called a pyelosebaceous unit), and sweat ducts and their glands. These appendages are derived from ectoderm and retain the ability to transform to squamous epithelium, a process known as *squamous metaplasia*. Therefore, if viable epidermal appendages remain after injury and their viability can be preserved, the wound will reepithelize by squamous metaplasia.

Very superficial burns (commonly known as first-degree) are char-

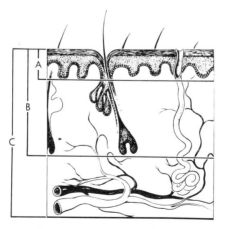

Fig. 37-1. Diagram of skin showing a practical classification of depth of injury. **A,** Injury down to this level is known as superficial partial thickness burn. **B,** Deep partial thickness burn. **C,** Full thickness burn.

acterized by erythema. Only the upper portion of the surface epithelium is destroyed, and rapid healing without scar occurs.

In superficial partial thickness burns (superficial dermal burns or superficial second-degree burns) the entire surface epithelium is destroyed. However, a major portion of each epidermal appendage remains alive. Therefore the likelihood of spontaneous healing is excellent, usually in 3 weeks or less. Because of only slight disturbance to the collagen in the dermis, there is rapid return of skin tone and texture, and scarring is minimal.

In deep partial thickness burns (deep dermal burns or deep second-degree burns) the surface epithelium, pyelosebaceous units, and a large portion of the sweat ducts are destroyed. Only the deep-seated sweat glands are preserved. These cells undergo squamous metaplasia and appear in the granulation tissue as islands of epithelium which expand and coalesce to resurface the wound (Fig. 37-2). In burns of this depth, healing takes much longer and may occur as late as 120 days after injury. The existence of these sweat glands is tenuous.

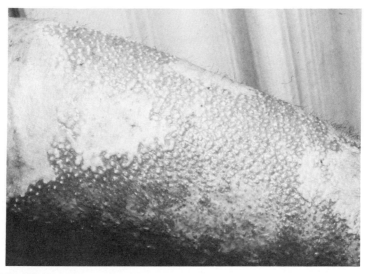

Fig. 37-2. Healing partial thickness burn showing islands of squamous epithelium that have emerged from epidermal appendages. The epithelium will expand to resurface the wound.

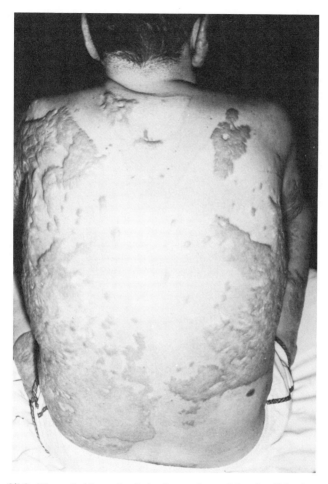

Fig. 37-3. Most of this patient's back was burned but it all healed without skin grafting. Adjacent to the unburned skin (outlined by straps of overalls), are unscarred areas intermixed with irregular raised areas, which constitute hypertrophic scarring. Superficial partial thickness burns usually heal with minimal scarring, but the deeper the partial thickness burn the more likely the chance of hypertrophic scarring.

Their destruction by infection is probably a frequent occurrence and is a mechanism by which partial thickness burn is converted to full thickness injury. In deep partial thickness burns there is also extensive disturbance of dermal collagen fibers. As healing progresses, the re-formed collagen fibers are often in disarray and irregular whorls are seen histologically. A *hypertrophic scar* forms. This kind of scar is erythematous, raised, and indurated (Fig. 37-3). This is not to be confused with a *keloid,* which has a neoplastic connotation.

In full thickness (third-degree) burns, surface epithelium as well as all epidermal appendages are destroyed. Spontaneous healing from the depth of the wound is impossible. Coverage of the wound occurs

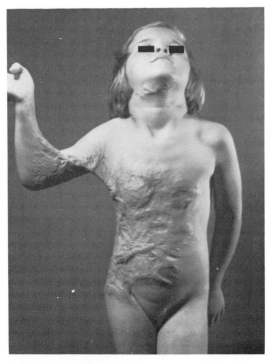

Fig. 37-4. Burn contracture of axilla and antecubital fossa, severly limiting motion of right upper extremity.

only by epithelial ingrowth from the edges or by autogenous skin grafting.

The identification of burn depth by gross inspection is unreliable. Depth can be determined with certainty only by biopsy. To await spontaneous healing is not accurate, because partial thickness burns may be converted to full thickness.

Burn tissue is a foreign body that must be autolyzed and digested or cast off as a sequestrum. The sequestrum is known as an *eschar*. Inflammation occurs at the interface between the eschar and viable tissue which, by liquefaction and suppuration, eventually separates the eschar. If this zone of inflammation is colonized by bacteria, several devastating events can occur. (1) An abscess may form. If the abscess is not drained, invasive infection of the underlying viable tissue may follow. (2) Infection also causes rapid separation of eschar; but as pointed out before, it also can destroy viable epidermal appendages and convert partial thickness burns to full thickness. (3) Finally, septicemia is a likely sequela. All these events are enhanced by depressed natural immunity against infection, of which there is ample evidence in severely burned patients.

Although many bacteria, fungi, and even viruses can cause invasive infection of burns, currently the most troublesome organism is *Pseudomonas aeruginosa*. When the concentration of these microorganisms exceeds 100,000 per gram of tissue, bacterial invasion and devitalization of tissue occurs. The process is self-perpetuating.

Contraction plays an important role in the healing of all burns and contributes to much of the deformity after a burn has healed. The resulting *contracture* is defined as epithelized scar which inhibits normal range of motion (Fig. 37-4).

Fluid shifts and burn shock

Thermal injury causes translocation of body fluids, the net result of which is hypovolemia. If the burn is large enough and the patient is not properly treated, circulatory and renal failure occur; this is known as *burn shock*. The lesion responsible for the shift of body fluids lies in the microcirculation, where capillaries become abnormally permeable. This lesion may arise from hypoxia, direct thermal injury, biologically active substances produced in heated tissues, released intracellular enzymes, or a combination of these factors. Obligatory sequestration of fluid into the extravascular space, containing an ultrafiltrate of plasma, occurs in both injured and uninjured tissues. This produces edema, which at times is massive (Fig. 37-5). The shift of fluid from the intravascular space progressively diminishes plasma volume, blood volume, and cardiac output, and leads to hemocon-

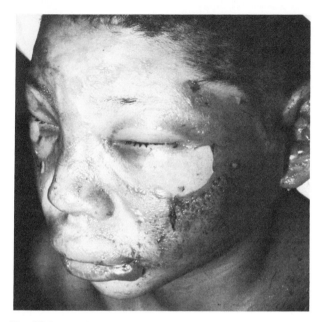

Fig. 37-5. Swelling caused by burn that healed without scar.

centration, hypotension, poor tissue perfusion, lactic acidemia, and metabolic acidosis. If treatment is inadequate or the patient does not respond to the resuscitative effort, acute renal failure supervenes and intravascular thrombi form as blood flow slows. Death ensues.

The rate of obligatory sequestration of fluid, maximal soon after injury, follows a descending parabolic curve. Sometime between 18 and 30 hours after injury microcirculatory integrity is restored. At this point edema is maximal. Then there is gradual resorption of edema concurrent with an increase in the intravascular volume, cardiac output, and urine. The diuresis continues at a steady pace until the patient returns to water balance, which occurs in 4 to 14 days depending upon the size of the burn. Some fluid is also lost from the body through the wound. During the period of resorption, there is an increased risk of congestive heart failure and pulmonary edema.

Urinary output is an important index of the adequacy of fluid resuscitation. Patients with biologically significant burns become oliguric unless they receive adequate fluid. Even with clinically acceptable urine flows, there is depression of renal plasma flow and a slight decrease in the glomerular filtration rate.

Although some of the red cell mass is destroyed during the injury, the hematocrit level and hemoglobin concentration are elevated because of the aforementioned hemoconcentration. Hemoglobinuria may occur. The serum potassium and sodium levels are usually normal. The serum bicarbonate and pH and Pco_2 of arterial blood are usually low, reflecting metabolic acidosis. If the Pa_{CO_2} is normal or elevated, it suggests either an associated inhalation injury or preexisting pulmonary insufficiency, and the prognosis is worse. The Pa_{O_2} is usually low to normal. The serum levels of BUN and creatinine are usually normal; an elevation suggests preexisting renal disease or a delay in treatment, implying a poorer prognosis.

Many systemic effects are associated with large surface and deep burns, for example, a circulating myocardial depressant factor, alterations in clotting mechanisms, suppression of leukocyte function, and alterations in immunological mechanisms. Some of these systemic effects are a consequence of released intracellular enzymes or "toxins" produced in heated tissues.

KINDS OF BURN
Solar (sunburn)

Sunburn is the result of a complex photochemical reaction caused by exposure to sunlight or an ultraviolet lamp. The burn is superficial and usually not biologically significant. An occasional patient will need to be admitted to the hospital for control of pain with analgesics and cool dressings. The worst cases result from sunlamps, especially when the victim falls asleep during exposure.

Flame

Injury by flame causes the greatest number of significant burns. When clothing burns, the exposure to heat is prolonged. This enhances the extent of injury, depth of injury, amount of skin grafting required, and mortality.

The pattern of burn sustained from a clothing fire is predictable and depends upon the flammability of cloth and style of clothing worn. For instance, the burn from a dress or nightgown classically extends from midthigh to the midportion of the face, whereas the major damage from a fire involving pants is below the level of the belt.

Scald

Patients with scalds have the same mortality rate as those with flame burns of the same extent. However, it is unusual for the surface area involved by a scald to be greater than one-third of the body.

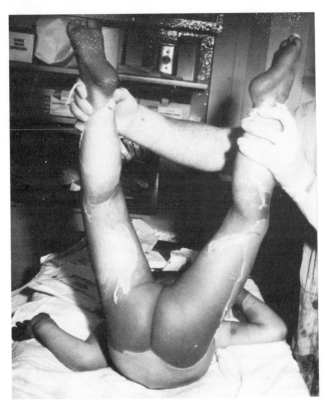

Fig. 37-6. Deep burn sustained while seated in bathtub when a sibling turned on hot water tap.

There are patterns of scalding that are easily recognized. Infants inadvertently placed in scalding bathwater sustain a burn of the lower portion of the body (Fig. 37-6). Toddlers who spill scalding liquids upon themselves sustain a unilateral burn. Occasionally, scalding liquids are thrown in the face for punishment; if they are laced with chemicals, devastating injuries to the eyes are a frequent result.

Heat contact

Except for immersion in molten metals, burns from heat contact are usually limited in extent and therefore are not an important cause of death. However, these burns are usually deep and often require skin grafting.

Chemical

The majority of serious chemical injuries occur in industrial accidents. The list of potentially injurious agents is infinite. They damage tissue in a variety of ways: coagulation of protein by reduction/oxidation, salt formation, corrosion, protoplasmic poisoning, metabolic competition, metabolic inhibition, desiccation, or ischemia. These agents can also be classified in chemical classes, i.e., acids, alkalis, and vesicants.

As long as the chemical is in contact and active, injury continues, increasing the depth. Therefore, as soon as practical, it is important to either wash the chemical away or neutralize it. The most beneficial first aid treatment is copious lavage with water. Lavage rather than soaking should be done, because if the diluent containing active chemical is not removed, the chemical may again come into contact with the patient. Beyond these principles, management of chemical burns is the same as for any other burn.

Electrical injury

Electricity causes a specialized form of thermal injury. Tissue damage is based on the amperage generated by the voltage delivered against the resistance of that tissue. Bone has the highest resistance, nerve tissue the least, and skin is in between. Damage also depends upon the course the electricity takes through the body. Entry is most often in the upper part of the body and exit through the feet.

Because the current frequently passes through the brain, temporary unconsciousness is common. Passage through the midbrain may result in respiratory or cardiac arrest or both. Electrical injury to the heart may cause ventricular fibrillation. In any event, cardiopulmonary resuscitation should be done because if it is successful the prognosis for life is good even among those with extensive electrical injury.

There are three categories of electrical injuries: those caused by low voltage (less than 1,000 volts), those caused by high voltage (1,000 volts or greater), and lightning.

In low voltage injury, which commonly occurs in the home, tissue damage is usually of small extent. However, when children chew on defective electrical cords and sustain full thickness necrosis of the lips, unsightly deformity may result. Cardiopulmonary arrest may occur during low-voltage accidents.

Young adult males at work are those almost exclusively involved in high voltage accidents. Tissue damage is usually great, especially at

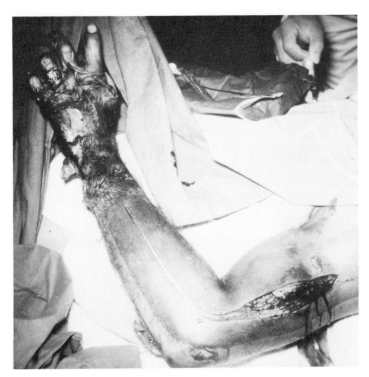

Fig. 37-7. High-voltage electrical injury. Obvious charring of hand and wrist. Incision through skin caused bleeding only in the mid-arm. The muscle in both arm and forearm was necrotic; shoulder disarticulation was necessary. The patient survived.

the site of entry (Fig. 37-7). Underlying muscle damage may be extensive and extend far beyond the area of skin injury; therefore, major amputation is often necessary. Extensive muscle injury results in high levels of myoglobinemia; therefore these patients are at risk for acute renal insufficiency.

The proper time to debride patients with deep necrosis is a matter of controversy. We believe the risk of, and the sequelae from, bacterial and clostridial myonecrosis are too great to treat these wounds expectantly. We advocate the following plan. Soon after admission the wounds are incised and the underlying muscle examined

Table 37-1. Burn mortality*

	Age in years		
Percent burn	*0-39*	*40-59*	*60-100*
10-29	2/138 = 1%	1/32 = 3%	1/30 = 23%
30-59	1/63 = 2%	5/15 = 33%	9/10 = 90%
60-79	10/25 = 40%	2/2 = 100%	7/7 = 100%
80-100	13/13 = 100%	7/7 = 100%	4/4 = 100%

*Burn mortality for 346 patients with burns of 10% of body surface or greater treated at the University of Iowa between April, 1970, and December, 1974. Number of deaths in numerator; number of patients in denominator.

(Fig. 37-7). If the muscle is viable, the wound is managed as any thermal burn. If the muscle is necrotic, plans are made for debridement in the operating room. We usually do not debride until the danger of acute renal failure is past. It may take several procedures to remove all the dead tissue.

Electrically injured patients have a high incidence of cataracts and neurological changes, although any organ or part of the body may be involved.

FACTORS THAT INFLUENCE PROGNOSIS
Depth of burn

Classification of depth of burns was discussed in the section on pathophysiology of the burn wound. The deeper the burn, the greater the mortality. If partial thickness burns are converted to full thickness by infection, the prognosis is much worse because of the increased risk of septicemia.

Age of the patient

Table 37-1 emphasizes the importance of age as a function of survival for burned patients. Although not shown in the table, burns are poorly tolerated by infants because of immature organ and immunological systems. Among the aged, the prognosis is poor because of associated degenerative disease and diminished properties of healing inherent in the aging process.

Surface area involved by burn

The greater the body surface area burned, the greater the mortality.

A rapid estimate of the surface area burned can be obtained by

674 *Synopsis of surgery*

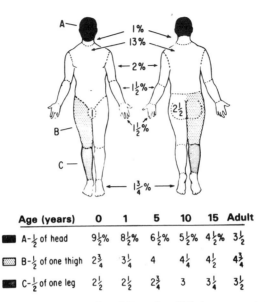

Age (years)	0	1	5	10	15	Adult
A-½ of head	9½%	8½%	6½%	5½%	4½%	3½
B-½ of one thigh	2¾	3¼	4	4¼	4½	4¾
C-½ of one leg	2½	2½	2¾	3	3¼	3½

Fig. 37-8. Modified from Lund and Browder. This is an accepted method to calculate surface area involved by burn. It takes into account that as one grows from infancy to adulthood the surface area of the head becomes relatively less and the surface area of the lower extremities becomes relatively greater.

applying the "rule of nines,"* but this rule is not accurate. The method of Lund and Browder (Fig. 37-8) gives a more accurate assessment.

Table 37-1 clearly illustrates the relationship between percent of burn and mortality. In general, patients with burns of less than 30% of the body surface survive if they are not too old. Furthermore, patients previously in good health and under 40 years of age with burns up to 80% of the body surface or under age 60 years with burns of less than 60% of the body surface have a good chance of survival. Survival beyond these ages and extents of injury may be possible, but is unusual. To try to improve survival, newer techniques are being

*Rule of nines: The body is divided into areas, each representing 9 or 18% (twice 9) of the body surface area: head and each upper extremity are 9%; anterior torso, back, and each lower extremity are 18%.

investigated, including staged excision of the burn with immediate coverage by donor related skin grafts, immunosuppressants to prolong homograft survival, new agents to control infection caused by gram-negative bacteria, fungi, and viruses, and improvements in nutritional and supportive care.

Preexisting medical conditions

Although patients with advanced degenerative, neoplastic, and other serious medical conditions have been successfully treated for burns, these conditions generally indicate a poorer prognosis. Burned patients with chronic renal disease, or those who develop renal impairment from whatever cause, have a poor prognosis. Burns are also poorly tolerated by the morbidly obese, primarily because of their diminished pulmonary reserve and the fact that obese people are not truly well nourished.

TREATMENT OF BURN SHOCK

Prevention of or resuscitation from burn shock is the most important item in the early management of a seriously burned patient. The timely administration of fluids to patients with large surface burns prevents death from burn shock. These fluids must contain sodium, but whether colloids are needed or even desirable is controversial.

Several formulas have been devised for calculating fluid requirements of the burned patient. These formulas are only guides, and each patient's response to treatment must be assessed repeatedly and adjustments made in fluid therapy.

The Brooke formula, published in 1953, is a modification of the Evans formula, which was described in 1952. According to the Brooke formula, the volume of fluid recommended for each of the first two 24-hour postburn periods is calculated from the body weight and the percent surface area of burn. A percentage of this fluid is given as crystalloid and a percentage as colloid.

Brooke formula

First 24 hours:
Crystalloid: 1.5 ml./kg. body weight/% burn as lacated Ringer's solution
Colloid: 0.5 ml./kg. body weight/% burn as plasma, Plasmanate, or Dextran
Maintenance: 2,000 ml. as 5% dextrose in water
Half the calculated volume is given during the first 8 hours, the other half during the next 16 hours
Second 24 hours:
Half of the first 24 hours calculated colloid and crystalloid
Maintenance: 2,000 ml. as 5% dextrose in water

To avoid fluid overload, the authors of these two formulas recommended that the initial estimate should not exceed the volume estimated for a 50% surface area burn. However, in actual practice, the calculation accurately predicts the fluid requirement for a burn of up to 50% of the body surface; above that the volumes increase linearly as the extent of burn increases.

Many patients are successfully resuscitated with balanced salt solution alone. This technique is based on the premise that the amount of sodium needed is the common denominator for successful resuscitation, and that colloid given during the first 18 to 24 hours after injury does not augment the plasma volume. However, after the leaky capillaries seal, colloid then augments the plasma volume by the amount of colloid given. The original technique of using balanced crystalloid developed by Moyer and co-workers has been modified by Baxter. The latter recommends 4 ml. lactated Ringer's solution/kg. body weight/% body surface burn, half of the calculated volume to be given in the first 8 hours and the rest over the next 16 hours. After all the calculated fluid has been given, the patient is evaluated for adequacy of resuscitation; if signs are less than optimal, the patient is cautiously given colloid (plasma) to expand the plasma volume.

By prospective study, we have found that adding albumin to lactated Ringer's solution to make a 2.3% solution of albumin reduces by one-third the amount of fluid and sodium needed for successful resuscitation when compared with lactated Ringer's solution alone (Table 37-2). Children require more fluid than adults with the same percent body surface burn. We did not find a difference in mortality among patients treated with the two solutions. However, there was a statistically significant reduction in complications of fluid therapy among those treated with the albumin in lactated Ringer's solution.

Table 37-2. Average volumes of fluid given in first 24 hours*

Age (years)	LR† ml./kg./% burn	LR + A‡ ml./kg./% burn
2-12	5.2	3.4
13-59	2.9	2.0

*Fluid volume data derived from 29 patients with burns in excess of 30% of the body surface who were successfully resuscitated and whose urinary output was maintained between 30 and 50 ml. per hour.
†Lactated Ringer's solution.
‡2.5% albumin in lactated Ringer's solution.

Most previously healthy young adults with burns of less than two-thirds of the body surface are successfully resuscitated by a variety of regimens. However, the following circumstances make treatment difficult: burns in excess of two-thirds of the body surface, extremes of age, premorbid impairment of the cardiovascular, respiratory, and renal systems, and delay in treatment. *It is also apparent that those physicians who attend their patients with frequent, careful, and knowledgeable assessment, making the necessary adjustments in therapy, have the best results.*

Our technique of fluid resuscitation

As soon as the patient is admitted, the extent of injury and the patient's overall condition are rapidly assessed. Children with burns of greater than 10% of the body surface and adults with burns of greater than 15% of the body surface receive intravenous fluids to prevent burn shock.

Immediately, a large-bore cannula is placed in a vein. If no practical unburned site is available, the cannula is inserted through burned tissue. Venous blood is obtained for laboratory studies and cross matching of blood. Arterial blood is obtained for measurement of pH and blood gases.

The urinary bladder is catheterized and the hourly urine volume is recorded. Because many burn patients develop paralytic ileus, a nasogastric tube is inserted to decompress the stomach and prevent vomiting and aspiration.

The fluid given intravenously is lactated Ringer's solution, to each liter of which is added 25 Gm. of albumin. Sodium bicarbonate is used to correct the inevitable metabolic acidosis.

Fluid is administered rapidly until urine flow is established and then is adjusted to maintain a urine flow of 30 to 50 ml. per hour, with corresponding but lesser amounts for children. The amount of fluid required to maintain circulation and the desired urine flow decrease gradually during the first day after injury. Our data on the volumes of fluid required during the first 24 hours are given in Table 37-2. These are averages; the actual amount needed varies with the individual.

Hourly assessments are made of urinary output, pH, and specific gravity; blood pressure; pulse rate and rhythm; respiratory rate; ease or difficulty of breathing; and the level of consciousness. From these observations and reexamination of the patient, the physician adjusts the rate of fluid administration and determines whether additional kinds of therapy or laboratory tests are needed.

Between 18 and 30 hours after injury the patient should be satisfactorily resuscitated. Shock persisting beyond this time is usually not the result of the burn and other causes should be sought, e.g., heart failure or renal failure. When the need for the intravenous cannula and urinary bladder catheter has been met, these should be removed to prevent infection. When the patient regains gastrointestinal function, oral alimentation is instituted.

COMMON EARLY BURN COMPLICATIONS
Edema

The circumferential eschar of a full thickness burn prevents expansion of fluid-laden tissues. If this occurs in an extremity, the blood vessels become compressed, leading to ischemia distally. This complication is heralded by cool, pale, painful, immobile digits with poor capillary refill and altered flow characteristics, or absent pulse signals by examination with a Doppler flowmeter. Treatment is by escharotomy, an incision through the eschar. This incision is painless because it is through full thickness burn, and bloodless because the deeper viable tissues are not incised. As the tissues are released the subcutaneous fat bulges through the incision, tension is relieved, and effective blood flow is usually restored.

A dense eschar surrounding the abdomen and chest may compromise ventilation as underlying edema increases. Relief of respiratory distress often follows release of the chest by escharotomy, permitting full respiratory excursions.

As a consequence of edema beneath a burn involving the neck, obstruction of the upper airway may occur. The symptoms are inspiratory stridor, intercostal retraction, tachypnea, and hypoxia. Although this may be treated successfully by escharotomy of the neck, an endotracheal tube or tracheostomy is usually necessary. When the edema resolves in 2 or 3 days, the tube is removed.

Inhalation injury

Inhalation injury is a devastating complication associated with high mortality. It is caused by inhaling noxious gases and most frequently occurs among those burned in closed spaces. Usually there is a symptom-free interval, then the onset of clinical manifestations may occur as late as 72 hours after the accident. The first signs and symptoms are tachypnea, dyspnea, and wheezes caused by bronchospasm. The arterial blood gases indicate slight respiratory acidosis and hypoxia. The chest roentgenogram is normal. Suggested treatment for this stage consists of humidified oxygen and large doses of steroids, although the therapeutic efficacy of steroids has not been proved.

If the attack is not aborted or if the exposure was severe, a chemical pneumonia manifested as pulmonary edema occurs, leading to progressive pulmonary insufficiency. If indicated, positive pressure ventilation is instituted. It may be as long as 3 weeks before the patient can be weaned from the ventilator. The principal complication of inhalation injury is superimposed bacterial pneumonia from secondary invading organisms. Since this occurs in virtually every patient, our treatment program includes antibiotics effective against both gram-positive and gram-negative bacteria.

TREATMENT OF THE BURN

After fluid resuscitation is begun and a complete history and physical examination are completed, attention is directed to the burn. The burn is gently cleansed, with removal of debris and dead skin. Topical therapy is then started.

Topical antibacterial therapy

The three most commonly used topical antibacterial agents are 0.5% silver nitrate solution, mafenide (Sulfamylon), and silver sulfadiazine. Each agent has advantages and disadvantages; however, each improves survival by reducing invasive infection of the wound, septicemia, and conversion of partial thickness to full thickness burns. Among the three agents there is no statistically significant difference in patient survival.

Silver nitrate

Ionic silver inhibits bacterial growth by binding with sulfhydryl and other chemical groups in bacterial enzyme systems and with deoxyribonucleic acid. Silver in 0.5% concentration has no appreciable adverse effect on regenerating epithelium or skin grafts. When the concentration of silver approaches 0.1%, it is bacteriologically ineffective; when it approaches 1.0%, it produces tissue damage (escharotic agent).

Silver nitrate is not a universal bacteriostatic agent; it has little if any effect on the paracolon, *Klebsiella-Aerobacter,* and clostridial species. It is effective against *Staphylococcus aureus,* hemolytic streptococcus, *Pseudomonas aeruginosa,* and *Escherichia coli.*

The dressings consist of approximately 20 thicknesses of coarse mesh gauze, held in place with elastic gauze bandage, which is then covered with stockinette (Fig. 37-9). The dressings are saturated and kept continuously wet with 0.5% silver nitrate solution. The patient is covered with a dry blanket to reduce heat loss by vaporization. This keeps the patient comfortable. In most instances, the dressings are changed once each day.

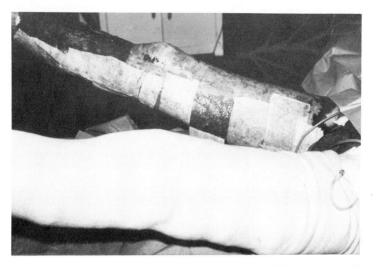

Fig. 37-9. Clean granulation tissue on posterior medial aspect of right thigh and leg covered with biological dressing of pigskin. The left leg shows completed dressing used for 0.5% silver nitrate.

Since silver nitrate in a concentration of 0.5% is hypotonic (29.4 mEq./L.), the principal biological danger is depletion of salt by diffusion across the burn. In children this may occur rapidly. This complication is prevented by administration of sodium (sodium chloride), potassium (potassium gluconate), and bicarbonate (sodium bicarbonate), usually by mouth. Depletion of serum calcium and magnesium may occur in large burns. Argyria does not develop. Instances of methemoglobinemia have been reported. Another problem with silver nitrate solution is the large number of dressings it requires; in addition, it imparts a black stain to floors, walls, clothing, and skin when exposed to light.

Mafenide (Sulfamylon)

Mafenide acetate is used in 10% concentration in a water-soluble ointment. In this concentration it has a wide bacteriostatic effect against many gram-positive and gram-negative organisms, including *Pseudomonas aeruginosa* and clostridia. This drug is unique among sulfonamides, inasmuch as its efficacy is not reduced by blood or exudate. It is not an effective systemic antibiotic; crystalluria does not occur.

The patient is treated by the open technique. Mafenide is spread in a layer, 0.5 mm. thick, twice daily. If a burn covered with mafenide is not exposed to air, maceration and invasive infection may occur. Therefore, patients with burns on both sides of the body must be turned frequently. Since this drug inhibits healing, application is stopped when all necrotic tissue has been removed.

Mafenide permeates the eschar and is continuously absorbed. It is a strong carbonic anhydrase inhibitor, which accounts for its biological danger. Mafenide induces a bicarbonate diuresis and impairs renal tubular function in maintaining normal pH of blood. Hence the lungs assume the primary role in maintaining normal pH by expelling carbon dioxide. Most patients are hyperpneic. If pulmonary function is impaired by atelectasis or pneumonia, a dangerous acidosis may ensue. If this occurs mafenide must be stopped and measures taken to improve pulmonary function. Patients often complain of a transient burning sensation when the drug is applied. The incidence of allergic skin reaction is approximately 6%, but these reactions are usually controlled with antihistaminics, permitting treatment to continue.

Silver sulfadiazine

Silver sulfadiazine was approved by the Food and Drug Administration for topical burn therapy in 1974. The binding of silver to sulfadiazine apparently prevents inactivation of sulfadiazine in the wound. As the silver binds with DNA of a bacterium, the sulfonamide moiety is released.

Silver sulfadiazine has wide antibacterial activity. Although the current major pathogens—*Pseudomonas aeruginosa, Enterobacter aerogenes, Escherichia coli,* and proteus species—can be cultured from biopsy samples of wounds treated with this agent, it is as effective in inhibiting bacterial growth and invasive infection as the other topical agents in use. Early colonization of wounds with penicillinase producing *Staphylococcus aureus* requires systemic treatment with a penicillinase-resistant antibiotic.

Silver sulfadiazine can be used by the semiopen or closed technique. The agent is usually applied twice a day. The major advantage of silver sulfadiazine is absence of the biological dangers that exist with 0.5% silver nitrate and mafenide.

Other topical agents

Gentamicin sulfate cream, silver lactate ointment, silver nitrate cream, and Betadine are occasionally used as topical antibacterial agents for treating burns.

Surgical care of the burn

Topical antibacterial agents are adjuncts in the therapy of burns and are not substitutes for meticulous care of the wound based on well-established surgical principles.

Several days after the burn injury, when the patient's condition is stable, daily hydrotherapy is begun. The patient is immersed in tepid water to loosen eschar and to aid in physical therapy. Because of danger of fluid and electrolyte imbalance from diffusion across the burned surface, the period of immersion should not exceed 20 minutes. Many agents, including a variety of detergents, dilute sodium hypochlorite, etc., have been used in the bath water to prevent growth of bacteria. There is no evidence that these agents or hydrotherapy improve survival.

During the bath, or immediately after, the burn is debrided. Only loose, necrotic tissue is removed, and this debridement should not

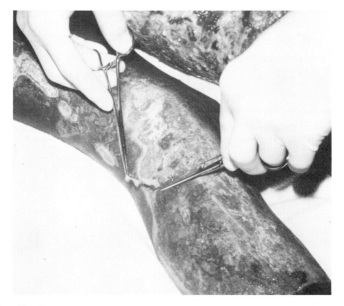

Fig. 37-10. Debridement of loose eschar should not produce pain or bleeding. The wound is debrided daily until all necrotic material is removed, leaving a clean granulation tissue surface, as shown in Fig. 37-9.

produce pain or bleeding (Fig. 37-10). It usually takes 3 to 5 weeks
for the eschar to completely separate. In many instances the debridement is completed in the operating room with the patient anesthetized.

After removing the eschar there remains a base of granulation
tissue, which is an excellent barrier to invasive infection. A decision is
now made whether a particular area will reepithelize from epidermal
appendages or whether it requires autogenous skin grafting. This
decision requires judgment based on experience. Many burn surgeons
use a biological dressing to protect surfaces that will epithelize spontaneously or to prepare surfaces for skin grafting.

Biological dressings

Biological dressings consist of allograft or xenograft and are used
to temporarily cover wounds in place of conventional dressings. Commonly employed materials are human cadaver skin, human fetal membranes, and pigskin.

Viable allograft of split thickness skin has been used for many years
in treating burn patients. The skin, usually from a cadaver, is placed on
a clean surface of granulation tissue. This in effect closes the wound
and improves the patient's overall condition.

Advantages of a biological dressing include:
1. It reduces fluid and protein loss from the wound to improve
   the patient's nutritional condition
2. Wounds become pain free
3. It inhibits bacterial growth
4. It enhances healing of partial thickness burns
5. Adherence of the biological dressing ensures a favorable wound
   for autografting

If the allograft skin is allowed to adhere it will then become
vascularized, followed by rejection in 1 to 3 weeks; not only must the
wound be prepared again for skin grafting, but the patient's overall
condition worsens because of the physiological sequelae of rejection.
However, if the allograft skin is used only as a temporary dressing,
all the benefits derived from closing the wound can be realized without any of the adverse effects of rejection. The technique is as follows.
After removing the eschar, allograft skin is placed on the granulation
tissue. If adherence does not occur, new allograft is placed. When
adherence does take place, the allograft is changed every 2 to 5 days
until it becomes feasible to use autogenous skin grafts (Fig. 37-9).
The allograft is allowed to remain on a partial thickness burn since
it protects the viable epidermal appendages; as epithelization occurs,
the allograft will slough.

The demand for allograft skin is great and at times the supply is limited. An effective alternate is porcine xenograft skin. This material in the nonviable form is available commercially and is in wide use. Fetal membrane is a readily available material used by some burn surgeons as a temporary biological dressing. Fetal membrane is thought to be superior to nonviable porcine skin and as efficacious as viable cadaver skin.

Excision of burns

Some surgeons excise and graft burns immediately (autograft or biological dressing) to rapidly close the wound and shorten the hospital course. This principle has been employed with some success in patients with large surface burns whose mortality is essentially 100% when treated by conventional means. This management has merit, provided the patients are carefully selected.

Usually it is difficult to determine accurately the depth of injury in the immediate postburn period, and immediate excision may unnecessarily remove skin that is not burned deeply. Furthermore, there is a limit to the area that can be safely excised at one sitting, believed to range from 15 to 20% of the body surface. Generally, excision is performed down to the fascia; however, excision by shaving down to the point of bleeding (tangential excision) is advocated by some.

Considerations for operations on burn patients

Hypothermia is a major factor limiting the duration of operations done on burn patients. To prevent this complication a warm operating room or heat shield is employed, parts of the body not being operated upon are covered, blood is given through a warmer, and every effort is made to limit the operation to 2 hours.

The recent development of dissociative anesthetics (e.g., ketamine hydrochloride) is an important advance for burn patients, especially the critically ill. These agents depress respiration much less than inhalation anesthetics and consequently lessen postoperative pulmonary complications. Also, because vital reflexes (e.g., gag reflex) are better maintained, aspiration is rare. Patients do not develop ileus from dissociative anesthetics and oral alimentation can be restarted as soon as the patient emerges from the ansethetic. Operations on the face and neck are facilitated because this anesthetic technique does not require an endotracheal tube, airway, or mask. A disadvantage is the hallucinogenic potential, which is minmized with proper preanesthetic medication.

Most seriously ill burn patients require blood replacement during operation.

Failure of skin graft to "take" is disastrous. Not only does the grafted wound remain open but the partial thickness skin injury created in the donor site adds to the area of open wound. Skin grafts fail because of (1) slippage of the graft; (2) foreign material under the graft (blood, serum, necrotic tissue, suture material); or (3) infection: (a) streptolysin produced by the group A beta hemolytic streptococcus dissolves skin grafts, or (b) 100,000 organisms or greater per gram of tissue usually signifies invasive infection.

Donor sites must be properly healed and free of foreign material such as AgNO$_3$ crusts. Donor sites can be treated in a variety of ways but are best managed the same way the patient's burns are being treated. Currently the most popular dermatomes used to obtain split thickness skin grafts are those driven by air or electricity. Grafts are cut as thin as possible, yet thick enough so as not to tear with careful handling. There are several methods to expand available skin to cover large surfaces. The most popular instrument for this purpose is the Tanner-Vandeput mesh machine, which makes a series of cuts in the donor skin so that it is stretched out as lace.

COMMON LATE BURN COMPLICATIONS
Infection

Infection is the most frequent cause of death in burn patients; pneumonia and septicemia account for over half the deaths.

The responsible organism causing death in burn victims has changed in recent decades. Prior to the 1940's, the *group A beta hemolytic streptococcus* was the primary offender. This organism colonized the edematous tissues within a few days after injury and death rapidly ensued. Death from this organism has been virtually eliminated by penicillin.

In the 1950's hemolytic *Staphylococcus aureus,* especially those which produce penicillinase, emerged as the most dangerous organisms to the burn patient. However, penicillinase-resistant penicillin has greatly reduced this threat.

During the 1960's organisms once thought to be of low-grade pathogenicity emerged as serious threats to burned patients. The most important group is the gram-negative bacilli, especially *Pseudomonas aeruginosa.* However, any bacterium, fungus, or virus can gain a foothold in a burned patient to produce clinical infection. As a matter of fact, since more effective measures against the gram-negative bacilli have been developed, fungi (particularly *Candida albicans*) have become more important.

The risk of invasive infection varies with the extent of burn and the age of the patient. That is to say, each patient has the immunological capability and metabolic reserve to tolerate a certain amount of thermal injury and when that limit is exceeded the patient is at high risk for infection. When the burn is less than 30% of the body surface the risk of septicemia is small; but when the burn exceeds 30% of the body surface the risk is great and increases exponentially thereafter. The aged and infants are at much greater risk for septicemia than are older children and young adults.

Within several days of injury, pathogens can be cultured from the wounds of patients who are not treated with effective topical chemotherapeutic agents. However, if effective agents are used, colonization of the wound is delayed, colony counts are reduced, and different organisms are recovered.

Serious infection occurs much earlier and in a more insidious fashion than is generally appreciated. Among burn patients who eventually die of septicemia, gram-negative bacteremia is common during the first week. The clinical manifestations of the septicemia are at first subtle, but then become overwhelming during the second week. If treatment is ineffective, death will likely ensue during the third week.

It is crucial to recognize the early, subtle manifestations of septicemia, because if one waits for overt signs before obtaining blood cultures, and then waits for positive bacteriological proof before starting appropriate therapy, the patient will be irretrievable. Therefore, treatment is instituted on the clinical suspicion of septicemia and a reasonable prediction of the most likely offending organism or organisms.

Important early manifestations of septicemia are:
1. Core temperature greater than $39°$ C., or hypothermia
2. Leukocyte count of greater than 20,000 cells per mm.^{3}, or leukopenia
3. Gastroduodenal bleeding or perforation
4. Azotemia with blood urea nitrogen level greater than 30 mg.%
5. Anemia, or failure to maintain a normal hemoglobin
6. Change in sensorium
7. Ileus, often heralded by anorexia
8. Gain of body weight in conjunction with a decrease in caloric intake

Presence of two of these eight manifestations provides enough suspicion of septicemia to justify obtaining the necessary cultures and beginning appropriate therapy.

The more common sources of burn sepsis are: the burn wound (invasive infection), veins (septic thrombophlebitis), lungs (aspiration pneumonia, hypostatic pneumonia, tracheobronchitis from tracheostomy), and urinary tract (inlying urinary bladder catheter, pyelonephritis).

Prevention and treatment of burn infection

Burns are tetanus prone wounds; burned patients should be immunized.

The burn wound should be covered with one of the topical antibacterial agents. There is no statistical evidence that any one is superior to another.

Since the major contributing factor to burn sepsis is the large volume of necrotic tissue in the wound, daily inspection and debridement are mandatory.

All burn patients should receive penicillin for several days to prevent infection from *group A beta hemolytic streptococcus,* but beyond this the role of antibiotics is controversial. Most authorities advocate antibiotics for a specific indication of infection. All agree that every patient with burns of more than 30% of the body surface demands one or more antibiotics during treatment. Burn therapists must keep current with developments in the field of antibiotics, and know the contemporary indigenous microorganisms of their burn unit or hospital.

Curling's ulcer

Hemorrhage from "stress," or Curling's ulcer, is a classical complication of a severely burned patient. The ulcers, located in either stomach or duodenum, are usually multiple, round, punched out, and often painless. Frequently ileus precedes massive bleeding; septicemia predisposes to stress ulcer. Often there is no prior history of acid-peptic disease. Preventive measures are of questionable value, and are those commonly prescribed for patients with peptic ulcer disease. Those who use large volumes of milk for nutritional purposes believe their patients have a lower incidence of this complication. Perforation and excessive bleeding are indications for operative treatment.

Scars and contractures

The principal late complications of burns are hypertrophic scars and contractures. These entities are defined in the section on pathophysiology of the wound.

Hypertrophic scars (Fig. 37-3) are dynamic lesions in which the disordered collagen tends to realign into a more orderly and linear pattern. With time the scar gradually loses its erythema, becomes softer and more pliable, and usually flat. This process is known as *maturation* of the scar. At times, all the hypertrophic qualities do not disappear and the scar remains raised. Maturation is thought to be hastened by applying pressure, usually via a rubber elastic bandage or a custom-made elastic garment.

Recently healed or grafted burns often itch, frequently to an annoying extent, because of a mild sterile inflammatory reaction.

Symptoms are relieved by antipruritic medication and aspirin. The itching gradually disappears within 18 months.

Contraction is a factor in the healing of all wounds, and burns are no exception. When preventive care is inadequate and at times even when preventive care seems adequate, contractures occur. The major sites of contracture are the neck, axilla, antecubital fossa (Fig. 37-4), and hand; however, any joint may be involved. Contractures of the face are particularly dangerous: eyelid contracture may expose the cornea with all its horrible sequelae; mouth contracture may produce microstomia, which makes eating, oral hygiene, and dental manipulations difficult and the conduct of anesthesia excessively dangerous.

Prevention of contractures is the key. This includes proper splinting in the anticontracture position (e.g., elbows extended) and conscientious physical exercise until the danger of contracture is past. If a contracture develops, splinting may reverse the process, but in most instances operative release of the contracture is needed.

Among the severe and extensively burned, it takes about 2 years to complete scar maturation and necessary reconstructive procedures.

A late and infrequent complication of burns is a *Marjolin's ulcer*-- a cancer arising in an old scar.

Emotional problems

A severe burn is emotionally devastating. This is true not only for the patient but for his family as well.

Virtually all patients with burns manifest emotional symptoms, including depression, regression, anxiety, excessive sensitivity, emotional lability, insomnia, and phobias. The severity of symptoms depends upon the patient's premorbid emotional maturity and the length of hospitalization, i.e., the symptoms are worse among those with the larger burn and more immature personality. Delirium and frank psychosis are common among the severely burned, especially during septicemia. In most instances the psychosis abates as the patient's burns heal and his condition improves.

During fluid resuscitation, edema of the eyelids frequently prevents the patient from opening his eyelids, and the patient believes that he is blind. The patient must be reassured that in a few days he will be able to open his eyes and see again. Males with scrotal edema often believe themselves to be impotent; this, of course, is not true. The greatest fear among the burned is deformity and mutilation. In many instances this is justifiable, and professional psychiatric help may be needed.

The overall emotional prognosis for adults is not as poor as previously thought. For instance, if an adult is emotionally mature prior to his injury, he likely will reattain emotional maturity again. The traumatic neurosis from the burn usually resolves by 1 year after injury. However, individuals with pathological emotional symptoms prior to injury often develop a permanent traumatic neurosis, and their emotional problem is compounded. The prognosis among children is not good, especially among those with noticeable disfigurement. They do poorly because their emotional development is interrupted by the burn and they must face life with the emotional problems that attend deformity.

In dealing with the burn patient's family it is essential that they be realistically appraised of the prognosis, both for life and for deformity. Unrealistic encouragement should not be given. We believe it important that the family visit the patient frequently and help with the nonprofessional aspects of the patient's care, especially feeding. This assures the patient that he has not been abandoned by his loved ones.

Nutrition

A large surface burn probably causes a greater catabolic stress than any other disease or injury. Tissue breakdown and exhaustion of body stores occur extremely rapidly unless measures are taken to preserve nutritional integrity. The metabolic activity of a burned patient is reset at a higher level and does not return to normal until after the wounds are closed. Contributing factors include an increase in metabolic rate, core temperature, and wound temperature, increased levels of glucagon, catecholamines, and free fatty acids, and loss of body weight.

The catabolic process is augmented by a variety of stimuli, the most serious of which is infection. Cold, pain, anxiety, and hypovolemia are all potent catabolic stimuli mediated through augmented catecholamine response. Much has recently been written about vaporizational heat loss contributing to the metabolic demands of the burned. This is minimized by nursing these patients in a temperature environment similar to that of the wound by using heat lamps or shields, and by dressing techniques similar to those described for 0.5% silver nitrate.

An adult with a large surface burn requires approximately 2,000 kilocalories per square meter of body surface area each day. Infants and young children require more. Most patients refuse to eat this much food because of anorexia, making tube feedings necessary. Some advocate central venous hyperalimentation, but the risk of infection with this technique is great.

In actual practice, the patient's nutritional situation must be repeatedly assessed. When the initial ileus has resolved, the proper number of calories is given by mouth. If the patient's body weight and nutritional integrity cannot be maintained on the prescribed diet, the diet or method of delivery or both should be altered. If the patient does not gradually excrete the fluid load given for resuscitation or subsequently gains weight in the face of a decrease in caloric intake, one should suspect septicemia.

COLD INJURIES

Freezing induces tissue injury equally severe to that produced by burns. Exposure to cold induces vasoconstriction of arterioles and small arteries with consequent local tissue hypoxia. In addition, cold produces direct tissue injury. As with burns, frostbite injury can be quantitated by the degree of damage provoked: superficial damage (first-degree), partial damage to the dermis (second-degree), and complete damage to the dermis (third-degree).

Frostbitten tissue initially feels numb and begins to ache in the rewarming process. The feet, nose, ears, and hands are most commonly involved because these parts are exposed most to cold and are located peripherally in the circulatory system. Initial redness of the skin is followed by a pale or waxy whiteness in a few hours. The area then becomes bluish-red and swollen. Vesicle formation and areas of eschar indicate severe damage; a thick black eschar marks third-degree stages. Wetness of the area, such as immersion of the extremities, exaggerates the damage. However, since most civilian cold injuries occur in a dry atmosphere, actual freezing is uncommon, except in alcoholics who fall asleep in the cold.

Treatment

The emergency management requires removing all clothing, with rapid rewarming of the injured part by immersion in water at 34° to 40° C. Blisters are covered with a dry dressing to prevent contamination. Silver nitrate (0.5% solution) achieves the same end. Bed rest is mandatory until edema resolves and demarcation of tissues has occurred. Areas of gangrene either undergo autoamputation or the surgeon anticipates the demarcation line and amputates to save hospital time. During this period necrotic tissue is debrided. Antibiotic therapy helps prevent massive infection.

CHAPTER 38

Orthopedics

REGINALD R. COOPER

Orthopedics encompasses the investigation, preservation, and restoration of form and function of the musculoskeletal system and related structures. Orthopedists employ medical, surgical, and physical methods of treatment.

Numerous conditions affect the musculoskeletal system, but I will discuss only the common ones that involve most orthopedic patients seen in clinical practice. These disorders can be categorized according to etiology as follows:

1. Congenital and developmental
2. Infectious and inflammatory
3. Traumatic
4. Metabolic
5. Neoplastic
6. Neuromuscular
7. Degenerative
8. Mechanical and postural
9. Idiopathic

Some disorders involve only one region, but others are not so restricted.

ORTHOPEDIC EVALUATION OF A PATIENT

Medical, emotional, social, and economic factors influence the patient with an orthopedic disorder. The astute physician considers each of these in its proper perspective.

The patient who seeks the advice of an orthopedist usually complains of one or more of the following: (1) something feels wrong (pain, numbness, tenderness); (2) something looks wrong (deformity, limp, bump); or (3) something moves wrong (limp, weakness, stiffness, instability).

If the disorder is localized, complaints often remain in the involved part; however, pain can be referred to a remote site (knee pain from hip disease). A lesion that irritates a peripheral nerve produces pain in the area supplied by the nerve (pain in the lower extremity from a herniated lumbar intervertebral disc). In the back and extremities, protective muscle contraction frequently produces symptoms at a distance from the disease.

With the doctor's guidance, the patient must relate a pertinent, integrated, chronological history of all complaints. Important questions about pain include the following: What are the circumstances surrounding its onset? What is its progression? Was the onset associated with injury? Was it sudden or gradual? Was this the first episode? Has the pain been continuous? Is it sharp or dull, superficial or deep? What relieves it? What makes it worse? Does it interfere with function or sleep?

A similar chronology must be documented for complaints other than pain.

A normal opposite part serves as a valuable comparison during an examination of a patient with a musculoskeletal problem. Depending on the involved region, the physician can modify the following physical examination outline:

Joints

Inspection: In what position is the joint held? Is this normal? What is the joint contour? Is it swollen? Is the overlying skin normal? Are there discolorations, venous distensions, trophic changes, cuts, scars?

Palpation: Is there tenderness? Does it feel hot or cold? Is there excessive joint fluid? Can a fluid wave be balloted? Is the synovium thickened? Are all the ligaments intact? Is there unstable, abnormal motion?

Range of motion:

Active: Is it limited? If so, why? Is there pain, muscle spasm, contracture (fixed, spasm), bony block? In what direction is the limitation? Record range of motion in degrees.

Passive: Can you move the joint through a greater range than the patient can? If so, is muscle torn, paralyzed, or reflexly inhibited? Record range of motion in degrees.

Muscles

Does each one contract?

What is its strength?

Grade 5, normal, 100%—range of motion against full resistance

Grade 4, good, 75%—range of motion against some resistance

Grade 3, fair, 50%—range of motion against gravity
Grade 2, poor, 25%—range of motion with gravity eliminated
Grade 1, trace, 10%—slight contraction, no motion
Grade 0—no contraction
Is there measurable atrophy or enlargement?
Compare limb circumference with the opposite side. Find the same level on two sides by measuring from a *fixed* part to a given site. *Example:* To find thigh circumference, measure 6 or 7 inches proximal to the tibial tubercle (a fixed part), not from the patella (a movable part).

Does the tendon glide freely? Is it tender? Is it intact?

Are there masses in muscle or tendon?

Bone

Is the integrity maintained? Stability, crepitus (grating of bone fragments on each other).

Is it obviously deformed? Angulated, curved.

Is it of normal size? Length, width.

Is it in proper relation to other bones?

Is it tender?

Is the overlying skin normal?

Are any masses present? If so, note type, location, size, consistency, fixed or free, pulsatile, bruit, transillumination.

Neurological examination

Motor, sensory, reflexes.

Vascular: Skin changes of vascular insufficiency, pulses, veins, masses, bruit.

Function

Put the part through voluntary motions of everyday activities.

Gait: Is it normal? If not, what abnormal components are present? (Short leg limp, hip abductor weakness—lurch to involved side, hip dislocation, waddle.)

Roentgenograms are usually necessary, if not mandatory, for complete evaluation of a complaint related to the musculoskeletal system. Comparable views of the opposite normal side sometimes aid in making a diagnosis.

REGIONAL ORTHOPEDICS
Neck (Table 38-1)
Torticollis (wry neck, congenital muscular torticollis)

A fibrotic, contracted sternocleidomastoid muscle tilts the head to the ipsilateral side and turns the face to the contralateral side (Fig.

Table 38-1. Disorders of the neck

Age	Disorder	Etiology
Birth to 2 yr.	Torticollis	Developmental
4-8	Acute wry neck	Trauma or inflammatory
Adult	Stiff neck	Inflammatory?
	Degenerative joint disease (cervical spine arthritis, degenerative disc disease, cervical spondylosis)	Degenerative
	Acute sprain	Traumatic

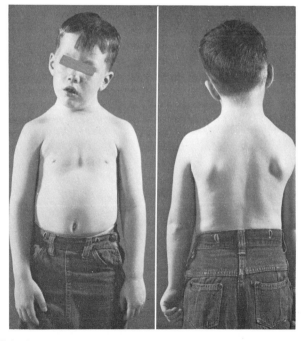

Fig. 38-1. Congenital torticollis. The head tilts to the side of the fibrotic sternocleidomastoid muscle, and the face turns to the opposite side.

38-1). Etiology remains unknown. Theories include birth trauma, muscle fibrosis, and abnormal muscular development. Many involved babies were breech presentations. About 3 weeks after birth, the parents find a lump in the child's sternocleidomastoid muscle. The mass disappears in a few weeks, and some of these infants later develop torticollis. Some afflicted children had no noticeable mass. Asymmetry of face and skull bones accompanies torticollis.

The parents should stretch the tight muscle gently each day. They should position the bottle and toys so that the baby turns to them in a way that stretches the tight sternocleidomastoid muscle. Many cases correct spontaneously and do not develop a wry neck. Marked persistent deformity at age 2 or 3 warrants excision of a segment of the contracted muscle. Much of the asymmetry disappears with subsequent face and head growth.

Any of the following can produce torticollis: hemivertebra and other cervical spine abnormalities, visual disturbances in which the patient tilts his head to see better, acute cervical lymphadenopathy that causes the patient to tilt his head to relieve pain.

Acute wry neck

Children develop acute wry neck because of cervical lymphadenopathy associated with acute pharyngitis or because of rotatory subluxation of the cervical spine. A history of acute onset differentiates either from congenital muscular torticollis.

At times during acute pharyngitis, hyperemia and inflammation around cervical spine ligaments allow rotatory subluxation of cervical spine facets. Treatment consists of appropriate therapy of the primary disorder, head halter traction to realign facets, and postreduction immobilization for 2 or 3 weeks in a cervical collar.

Occasionally a child suddenly twists his neck, hears a click, experiences sharp neck pain, and locks in a twisted position. An open mouth roentgenogram of C1-C2 demonstrates a subluxated facet of C1 on C2. Head halter traction with the spine in neutral or slight flexion reduces the subluxation. The child should wear a collar or brace for 3 weeks.

Stiff neck

A person who has slept with his neck twisted or one who has been in cold air often complains of a stiff neck. He holds his head rigidly inclined to the involved side and complains of sore, tender neck muscles. Neck motion produces pain. Etiology is unknown. Some believe an inflammatory myositis produces stiff neck. With heat, analgesics, rest, and support by a collar or traction, symptoms subside in 5 to 10 days.

Degenerative joint disease (cervical spine arthritis, degenerative disc disease, cervical spondylosis)

In this disorder, intervertebral discs and cervical facets degenerate. Spurs of bone and inflammation adjacent to discs, intervertebral body joints, and facets impinge cervical nerve roots at one or more levels. At times, degeneration occurs after trauma, but it can arise spontaneously. Symptoms vary from mild to severe. Frequently, pain radiates from the neck to the head or upper extremities. Pain and paresthesias can follow a nerve root distribution. Persistent nerve root irritation causes reflex sympathetic nerve stimulation with blurred vision, loss of balance, and headaches. Often, the patient inclines the head away from the painful side to get temporary relief. Neck motion decreases.

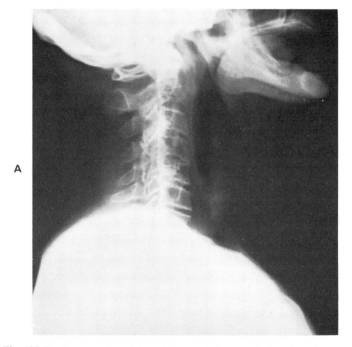

Fig. 38-2. Degenerative joint disease of the cervical spine. **A,** Lateral view. The normal cervical curve is gone, and the C4-C5 disc space is narrow. **B,** Oblique view. Degenerative spurs have narrowed intervertebral foramina.

Pressure over spinous tips and longitudinal compression of the spine produce pain. Reflexes and sensation decrease. Radiographic examinations help in localizing the level(s) of disc narrowing and spur formation (Fig. 38-2).

Periods of rest, pillows designed to support the cervical spine in neutral position or extension, moist heat, salicylates, intermittent head halter traction (7 pounds, 15 minutes, 3 times a day), and night head halter traction often relieve symptoms. If conservative measures fail, the patient might need surgery. Depending on the severity and location of the disorder, surgeons can remove the disc, enlarge the foramina, and/or fuse the cervical spine.

Cervical disc herniation can produce motor loss, decreased reflexes, and sensory loss that follows a definite nerve root pattern. Myelograms help confirm the diagnosis and localize the level. (See discussion on disc herniation, Chapter 40.)

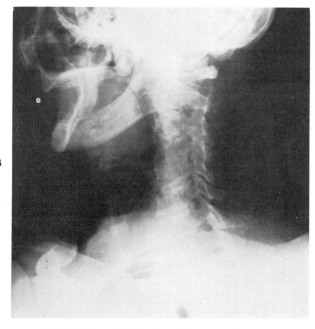

B

Fig. 38-2, cont'd. For legend see opposite page.

Acute sprain

Cervical sprains concern the legal profession about as much as they concern the medical profession. The occupant of an automobile struck from the rear often sustains neck injury. Some patients have immediate neck pain, but others have none for 12 to 36 hours. Patients complain of diffuse pain over the posterior surface of the neck and head. Protective muscle contraction decreases neck motion in an attempt to prevent pain. At times, patients develop sore muscles, stiff neck, severe pain, vertigo, nausea, headache, and paresthesias. Symptoms tend to be intermittent and frequently persist for months but subside eventually in most instances.

Interspinous ligaments and neck and shoulder muscles are tender. Cervical spine motion decreases. Decreased sensation in the upper extremities usually does not follow a well-defined nerve distribution and varies from examination to examination. Definite, severe, and persistent neurological signs should lead one to suspect more than ligamentous and/or muscular damage. Roentgenograms are usually normal but *must be taken* to rule out fracture and/or dislocation.

Analgesics, heat, rest, massage, and mild head halter traction for 2 to 10 days often relieve acute symptoms. If so, the patient should gradually increase neck motion as symptoms decrease. Many patients with persistent symptoms have pending lawsuits. Doctors often speculate about the relation of symptoms to insurance settlements.

Shoulder (Table 38-2)
Fractured clavicle

The clavicle is the bone most frequently fractured during delivery. It begins ossification before other long bones, and the shoulders are the widest part of a newborn's body. When an examiner attempts to

Table 38-2. Disorders of the shoulder

Age	Disorder	Etiology
Birth to 2	Fractured clavicle	Trauma
	Brachial palsy (obstetric palsy)	Trauma
2–4	Pulled shoulder	Trauma
Adult	Rotator cuff degeneration (acute bursitis, noncalcific or calcific; rotator cuff disease)	Degenerative
	Frozen shoulder (adhesive pericapsulitis)	Degenerative
	Acute rupture of the rotator cuff	Trauma and degenerative
	Snapping scapula	Inflammatory (?) Degenerative (?)

elicit a Moro reflex, the baby with a fractured clavicle does not move the arm on the involved side. Brachial plexus injury, fracture of the humerus, and dislocated shoulder produce a similar sign.

No reduction is necessary. Strapping the baby's arm to his chest for 7 to 10 days relieves discomfort. A lump of callus appears within a few days, disappears during the ensuing weeks, and full function returns.

Brachial palsy (obstetric palsy)

Mechanical stretch of the brachial plexus during delivery paralyzes various muscles of the upper extremity and produces loss of sensation in the distribution of involved nerves. Nerves remain intact but stretched, or they rupture completely. The infant does not move the involved arm or forearm. Signs depend upon anatomic location of the lesion. In the common upper arm type of Erb-Duchenne (caused by downward traction on the shoulder), an injury of C-5,6 nerve roots paralyzes deltoid, supraspinatus, infraspinatus, and biceps muscles. The arm adducts and internally rotates, and the forearm pronates. In the lower arm paralysis of Klumpke (caused by upward traction with the arm overhead), an injury of C-8 and T-1 paralyzes intrinsic muscles of the hand and/or the long finger flexors. In the whole-arm type, various combinations of paralyses lead to severe dysfunction.

During the months after birth, the infant usually improves but seldom recovers completely. Prognosis is best in the upper-arm type. Treatment soon after birth prevents contractures. Each day the child's shoulder should be moved passively into abduction and external rotation, and the forearm into supination. In older cases, release of contractures, transfer of tendons, and osteotomies might improve function.

Pulled shoulder

Occasionally a parent grabs a child by the hand and pulls him onto a curb or in a given direction. The infant has immediate pain and refuses to move his arm. His shoulder is tender. If roentgenograms reveal no fracture, the child probably has a partial tear of the shoulder capsule and bleeding into the joint. Rest of the part for a few days by strapping the arm to the body relieves symptoms. If left to his own devices, with pain as his guide, the child will regain motion in his arm. No physical therapy is needed.

Rotator cuff degeneration (acute bursitis, noncalcific or calcific; rotator cuff disease)

The rotator cuff, composed of the supraspinatus, infraspinatus, teres minor, and subscapular muscles, holds the head of the humerus downward and medially against the glenoid, thereby producing a stable fulcrum for arm abduction. The floor of the subdeltoid (subacromial) bursa covers the superior surface of the rotator cuff, and a disorder of one involves the other. Frequently cuff degeneration of unknown etiology produces pain and limits shoulder motion. The supraspinatus usually degenerates near its insertion into the greater tuberosity of the humerus. If the degenerated area and surrounding repair tissue extend to the external surface of the tendon, subacromial bursitis develops. If the degenerated tendon calcifies, this calcium can rupture into the bursa. Degeneration can partially rupture the rotator cuff. Symptoms vary with the following syndromes.

Acute degeneration and bursitis. The patient notes sudden, sharp, severe pain in the subacromial region. Pain radiates down the arm. Shoulder motion, especially abduction and external rotation, decreases. Examination discloses point tenderness over the greater tuberosity, and active and passive motion produce pain. As the greater tuberosity passes beneath the acromion during abduction from 30 to 80 degrees, the patient experiences his most severe pain (painful arc syndrome). Roentgenograms either reveal no abnormality or show calcification in the tendon or bursa.

The patient should rest and use analgesics and hot packs to relieve pain. Oral analgesics and anti-inflammatory drugs or local injection of an anesthetic and/or steroids into the bursa often help. Pain should decrease in 48 to 72 hours. If it does not, the physician might wish to aspirate calcium or remove it by operative incision. When pain subsides, the patient must begin shoulder circumduction, abduction, and external rotation to prevent a frozen shoulder. (See section on frozen shoulder, p. 701.)

Chronic degeneration and bursitis. With or without a previous acute episode, the patient with rotator cuff disease complains of intermittent aching in the shoulder, tenderness over the cuff insertion, and pain on motion. If the cuff ruptures, shoulder abduction weakens. Patients with chronic and recurrent rotator cuff disease should use heat and analgesics to decrease pain. Between acute episodes, they should initiate active range of motion exercises. If calcium produces a mechanical obstruction to motion, it should be excised.

Tenosynovitis of the long head of the biceps. This produces symptoms much the same as those of acute rotator cuff tendinitis except tenderness is over the biceps groove. Supination of the forearm against resistance produces shoulder pain. Conservative treatment is the same as in acute bursitis. If the process continues and motion gradually decreases, the patient might need surgical release of the long head of the biceps.

Frozen shoulder (adhesive pericapsulitis)

Adhesions form in the gliding planes about the shoulder after trauma, shoulder disease, or any disorder that limits shoulder motion. Patients, usually 40 to 60 years old, complain of severe pain. Motion decreases markedly. Roentgenograms usually disclose no abnormalities. Occasionally they show signs of previous shoulder disease. Heat and active circumduction exercises help restore shoulder function. If the range of motion is not improving, manipulation under anesthesia might be necessary. This disorder tends to subside in 12 to 18 months, and motion increases.

Acute rupture of the rotator cuff

A force applied during lifting or during a fall can rupture a normal rotator cuff or a previously degenerated one. With a complete tear, the patient experiences severe pain, feels a sharp snap, and loses active abduction and external rotation of the shoulder. If his arm is passively elevated above his head, he might be able to hold it there by use of his deltoid muscle. Immediate surgical repair of a complete tear produces a good chance for recovery of function. Partial tear is common. The patient complains of mild pain, and he moves the shoulder to a limited extent. With symptomatic treatment, the patient regains function.

Snapping scapula

The patient complains of grating, snapping, and/or pain as the scapula rotates over the chest wall. Persons in certain occupations have difficulty working. Although a subscapular exostosis can produce symptoms, snapping is usually caused by poor posture, an abnormally formed scapula, subscapular bursitis, or inflammation in fascial planes. The physician should obtain roentgenograms to rule out lesions of the scapula. Usually, attempts to correct poor posture, injection of tender areas with local anesthesia, and exercises to strengthen the scapular muscles relieve symptoms. Rarely pain persists and is severe enough to warrant surgical removal of the medial edge and superior angle of the scapula.

Elbow

Pulled elbow (nursemaid's elbow)

The history of a child with a pulled elbow is similar to that of one with a pulled shoulder. Pulled elbow is more common. The child holds the forearm pronated and the elbow flexed 30 to 40 degrees. Roentgenograms are normal. In this disorder, the radial head subluxes through the annular ligament. In a child over 6 years of age, the larger radial head does not sublux. If the doctor quickly manipulates the child's forearm into supination and extension, he will often hear a click as the radial head reduces. To prevent recurrent subluxation, he should splint the forearm in supination and extension for 7 to 10 days. The patient then initiates motion as he desires. No physical therapy is needed.

Tennis elbow (lateral humeral epicondylitis, tendinitis)

The patient complains of pain over the lateral humeral epicondyle. This often follows injury or activities wherein the forearm repeatedly supinates and extends (a backhand in tennis). The cause of symptoms is debatable. Some attribute complaints to a disrupted common extensor origin at or immediately distal to the lateral humeral epicondyle. Others believe that the radiohumeral bursa beneath the common extensor origin becomes irritated. In any case, the lateral humeral epicondyle is tender. The patient complains of pain during attempts at forearm supination or wrist extension against resistance. Warm, moist packs, rest, analgesics, and injections of local anesthetic and/or steroids usually resolve symptoms. Some patients have recurrence that again responds to conservative therapy. In 5 to 10% of the cases, persistent symptoms warrant surgical exploration and excision of the degenerated and torn extensor tendon.

Table 38-3. Disorders of the elbow

Age	Disorder	Etiology
2–4	Pulled elbow (nursemaid's elbow)	Trauma
Adult	Tennis elbow (lateral humeral epicondylitis, tendinitis)	Degenerative, trauma

Table 38-4. Disorders of the hand

Age	Disorder	Etiology
Birth to 2	Syndactyly	Congenital and developmental
	Polydactyly	Congenital and developmental
	Congenital bands	Congenital and developmental
Adult	Dupuytren's contracture	Idiopathic
	de Quervain's disease	Developmental, inflammatory
	Trigger finger	Developmental, inflammatory

Hand

The age and etiology for disorders of the hand are given in Table 38-4 and are discussed in Chapter 39.

Spine (Table 38-5)
Spina bifida and meningomyelocele

In spina bifida, a development disorder, one or more vertebral arches fail to fuse in the posterior midline. At times, the incomplete neural arch allows the contents of the spinal canal to herniate. Spina bifida occurs in about one out of every 1,000 births. It most frequently involves lumbar and sacral vertebrae but can affect others. In many children with meningomyelocele, extensive defects lead to death at birth or soon thereafter. Within the last few years medical teams have improved prospects for increasing the life-span of these children.

The several types of spina bifida depend on the anatomic defect. In spina bifida occulta, the neural arch is defective, but neural contents do not herniate or at least not enough to cause neurological symptoms. In some instances, the overlying skin is pigmented, indented, or hairy. Later in life, some of these children gradually develop incomplete paralysis, sensory loss, weakened intrinsic foot muscles, cockup toes, and cavus feet. In spina bifida with meningocele, one or more layers of the meninges herniate through the neural arch defect. In spina bifida with meningomyelocele the hernial sac contains

Table 38-5. Disorders of the spine

Age	*Disorder*	*Etiology*
Birth to 2	Spina bifida and meningo-myelocele	Congenital and developmental
2–4	Scoliosis	Idiopathic, infantile, congenital
4–8	Scoliosis	Idiopathic and paralytic
8–14	Scoliosis	Idiopathic and paralytic
	Juvenile round back (vertebral epiphysitis, Scheuermann's disease)	Developmental—osteochondritis, epiphysitis (?)
Adult	Spondylolysis and spondylolisthesis	Developmental defect; trauma (?)
	Acute back sprain	Trauma
	Intervertebral disc degeneration and herniation	Degenerative
	Coccygodynia	Trauma (?), unknown (?)

meninges, cerebral spinal fluid, spinal cord, and/or nerve roots. Frequently these children have extensive paralysis, sensory loss, lack of bowel and bladder control, and associated hydrocephalus.

Symptoms and signs in spina bifida are produced by the protruding mass, neurological loss, and resulting deformities. Frequently the skin over the hernial sac ulcerates and becomes infected. Meningitis follows. Neurological defects vary with extent and location of the lesion. Sensory loss and skin ulcerations are common (Fig. 38-3). Paralyzed muscles are usually flaccid. Deformities depend on the level of nerve root involvement. Many children have hip flexion contractures, dislocated hips, knee contractures, and equinovarus feet.

The complex treatment of the child with spina bifida is best done by a team that includes parents, pediatrician, neurosurgeon, orthopedic surgeon, urologist, orthotist, physical therapist, occupational therapist, and social worker. The neurosurgeon closes the hernial sac and treats hydrocephalus. Urologists prevent and treat urinary tract infections

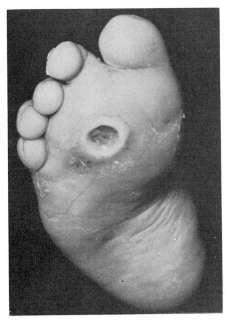

Fig. 38-3. Chronic foot ulcer in a patient with spina bifida and meningomyelocele.

and provide proper emptying of the urinary collecting system. Orthopedic surgeons prevent and correct deformities by physical therapy, manipulation, splints, braces, and surgery. Therapists help in gait training and instruct the child in self-care. The child needs nursing care to prevent ulcers. Parents must understand the magnitude of the problem and be willing to help with therapeutic programs.

Scoliosis

Lateral curvature of the spine can result from neuromuscular disorders (polio, muscular dystrophy, spinal cord tumor, neurofibromatosis), congenital defects (wedge vertebra or failed segmentation), or any disorder producing muscle spasm (disc herniation). However,

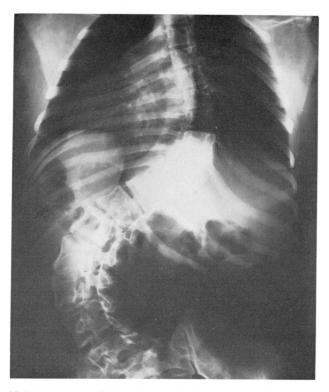

Fig. 38-4. Postpolio scoliosis with a right thoracic and left lumbar curve. Note rotation of vertebral bodies.

most cases of idiopathic scoliosis develop during rapid spine growth at adolescence.

Idiopathic scoliosis is more frequent in girls aged 8 to 14 and often consists of one main thoracic or lumbar curve and one or two compensatory curves. In thoracic curves, the spine and chest not only deviate laterally but also rotate. The chest protrudes anteriorly on the concave side of the curve and posteriorly on the convex side of the curve to produce a hunchback. In lumbar curves the hip and pelvis on the side of the concavity appear prominent.

Patients with scoliosis usually have no symptoms. The patient or the parents note the curve, the high shoulder, or the prominent thorax or hip. The physician must rule out all known causes of scoliosis before he classifies it as idiopathic. Spinal roentgenograms (Fig. 38-4) with the patient standing up and lying down and bending to each side indicate the amount of curve flexibility. From these, the orthopedist measures the angle of the curve. If it is over 20 or 30 degrees, he should start treatment at once. If not, he might observe the patient carefully to see if the curve increases. If roentgenograms 3 months later show an increased curve, the patient needs treatment. In general, the thoracic curves progress rapidly, especially if the patient is young. After spine growth stops, curves progress slowly if at all.

A Milwaukee brace distracts the head from the pelvis and applies corrective lateral and rotatory forces to the spine by means of pads against the ribs. The orthopedist must check the brace frequently to be sure it fits well. As the curve corrects and as the child grows, the orthotist must adjust and lengthen the brace. Some curves, if treated early by the brace, improve markedly or correct almost completely. If a curve progresses despite a brace or if a severe curve remains, the orthopedic surgeon can correct the curve and fuse the spine. Postoperatively, the patient remains in a body cast for 8 to 10 months and wears a brace for many more months. Even then, pseudoarthrosis may develop. This break in the fusion usually produces no pain but might allow progression of the curve and necessitate refusion.

Juvenile round back (vertebral epiphysitis, Scheuermann's disease)

Occasionally the secondary ring epiphyses and the upper and lower margins of vertebral bodies ossify poorly. Boys between 12 and 16 years of age develop epiphysitis more often than girls. Thoracic vertebrae are most commonly involved. Anterior vertebral body growth is decreased. The patient at times has mild backache. Thoracic kyphosis increases to give a round back and stooped shoulders. Roentgenograms disclose an irregular upper and lower vertebral surface and an anterior wedging of the vertebral body (Fig. 38-5). The patient should limit

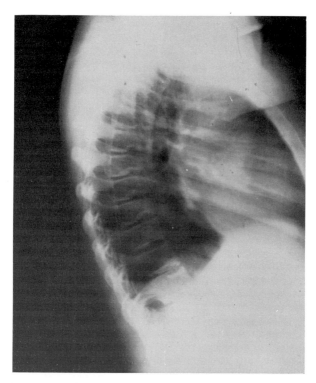

Fig. 38-5. Scheuermann's disease. Dorsal kyphosis is increased, vertebral bodies are wedged anteriorly, and epiphyseal rings are irregularly ossified.

activities to the point where he is free of pain. In case of rapid progression of dorsal kyphosis, a Milwaukee brace helps prevent and correct deformity. The disorder is self-limiting.

Spondylolysis and spondylolisthesis

In spondylolysis, the pars interarticularis of the neural arch is defective and the posterior portion of the arch has no bony continuity with the remainder of the vertebra. In spondylolisthesis, the neural arch is defective, and one vertebral body, usually L5, slides forward upon another, S1 (Fig. 38-6). The defect is probably congenital, but

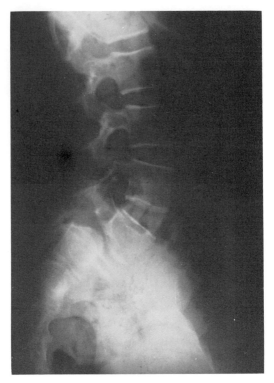

Fig. 38-6. Spondylolisthesis. L5 has slipped anteriorly on S1. The neural arch is defective.

the actual slip tends to occur between the ages of 6 and 12. Once established, the slip usually does not progress; however, the intervertebral disc degenerates sooner than normal at the involved site. Spondylolisthesis is usually not so painful unless the disc degenerates. The patient might then have low back pain with radiation into the posterior aspect of the lower extremities. The patient must be taught to lift properly. He should stoop so that his spine does not bend but his hips and knees do. He builds up abdominal muscles by sit-up exercises with his hips and knees flexed. If pain persists, spinal fusion might be necessary.

Acute back sprain

Acute flexion during a fall or while lifting frequently tears ligaments, fascia, and muscles of the low back. Patients experience sudden, sharp pain. Upon examination, muscle spasm and tenderness are found. Spine motion decreases. Roentgenograms may reveal no abnormalities. Rest, heat, and protection against extremes of motion relieve symptoms in 1 or 2 weeks.

After a sudden twist or bend, the spine at times locks in one position. Patients have severe pain. Based on the theory that facets lock in a subluxed position, doctors have called this a facet syndrome. Roentgenograms commonly show asymmetry of lumbosacral facets. Bed rest and sedation relieve acute symptoms. To prevent attacks, patients should then avoid sudden twisting and bending.

Intervertebral disc degeneration and herniation

Because of its ability to retain fluid and its intradiscal tension, the intervertebral disc gives the spine both flexibility and stability. As individuals age, intervertebral discs lose their elasticity and ability to retain fluid. Some discs then consist of nonelastic connective tissue, and others have clefts. Whether degeneration represents a variation of normal aging or is a disease is debatable. Disc degeneration often produces spine instability in the involved segment. This places abnormal stresses on ligamentous structures and spinal facet joints. In an attempt to repair and stabilize the spine, the body produces bone spurs. The inflammatory process often involves nerve roots. Frequently the patient complains of back pain and pain radiating into the thigh along the sciatic nerve. Pain is usually mild and intermittent for several months. Lifting, bending, and twisting increase pain, and rest relieves it. In some, pain starts in the low back and later radiates into one lower extremity. Motion of the involved segment of the spine decreases. The doctor sees this best if he views the patient from the side and asks him to bend forward. Normally, motion starts at the neck and continues smoothly until the entire spine forms a continuous curve. In a patient with disc degeneration, involved segments remain flat. Hyperextension causes discomfort. Pressure over the spinous tip at the involved site produces pain. If the patient then hyperextends the back by lifting his head and shoulders off the table and pressure produces less pain, this is a positive instability test that helps localize the level of degeneration. Straight leg raising test is positive when it reproduces radiating pain or back pain. Reflex, sensory, and motor activity vary from patient to patient. Roentgenograms often reveal a narrowed interspace and degenerative changes, most often at L5-S1 or L4-L5. Flexion and extension lateral views of the spine at times show sliding of one vertebral body upon the other or tilting open of a disc space anteriorly on hyperextension.

During the acute stage of pain, bed rest usually relieves symptoms. The patient must then use his back properly. He should avoid bending, lift only by bending his knees, and avoid soft chairs and beds that allow the spine to sag. In the early stages of treatment, a low back brace reminds the patient of the proper position for his spine. Later, the patient should start on progressive resistance exercises (sit-ups) to build up the abdominal muscles and spine flexors. He should do sit-ups with the hips and knees flexed. Nearly all patients improve on this therapy.

If the annulus tears, the nucleus pulposus can herniate and press on a nerve root. This causes radiating pain and often interferes with reflex, motor, and sensory function in the lower extremity. The patient usually gives a history much like one with a degenerated disc. In many instances, the most recent episode is severe and unrelenting. On physical examination, the physician often finds changes similar to those in a person with degenerative disc disease. In addition, the patient's reflexes decrease (ankle or knee jerk), muscles lose strength (toe extensors), and sensation in the L5 or S1 dermatome decreases.

Bed rest and medication for relief of pain lead to improvement in most patients. If so, the patients are then treated as outlined for disc degeneration. A few patients need surgical removal of the intervertebral disc if (1) they fail to improve in 3 or 4 weeks on a conservative therapeutic regime, or (2) neurological loss progresses. The physician should do a myelogram if he is not sure of the level of herniation or if he has a question about the diagnosis. After disc removal, some surgeons fuse the involved level of the spine. Others do not. After surgery, the doctor should treat the patient just as he would a degenerated disc until the intervertebral region stabilizes. Fusion is probably indicated if the patient has a defect such as spondylolisthesis.

Coccygodynia

Women develop a painful tailbone more often than men do. Some give a history of an acute injury to the coccyx. In others, trauma seems to play no role. Sitting and motion of the coccyx increase the pain. The physician must rule out psychoneurosis, spine disease (bone tumors), and spinal cord and nerve lesions with pain referred to the coccyx. Rectal examination is mandatory. Roentgenograms help rule out bone lesions. Rest and heat often relieve acute coccygodynia. The patient is instructed to sit on a soft pillow or ring. Excision of the coccyx is rarely warranted since most patients continue to have pain despite surgery.

Hip (Table 38-6)
Congenital dislocation

The physician must diagnose congenital dislocation of the hip soon after birth of the affected infant. If he does not, he often commits the child to a life of disability. Hip joint capsule relaxation and acetabular dysplasia of unknown etiology produce congenital dislocation of the hip. Girls are affected seven times oftener than are boys. The disorder is at times familial. The doctor should warn parents of an

Table 38-6. Disorders of the hip

Age	*Disorder*	*Etiology*
Birth to 2	Congenital dislocation	Developmental
4–8	Legg-Calvé Perthes disease (coxa plana)	Metabolic (?)
	Synovitis	Viral (?)
8–14	Slipped capital femoral epiphysis	Metabolic (?)
Adult	Snapping hip	Anatomical variation

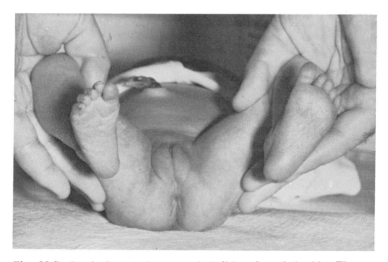

Fig. 38-7. Ortolani's test for congenital dislocation of the hip. The examiner's thumb pushes posteriorly on the baby's knee while the examiner's fingers lift the greater trochanter anteriorly and push medially to snap the femoral head into the acetabulum.

affected child to have all subsequent children examined carefully. The degree of involvement varies from mild dysplasia (shallow acetabulum) to complete dislocation. In some babies, the hip is dislocated before birth. In others, the femoral head slips out of the acetabulum after birth. For clinical purposes, the disorder is classified as a dysplastic hip, subluxation, or dislocation.

The doctor examining a newborn must look for signs of hip dislocation. The most common reliable sign is a slight jerk and snap as the femoral head slides in and out of the acetabulum (Ortolani's sign). This is produced when the thighs, in flexion and slight abduction, are alternatively pushed posteriorly and pulled anteriorly

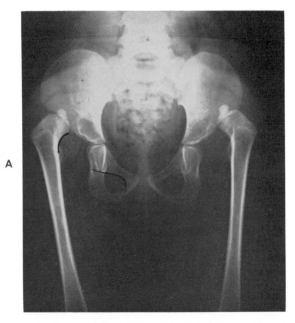

Fig. 38-8. Bilateral congenital dislocation of the hips. **A,** Note the shallow, sloping acetabular roofs, the superior lateral displacement of the femoral heads, and the broken Shenton's line. **B,** Roentgenograms through plaster after traction, adductor tenotomy, and closed reduction. **C,** Roentgenograms 8 months later. The femoral heads are centered in the acetabulum, and Shenton's line is unbroken.

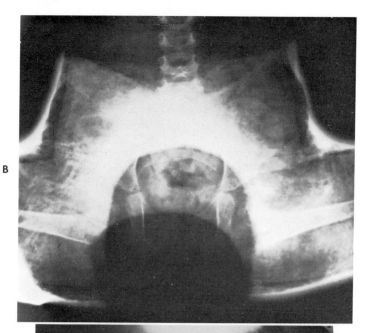

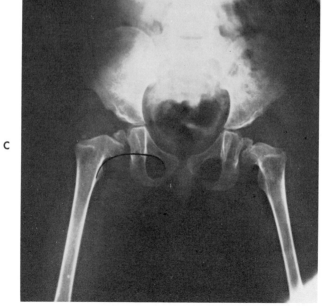

Fig. 38-8, cont'd. For legend see opposite page.

(Fig. 38-7). Other signs include: limited abduction while the hip is flexed, posterior and lateral displacement of the greater trochanter, an extra fold or asymmetric gluteal folds, and telescoping (abnormal cephalocaudad motion of the femur with push and pull). If diagnosis and treatment are delayed until the child walks, he waddles. The involved leg is shorter. When the patient stands on the involved extremity, the pelvis drops toward the opposite side (positive Trendelenburg test).

Initial roentgenographic examination often reveals only lateral displacement of the proximal femur. Later roentgenograms (Fig. 38-8) show a shallow, sloping acetabular roof, a laterally displaced proximal femur (if the acetabular region is divided into quadrants by a line passing through the triradiate cartilage of both acetabulae and a line dropped from the superior acetabular edge, the femoral head should lie in the lower inner quadrant), a delay in ossification of the femoral head, a break in Shenton's line (the normal continuous arch formed by a line drawn along the inferior border of the femoral neck and head and continued along the superior border of the obturator foramen), and an acetabular angle over 30 degrees (the acetabular angle is formed by one horizontal line that goes through the triradiate cartilages and another that goes from the superior acetabular edge to the triradiate cartilage on the involved side).

A child who remains undiagnosed has abnormal hip mechanics and develops early degenerative changes in the hip. To prevent crippling sequelae, the doctor must diagnose and treat congenital hip dislocation soon after birth. If he applies the appropriate treatment, results are gratifying.

Treatment in the newborn depends on the degree of hip involvement. If the patient has a mild dysplastic hip, the mother should keep the child's legs abducted by pillows designed for this purpose. If the femoral head is well centered, a dysplastic acetabulum deepens and develops as the child grows. If the femoral head is subluxed or dislocated, the orthopedist can do a gentle, manipulative reduction after a few days of skin traction. Tight hip adductors might necessitate a subcutaneous adductor tenotomy. A plaster cast then holds the child's hips in 90 degrees of flexion and 70 degrees of abduction for 3 to 4 months. After this, the patient wears a brace to hold the extremities in this position. As the acetabulum deepens, the brace is gradually worn less, but it is worn at night for several years. In children over 2 or 3 years, closed reduction is at times impossible. Operative measures might be needed, but frequently results are not satisfactory. The doctor must follow a child with congenital dislocation during his growth years to be sure that the hip does not displace again.

Legg-Calvé-Perthes disease (coxa plana)

Avascular necrosis of the femoral head of unknown etiology is more common in boys aged 4 to 9 than in girls. Biopsy of the epiphyseal plate shows derangement of chondrocytes and clefts in the cartilage. These probably interfere with blood vessels passing through the periphery of the epiphyseal plate and supplying the femoral head.

The child first complains of mild pain in the medial aspect of the knee and thigh or in the anterior part of the hip. The parents notice a limp. Upon examination, the physician finds limited motion of the child's hip. Abduction and internal rotation decrease markedly. The child complains of tenderness and pain on motion. Muscle spasm is frequently severe. In early stages of the disorder, radiographic examination shows a distended joint capsule and slight flattening of the femoral head. Later, the femoral metaphysis widens, and the epiphyseal plate becomes irregular. The necrotic portion of the femoral head is radiopaque as compared to surrounding bone that has undergone disuse atrophy (Fig. 38-9). If the child bears weight, the femoral head collapses, widens, and leads to joint incongruity that can produce degenerative joint disease.

Treatment does not always restore a normal hip joint. Early treatment includes rest or a cast with the thighs in abduction to relieve the pain of muscle spasm and acute synovitis and to center the femoral head in the acetabulum. The child walks with crutches or a brace to limit weight bearing on the involved extremity until new bone replaces necrotic bone. After this, the child gradually increases the amount of weight bearing. A differential diagnosis in Legg-Calvé-Perthes disease should include tuberculosis, rheumatoid arthritis, and idiopathic synovitis.

Synovitis

Occasionally children complain of hip and/or knee pain and limp to protect the involved extremity. Past history is noncontributory. Hip motion decreases. The child holds the hip flexed, externally rotated, and abducted. Pressure over the hip anteriorly produces discomfort. The doctor must do laboratory and roentgenographic studies to rule out pyogenic arthritis, osteomyelitis, and rheumatoid arthritis. By exclusion, he diagnoses idiopathic (viral) synovitis, treats the child by rest with traction, bed, or crutches, and follows the patient at frequent intervals. If, in fact, the child has idiopathic synovitis, he improves in 2 or 3 weeks and has no residual difficulty.

Slipped capital femoral epiphysis

Slipping of the capital femoral epiphysis is usually a gradually progressive displacement of the femoral neck anteriorly and superiorly

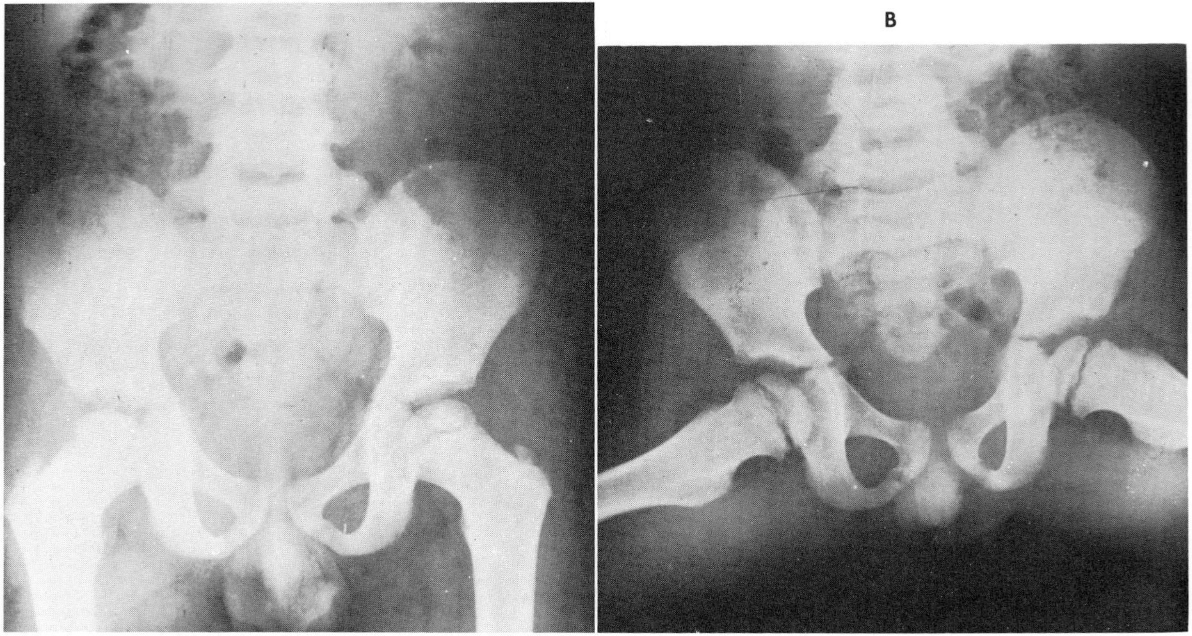

Fig. 38-9. Legg-Calvé-Perthes disease. **A** and **B**, Anteroposterior and lateral roentgenograms a few weeks after the child limped and complained of mild right hip discomfort; the right femoral head is somewhat irregular and smaller than the left.

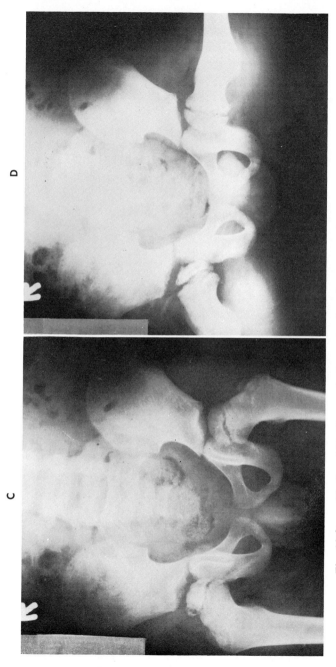

C

D

Fig. 38-9, cont'd. C and **D,** Six months later, the flat, dense, necrotic femoral head is obvious. *Continued.*

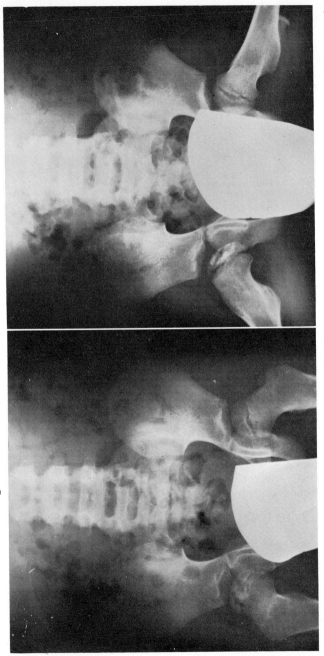

Fig. 38-9, cont'd. E and F, In another 6 months, new bone is replacing dense, dead bone; the femoral head is still flat, and the metaphysis is wide.

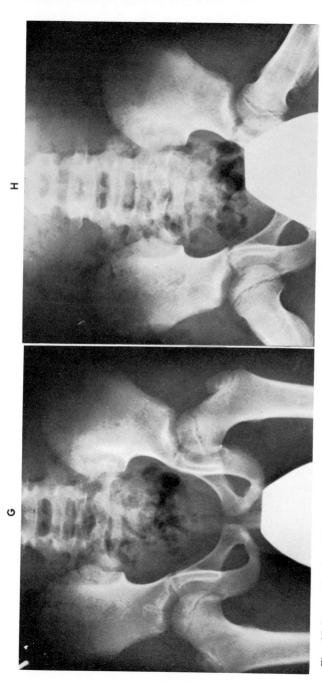

Fig. 38-9, cont'd. G and H, Two years later, new bone has replaced dead bone, and the femoral head has only mild residual flattening.

in relation to the femoral head. Etiology is unknown, but the disorder involves epiphyseal plate cells. The changes in the cartilage cells of the plate are similar to those in Legg-Calvé-Perthes disease. Slipped epiphysis develops between the ages of 10 and 16. The patient complains of discomfort in the knee, thigh, and/or hip. His discomfort, although mild and intermittent at first, usually persists and becomes more pronounced. The parents notice that the child limps. Slipped epiphysis commonly affects one of two types of children. The child is either fat and physically and sexually immature, or he is tall and thin. In the latter instance, he has recently grown rapidly.

The patient holds the involved hip externally rotated and adducted. He complains of pain on motion and limits internal rotation

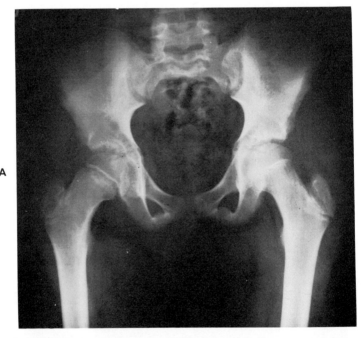

Fig. 38-10. Slipped capital femoral epiphysis. **A,** Anteroposterior roentgenograms showing early slip of the right femoral epiphysis; the epiphyseal plate is widened, and the femoral neck is displaced superiorly and anteriorly in relation to the femoral head. **B,** Lateral view; the slip is more obvious. **C,** Roentgenogram 6 months after internal fixation.

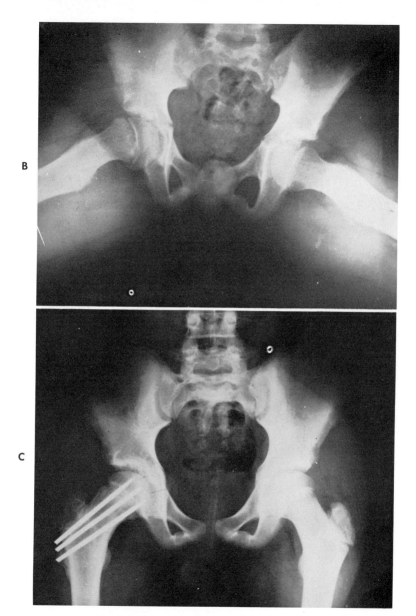

B

C

Fig. 38-10, cont'd. For legend see opposite page.

and abduction as compared to the normal side. Characteristically the leg goes into external rotation upon flexion of the hip with the knee flexed. Often anteroposterior roentgenograms show slight widening of the epiphyseal plate and metaphysis, but lateral views reveal anterior displacement of the femoral neck (Fig. 38-10). This varies from minimal displacement to complete separation of the femoral head from the femoral neck.

To prevent further displacement and serious hip disability, the child should bear no weight. A patient with a mild displacement should have the epiphysis fixed to the femoral neck by means of threaded pins. He then uses crutches until the femoral head unites by bone to the femoral neck. In an individual with marked displacement, the physician applies skin or skeletal traction to the limb over a period of several days to abduct and internally rotate the leg in a manner that reduces displacement to the point where the head can be fixed to the femoral neck by pins. Vigorous manipulative reduction damages the blood supply to the femoral head and produces aseptic necrosis.

A few children with slipped capital femoral epiphysis develop one of the following complications: acute arthritis of the hip, chondrolysis, residual joint incongruity, or aseptic necrosis. These can produce a degenerative joint that later needs reconstructive surgery.

Snapping hip

Flexion, abduction, or internal rotation of the hip produces an audible, palpable, or visible snap located over the greater trochanter of the femur. A thickened band of fascia snaps over the trochanter. Differential diagnosis includes loose bodies in the hip or subluxation of the hip. In case of a fascial band, pain is usually not severe enough to warrant treatment. If it is, the surgeon can divide the tight fascial band.

Knee (Table 38-7)
Bowlegs (genu varum)

Bowlegs are most often a variation of normal, but the doctor must be sure that the child does not have rickets or an epiphyseal disorder.

Most newborns have bowlegs. This physiological bowing persists for several years, but the majority correct spontaneously with growth. No one has proved that shoe corrections help. A few severe and persistent bowlegs need treatment with a long leg brace designed to apply pressure laterally at the knee and medially over the thigh and lower leg. An even fewer number persist to the point of needing osteotomy to correct the bowing.

Table 38-7. Disorders of the knee

Age	Disorder	Etiology
Birth to 2	Bowlegs (genu varum)	Developmental or metabolic
	Knock knees (genu valgum)	Developmental
	Congenital pseudarthrosis of the tibia	Developmental (?)
8–14	Osgood-Schlatter disease	Trauma (?)
	Recurrent dislocation of the patella	Developmental
	Osteochondritis dissecans	Trauma (?)
	Baker's cyst (popliteal cyst)	Developmental or inflammatory
Adult	Bursitis	Bursal inflammation
	Chondromalacia	Degenerative (?)

In this country, bowlegs caused by vitamin D–deficient rickets are infrequent. An occasional patient with vitamin D–resistant rickets may develop bowlegs. Roentgenograms of a child with rickets show the widened epiphyseal plate and metaphysis wherein cartilage and bone matrix are produced but fail to mineralize. The physician must treat the primary disorder. Some of these children need osteotomies to straighten the legs.

Tibia vara (Blount's disease) produces bowlegs by delay in growth and irregular development of the medial and posterior epiphyseal plate of the proximal tibia. The deformity increases until the epiphyseal plate disturbance subsides. A child with severe deformity needs tibial osteotomy.

Knock knees (genu valgum)

Knock knees are usually a variation of normal. Probably because of their wider pelvis, girls have knock knees more frequently than boys do. Most children need no treatment. The legs straighten as the child grows. The physician must rule out an underlying bone disorder. A few children with severe knock knees need a long leg brace or an osteotomy. Again, shoe corrections are probably of no value.

Congenital pseudarthrosis of the tibia

The term *congenital pseudarthrosis* is a misnomer for this rare condition of unknown etiology. Most children who develop this disorder are born with an intact tibia that is thin at the junction of its middle and distal one-third and bowed anteriorly (Fig. 38-11). Some of the children have manifestations of neurofibromatosis. The bone

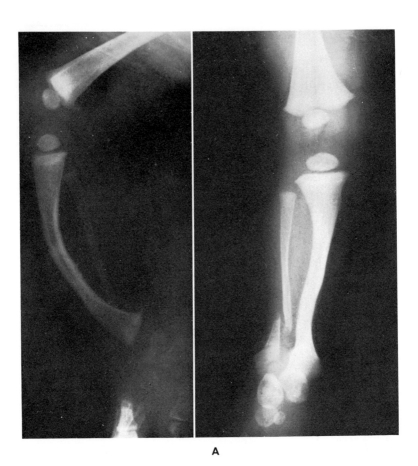

A

Fig. 38-11. Congenital "pseudarthrosis" of the tibia. **A,** Lateral and anteroposterior roentgenograms soon after birth show anterior bowing of the tibia and the fractured fibula. **B,** Five months later the tibia has broken.

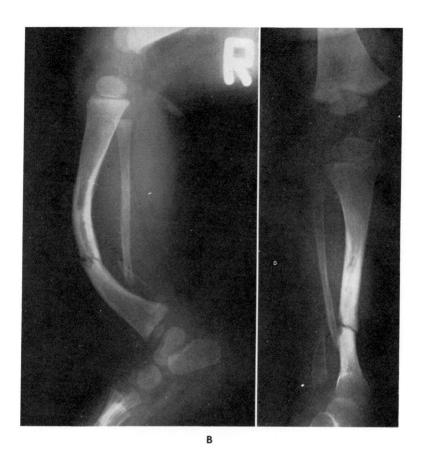

B

Fig. 38-11, cont'd. For legend see opposite page.

breaks soon after birth and resists healing. Surgeons have used numerous operative procedures, most with bone grafts, to try and obtain
union of these defects. Often pseudarthrosis remains, the leg is short,
and is amputated.

Osgood-Schlatter disease

In this disorder, common in boys 10 to 15 years of age, the tibial
tubercle becomes fragmented. The patient complains of a tender bump
and has pain if he kneels or jumps. On examination, the physician
finds a swollen, hard, tender tibial tubercle. Extension of the knee
against resistance produces pain. Roentgenograms show a dense fragmented portion of bone separated from the underlying tibia (Fig.
38-12). This process is similar to "osteochondritis" in other areas. In
most cases, the fragment ossifies normally and complaints subside.

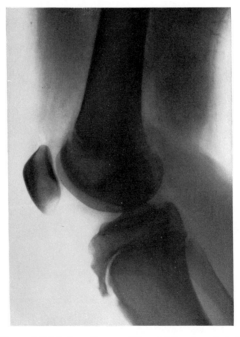

Fig. 38-12. Osgood-Schlatter disease. The tibial tubercle is irregular and
fragmented. A small, dense piece of bone remains ununited.

The child should limit activity during the acute painful stage in order to relieve strain on the tibial tubercle. A cylinder cast relieves severe pain. The child resumes activity as symptoms subside. In a few children, the fragment does not heal, and a small separate dense piece of bone remains surrounded by fibrous connective tissue and/or a bursa. These may remain symptomatic and necessitate removal of the fragment.

Recurrent dislocation of the patella

Recurrent dislocation of the patella is more likely to occur in girls 8 to 16 years old than in boys. One or more of the following predisposing developmental defects causes this disorder: high-riding patella, knock knees, flattened lateral femoral condyle, lax medial patellar retinaculum. The patient gives a history that during vigorous physical activity while the knee was flexed, the leg gave way. This produced severe knee pain, and the knee locked in flexion. Some astute observers tell the doctor that the knee cap slid to the outside of the knee, and the knee was swollen and tender for a week or so. Young girls with such a history often have subsequent episodes of subluxation wherein the kneecap slides over and back without locking in complete dislocation.

Upon examination, the physician often finds the patella higher than it should be, and it does not lock against the femur when the knee is flexed 30 degrees as it normally should. Often roentgenograms show no abnormalities, but they might disclose a high-riding patella, valgus knees, or an underdeveloped lateral femoral condyle. At times, they show a chip fracture of the lateral femoral condyle produced by the patella sliding over the condyle. A patient who has repeated episodes of patellar dislocation usually wants treatment. The older the patient, the less is the likelihood of subsequent dislocation. The physician might advise girls 16 or 18 to wait and see if the frequency of dislocation decreases. In other instances, he will advise surgical repair. The orthopedic surgeon reconstructs the extensor apparatus by transferring the patellar tendon insertion distally and medially on the tibia, reefing the medial patellar retinaculum, and releasing the lateral retinaculum. In some patients who have had multiple dislocations, patellar cartilage degenerates. In such cases the orthopedist might remove the patella and transfer the extensor apparatus to prevent it from dislocating.

Osteochondritis dissecans

In osteochondritis dissecans of the distal femur an osteochondral fragment, usually on the lateral surface of the medial femoral condyle,

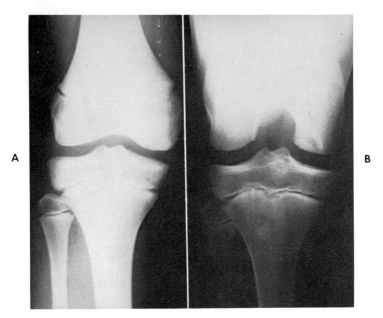

Fig. 38-13. Osteochondritis dissecans. **A,** Routine anteroposterior roentgenogram does not outline the defect well. **B,** An anteroposterior roentgenogram with the knee flexed shows the fragment in its most common location on the lateral surface of the medial femoral condyle.

loses its blood supply and separates from the rest of the femur. No one knows the cause. The fragment can revascularize and be replaced by new bone but frequently detaches and becomes a "joint mouse." If the fragment is not detached, the patient usually complains of vague knee pain and swelling made worse by activity. If the fragment becomes a loose body, the knee frequently locks and gives way. At times the patient feels loose bodies sliding about in the joint.

Roentgenograms show the fracture line with the overlying dense bone, if the fragment does, in fact, contain much bone (Fig. 38-13). Roentgenograms show a free fragment only if it contains bone or mineralized cartilage. The defect on the femoral condyle is often visible.

If the physician sees a patient with an intact fragment, he should advise non–weight bearing and observation to see if the fragment revascularizes. If a free body produces symptoms, it should be removed.

Baker's cyst (popliteal cyst)

Baker's cyst is not unusual in children. The cysts result from enlargement of the semimembranous bursa or the bursa beneath the medial head of the gastrocnemius muscle. Herniation of knee joint synovium through the posterior capsule of the knee also produces popliteal cysts. Symptoms consist of dull aching, swelling that fluctuates in size, and at times constant pain. If the patient has severe symptoms, the surgeon can excise the bursa and close any defect in the posterior knee capsule.

Bursitis

Bursae, synovial-lined sacs located between tendons, muscles, and fascia in gliding areas, reduce friction. Adventitious bursae are produced by constant friction or repeated trauma. There are many bursae about the knee. Bursae can be acutely or chronically inflamed, infected, or involved by a systemic disorder like rheumatoid disease or gout. Pain is the most prominent symptom, and swelling and tenderness are the prominent signs. Treatment depends on the underlying cause. Any systemic disorder must be treated. Locally, trauma and irritants should be eliminated. Rest, hot packs, elevation, and compression help relieve symptoms. In noninfected cases, bursae can be aspirated. To avoid infection, the physician must use extreme care. If an aspiration is to be done, the skin must be prepared as if one were going to do an open operation. One should avoid injecting directly through the skin over the bursa. Instead of this, the needle should start at a distance from the bursa in normal skin and subcutaneous tissue and enter the bursal sac from its deep surface. In this way, infection is less likely to be introduced. Incision and drainage and antibiotics usually cure an acutely infected bursa. Excision of a chronically infected bursa might be necessary.

Chondromalacia

Chondromalacia, of unknown etiology, consists of softening, yellow discoloration, fraying, and degeneration of the articular surface of the kneecap. Women 14 to 28 years of age frequently acquire chondromalacia. They complain of knee discomfort that is mild at first but later is severe. Activities like stair climbing that produce forcible knee flexion increase the pain. The joint swells, and patellar compression produces pain and crepitus. Joint fluid increases, and patellar margins become tender. Roentgenograms often show no abnormalities. Straight leg raising exercises to increase quadriceps strength and avoidance of strenuous activities that aggravate symptoms usually relieve discomfort. In some patients, conservative treatment does not control symptoms. In these instances, the surgeon might explore the knee joint and either skive the diseased cartilage or remove the patella.

Foot (Table 38-8)
Clubfoot

Congenital defects or neurological disorders (myelodysplasia, cerebral palsy) produce clubfeet. The name of the most frequent congenital variety, talipes equinovarus, describes the position of the foot. The heel cord is tight, the ankle (talipes) is plantar-flexed (equinus), and the foot is inverted (varus) (Fig. 38-14). The forefoot is adducted. Talipes equinovarus affects boys much more frequently than it does girls. In most instances, no one knows the cause of clubfoot. The heel cord and the structures on the medial side of the foot contract. This pulls the calcaneus into plantar flexion, the navicular medial to the talus, and the cuboid medial to the os calcis. Children

Table 38-8. Disorders of the foot

Age	Disorder	Etiology
Birth to 2	Clubfoot	Developmental
	Metatarsus adductus (metatarsus varus)	Developmental
	Calcaneovalgus	Developmental
	Congenital bands (constriction rings)	Developmental
	Toeing in	Developmental
	Toeing out	Developmental
	Flat feet (pes planus)	Developmental
2–4	Köhler's disease	Osteochondritis
8–14	Sever's disease	Osteochondritis
	Freiberg's disease	Osteochondritis
Adult	Bunions (hallux valgus)	Developmental (?)
	Hallux rigidus	Arthritic (?) developmental (?)
	Metatarsalgia	?
	Corns	Traumatic
	Heel spur	Traumatic (?)
	Ingrown toenail	Traumatic (?)
	Digital neuroma (Morton's neuroma)	Traumatic (?) and developmental
	Cockup toes and hammer toes	Congenital, neuromuscular, arthritic

do not outgrow talipes equinovarus, and, in fact, the older they get, the more the foot bones deform. The orthopedist must institute treatment soon after birth while contracted soft tissues are more easily stretched. Long leg casts are changed at 5- to 7-day intervals. Each cast produces a corrective force that slides the foot beneath the talus, thereby correcting forefoot adduction and inversion. The casts extend above the knee to prevent rotation of the cast. Some of the deformity corrects with each cast until the foot overcorrects except for the

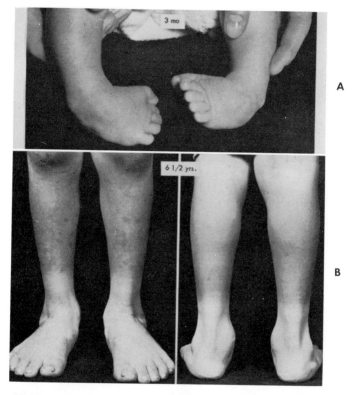

Fig. 38-14. Congenital talipes equinovarus. **A** shows the feet at the beginning of treatment when the child was 3 months old. **B** shows the feet at the age of 6½ after treatment with corrective casts and night splints.

equinus. At this stage, subcutaneous section of the heel cord (Achilles tendon) corrects equinus immediately. After this, the child wears a cast in a corrected position for 5 weeks while the tendon heals. (Some use casts to correct the equinus. Extreme caution is needed to avoid pressing up beneath the forefoot while the heel cord holds the os calcis in equinus. Such pressure "breaks" the foot and produces a rocker bottom foot.) After correction of deformity, the infant should use night splints to hold the feet corrected until the age of 5 to 7 years. Such treatment instituted soon after birth leads to satisfactory results in 90% of cases. However, the foot tends to redeform until maturity. The doctor must stress this point to parents. Frequently, neglected or recurrent clubfeet require surgery of soft tissues and/or bones of the foot. Such surgery often leaves the foot more rigid than normal.

Metatarsus adductus (metatarsus varus)

In this congenital disorder, the child's forefoot adducts (Fig. 38-15). Upon examination, the doctor might be able passively to correct the forefoot to neutral. If so, he advises the parents to hold the child's heel fixed in one hand and stretch the forefoot into a corrected position several times daily. If the infant is walking he might also

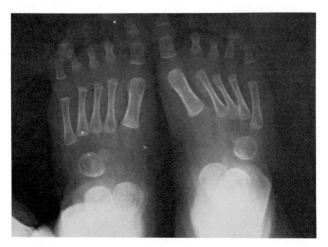

Fig. 38-15. Metatarsus adductus. Roentgenograms show adduction of the right forefoot.

wear straight-last shoes. If, however, the doctor finds that a child's foot is too rigid to correct to neutral, he should apply a series of casts and obtain gradual correction. This should be done between 3 and 6 months of age. The child wears straight-last shoes to keep the feet out of a deformed position.

Calcaneovalgus

Occasionally newborn babies' feet dorsiflex in front of the tibia and evert (valgus). In contrast to talipes equinovarus, these feet improve with time and need only gentle daily stretching. Calcaneovalgus must be differentiated from vertical talus, a rare disorder in which the foot is rigid and which must be corrected surgically.

Congenital bands (constriction rings)

Tight fibrous connective tissue bands that surround a digit or extremity involve the skin and subcutaneous tissues and constrict underlying muscle and vessels (Fig. 38-16). Occasionally edema and vascular insufficiency distal to the band produce gangrene. These bands, once thought to be amniotic remnants, probably represent developmental defects. Frequently, the patient has associated congenital anom-

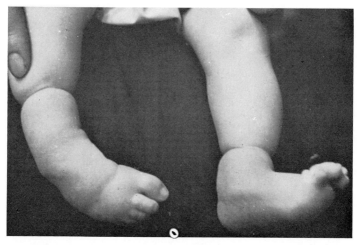

Fig. 38-16. Congenital bands (constriction rings) of both legs. (From Kenney, W. E., and Larson, C. B.: Orthopedics for the general practitioner, St. Louis, 1957, The C. V. Mosby Co., p. 27.)

alies (syndactyly and polydactyly). The surgeon should excise bands
by multiple Z-plasties several weeks apart to avoid interruption of circulation to the extremities. Z-plasties prevent circumferential scarring
with subsequent recontracture. (See Chapter 34.)

Toeing in

Parents frequently bring pigeon-toed children to the doctor. Usually, toeing in results from one of three disorders: (1) metatarsus
adductus, (2) internal tibial torsion, (3) medial femoral torsion, or
femoral neck anteversion. The physician often obtains a clue as to
which of these is present by observing the child walk. He diagnoses
metatarsus adductus when the forefoot, in fact, adducts in relation
to the hindfoot. If the child has no foot deformity and if the kneecaps point straight ahead when he walks, the problem is probably
internal tibial torsion. Normally, the lateral malleolus is 15 to 20 degrees posterior to the medial malleolus. In internal tibial torsion, this
angle decreases or reverses. If, on the other hand, the kneecaps point
medially when the child walks, femoral torsion or anteversion of
the femoral neck is likely. Sitting and sleeping with the feet turned
in aggravates tibial and femoral torsion. As the child grows and
sitting and sleeping positions change, femoral and tibial torsion usually
correct. Although thousands of dollars are spent each year on shoe
corrections, they probably do not influence toeing in caused by bone
torsion. The physician should follow the patient as he grows, and if
the disorder is not correcting, the child should wear a night splint
to hold the feet externally rotated. This splint consists of a metal bar
fixed to the shoe soles in a manner that holds them rotated to the
desired position. A few individuals with severe residual torsion need
corrective rotational osteotomy.

Toeing out

Toeing out, too, is produced by intrinsic foot deformity, external
tibial torsion, or external femoral torsion. A child just learning to
walk frequently toes out to obtain a wider base for balance. External
femoral or tibial torsion tends to correct with growth.

Flatfeet (pes planus)

The physician should exercise caution in diagnosing flatfeet in
a child under 2 or 3. Before this age, a fat pad in the foot obscures
any arch that might be present. Flatfeet in children are either flexible
or rigid. In the common, flexible type, the arch flattens, and the heel
goes into valgus during weight bearing. These correct when body
weight is removed. These feet are not painful in childhood, and most
of them correct as the child gets older and foot ligaments tighten.

Even if a flexible flatfoot does not correct, the child has no functional handicap. Shoe corrections probably do nothing to help these feet. Medial heel wedges and arch pads keep shoes from running over and wearing out rapidly. These inexpensive corrections save the parents the cost of buying new shoes at frequent intervals.

Bone defects such as congenital fusion of tarsal bones (tarsal coalition) produce most rigid flatfeet. These feet are not passively correctable. If the child has foot and leg pain, an orthopedic surgeon should see him. Surgery might be necessary to relieve pain and deformity.

Köhler's disease

Aseptic necrosis of the tarsal scaphoid usually affects children 2 to 4 years old. Activity accentuates foot pain and rest relieves it. The physician finds tenderness in the medial side of the foot arch. Roentgenograms show a dense, narrow scaphoid. Limiting the child's activity controls discomfort. Osteochondritis is self-limiting, and the scaphoid usually revascularizes.

Sever's disease

A child 7 to 12 years of age with fragmented ossification of the os calcis apophysis complains of pain over the posterior aspect of the heel. The doctor finds tenderness in this area. Roentgenograms show a dense fragmented os calcis apophysis. Shoes that raise the heel and relieve pressure over the tender area and limitation of activity decrease symptoms. The disease is self-limited.

Freiberg's disease

Osteochondritis of the second metatarsal head affects girls 10 to 15 years of age more often than it does boys. Symptomatic treatment is instituted until the area revascularizes. Occasionally the articular surface of the metatarsal phalangeal joint collapses, and pain continues. In such an instance, excision of the metatarsal head or arthroplasty might be necessary.

Bunions (hallux valgus)

A painful bunion results when the great toe deviates laterally at the metatarsal phalangeal joint (hallux valgus), the head of the first metatarsal bone becomes prominent medially, and a callus and/or bursa develops over the metatarsal head (Fig. 38-17). Congenital adduction of the first metatarsal or lax ligaments produces deviation of the great toe. Because of the ridiculous shoes they tolerate, women develop bunions much more often than do men. Some bunions produce slight discomfort. In such an instance, shoes fitted to relieve

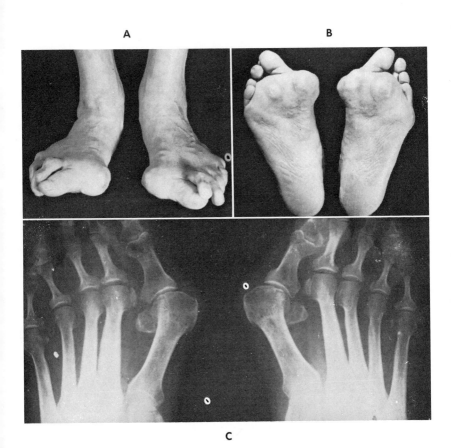

Fig. 38-17. Bunions. **A,** Dorsal view, showing lateral deviation (hallux valgus) of the great toe and overlapping second toes. **B,** Plantar views showing callosities beneath prominent metatarsal heads. **C,** Roentgenograms showing bilateral hallux valgus.

pressure, or cut out over the bunion, relieve pain. The patient with severe pain often needs surgical correction including arthroplasty to remove overgrowth on the metatarsal head, decompression of the metatarsal phalangeal joint, and correction of angulation between the great toe and first metatarsal bone.

Hallux rigidus

In hallux rigidus, the great toe fails to dorsiflex at the metatarsal phalangeal joint. A bunion of long duration or any process that destroys the metatarsal phalangeal joint can cause hallux rigidus. The patient who lacks dorsiflexion at the first metatarsal phalangeal joint develops pain and walks in a protective manner to relieve this pain. Surgical treatment consists of resection of the bunion and decompression of the metatarsal phalangeal joint by removal of the proximal half of the proximal phalanx of the great toe.

Metatarsalgia

Pain beneath metatarsal heads develops in a foot that loses the transverse metatarsal arch. Weight bearing increases pain. Painful calluses develop over a prominent metatarsal head. Proper shoes and a pad in the shoes decrease pain. The pad must support weight in the region posterior to the metatarsal heads. Removal of a prominent metatarsal head beneath a persistent callus might be necessary.

Corns

Pressure on the skin against an underlying bony prominence produces corns that frequently become exquisitely painful. Treatment consists of proper shoes, pads, and cutouts to relieve pressure, and gentle trimming of the superficial dead skin. If conservative measures fail, the underlying bony spike can be removed.

Heel spur

A heel spur per se is not a disease but is a manifestation of bone repair reaction at the site of degeneration of the plantar ligaments near the os calcis. The patient, at times, gives a history of a recent change from one type of shoe to another or of walking a prolonged distance. The doctor should treat the heel spur with a pad cutout to relieve pressure. This disorder tends to repair itself after several months. In general, excision of the spur does not hasten repair time.

Ingrown toenail

An abnormal shape of the great toenail, an infected area along the toenail, pressure from tight shoes or socks, and trimming the nail too close at its corners all contribute to an ingrown toenail. The patient develops intermittent acute inflammation of soft tissues at the medial side of the great toenail (Fig. 38-18). During the acute stage, warm soaks, elevation, and antibiotics help control infection. After the acute episode, the patient should let the nail grow out, trim it straight across, not back at the corners, and avoid shoes and socks that cause pressure on the toe. At times, elevating the nail edge and packing sterile cotton beneath it help the nail to grow out. If a deformed nail causes continued symptoms, the patient might want surgical treatment. The surgeon can remove the medial one-third of the nail, curet the nail base, and suture the skin beneath the nail bed to close the defect and create a new nail groove. If this fails, he can remove the entire nail, nail bed, and distal portion of the phalanx.

Digital neuroma (Morton's neuroma)

The patient, usually a woman, with a neuroma of the common digital nerve to the contiguous sides of the third and fourth toe gives a classic history of episodes of severe, sharp, knifelike pain and

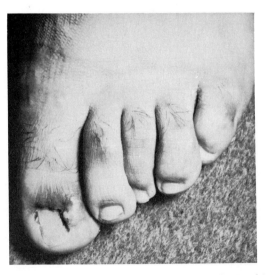

Fig. 38-18. Ingrown toenail. Soft tissues at the lateral edge of the great toenail are hypertrophied and infected.

paresthesias radiating into the adjacent sides of two toes. She removes the shoe and rubs the foot to relieve discomfort. Metatarsal pads may relieve pressure. If symptoms are severe enough, the patient usually wants surgical excision of the neuroma.

Cockup toes and hammer toes

Cockup toes hyperextend at the metatarsal phalangeal joints and flex at the proximal interphalangeal joints. A variety of disorders (congenital, neuromuscular, arthritic) cause them. Any muscle imbalance that produces relatively strong extrinsic toe extensors and weak intrinsic toe extensors might produce cockup toes. These toes correct passively in contrast to hammer toes, which are fixed in their deformed position. Painful callosities develop over the proximal interphalangeal joints of hammer toes or cockup toes. During the flexible stage, deformity is corrected by restoring muscle balance through the use of intrinsoplasties—the restoration of intrinsic muscle function by transplantation of the extrinsic toe flexors into the extensor hood. If deformities are fixed, excision or fusion of the proximal interphalangeal joint relieves symptoms.

INFECTION

In osteomyelitis, an infection of bone, offending organisms migrate via the bloodstream from a remote soft tissue infection to the bone (acute hematogenous osteomyelitis), or they invade bone directly through an open wound or extend from an adjacent infection. Pyogenic bacteria induce the majority of bone infections. *Mycobacterium tuberculosa, Treponema pallidum,* and fungi infect bone infrequently.

Acute hematogenous osteomyelitis

Acute hematogenous osteomyelitis is one of the few orthopedic emergencies. Bacteria invade the bloodstream from a boil, a cellulitis, a sore throat, etc. They travel to bone and lodge in the metaphysis where bone blood flow is greatest but where *rate* of flow is slow and capillaries are open. The bacteria invoke an inflammatory reaction, suppuration, bone erosion, and bone death. A piece of dead bone surrounded by pus or infected granulation tissue is a *sequestrum.* If phagocytosis, body defense mechanisms, and antibiotics do not destroy the bacteria, the abscess takes one or more of the following routes:

1. Pus extends into the medullary cavity of the bone, and its pressure compromises the blood flow in nutrient vessels that enter the endosteal surface of the cortex and supply its inner half to two-thirds. Much of the bone shaft sequestrates.

2. The abscess perforates the cortex, dissects beneath the periosteum, strips it from the bone, destroys the periosteal blood supply, and sequestrates the outer third of the cortex. Subperiosteal and endosteal new bone form around the sequestra. This new bone is an *involucrum*. If the infection subsides, granulation tissue erodes sequestra and replaces them with new bone.
3. The infection perforates the periosteum and forms a soft tissue abscess.
4. Pus enters the adjacent joint, especially if the metaphysis is intracapsular as in the hip.
5. Although the epiphyseal plate acts as a barrier to infection, granulation tissue occasionally destroys it and alters growth.

Occasionally bacteria reenter the bloodstream, perpetuate septicemia, and establish metastatic foci in other sites including bone.

Acute hematogenous osteomyelitis usually affects children, boys more than girls, and most commonly attacks the upper tibia or the distal femur. The most common offending organism varies somewhat with the patient's age. In the child under 1 month of age, a gram-negative rod enters the bloodstream from an infected umbilicus and produces osteomyelitis. In the infant *Streptococcus* is common, but in the older child and adult *Staphylococcus* causes most bone infections.

In most instances, the child has an infected cut, a boil, or a sore throat; 2 to 10 days later, he suddenly develops bone pain and loses function of the involved part. Generalized symptoms vary with the severity of the septicemia. If the organism is of low virulence or if antibiotics have been used, the temperature often increases only slightly. At times, antibiotics suppress clinical symptoms while underlying destruction continues. In an infant with severe septicemia, the temperature frequently rises to 104 or 105° F. The child is warm, dry, restless, and sometimes develops toxic myocarditis and pericarditis.

Upon examination, the physician finds heat, redness, and well-localized tenderness. By using a small object such as a pencil eraser to press on various parts of the bone, one can demonstrate circumscribed point tenderness in the infected portion of the bone. A fluctuant mass indicates subperiosteal or soft tissue abscess. If the infection involves only bone, the child moves adjacent joints slowly without pain. Usually the sedimentation rate and white blood count rise, and the differential count shifts to the left. During septicemia, offending organisms can be grown from a blood culture.

The doctor must make the diagnosis clinically because during the first several days roentgenograms show nothing but soft tissue swelling. Only after 8 to 10 days do roentgenograms disclose periosteal

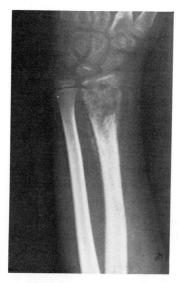

Fig. 38-19. Acute hematogenous osteomyelitis of the radius 3 weeks after onset of symptoms. The infection has destroyed metaphyseal bone. Periosteal new bone is forming.

new bone (Fig. 38-19). To avoid disastrous sequelae, the physician must make the diagnosis before this while the infection remains confined in metaphyseal bone. The orthopedist should treat the child with acute hematogenous osteomyelitis by general supportive measures, correct dehydration, restore adequate hemoglobin level, start antibiotics, surgically drain bone abscesses, culture the pus, obtain sensitivities, and institute appropriate antibiotic treatment. The patient improves dramatically within a few hours. Postoperatively, rest with a cast or plaster splint prevents pathological fracture until new bone replaces dead bone and areas of bone destruction. The patient takes antibiotics for 4 to 6 weeks after all symptoms and signs have disappeared. With this treatment, the child has the best chance to control the infection and avoid chronic osteomyelitis.

Chronic osteomyelitis

Chronic osteomyelitis is difficult to cure. It follows one of several courses. Some patients develop intermittent acute exacerbations. In some, the infection remains dormant only to flare years later, whereas

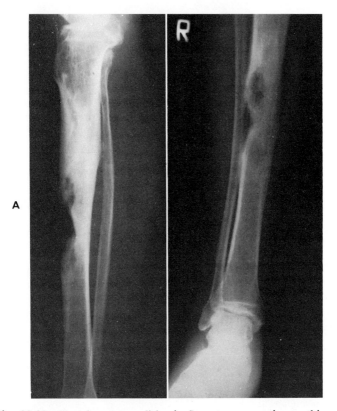

Fig. 38-20. Chronic osteomyelitis. **A,** Seventy years prior to this roentgenogram, the patient had acute hematogenous osteomyelitis; since then, the recurrent chronic infection had drained intermittently; for 2 years, drainage had been continuous; multiple lytic areas are surrounded by sclerotic bone. **B,** Eight months later, the patient had increased drainage and pain and a foul-smelling wound; roentgenograms reveal extensive destruction from the epidermoid carcinoma that developed in the draining sinus.

in others, draining sinuses persist. After years of drainage, a few of these patients develop epidermoid carcinoma in sinus tracts.

Unresorbed sequestra and unobliterated cavities surrounded by sclerotic bone perpetuate chronic infection (Fig. 38-20). Patients with acute exacerbations need appropriate antibiotics and drainage of abscesses. In those with chronic draining areas, surgeons remove underlying diseased bone, collapse cavities, and use appropriate antibiotics in an attempt to close wounds.

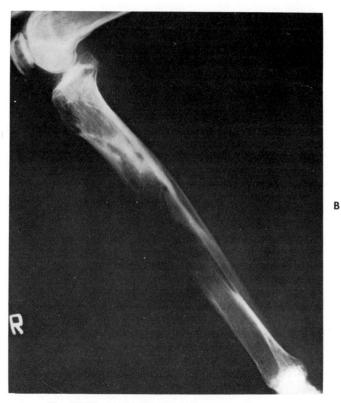

B

Fig. 38-20, cont'd. For legend see opposite page.

Osteomyelitis secondary to open wounds

This type of bone infection usually localizes and gives fewer generalized symptoms than does acute hematogenous osteomyelitis. Surgeons can prevent most of it by thoroughly debriding wounds and using antibiotics if indicated. A patient with this type of infection needs drainage of abscesses, removal of diseased bone and dead tissues, and antibiotics.

Acute pyogenic arthritis

Bacteria enter a joint from underlying osteomyelitis, from an open wound, or directly from the bloodstream. Infected synovium and purulent joint exudate interfere with proper nutrition of articular cartilage by synovial fluid. This, and perhaps proteolytic enzymes, destroys cartilage in the weight-bearing area. The infection extends to subchondral bone. Capsular and intra-articular adhesions combined with incongruous joint surfaces limit joint motion.

The patient with acute pyogenic arthritis develops acute joint pain. The joint swells, and the part loses function. Often generalized symptoms of infection prevail. Upon examination, the doctor finds a swollen joint with excessive joint fluid. Joint motion triggers pain.

Roentgenograms reveal a distended capsular outline. After several days, the joint space narrows. If uncontrolled, infection destroys bone. In many instances at 8 to 10 days, a focus of osteomyelitis becomes evident.

The physician confirms the diagnosis by aspirating purulent, synovial fluid and finding bacteria upon microscopic examination. The patient should have (1) general supportive measures, much the same as in acute hematogenous osteomyelitis, (2) surgical drainage of the joint and underlying bone infection, and (3) appropriate antibiotics. To avoid permanent joint damage, treatment must be started at once.

Acute idiopathic synovitis (viral synovitis) of children presents one of the most confusing differential diagnostic problems. The child holds the joint, usually the hip, immobile, complains of tenderness, and cries with pain on motion. He usually has no generalized symptoms. The patient often gives no history of prior infection; joint fluid contains no bacteria; roentgenograms show no abnormalities; and the condition subsides spontaneously with rest.

Cellulitis overlying the metaphysis of a child must be considered osteomyelitis until proved otherwise. The patient with cellulitis has fewer generalized symptoms, less pain than one with osteomyelitis, and more diffuse tenderness.

Acute rheumatic processes often begin gradually. The patient gives no history of prior infection. He has fewer generalized symptoms and no bone tenderness. The process involves many joints. The white blood count and sedimentation rate rise less than in patients with osteomyelitis.

At times, neoplasm, especially Ewing's tumor, simulates an acute infection even to the extent of presenting with heat and tenderness, generalized symptoms, fever, and sedimentation rate and white blood count elevation. Roentgenograms usually reveal the bone involvement.

Tuberculosis

At times, tuberculosis involves bone without entering a joint, but more often it infects both. The bacteria from a pulmonary lesion (less often from an enteric lesion) travel via the bloodstream to subarticular bone or synovium. Synovium proliferates with a tuberculous, granulomatous pannus that grows across and erodes beneath articular cartilage. The pannus from opposing joint surfaces bridges the joint with fibrous tissue that limits joint motion. Sometimes this ossifies and fuses the joint. The infection frequently destroys joint capsule and forms a soft tissue abscess (cold abscess) of caseous material. This can penetrate skin and form sinuses that become secondarily infected with pyogenic organisms.

Bone tuberculosis often attacks the hip and spine of children. The patient notes gradual onset of pain, joint swelling, and loss of motion. Later, contractures ensue. Children with tuberculosis commonly perspire and cry at night. The temperature rises in the afternoon, and the white count increases. In early stages of the disease, roentgenograms show distension of capsular outlines and bone atrophy, especially of subchondral cortex. Later, marginal notching is visible. In advanced lesions, bone and joint are destroyed.

Pulmonary tuberculosis and a positive skin test support the diagnosis. Isolation of bacteria by culture or guinea pig inoculation proves the diagnosis.

The doctor should treat the patient with general supportive measures, continue appropriate antituberculous drugs for 12 to 18 months, and immobilize the part by a cast, splint, or traction. When the patient is in a good general condition, the orthopedist can excise localized lesions and attempt to restore function of the part, drain abscesses, excise advanced lesions, and fuse the involved joint.

TRAUMA
Fractures

A *fracture* is "a break in continuity of bone or articular cartilage."

Etiology. Fractures result from (1) a direct force at the site of fracture, or (2) an indirect force transmitted from a distance, i.e., fracture of the humerus from a fall on the outstretched hand.

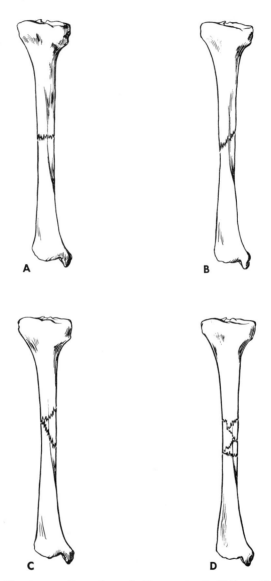

Fig. 38-21. Fracture configurations. **A,** Transverse. **B,** Oblique. **C,** Butterfly. **D,** Comminuted.

Types

Closed: No communication between the external surface of the body and bone.

Open: Communication between external surface of the body and bone via an open wound.

Pathological: A break, usually produced by less force than that required to break a normal bone, through a bone weakened by disease (infection, neoplasm, osteoporosis).

Avulsion: A fragment of bone pulled off by ligament or tendon at its attachment.

Epiphyseal separation: A break in the region of a child's epiphyseal plate (Fig. 38-22). Most involve subepiphyseal spongy bone, but some cross the epiphyseal plate or crush epiphyseal cells and result in subsequent growth dis-

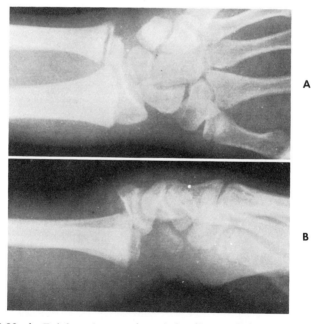

Fig. 38-22. A, Epiphyseal separation of the distal radial epiphysis. The lateral view, **B,** shows a triangular fragment of metaphysis that remained with the dorsally displaced epiphysis. (From Cooper, R. R.: J. Iowa Med. Soc. 54:689, 1964.)

turbance (angulation and/or length discrepancy) (Fig. 38-23).

Greenstick: One side of a child's bone "bends," and the other side breaks (Fig. 38-24).

Comminuted: A break with three or more fragments (Fig. 38-21).

Diagnosis. The physician should suspect a fracture in a patient who gives a history of injury and complains of pain, swelling, and loss of function. Displaced fragments produce obvious deformity. Point tenderness at the fracture line is demonstrable, and gentle motion produces crepitus—one bone fragment grates upon the other. Roentgenograms in at least two planes at right angles to each other are mandatory, and views of the opposite normal counterpart are valuable especially in children where epiphyseal plates, nutrient arteries, and irregular ossification centers might be confusing.

Before he treats a fracture, the doctor must examine and record the

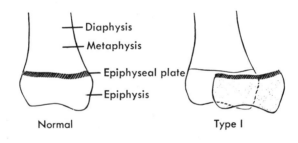

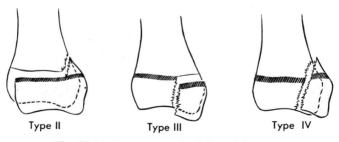

Fig. 38-23. Four types of epiphyseal fractures.

neurovascular status of the extremity distal to the fracture. He must document associated nerve, artery, ligament, or other soft tissue injuries.

Treatment. If he applies certain basic principles, the physician can treat the great majority of fractures satisfactorily, especially in children. If he deviates from these principles, he frequently produces disastrous sequelae. Many fracture complications result from poorly indicated and improperly applied therapy, usually in the form of overtreatment with nuts, bolts, rods, and various pieces of hardware. Before treating a fracture, the physician must diagnose and treat associated injuries that threaten life and that demand priority (airway obstruction, hemorrhage, shock, perforated viscus).

Goals in treatment of fractures are to (1) prevent further damage, (2) gain satisfactory position of involved bones, (3) obtain union as rapidly as possible, (4) use the safest method, and (5) preserve

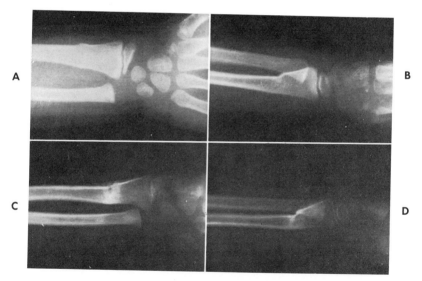

Fig. 38-24. Greenstick fracture. **A,** Anteroposterior view shows expanded cortex at the site of fracture. **B,** Lateral view shows the "buckle" of the dorsal cortex of the radius. **C,** Anteroposterior view after 3 weeks of treatment in a long arm cast; repair has made the fracture more obvious. **D,** Lateral view at 3 weeks. (From Cooper, R. R.: J. Iowa Med. Soc. **54:**689, 1964.)

and/or restore function of the involved part. Stages in fracture treatment are as follows:

1. *First aid:* Prevent further damage and relieve the patient's discomfort until institution of definitive therapy. The following two actions usually accomplish first aid of extremity injuries:
   a. Cover wounds with a pressure dressing of the cleanest bandage available to prevent further contamination and control hemorrhage. As a general rule, tourniquets are unnecessary and can be dangerous.
   b. Immobilize the involved part to relieve pain and prevent further damage—penetration of nerves, arteries, and muscles by bone ends and penetration of skin, thereby converting a closed fracture to an open one. One can immobilize the part effectively with simple splints of magazines, pillows, boards, and strips of cloth.
2. *Reduction:* Place bone fragments in proper relationship to each other. Before this can be done, the doctor must relieve the patient's pain by:
   a. Local injection of an anesthetic into the fracture hematoma. Two precautions are necessary: (1) use strict sterile techniques since a tract is established between a closed fracture and the body surface with the risk of subsequent infection; (2) to obtain satisfactory anesthesia, insert the needle into the hematoma as evidenced by aspiration of blood.
   b. Regional anesthesia (axillary block, sciatic block, etc.).
   c. General anesthesia. To minimize the risk of vomiting and aspiration, allow sufficient time to elapse after the patient ate or drank.

   Thoroughly and carefully debride (remove all devitalized tissue and foreign bodies) all open wounds. Decide whether to close the skin depending on time since injury, amount of contamination, site of injury, and degree of tissue damage. To make this decision, one needs clinical judgment that comes only with experience. If an open wound accompanies a fracture, tetanus prophylaxis must be instituted, and "prophylactic" antibodies are warranted.

   Three considerations in the reduction of a fracture are listed in order of importance as follows:
   a. *Alignment:* Malalignment of a fracture resolves into two components (Fig. 38-25):
      Rotary malalignment: Malposition of one fragment in relation to the other because of turning about an axis parallel to the long axis of the bone; e.g., if a patient fractures his tibia and his toes point posteriorly, one may reasonably assume

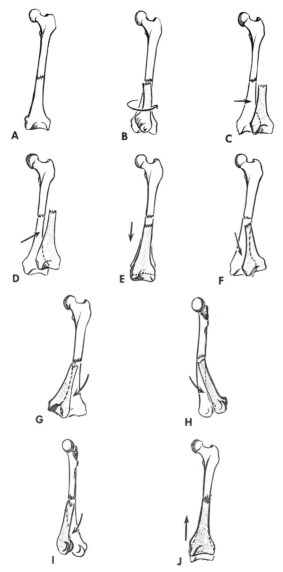

Fig. 38-25. Fracture deformities. A, No deformity. B, Rotation. C, Apposition loss. D, Overriding. E, Distraction. F, Angulation: valgus. G, Angulation: varus. H, Angulation: anterior apex. I, Angulation: posterior apex. J, Impaction.

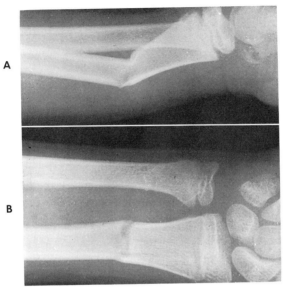

Fig. 38-26. Angulated fracture of distal third of a child's forearm. Lateral view, **A**, shows the angulation. Anteroposterior view, **B**, shows no loss of length or apposition. (From Cooper, R. R.: J. Iowa Med. Soc. 54:689, 1964.)

that rotatory malalignment exists. A fracture unites in a mal-rotated position and does not correct with time in either a child or an adult.

Angulation: Malposition of one fragment in relation to another because of rotation about an axis at 90 degrees to the long axis of the bone (Fig. 38-26). In certain instances, angulation is acceptable. In children, growth corrects angulation in some locations dependig on the child's age and the degree and directon of angulation. In general, the younger the child and the nearer the fracture to the end of a long bone, the more angulation permissible, provided that thet apex of the angle points in the direction of the plane of greatest motion of the adjacent joint (anteriorly or posteriorly in a fracture) near the knee. In no case should more than 25 degrees of angulation remain. Even in adults, in a bone deeply buried in muscle, some angulation does not mean an unsatisfactory result.

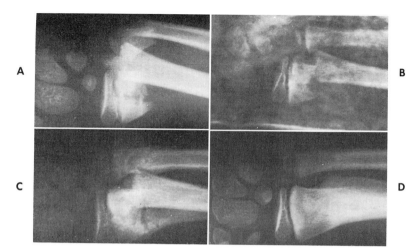

A

B

C

D

Fig. 38-27. Loss of apposition in a fracture of the distal third of a child's forearm. **A,** Anteroposterior roentgenograms showing loss of apposition and length. **B,** With manipulative reduction, length is restored; 50% loss of apposition remains. **C,** Four weeks later, new bone has united the fragments. **D,** Six months later, loss of apposition is being corrected by resorption of the bone on the medial side and bone deposition on the lateral side. (From Cooper, R. R.: J. Iowa Med. Soc. 54:689, 1964.)

b. *Length restoration:* In completely displaced fractures, fragments override because of muscle spasm. The physician must restore appropriate length. Anatomic reduction is not always necessary. In certain instances some overriding is not only acceptable but is even desirable. In a child with a completely displaced long bone shaft fracture, one can accept 1 cm. of overriding with side-to-side union. After such a fracture, blood supply to the limb increases and causes increased growth of the involved extremity. In an adult, side-to-side union of a deeply buried bone is permissible. One should err on the side of overriding rather than distracting the fracture, since distraction predisposes to delayed and/or nonunion.

c. *Apposition:* The amount of end-to-end contact of fragments ranks least important of the three factors, unless the fracture involves a joint surface or unless the bone is subcutaneous where the "stepoff" produced by appositional loss would be cosmetically undesirable. In side-to-side union, complete loss of cross-sectional apposition exists (Fig. 38-27).

When the preceding factors have been corrected, the fracture is reduced. In obtaining a reduction, the physician should always think in the following sequence:

"Can I manipulate the fracture and apply a plaster cast?"

If so, this is the best method yet devised for treatment of a fracture. If he cannot do this or if he knows from past experience that he cannot, he should next think:

"Can I apply traction either to the skin, by attaching adherent tapes to the skin, or to the skeleton, by placing a pin through bone distal to the fracture?"

Traction is retained until fracture fragments stick together sufficiently to go without immobilization or to maintain position in a cast. Both methods of tractions have advantages and disadvantages. Skin traction is easily applied and does not open a bone. In some patients, the skin reacts to tape. The amount of traction and the length of time it can be maintained are limited with skin tapes. Skeletal traction is comfortable and tolerates more weight for a longer time than does skin traction. It can be applied under local anesthesia, but strict sterile technique and a threaded pin must be used to decrease the risk of infecting the bone.

A physician should use no other methods in treating children's fractures except for a few rare articular fractures and the following three common elbow fractures: (1) most fractures of the lateral condyle of the humerus require open reduction; (2) fractures of the medial epicondyle need open reduction if the bone fragment is entrapped in the elbow joint or if the ulnar nerve is impinged; (3) a few fractures of the radial neck cannot undergo closed reduction.

"Must I do an open reduction?"

Only in instances in which the first two methods do not work. Fractures must have a blood supply in order to heal. Any open reduction destroys some vessels and delays healing. Open reduction must definitely be indicated and used only by one aware of all risks and one technically competent to do open reductions.

3. *Fixation:* Hold the fragments reduced by plaster, traction, or in certain instances internal devices.

4. *Immobilization:* The part must be as free of motion as possible until the fracture unites as determined by clinical examination (lack of tenderness and motion) and roentgenographically (obliteration of the fracture line by new bone). Union usually occurs more rapidly in children than in adults.

5. *Preserve and/or restore function to the involved part:* The physician must constantly remember this goal. It is useless to obtain a perfectly united fracture if, in so doing, function is lost. Children restore function well if left to their own devices with pain as their guide to activity. Some adults need physical therapy to help restore function during and after fracture treatment. After an epiphyseal injury, the doctor must follow the child to see if the bone deforms.

Specific fractures
Clavicle fractures

Children and young adults frequently fracture the clavicle, usually by indirect force transmitted up the arm from a fall on the outstretched hand or through the acromion from a fall on the shoulder. Less frequently, a direct blow breaks the clavicle. After fracture, the weight of the upper extremity displaces the distal fragment caudad and the sternocleidomastoid displaces the proximal fragment cephalad (Fig. 38-28). Despite its subcutaneous location, the fractured clavicle usually fails to perforate the skin.

Children commonly sustain a greenstick fracture of the clavicle.

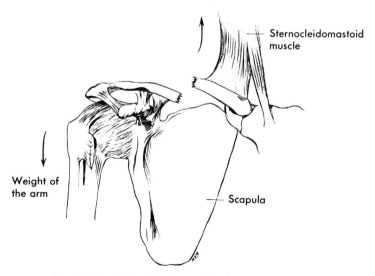

Sternocleidomastoid muscle

Weight of the arm

Scapula

Fig. 38-28. Deforming forces in clavicular fractures.

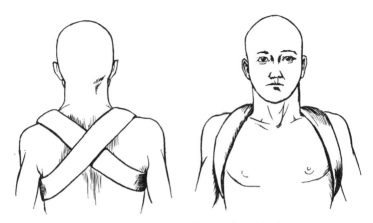

Fig. 38-29. Figure-of-eight splint dressing.

In adults, brachial plexus, vessel, rib, and pulmonary injuries infrequently accompany clavicle fractures.

A figure-of-eight dressing relieves pain, lifts the distal fragment, and pulls it posteriorly to appose the proximal fragment (Fig. 38-29). In children, the dressing consists of a stockinette filled with padding. In adults, plaster over padding effectively holds the clavicle.

Clavicle fractures nearly always unite, and excellent function returns even if moderate displacement remains. Anatomic reduction becomes a goal only if cosmesis is the primary concern.

Humerus fractures

Usually a force transmitted upward through the hand and forearm fractures the humerus. Although shaft, lateral condyle, and medial epicondyle fractures and proximal epiphyseal separations are not uncommon in children, the bone breaks most often at the supracondylar level. In adults the shaft or surgical neck fractures most frequently.

Humerus fractures usually remain closed. Associated injuries include radial nerve injuries, either at the time of fracture or by entrapment in callus during healing. In adults, arterial damage is uncommon. Brachial artery injury must always be considered during treatment of supracondylar fractures in children.

A supracondylar fracture of the humerus constitutes perhaps the most dangerous common fracture in a child's extremity. The distal fragment usually displaces posteriorly and proximally and compresses the brachial artery and median nerve between swollen soft tissues and the sharp distal end of the proximal fragment. Most children with this fracture should be hospitalized and the fracture reduced as soon as possible with skin traction applied to the forearm or with skeletal traction by a pin in the proximal ulna. The hand must be observed carefully and frequently for signs of neurovascular compression (pain, pallor, paresthesias, paralysis, lack of capillary refill, and disappearance of a radial pulse). Progression of any of these signs may necessitate surgical exploration of the brachial artery to prevent the dread complication of Volkmann's ischemic contracture. (See Complications, p. 768.) After 5 to 10 days in traction, the elbow can be held safely in flexion during immobilization in a posterior splint or Velpeau dressing for 3 or 4 weeks.

Treatment of humeral shaft and surgical neck fractures usually consists of a spica cast (one that immobilizes the upper extremity to the body) or a long arm hanging cast. The latter acts as a weight on the arm to prevent overriding and to align fragments during healing. The hanging cast allows early shoulder joint motion, an important consideration in the elderly. Most humeral fractures unite readily. Radial nerve defects occurring at the time of fracture usually resolve. Late entrapment of the radial nerve by callus may require neurolysis.

A lateral humeral condyle fracture in a child extends into the articular surface. Usually, the common extensor muscle origin rotates the fragment 180 degrees so that the articular surface of the distal humerus contacts the fractured surface of the proximal fragment. These fractures fail to reduce by closed methods and if left alone become nonunited, with a subsequent progressive cubitus valgus deformity. This produces delayed ulnar nerve paralysis from stretching the ulnar nerve around the increased valgus angle of the elbow. Appropriate treatment consists of open reduction of the fragment and fixation with one or two pins in an anatomically reduced position. Care must be taken not to strip the common extensor origin from the fragment since this constitutes its only blood supply. After reduction, the child remains in a posterior splint or cast for 5 or 6 weeks, at which time the pins are removed.

A medial humeral epicondyle fracture in a child results when the common flexor muscle origin avulses the epicondyle. The fracture remains extra-articular. It requires open reduction if (1) the fragment displaces and becomes entrapped into the joint, or (2) signs of ulnar nerve compression exist. Open reduction may also be indicated if there is marked displacement especially in a boy, since a fibrous union or a lack of union might weaken forearm muscles. The fragment is fixed to its original position either with sutures or a wire.

Forearm fractures

Radial neck fractures in children ordinarily angulate only mildly and reduce by pressure applied directly over the radial head as the forearm is rotated into pronation and supination. Occasionally a radial neck fracture angulates nearly 90 degrees and fails to reduce by closed methods. In this instance, open reduction and replacement of the radial head onto the radial shaft becomes necessary. Postoperatively, the part is immobilized for 3 or 4 weeks until the fracture unites firmly.

Unlike children, adults frequently fracture the radial head. This, at times, is severely comminuted and if left in place leads to degenerative changes in the radiohumeral joint. In adults, an injured radial head can be safely excised.

Olecranon fractures in adults frequently result from a fall on the elbow with application of direct force to the proximal ulna. If the proximal fragment includes less than one-third of the ulnar articular surface, the fragment may be excised and the triceps tendon attached to the remaining portion of the ulna. If the olecranon fragment is

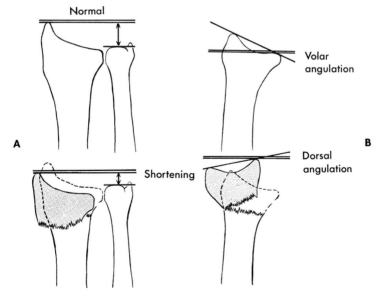

Fig. 38-30. Distal radial fracture. **A,** Anteroposterior. **B,** Lateral.

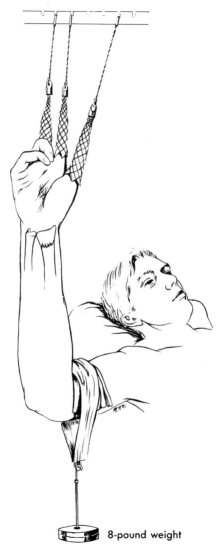

8-pound weight

Fig. 38-31. Traction using finger traps and counterweight.

larger, it can be replaced and fixed to the ulnar shaft by means of an intramedullary screw. Postoperatively, the elbow is immobilized in a posterior plaster splint for 3 to 6 weeks and then progressive active motion begins.

A direct blow or a fall on the outstretched hand may fracture the radius and/or ulna. In children, forearm fractures are commonly greenstick. In older children, distal radial epiphyseal separations are not unusual. Older adults frequently fracture the distal 3 cm. of the radius and the ulnar styloid (Colles' fracture). The mechanism of injury, a fall on the outstretched hand, displaces the distal fragment dorsally, proximally, and radially (Fig. 38-30). Surrounding tissues usually remain uninjured.

Local anesthesia affords satisfactory relief of pain for closed reduction of many forearm fractures in adults and children. After the fracture hematoma is injected, distraction accomplished by finger traps and a counterweight on the upper arm (Fig. 38-31) often corrects angulation, overriding, and displacement. In children, a long arm cast then holds the fracture until it unites. In the older patient with Colles' fracture, a plaster cast from metacarpophalangeal joints to elbow for 3 to 4 weeks often suffices. This allows elbow, shoulder, and finger motion so necessary to avoid crippling stiffness of the arm and hand.

In adults with a radial and ulnar shaft fracture, closed reduction may be impossible, thereby necessitating open reduction and internal fixation.

Hand fractures
(See Chapter 39.)

Vertebral fractures
Vertebral fractures may be classified into (1) vertebral body fractures, usually with anterior wedging and compression, and (2) fractures that involve the neural arch, often with a shift of one vertebral body upon the other. The mechanism of injury in the first type is usually compression of the vertebral body as in a fall from a height onto the legs or buttocks or from striking the top of the head as in diving into shallow water. The second type of fracture may also occur by these mechanisms but often follows severe rotational and displacement forces such as those produced in an automobile accident.

Vertebral fractures usually remain closed. Frequently spinal cord and/or nerve injuries accompany these fractures. Usually no external deformity is seen in vertebral fractures, although with marked compression there may be visible angulation. Radiographs show anterior wedging of the vertebral body or fractures of the neural arch with displacement of one vertebral body upon the other. Treatment is aimed at preventing spinal cord damage or at preventing further cord damage in patients demonstrating initial neurological deficit.

Fracture dislocations of the cervical spine require reduction by tongs placed in the skull followed by further immobilization in plaster and/or by operative fusion of the involved vertebral bodies. Mild dorsal and lumbar compression fractures may be treated by bed rest with walking as soon as pain disappears. Residual deformities do not usually limit function and late results often depend on the degree of spinal cord injury.

Fracture with spinal cord and/or nerve injury, especially if the loss progresses, requires early neurosurgical care.

Pelvic fractures

Pelvic fractures result from direct trauma or from forces transmitted to the pelvis through the femur. Some fractures pass through weight-bearing portions of the pelvis and some do not (Fig. 38-32). Pelvic fractures usually remain closed. Associated bladder, urethral,

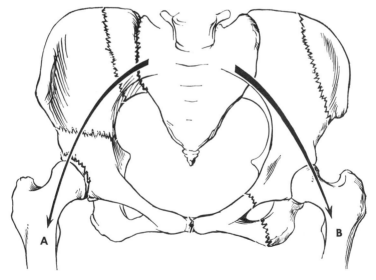

Fig. 38-32. Pelvic fractures. **A,** Fractures through the weight-bearing line. **B,** Fractures not through the weight-bearing line.

or rectal injuries must be suspected. Sacral fractures may lacerate nerves emerging through sacral foramina. Displacement in pelvic fractures is often minimal. Displaced fractures in one part of the bony pelvic ring usually signify fractures through opposite portions of the ring. In some fractures, the hemipelvis displaces cranially (Fig. 38-33). Treatment in this situation consists of traction through the corresponding leg to attempt restoration of alignment. Nondisplaced fractures warrant ambulation as early as symptoms permit.

Acetabular fractures that involve displacement with incongruity between the femoral head and the weight-bearing acetabular dome often require open reduction and fixation. These frequently result in subsequent degenerative joint changes and hip pain.

Other pelvic fractures usually produce no residual severe deformity. Appreciable displacement in women of child-bearing age may mitigate against future vaginal delivery.

Hip fractures (femoral neck and intertrochanteric)

These injuries usually occur from minor trauma in aged patients with osteoporosis. Pathological fractures from metastatic carcinoma often involve these locations. The deformity in both femoral neck and intertrochanteric fractures consists of shortening and external rotation of the extremity, a deformity usually obvious clinically and radiographically.

Treatment of femoral neck fractures consists of closed reduction by traction, internal rotation, and abduction of the limb followed by

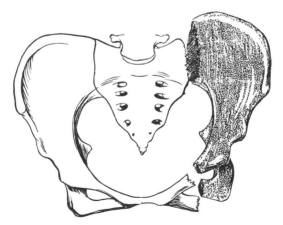

Fig. 38-33. Double vertical fracture of the pelvis.

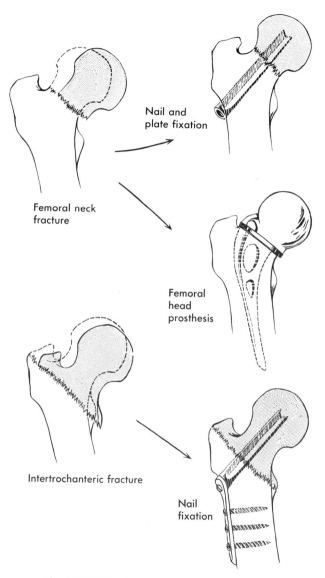

Fig. 38-34. Hip fractures and their treatment.

Nail and
plate fixation

Femoral neck
fracture

Femoral
head
prosthesis

Intertrochanteric fracture

Nail
fixation

internal fixation with multiple threaded pins or a nail through the femoral neck and head (Fig. 38-34). The femoral head is replaced by a prosthesis in selected cases. Intertrochanteric fractures are treated by closed reduction and internal fixation with a nail and side plate (Fig. 38-34). Fixation permits patients to sit by 1 or 2 days postoperatively and walk in a walker or on crutches without bearing weight if they have sufficient strength. This prevents a multitude of complications (thrombophlebitis, pulmonary emboli, pneumonia, renal stones, pressure ulcers) that often lead to death.

Results in hip fractures leave much to be desired. Many patients die during the first year after treatment. Intertrochanteric fractures usually heal, but nonunion with aseptic necrosis frequently accompanies femoral neck fractures. Replacement prostheses eliminate nonunion, but introduce unique problems of their own.

Femoral shaft fractures

The injuring force may be a direct blow or transmission of stress upward through the foot and tibia. Most femoral shaft fractures remain closed. Marked blood loss (up to 3 liters) accompanies femoral shaft fractures. Associated femoral artery injuries must be treated promptly and correctly to save the limb. Varying degrees of muscle injury, especially to the quadriceps, may produce fibrosis with subsequent functional loss.

The clinical examination usually reveals shortening of the extremity and swelling of the thigh, both from the fracture hematoma and the shortened musculature. The fracture fragments almost always override, angulate, and rotate. Distraction, because of excessive traction, greatly increases chances of nonunion. A small amount of overriding is desirable especially in the growing child since the stimulus of increased blood supply to epiphyseal plates increases linear bone growth. Rotational deformities must be avoided since even the child's growing bone will not correct rotational malalignments spontaneously.

Femoral shaft fractures in adults are commonly treated with 8 to 20 pounds of traction through a skeletal traction pin for 8 weeks followed by a hip spica until union is solid. Recently the use of a cast brace has been adopted by many physicians for treatment of femoral shaft fractures. With this method, the patient remains in traction for 1 to 6 weeks and is then placed in a well-fitted cast brace. This is designed to permit knee motion and to take partial weight bearing through the fractured bone and partial weight bearing on the ischial tuberosity and through the soft tissues of the thigh. This method has the advantage of allowing healing to be stimulated by some forces being transmitted through the bone, and it allows earlier walking. In children, skin traction often suffices. Toddlers may bear full weight with solid bony union in about 4 weeks. Certain femur shaft fractures in adults can be treated by an intramedullary rod. This shortens hospitalization but adds formidable risks of operation and infection.

Patellar fractures

Fracture of the patella includes two general types that often differ in mechanism of injury, associated damage to surrounding structures, and treatment.

Transverse fractures occur with violent sudden contraction of the quadriceps muscle (when one slips and attempts to prevent a fall). Less often, a direct blow produces a transverse fracture. The two fragments may be equal or the fracture line can occur toward either pole of the patella, producing dissimilar fragments. If the fragments retain opposition, physical examination shows only mild local swelling and tenderness with pain on knee extension. Wide separation of the fragments produces a palpable sulcus. This also indicates medial and lateral tearing of the quadriceps expansion and the joint capsule.

If the fragments do not separate, treatment consists of a posterior plaster splint or cylinder cast with graduated quadriceps exercise started at 2 to 3 weeks and with progressive weight bearing soon thereafter. Wide separation of fragments demands operative realignment, suture of the torn quadriceps expansion, and 6 to 10 weeks of plaster immobilization. Marked disparity in fragment size justifies removal of the smaller one and repair of tendon or muscle attachments to the retained fragment.

Comminuted patellar fractures generally result from a direct blow. Associated lacerations of the joint capsule or quadriceps expansion are less severe; however, damage of the articular surfaces of femur and patella is frequently extensive. Treatment then consists of patellectomy and suture of the patellar tendon to the quadriceps tendon. A plaster cast immobilizes the extremity in extension for 4 to 6 weeks.

Tibial fractures

Tibial shaft fractures result from torsional force or from a direct blow (bumper fracture), and tibial plateau fractures result from a force transmitted up the tibia and to the femoral condyles (body weight). Bone fragments from the subcutaneous tibia frequently protrude through skin lacerations. Tibial fractures may injure the posterior tibial artery. Skin injuries often result in difficulty of obtaining soft tissue closure over open tibial fractures. Lateral displacement sufficient to cause overriding is uncommon in transverse fractures, but common in oblique fractures. Rotational deformity must be suspected in displaced tibial fractures. Tibial plateau fractures angulate into varus or valgus.

Tibial shaft fractures can usually be treated by closed reduction and a long leg plaster or by skeletal traction distal to the fracture until the fragments unite sufficiently to prevent displacement in a cast. Solid union may not occur for 3 to 8 months.

Tibial plateau fractures may be comminuted and require splinting with subsequent early motion, or they may consist of one large fragment that can be openly reduced and fixed to the remaining tibia.

Ankle fractures (medial and lateral malleoli and ankle ligaments)

The medial malleolus (tibia), posterior malleolus (posterior lip of the distal articular surface of the tibia), and lateral malleolus (fibula) fracture alone or in various combinations. Ligament injuries may accompany one or more of these fractures and often demand as much or more attention than the fracture itself. The mechanism of injury is excessive movement of the mobile leg upon the fixed foot or of the mobile foot upon the fixed leg. The injuring force frequently externally rotates and/or abducts the foot, talus, and distal tibia and fibula. Certain combinations of force produce characteristic fracture patterns. Ankle fractures remain closed unless a direct injury lacerates the skin or the injuring force dislocates the talus from the tibia with resulting skin loss or subsequent necrosis.

The deformity of a fracture dislocation of the ankle is obvious on inspection (gross loss of the relationship between the foot and leg). Without dislocation, the injury produces swelling and tenderness over the injured malleoli. Final distinction between bony and ligamentous injuries requires roentgenograms in the anterior, posterior, lateral, and oblique projections.

Adequate reduction demands reconstitution of the forklike configuration of the medial and lateral malleolus (closing the ankle mortise). Interposition of a flap of soft tissues (deltoid ligament) between the medial malleolus and talus may necessitate open reduction to restore normal congruity between the articular surfaces of the talus and tibia (Fig. 38-35). Many ankle fractures can be reduced closed and immobilized 6 to 8 weeks in a short leg walking cast. More complicated fractures and fracture dislocations may require a long leg cast and no weight bearing for varying periods or open reduction with ligament repair and internal fixation of the fracture.

The results of treatment are usually good if (1) tibiotalar congruity is restored (the ankle mortise is closed) and (2) ligamentous injuries are recognized and treated adequately. Delayed union or nonunion occasionally occurs in medial malleolar fractures.

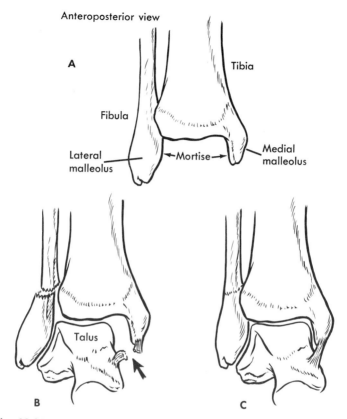

Fig. 38-35. Ankle mortise. **A,** Normal. **B,** Fracture of lateral malleolus and tear of deltoid ligament *(arrow)* opens mortise. **C,** Mortise closed with restored congruity of talus and tibia.

Foot fractures

Talus. Fractures often involve the neck of the talus and are frequently accompanied by ankle and/or subtalar dislocation. These fractures reduce with difficulty and may require surgical reduction. Because of the source of blood supply, aseptic necrosis of the body of the talus frequently develops and adds to morbidity and produces long-term complications.

Calcaneus. Fractures of the calcaneus usually occur after a fall from a height. These falls crush the bone and frequently extend into the subtalar joint. The foot becomes extremely swollen. Initial treatment consists of rest, elevation, and compression. After swelling decreases, many fractures can be managed with a short leg cast and weight bearing as tolerated. Several operations are designed to attempt reconstruction of various calcaneal fractures. After treatment, subtalar joint motion often remains decreased.

Metatarsal and phalangeal. These fractures usually require closed reduction and plaster immobilization for 3 to 4 weeks. Some, with marked displacement, demand open reduction and internal fixation.

Complications of fractures
Complications of casts

Improperly applied plaster or subsequent swelling produces pressure of the cast against underlying soft tissues over bone prominences. Skin circulation decreases, and necrosis results. In applying a cast, the physician should expose the tips of the patient's toes or fingers in order to observe the parts for signs of neurovascular compression. Pressure from a tight cast or padding, or hemorrhage and swelling into a muscular compartment compromises circulation to the extremity. Persistent neurovascular interference invokes Volkmann's ischemic paralysis, especially after humeral supracondylar fractures and fractures or dislocations near the knee. In this syndrome, muscular

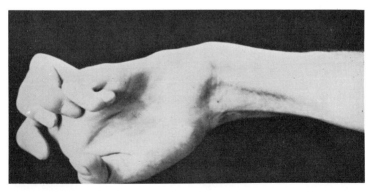

Fig. 38-36. Volkmann's ischemic contracture. The clawhand is rigid and useless. (From Steindler, A.: The traumatic deformities and disabilities of the upper extremity, Springfield, Ill., 1946, Charles C Thomas, Publisher, p. 296.)

circulation decreases, necrotic and fibrotic scar replaces muscles, and permanent contractures ensue (Fig. 38-36). Associated sensory loss further impairs function.

Because of these disastrous sequelae, the doctor must investigate and correct complaints of pain and numbness beneath a cast. Pain, pallor, swelling, discoloration, and lack of capillary refill indicate circulatory embarrassment. The doctor must treat a patient with any of these immediately by splitting the cast and the underlying padding, elevating the part, and observing the patient carefully to see if surgical exploration of the involved vessel is indicated.

Malunion

If a fractured bone is improperly reduced or loses reduction as swelling decreases, the bone unites in an unsatisfactory position. To avoid this complication, the doctor must reduce the fracture properly and follow the patient to be certain that reduction is *maintained*. If a malunion is cosmetically or functionally unacceptable to the patient, an orthopedic surgeon can rebreak the bone (osteotomy) and restore satisfactory position.

Delayed union

At times a bone fails to heal solidly after a reasonable period as determined by location of the fracture, type of fracture, and method of treatment. Continued adequate immobilization corrects most delayed unions.

Nonunion

Some bones fail to unite. Gross motion is generally demonstrable. Roentgenograms reveal sclerosis of adjacent bone ends and obliteration of the medullary canal. Fibrous scar tissue or a false joint (pseudarthrosis) fills the gap between bone ends. Bone grafting stimulates repair at these sites.

The causes of delayed and nonunion are not always immediately apparent and usually include a combination of inadequate reduction, inadequate fixation, inadequate immobilization, severe trauma to soft parts, improper operative treatment, distraction of fragments, infection, and location of the fracture. The femoral neck, carpal scaphoid, and junction of the distal one third and middle one third of the tibia unite slowly.

Shock

Bone is extremely vascular. At the time of fracture, large volumes of blood escape from the circulating blood into soft tissues or externally through an open wound. Neurogenic shock from pain aggravates shock from blood loss. For the patient in shock, the physician must provide an adequate airway and oxygen, control hemorrhage and pain, and restore blood volume.

Fat embolism

Patients who sustain massive trauma occasionally develop clinical signs and symptoms of fat embolism. This syndrome results from vascular impaction by fat, especially in the lungs, brain, and kidney. After massive trauma to long bones, marrow fat may contribute to intravascular aggregation of lipoproteins.

Classically, the patient begins to recover from the initial acute trauma and then regresses clinically. This occurs on the average of 24 hours after the acute injury and consists of an increase in the pulse, temperature, and respiration. The patient becomes apprehensive, delirious, may eventually exhibit focal neurological signs, convulse, and lapse into stupor and coma. Cyanosis may accompany these signs and symptoms. Frequently, petechiae at or before the development of other signs and symptoms appear, especially over the upper chest wall and in the conjunctivae. Chest roentgenograms often reveal diffuse cloudlike densities in the lungs. Fat may be demonstrated in the urine of some patients. Blood gas studies are of critical importance in monitoring the status of a patient with fat emboli. Therapy must be instituted promptly if the patient's life is to be saved. Further manipulation of injured extremities should be avoided. The patients need appropriate blood, fluid, and electrolyte replacement therapy. They should be digitalized if they develop cardiac failure. Blood gases serve as a guide to the need for and the use of oxygen therapy. The degree of pulmonary damage may necessitate positive pressure oxygen by means of tracheotomy and a respirator.

Some have advocated the use of steroids, alcohol, and heparin in management of fat embolism, but their status is more debatable than that of the critical need of oxygen by the patient with this syndrome.

Peripheral nerve injuries

At the time of fracture or during reduction, bone ends might injure nerves. Prior to attempts at reduction, the physician must evaluate motor and sensory nerve function distal to the fracture and record these observations. Closed fractures occasionally contuse nerves. These usually recover fully. Immediate open exploration is not warranted. In open fractures with nerve injuries, the surgeon inspects the nerve at the time of wound debridement, and if it is severed, plans appropriate surgical repair.

Infection

Bacteria can enter bone from an open fracture or from implantation during surgery. (See section on treatment of osteomyelitis, p. 739.)

Posttraumatic degenerative joint disease

After articular fractures, incongruous joint surfaces can subsequently develop degenerative joint changes. At times, the physician can minimize this by adequate apposition of fragments. If trauma is extensive, subsequent degenerative changes cannot be prevented. Patients with degenerative changes must be treated with appropriate measures depending on the severity of their symptoms. (See degenerative joint disease, p. 789.)

Acute atrophy (reflex dystrophy, postimmobilization atrophy, Sudeck's atrophy)

In certain patients, a part that remains immobile undergoes acute atrophy, including bone atrophy (Sudeck's atrophy). Patients who do not use portions of the extremity that are free of a cast develop atrophy more frequently than others. They complain of pain, motion decreases, edema develops, and the skin atrophies and becomes shiny. If the disorder progresses, contractures develop, adhesions limit joint function, and a useless part results. To prevent or treat this disorder, patients must use the part actively and institute range-of-motion exercises.

Aseptic necrosis

When a fracture isolates bone from its blood supply, the bone dies. Necrosis most often develops after fracture of the femoral neck, carpal navicular, and neck of talus. Dead bone appears radiopaque in contrast to surrounding normal bone that atrophies from disuse. Dead bone is slowly destroyed by granulation tissue and replaced by new bone. If force is transmitted before repair is complete, the bone fractures in the zone of replacement at the junction of dead and new bone. Bone grafting hastens repair of necrotic areas and, by supporting bone, prevents collapse.

Joint injuries
Sprains

A sprain is a tear in ligament and capsule fibers. Sprains are classified clinically and treated as follows:

Mild (first-degree). A few fibers separate. The region is tender, swollen, and bruised. The joint retains stability. The patient is treated with analgesics, rest, elevation, and cold packs for the first 12 to 24 hours. He then needs warm packs, a compression wrap or taping, and rest of the part for 7 to 10 days.

Moderate (second-degree). Several fibers tear. The patient complains of more tenderness, the part swells and becomes ecchymotic. On examination, the doctor notes some effusion and slight instability of the joint. Immobilization in a plaster cast for 3 to 6 weeks, depending on the joint involved, permits healing.

Severe (third-degree). The ligaments disrupt completely, and the joint loses stability. An orthopedic surgeon should repair these ligaments.

Without proper treatment, ligaments heal in an elongated position with residual laxity that predisposes to further episodes of injury and eventual need for surgical reconstruction.

Dislocations

During a dislocation, articular surfaces of opposing bones completely and persistently separate. During subluxation, opposing articular surfaces partially and temporarily separate. A dislocation damages joint capsule and ligaments. Prior to reduction of a dislocation, the physician should obtain roentgenograms for diagnostic and legal purposes. Fractures accompany many dislocations, and if a fracture is found after reduction, some might assume that the doctor produced it. Only if dislocation compromises vascular supply must reduction be done on an emergency basis before roentgenograms are obtained.

Before a dislocation is reduced, the patient needs proper anesthesia or analgesia. Complicated maneuvers are unnecessary to reduce most dislocations. Simple traction reduces many of them. Some must be reduced surgically.

The physician must obtain postreduction roentgenograms to be sure that he has reduced the dislocation. He then immobilizes the part for 3 to 6 weeks so that the ligaments heal properly. The patient restores function by using the part.

Torn ligaments that are not well protected heal in an elongated position with predisposition to recurrent dislocation that must often be treated by surgery.

Intra-articular derangement

Knee joint menisci are particularly prone to injuries. Medial menisci tear 10 to 12 times more frequently than do lateral menisci. The patient usually has the foot fixed and the knee partly flexed. He then forcibly rotates the body to the opposite side and notes sudden pain over the joint line. The joint *locks* (the knee will not fully extend and/or fully flex). An effusion develops over the next few hours. At times, traction unlocks the knee. Most meniscal tears do not heal but result in subsequent episodes of locking and giving way. Surgical removal of a torn meniscus alleviates these symptoms. Differential diagnosis includes osteochondral fractures and osteochondritis dissecans. During an osteochondral fracture, a piece of articular cartilage and subchondral bone breaks free from the underlying bone. In osteochondritis dissecans, common in teenagers, a piece of articular cartilage and underlying bone separates from the remainder of the bone. The bone fragments and dies. This disorder is usually located on the lateral surface of the medial femoral condyle. Frequently, the fragment revascularizes and heals, but it sometimes drops into the joint. In either of these disorders, a free fragment in the joint gives symptoms like those of a torn meniscus. Roentgenograms often reveal a defect in the femoral condyle where the fragment separated. If the fragment contains bone, a roentgenogram shows it. These free fragments should be removed.

Injuries of muscles and tendons

Excessive force produces separation of musculotendinous units at the junction of muscle and tendon, through the tendon, or at the site of tendon insertion into bone. The patient notes immediate pain, swelling, ecchymosis, and loss of function. Soon after disruption, the muscle or tendon should be restored surgically, especially if it is an important functional unit. If treatment is neglected, many units regenerate sufficiently to give adequate function. If not, surgical reconstruction is indicated.

Myositis ossificans

A direct blow to a muscle causes intramuscular hemorrhage that usually resorbs but that on occasion ossifies. Several days or even weeks after injury, the patient notices a lump. The mass enlarges and becomes firm during the next 5 to 10 weeks. In some instances, it is mildly tender and interferes with muscle function. Usually the mass then decreases in size and disappears after 6 to 8 months. Roentgenograms reveal increased ossification while the mass grows (Fig. 38-37). The bone becomes mature and usually resorbs. In a few instances, it remains. A thorough history helps differentiate myositis ossificans from a bone-forming tumor. Despite this, the doctor must observe the patient carefully. Excision of the mass soon after it develops leads to more hemorrhage and greater ossification. If, after a year or 18 months, the mass persists, one can safely excise it.

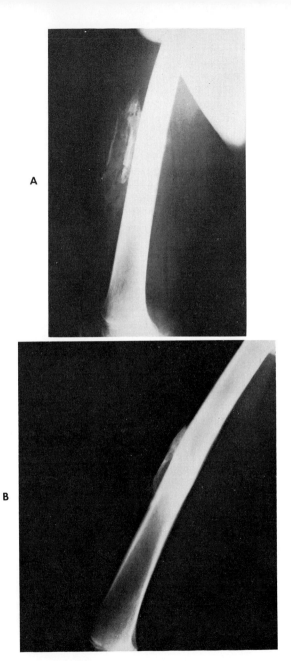

Fig. 38-37. For legend see opposite page.

BENIGN BONE TUMORS

To diagnose bone tumors, the physician must use a correlative approach wherein he integrates clinical facts, roentgenographic appearance, and histopathology, each in its proper perspective. Doing so is especially important in the diagnosis of a malignant tumor and perhaps even more important in prevention of misdiagnosis of malignancy in a benign lesion. Such an error would lead to unwarranted, mutilating overtreatment. Table 38-9 describes in detail benign lesions that are frequently misdiagnosed as malignancies.

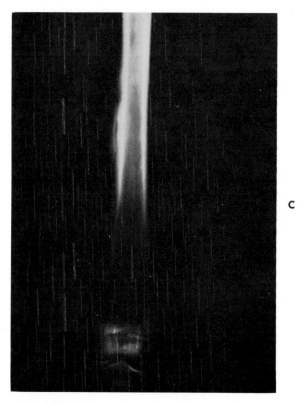

Fig. 38-37. Myositis ossificans. **A,** Roentgenogram of the thigh 1 month after injury showing ossification in the quadriceps muscle and beneath the periosteum of the femoral shaft. **B,** Twelve months later the myositis ossificans is resorbing. **C,** Two and one-half years after injury, some periosteal bone remains.

Table 38-9. Benign lesions often misdiagnosed as malignancies

Lesion	Common age	Sex distribution	Common location
Osteocartilaginous exostosis: a cartilage-capped projection of bone, enchondral ossification at the cartilage-bone junction continues until growth stops; developmental defect	6–10	Equal	Metaphysis, distal femur, proximal tibia
Metaphyseal fibrous defect: a developmental defect that consists of fibrous connective tissue, giant cells, and foam cells in the cortical and subcortical bone	4–10	Equal	Metaphysis, distal femur, proximal tibia
Bone cyst: a juxtaepiphyseal cavity lined by a thin layer of connective tissue and filled with yellow serum	4–14	Males	Metaphysis, proximal humerus, proximal femur
Osteoid osteoma: a reactive lesion consisting of a central nidus of osteoid and new bone in a fibrovascular stroma	10–25	Males	Femur and tibia
Osteoblastoma: a reactive lesion similar to but larger than osteoid osteoma	15–35	Equal	Vertebra, metacarpal, femur
Aneurysmal bone cyst: a reactive "blowout" of the cortex by a lesion composed of vascular lakes surrounded by fibrous connective tissue, foam cells, and giant cells	12–25	Females	Femoral metaphysis and vertebra
Enchondroma: A mass of hyaline cartilage within the confines of bone	10–50	Equal	Diaphysis phalanx of hand, metacarpal, humerus, femur

Symptoms	*Radiographic appearance*	*Treatment*
Mass; pain if: (1) bursa, (2) fracture, (3) nerve irritation	Sessile or pedunculated bony prominence projects from the metaphyseal cortex (Fig. 38-38)	Less than 1% become malignant (chondrosarcoma from the cartilage cap); remove for pain; neurological symptoms, or rapid growth especially after the epiphyseal plates close
None; incidental roentgen-ray finding	Eccentric metaphyseal lytic lesion surrounded by scalloped edge of reactive new bone (Fig. 38-39)	*DO NOT* ascribe pain to them; find the true cause of limb pain in a child
Pathological fracture	Metaphyseal central lytic and trabeculated cyst; the cortex expands on either side (Fig. 38-40)	Some heal after one or more fractures; others need treatment by curettement and bone grafting, preferably after the age of 10
Severe pain, worse at night; relieved by aspirin	Lytic lesion less than 1 cm. in diameter; a dense, central nidus surrounded by reactive new bone	Excision
Pain that is less severe than in osteoid osteoma	Central lytic lesion over 1 cm. in diameter surrounded by reactive new bone	Excision if possible
Pain and expanding mass	Lytic lesion with a "blown-out" distension of the cortex; frequently a thin layer of periosteal new bone surrounds the cyst	Curetting and bone grafting
Swelling, pain, fracture	Oval lytic area with "expanded" cortex, stippled calcifications	Curet and bone chips if fracture, rapid growth, or symptomatic; long bone enchondromas can become malignant (chondrosarcoma)

Continued.

Table 38-9. Benign lesions often misdiagnosed as malignancies—cont'd

Lesion	Common age	Sex dis-tribution	Common location
Fibrous dysplasia: a developmental error; certain regions of bone are replaced by a dense, fibrous connective tissue stroma from which trabeculae of new bone arise	5–25	Males	Diaphysis, ribs, femur, humerus
Giant cell tumor: a lesion of polyhedral stromal cells and many multinucleated giant cells within the confines of bone	20–50	Females	Epiphyseal, distal radius, distal femur, proximal tibia

MALIGNANT BONE TUMORS
Tumors primary in bone

Malignant bone tumors produce the same symptoms regardless of their histological type. Patients complain of pain, often mild and intermittent at first, but increasing to become severe and constant, especially at night. On examination the physician finds a mass, local tenderness, and warm skin with dilated subcutaneous veins. In more advanced cases, generalized symptoms include weakness and weight loss. Anemia is common. If a patient presents with these complaints suggestive of a malignancy, the physician must make the diagnosis. This usually involves a biopsy. The orthopedist, radiologist, and pathologist must maintain close liaison to make the correct diagnosis and outline the plan of treatment. Table 38-10 gives the characteristics of malignant tumors primary in bone.

Tumors metastatic to bone

Carcinoma commonly spreads to bone. In extensive autopsy studies of patients dying from carcinomatosis, pathologists find as many as 70% with bone metastases. Metastases most frequently involve vertebral column, pelvis, skull, humerus, and femur. They rarely spread to bones distal to the elbow and knee. Carcinomas of the prostate, breast, kidney, lung, and thyroid produce most bone metastases. Lesions can lyse bone (hypernephroma, thyroid), provoke an osteo-

Symptoms	Radiographic appearance	Treatment
Incidental finding; fractures or deformity	Lytic, ground glass–appearing lesions; cortex expands and bones deform	Curet and pack if symptomatic
Pain and mass	Central or eccentric epiphyseal destructive and/or trabeculated area surrounded by an expanded cortex	Excise if compatible with function of the part; if not, curet and graft; on recurrence, do a wide local excision or amputation since a strong potential for malignancy exists

blastic reaction (prostate), or be a mixture of these two (breast, lung).

Some metastases produce no symptoms. With others, the patient complains of pain and swelling. Frequently, the involved bone fractures. At times, the bone lesion causes symptoms before the primary tumor does. If, in such a case, the history, physical examination, and routine roentgenograms do not readily reveal the primary lesion, the orthopedist can biopsy a bone. This not only rules out a primary bone tumor, but in certain instances the histology of a metastatic lesion provides a clue to the primary site. Pathological fracture through a metastatic tumor usually heals. Orthopedists treat these fractures with internal fixation so that the patient is free of pain and can be ambulatory. Depending on the type of tumor, its size, and its location, treatment of the bone lesion consists of radiotherapy, chemotherapy, and hormonal therapy, or a combination of these. The physician strives to prolong life and to make the patient as comfortable and functional as possible.

Secondary invasion of bone by adjacent soft tissue tumors

Fibrosarcoma, synovial sarcoma, neurosarcoma, liposarcoma, and hemangioendothelioma at times erode adjacent bone. They produce symptoms like those of a malignant bone tumor. Roentgenograms

Table 38-10. Malignant tumors primary in bone

Lesion	Age	Sex	Common location
Osteosarcoma: a connective tissue tumor composed of malignant stromal cells that have osteogenic potential as manifest by the ability to produce tumor osteoid and bone	10–25	Male	Metaphysis, distal femur, proximal tibia
Juxtacortical sarcoma: an uncommon lesion that arises in relation to the periosteum and/or adjacent tissue; tends to form a deceptively benign-appearing fibrous stroma from which tumor bone arises; some areas contain clumps of cartilage	30–40		Distal femoral metaphysis
Chondrosarcoma: a tumor of malignant cartilage cells; *primary,* a chondrosarcoma arising at the site of no known preexisting defect; *secondary,* a chondrosarcoma arising from an osteocartilaginous exostosis or enchondroma; microscopically, chondrosarcoma is difficult to differentiate from a benign enchondroma; evidence for malignancy includes history, radiographic evidence of destruction, microscopic hypercellularity, plump nuclei, and double nuclei	30–50	Female	Diaphysis, ribs and pelvis, proximal femur and humerus
Fibrosarcoma: a tumor composed of malignant stromal cells that produce a fibrous, nonossifying matrix	10–40	Male	Distal femur, proximal tibia
Ewing's tumor: a highly malignant round cell tumor probably derived from primitive reticular cells of the bone marrow	10–25	Male	Diaphysis of femur or tibia, pelvis
Reticulum cell sarcoma: a round cell tumor composed of reticulum cells of the bone marrow	20–40	Male	Pelvis, femur
Multiple myeloma: a round cell tumor arising from primitive reticulum cells that have the capacity to differentiate into plasma cells	50–70	Male	Multiple sites, vertebra, skull, ribs, long bones

Radiographic appearance	*Treatment*	*Prognosis*
Metaphyseal osteolytic and/or osteoblastic; a triangle of subperiosteal reactive new bone, a sunburst appearance from striae of new bone, cortical destruction in a jagged manner (Fig. 38-41)	Amputation or disarticulation; chemotherapy	10 to 20% 5-year survival; tends to spread rapidly via the bloodstream
A sclerotic, lobulated mass extending from the cortex; tends to invade the underlying bone	Wide, local excision or amputation	30 to 50% 5-year survival
Mottled osseous destruction with fusiform expansion of the shaft; mottled calcification	Wide excision or amputation	25 to 40% 5-year survival; tends to spread locally and along veins; metastasize via the bloodstream
A lytic, destructive, nonbone-producing defect	Amputation	20 to 30% 5-year survival
A lytic, destructive process, reactive periosteal new bone in layers and occasionally marked reactive new bone much like osteogenic sarcoma	Irradiation, chemotherapy	0 to 4% 5-year survival
A lytic, destructive lesion with little tendency to produce reactive new bone	Irradiation or amputation	40% 5-year survival
Multifocal lytic lesions without much tendency to reactive new bone; osteoporosis (Fig. 38-42)	Irradiation, urethane, and antimetabolites	In most cases, eventually fatal

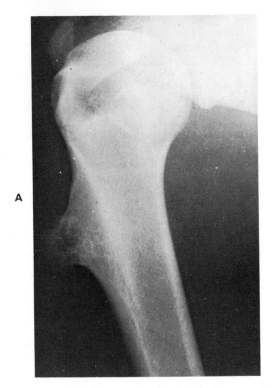

Fig. 38-38. Osteocartilaginous exostosis. **A,** Single exostosis of humeral shaft. **B,** Hereditary multiple exostoses.

reveal the soft tissue mass and an underlying lytic defect in the outer surface of the bone cortex. At times, the tumor destroys the entire cortex and invades the medullary canal. The physician uses the same diagnostic methods and treats the patient much the same as one with a primary malignant bone tumor.

NEUROMUSCULAR DISORDERS
Poliomyelitis

Poliomyelitis has disappeared as a major cause of neuromuscular disability in children. Vaccines have precipitously reduced the incidence of the disease. The polio virus attacks brainstem motor nuclei

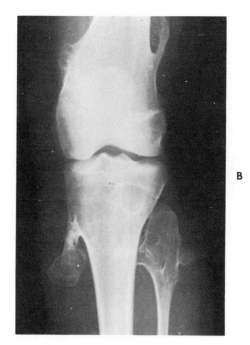

B

Fig. 38-38, cont'd. For legend see opposite page.

and spinal cord anterior horn cells in a spotty distribution. The virus kills some cells and temporarily inactivates others. The localization and severity of muscular paralysis vary from person to person. If motor neurons recover, weakened muscles regain function. Many patients improve for 1 or 2 years after their acute attack of polio. However, about 70% of muscle strength returns within 3 or 4 months.

Paralysis and deformity produce loss of function in patients who have polio. Various factors result in deformity: (1) muscle imbalance, (2) decreased growth of a severely paralyzed extremity, and (3) abnormal bone growth caused by irregular forces from muscle imbalance and gait disturbances.

Depending on the extent and location of postpolio residuals, orthopedists treat patients with a variety of measures:

1. Bracing to:
   a. Support body weight.
   b. Stabilize a joint—limit abnormal motion.

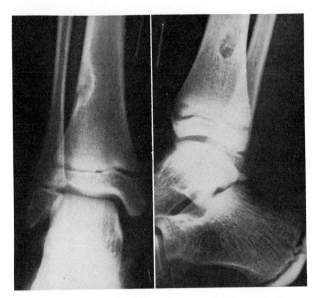

Fig. 38-39. Metaphyseal fibrous defect of the tibia. Reactive new bone surrounds the radiolucent defect.

    c. Counteract muscle imbalance—prevent a strong muscle from stretching a weak antagonist and deforming the part.

    d. Assist a weak muscle—a spring-loaded brace.

    e. Prevent deformity—distribute forces in muscle imbalance or gait disturbances.

2. Tendon transfers—restore muscle balance by moving one or more strong musculotendon units to replace function in a paralyzed muscle group.

3. Tendon lengthening—if a contracture develops.

4. Arthrodesis (fusion)—to control a frail, unstable joint.

5. Osteotomy—to correct bone deformities.

6. Leg length equalizations. An extremity with loss of muscle function grows slower than normal. Significant leg length discrepancy produces deformity and disordered gait mechanics, which strain the hips and spine and result in pain and further deformity.

Leg lengths are measured from the anterosuperior iliac spine to the tip of the medial malleolus. Orthoroentgenograms (roentgeno-

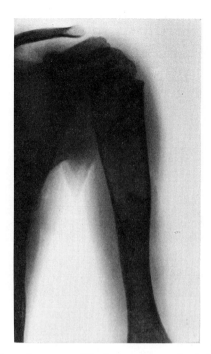

Fig. 38-40. Solitary bone cyst. The humeral metaphysis is expanded, and the cortex is thin. Ridges of bone on the cyst walls produce the trabeculated appearance.

grams of both lower extremities against a centimeter scale) (Fig. 38-43) disclose the exact discrepancy. Orthopedic surgeons correct discrepancy in one of three ways:

1. Lengthen the short limb:
   a. Osteotomy and gradual traction with extreme caution because of the distinct chance of neurovascular complications.
   b. Stimulate growth by ivory or metal pegs inserted near the epiphyseal plate or by stripping periosteum to increase epiphyseal plate blood supply. No one can predict the amount of length increase from these procedures.
2. Stop growth of the normal limb. Charts based upon studies of normal children show predicted growth from each epiphyseal plate at a given age. When a child with unequal leg lengths

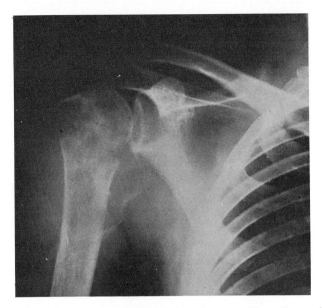

Fig. 38-41. Osteosarcoma of the proximal humerus. Bone destruction is extensive. A thin layer of new bone outlines soft tissue extension of the neoplasm. There is a pathological fracture of the neck of the humerus.

reaches an age where his expected leg growth equals his length discrepancy, orthopedists arrest growth of the normal limb by curetting the epiphyseal plate or by placing staples across the plate. The shorter limb continues to grow, and leg lengths equalize.

3. Shorten the normal limb.

Cerebral palsy

The term *cerebral palsy* denotes various syndromes that have in common nonprogressive neuromuscular dysfunction from brain damage. Causes are prenatal (fetal anoxia, German measles, developmental defects of the brain), associated with birth (prematurity and anoxia from drugs, prolonged labor), or postnatal (encephalitis).

Cerebral palsy is classified according to the type of neuromuscular dysfunction:

1. Spastic—stretch reflex, increased deep tendon reflexes, clonus.

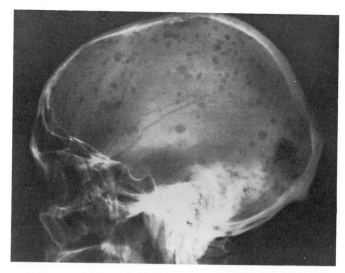

Fig. 38-42. Multiple myeloma. The roentgenogram shows multiple radiolucent lesions.

2. Athetoid—involuntary, writhing movements.
3. Ataxia—poor coordination, nystagmus, adiadochokinesis.
4. Rigidity—"lead pipe" resistance, absence of stretch reflex.
5. Tremor—intention or nonintention tremor.
6. Mixed—two or more of the preceding.

Cerebral palsy is also classified as to site involved:

Monoplegia—one limb
Hemiplegia—one arm and one leg
Paraplegia—both legs
Triplegia—three limbs
Quadriplegia—all four extremities

Many patients with muscular manifestations of cerebral palsy have associated defects of hearing, speech, and mentality. A team of physicians, physical therapists, occupational therapists, vocational counselors, speech therapists, and social workers should evaluate all aspects of the patient, establish realistic medical, social, and vocational goals based on motor and mental ability, and treat the patient with the proper modality:

1. Physical therapy—to aid in gait training, stretching tight muscles, sitting-and-standing balance, and muscle control.

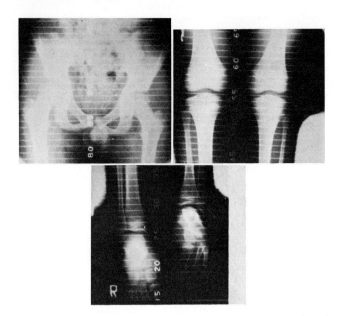

Fig. 38-43. Orthoroentgenograms showing that the left leg is 6.5 cm. shorter than the right.

2. Occupational therapy—to teach self-care.
3. Bracing to prevent deformity, prevent a spastic muscle from stretching a weak or normal muscle, give stability, help control involuntary motion, and give a solid base for walking.
4. Surgery:
   a. Release or lengthen spastic muscle contractures.
   b. Neurectomy—decrease spasticity.
   c. Arthodesis—stabilize deformed and uncontrolled joints in functional positions.
   d. Tendon transfer—restore muscle balance.

Myopathies and neuropathies

In certain stages of their disease, some patients with muscular dystrophy or Charcôt-Marie-Tooth and Friedreich's ataxia need orthopedic treatment. In early stages of a slowly progressive neuromuscular disorder, bracing relieves deformity and increases function. Tendon transfers and bone-stabilizing procedures are sometimes useful.

IDIOPATHIC DISORDERS
Rheumatoid arthritis

Rheumatoid arthritis, one of our great cripplers, is a part of a generalized disease that can involve almost any organ in the body. No one knows the cause of rheumatoid disease nor can its course be predicted in any individual. Rheumatoid arthritis attacks persons of all ages, but is most common in women 25 to 40 years of age. Arthritis usually begins as a synovial inflammation in smaller joints, is migratory, and can involve any joint. Synovitis often subsides without residual damage. If the disease continues, inflamed synovium extends as a pannus across the joint, destroys cartilage, and erodes underlying bone. The joint loses stability and motion and becomes deformed.

The afflicted patient complains of pain, deformity, and/or loss of function. Early in the disease, roentgenograms reveal soft tissue swelling and marginal destruction of the joint. Later progressive disease narrows and destroys the joint.

Rheumatologists and orthopedic surgeons, working together, should manage the rheumatoid patient with medical and surgical therapy used at the proper time for optimum results. The rheumatologist initiates appropriate drug therapy. The orthopedist aids in treatment by splinting involved joints in a position that avoids undesirable contractures. He also directs the active exercise program and passive stretching of contractures. If a particular joint does not respond and synovitis and joint effusion persist, a synovectomy may prevent further joint destruction. After synovectomy, the synovium regrows and at times resists rheumatoid disease. At various stages of the disorder, the surgeon might help the patient with one of several surgical procedures: release tight muscles and fascia, transfer muscles, perform arthroplasties (remolding of distorted joint surfaces with or without interposing metal or fascia over the reshaped bone surfaces), do arthrodeses (fusion of painful and destroyed joints), and replace joints with prostheses and total joint replacements (Fig. 38-44, *C*).

Degenerative joint disease

The term *degenerative joint disease* denotes changes wherein articular cartilage loses fluid, becomes less resilient, loses normal color, fragments, and thins. Weight-bearing portions of larger joints degenerate most often. The underlying bone contains cysts filled with fluid or granulation tissue. New bone production results in sclerosis of the bone ends and spurs at joint margins. Free pieces of cartilage and bone frequently displace into the joint.

Degenerative joint disease can arise after processes that produce incongruity of opposing joint surfaces (infection, trauma) with resultant abnormal joint mechanics. In most instances, however, no one knows the cause. Some view degenerative joint disease as part of normal aging, and others believe that it is a disease. Degenerative changes in the knees, hips, and spine are common in persons over 65. A person with clinical and roentgenographic signs of degenerative joint disease is not necessarily symptomatic.

Patients often relieve joint stiffness and discomfort by using rest, heat, and analgesics. Severe pain and loss of function necessitate one of the following surgical measures: joint debridement (excision of loose bodies and rough areas on the joint surface); release of tight muscles, fascia, and joint capsule; arthroplasty (Fig. 38-44); arthrodesis; prosthetic replacement; or total joint replacement.

Paget's disease (osteitis deformans)

Paget's disease, a disorder of unknown etiology, usually affects men over 55 years of age. Bone is destroyed and produced in an irregular

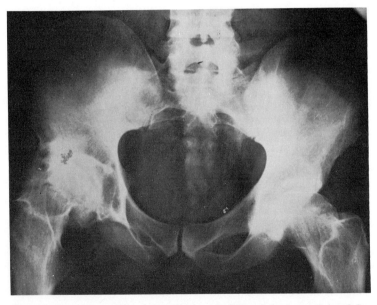

A

Fig. 38-44. Degenerative joint disease. A, The right femoral head has moved laterally, and the joint space is narrow; note osteophytic overgrowth of bone on the inferior margin of the femoral head and inferior acetabulum; acetabular cysts are surrounded by sclerotic bone.

manner. Microscopic examination shows many fragments of bone fitted together in a mosaic with blue "cement lines" between the pieces. A fibrovascular stroma fills spaces between bone trabeculae. Paget's disease commonly affects the spine, pelvis, and proximal femora. Roentgenographically, increased density from new bone production accentuates the major trabecular pattern. Bone destruction produces radiolucent areas. The involved bones often deform. At times, patients with Paget's disease have aches and pains. Often, however, the physician discovers the disorder when he obtains roentgenograms for other reasons. Patients obtain relief of discomfort by the use of aspirin. They occasionally develop osteosarcoma superimposed on the Paget's disease, and the doctor should follow them closely with this possibility in mind.

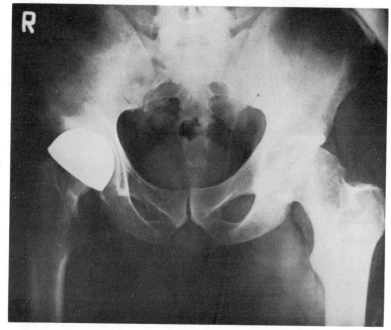

B

Fig. 38-44, cont'd. B, Joint surfaces have been remolded during a vitallium cup arthroplasty.

Continued.

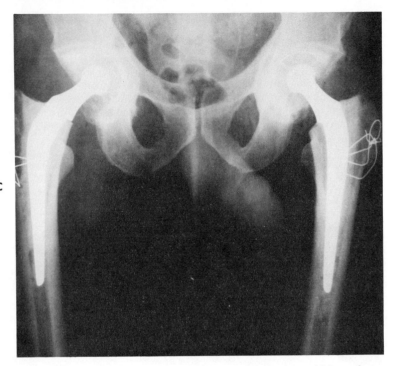

Fig. 38-44, cont'd. C, A recent method of treatment is total hip replacement with a metal femoral component and a polyethylene acetabulum.

METABOLIC DISORDERS
Rickets

In rickets, a disorder of growing children, skeletal manifestations develop from a continued production of bone matrix and epiphyseal cartilage matrix that fails to mineralize properly. A deficiency of sunlight or vitamin D or a lack of response to vitamin D produces this lack of mineralization. In the absence of vitamin D, the intestinal tract mucosa does not absorb calcium and phosphorus normally. In this country, lack of vitamin D intake combined with lack of exposure to sunlight occurs only rarely in lower economic groups. In the black patient, skin pigmentation interferes with vitamin D synthesis during exposure to sunlight. Patients with fat absorption disorders (celiac disease, sprue, and obstructive jaundice) lose vitamin D in the stool.

Children with rickets are restless and irritable. Their legs bow. The long bone metaphysis enlarges (trumpeting), the frontal and parietal bones protrude (craniotabes), costochondral junctions enlarge (rosary of rickets), the ribs sink in at the attachment of the diaphragm (Harrison's grooves), the pelvis collapses inward, and the spine curves. Roentgenograms reveal the wide, cupped metaphysis, a wide, irregular epiphyseal plate, an irregular hazy zone of provisional calcification, and bowing of the long weight-bearing bones. Serum phosphorus decreases, serum calcium remains normal, and serum alkaline phosphatase increases. Urine calcium decreases, and phosphorus remains normal or increases.

Vitamin D–deficient children heal rickets in 3 or 4 weeks if they take 3,000 to 6,000 units of vitamin D daily. If they are positioned properly during the active stage of the disease, they will not deform soft bones. The surgeon corrects severe, persistent deformities by osteotomy.

Vitamin D–resistant rickets

In some children, active rickets fail to respond to the usual doses of vitamin D. No one knows the exact cause of this disorder, which is often familial. An affected child often requires 10,000 to 1,000,000 units of vitamin D for treatment and 3,000 to 500,000 units for maintenance. The physician should use 24-hour urine calcium studies to determine the correct dosage of vitamin D.

Renal rickets

Patients who lose phosphorus or calcium because of renal defects frequently acquire rickets. Defective kidney tubules lose protein. If the glomeruli are defective, the patient frequently retains urea and sometimes becomes acidotic. The prognosis is not good in renal rickets. The physician must treat the associated defects.

Osteomalacia

Osteomalacia, the adult counterpart of rickets, is characterized by increased bone matrix and lack of mineralization. The bones soften and bend. In this country, physicians rarely see this disorder on a vitamin D deficiency basis. Steatorrhea or renal disease causes osteomalacia most frequently. The patients complain of weakness and deformity. Their bones fracture easily. Roentgenograms reveal a decrease in bone density, deformities, and Looser's zones (a fracture line surrounded by relatively dense bone). Serum and urine changes are similar to those in rickets. The physician must correct the underlying defect and use orthopedic measures to correct deformities.

Scurvy

Vitamin C deficiency is uncommon. Affected patients do not produce normal connective tissue. Increased capillary fragility produces painful subperiosteal hemorrhage with resultant pseudoparalysis. Roentgenograms reveal osteoporosis produced by a lack of bone matrix. The zone of provisional calcification increases; a lytic zone (scorbutic band) crosses the metaphysis; a dense ring of bone surrounds the epiphysis; spurs form at metaphyseal edges; and periosteal new bone is produced. Occasionally, an epiphysis separates from the metaphysis. Ascorbic acid, 100-120 mg. daily, corrects the disorder.

Hyperparathyroidism

Parathyroid hormone acts on kidney and bone to maintain normal serum calcium and phosphorus levels. Parathyroid adenoma or parathyroid hyperplasia produces hyperparathyroidism most frequently in women 25 to 45 years of age.

The following cause symptoms in hyperparathyroidism:
1. Increased serum calcium—lethargy, weakness, anorexia, constipation.
2. Bone destruction—pain or fractures.
3. Calcium increase in the urine—renal stones, renal insufficiency.

Serum phosphorus decreases, serum calcium increases, and serum alkaline phosphatase increases. Urinary phosphorus and calcium increase. Roentgenographically, bones demineralize, the cortex thins, the lamina dura of the teeth disappear, subperiosteal bone of the midphalanx of the fingers is resorbed, and the outer table of the skull thins and becomes indistinct. "Brown tumors" composed of fibrous connective tissue, hemorrhage, and giant cells appear as bone cysts.

After the offending portion of the parathyroid gland has been removed, the surgeon must observe the patient carfeully for postoperative tetany and must treat it promptly.

Osteoporosis

In a patient with osteoporosis, the total mass of bone matrix and mineral decreases. Osteoporosis results from one or more of the following:
1. Disuse—normal stress is needed to prevent loss of bone mass.
2. Endocrine:
   a. Cushing's disease—increased steroids and increased catabolism.

      b. Postmenopausal—decreased stress and decreased sex hormones.

      c. Hyperthyroidism.

      d. Acromegaly.

  3. Scurvy.

  4. Protein deficiency caused by decreased intake or excessive loss.

  5. Multiple myeloma and carcinomatosis.

  6. Idiopathic, senile, or post-menopausal.

No one knows exactly why the bone mass decreases. Most patients remain in the idiopathic group. Osteoporosis is most common in women over 60 in whom diet, disuse, and endocrine changes probably play a role.

The patients complain of bone pain and tenderness. Vertebral bodies and femoral necks frequently break. Calcium, phosphorus, and alkaline phosphatase usually remain normal. Some patients are in negative nitrogen and calcium balance. Roentgenograms disclose relatively radiolucent bone, thin cortices, and widened medullary canals. The vertebral bodies often collapse. Vertebral subchondral cortices curve, and vertebral bodies become biconcave.

Physicians diagnose idiopathic osteoporosis by excluding other disorders that give similar roentgenographic findings (osteomalacia, multiple myeloma, hyperparathyroidism, metastatic malignancies, Cushing's disease, and hyperthyroidism). Since one cannot determine the etiology in most instances, treatment is difficult. The patient should consume at least one quart of milk and 70 Gm. of protein each day. In addition to this regime, some physicians add vitamin D, 5,000 units a day for the first 3 months and then 1,000 units a day. The patient remains as active as possible. Estrogens and androgens improve nitrogen balance and make the patient feel better, but no one has evidence that they produce bone deposition. Some physicians use sodium fluoride to try to increase bone deposition. Physical therapy and spine supports sometimes provide symptomatic relief.

Gout

In gout, a metabolic disorder, the body produces excessive uric acid. Blood uric acid increases. Ureate crystals form deposits (tophi) in joints and para-articular structures. These crystals destroy the joint surface and erode underlying bone. During an acute attack, patients complain of severe pain in a joint or bursa. Uricosuric agents alleviate symptoms during the acute episode. Patients then use drugs to maintain a decrease in the blood uric acid. In some patients with gout, orthopedists excise tophi and do arthroplasties or arthrodeses on destroyed joints.

CHAPTER 39

The hand

DAVID W. FURNAS
ADRIAN E. FLATT
ROBERT Y. McMURTRY

Man's hands have allowed him to put human thought into action, exerting control over his environment. Sensation in the hand (an organ containing one fourth of all Pacinian [touch] corpuscles of the body) is the only sense among five in which man is clearly superior to animals. Pictures gained from earliest tactile and kinesthetic activities of the hand lay the groundwork for one's self-image and feelings of individuality. The hand also serves as a means of expression.

Thus, afflictions of the hand are of great significance to the patient and his physician; moreover, they are very common: approximately one-third of all industrial accidents and one-third of injuries seen in the emergency departments of metropolitan hospitals involve the hand.

NORMAL ARCHITECTURE

Everyday use of the hand demands a structure that has stability and power, combined with mobility, dexterity ,and precision. *Stability* is furnished by the rigid, *central pillar* of the hand (Fig. 39-1), formed by the firmly united carpal bones and the second and third metacarpal bones. Around this central pillar, in the manner of twin loading booms, rotate the two mobile units of the hand: (1) the extremely mobile first metacarpal invested with thenar structures and (2) the less mobile fourth and fifth metacarpals invested with hypothenar structures.

The *digits* with their two or three joints represent other highly mobile units. The *metacarpophalangeal joints* of the fingers have lateral *mobility* when they are *extended,* but lateral *stability* when they are *flexed* into grasp (where stability is required) because of the arrange-

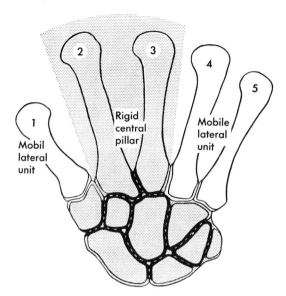

Fig. 39-1. Central pillar and lateral units of hand. The shafts of the second and third metacarpals are firmly united to the carpal bones, forming the stable central pillar. The two lateral units of the hand articulate freely with the carpal bones and are mobile.

ment of their collateral ligaments (Fig. 39-2). All of the *interphalangeal joints* have lateral *stability throughout* flexion and extension.

Three arches are formed by these units of the hand (Fig. 39-3): a *proximal transverse arch,* which is rigid, a *distal transverse arch,* which is flexible, and a *longitudinal arch* (the digital rays), which is rigid proximally and flexible distally.

Power to the wrist and hand is supplied by *five* groups of muscles (Fig. 39-4): two *extrinsic* (muscle bellies in the forearm) and three *intrinsic* (muscle bellies in the hand). The muscles are innervated by three nerves: median, radial, and ulnar.

Extrinsic muscle groups

The *flexor-pronator group* pronates the hand and flexes the wrist and digits. The flexor-pronator muscles (the three flexors of the wrist, the nine flexors of the digits, the pronators teres and quadratus) are supplied by the *median nerve (except* for the ulnar half of the flexor

Extension:
MP collateral ligaments

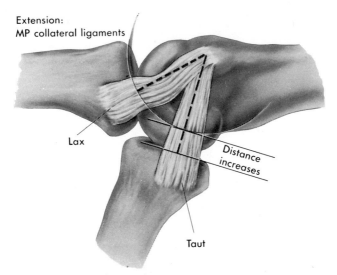

Lax

Distance
increases

Taut

Flexion: MP ligaments

Fig. 39-2. Stability of metacarpophalangeal (MP) joints. In flexion the collateral ligaments are placed under tension because of the eccentric profile and the lateral bulges of the metacarpal head; this prevents lateral motion of the joints. In extension the ligaments are flaccid, and lateral movements are possible. The position of flexion is usually chosen when immobilizing this joint, to prevent shortening of the ligament and deformity.

digitorum profundus, which is supplied by the ulnar nerve); the *extensor-supinator group* supinates the hand and extends the wrist and digits. The extensor-supinator muscles (the three extensors of the wrist, the four common and two proper extensors of the fingers, the two extensors and the long abductor to the thumb, and the supinator) are supplied by the *radial nerve*.

Intrinsic muscle groups

The *thenar muscles* (short flexor, short abductor, and opposing muscles of the thumb) are supplied by the *median nerve,* and the *hypothenar* muscles (abductor, short flexor, and opposing muscles of the little finger) are supplied by the *ulnar nerve.* These two groups work together to cup the palm and to oppose the thumb to the fingers. The *lumbricals, interossei,* and *adductor pollicis* are supplied by the *ulnar*

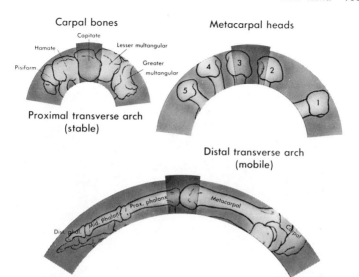

Fig. 39-3. Arches of the hand. The stable, immobile proximal transverse arch is composed of firmly knit carpal bones. The mobile distal transverse arch is made up of the metacarpal heads and the intervening tissues. The longitudinal arches, which are extremely mobile distally and stable proximally, are made up of the digital rays.

nerve (except for the first two lumbricals, which are median innervated). They furnish digital *adduction-abduction* movements, *flexion* at the metacarpophalangeal joints, and *extension* at the interphalangeal joints. (The *extrinsic flexors* are *also* able to flex the metacarpophalangeal joints, and the *extrinsic extensors* are *also* able to extend the interphalangeal joints.) The tendons of the intrinsic muscles interweave with the tendons and aponeuroses of the extrinsic muscles, forming a coordinated network (Fig. 39-5). This system of motors, superbly linked with input from the eyes and the sensory organs of the hand, lends precision and dexterity to movements of the hand.

ASSESSMENT OF THE HAND
Clinical
History

Intelligent assessment necessitates understanding the patient with whom one is dealing, including his personality, occupation, hobbies, and life expectations. Specific history relating to the hand should

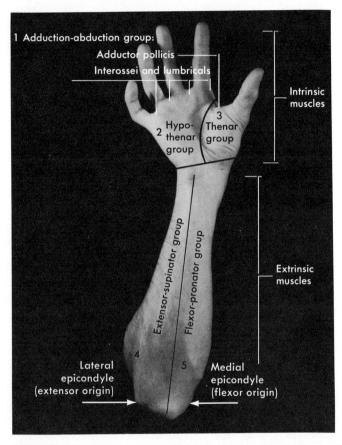

Fig. 39-4. Muscle power to the hand. Three groups of intrinsic muscles: 1 and 2 supplied by the *ulnar nerve* and 3 supplied by the *median nerve.* Two groups of extrinsic muscles: 4 supplied by the *radial nerve* and 5 supplied by the *median nerve.* Exceptions are *first* and *second lumbricals* supplied by the median nerve and *ulnar half of flexor digitorum profundus* supplied by the ulnar nerve.

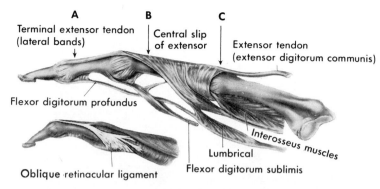

A Terminal extensor tendon (lateral bands)

B Central slip of extensor

C Extensor tendon (extensor digitorum communis)

Flexor digitorum profundus

Interosseus muscles

Lumbrical

Oblique retinacular ligament

Flexor digitorum sublimis

Fig. 39-5. Intrinsic and extrinsic networks for flexion and extension of the fingers. The distal interphalangeal joint is flexed by the *flexor digitorum profundus;* the proximal interphalangeal joint is flexed by the *flexor digitorum sublimis* (plus a transmitted increment from the *flexor digitorum profundus*); the metacarpophalangeal joint is flexed by the *interosseus muscles* through their direct osseus insertions and through their insertions into the wings of dorsal aponeurosis. (This flexion force is augmented by a transmitted increment from the *flexor digitorum profundus* and the *flexor digitorum sublimis*.) The distal interphalangeal joint is extended through the insertion of the lateral bands of the dorsal aponeurosis, powered by the extrinsic extensors and the intrinsics *(interossei* and *lumbricals)* (either or both may act); the proximal interphalangeal joint is extended by the central slip of the dorsal aponeurosis, powered in the same way as the distal phalanx; the metacarpophalangeal joint is extended by the extrinsic extensor tendons alone, acting through the dorsal aponeurosis. The *oblique retinacular ligaments* assist in coordination of these movements. For injuries at levels **A, B,** and **C,** see Fig. 39-18.

generate a clear understanding and documentation of the duration, nature, and onset of the complaint as well as the patient's definition of his disability. Exclusion of causes of hand disability arising proximally in the upper limb or higher neurologically should be routine.

Physical examination

As a part of hand examination consider the entire upper limb and a comparison of right and left sides at a minimum. *Look at, feel,* and *move* the hand to assess the five essential elements of function: *cover, mobility, stability, sensibility,* and *viability.* Initially look for abnormal postures. These occur because of an imbalance of forces with loss,

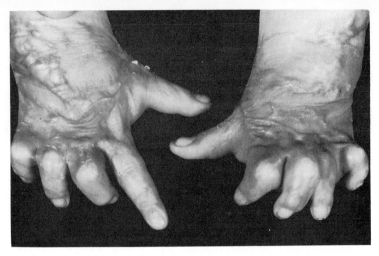

Fig. 39-6. "Intrinsic-minus" deformity or clawhand. Distal transverse arches are flattened. Metacarpophalangeal joints are hyperextended, proximal interphalangeal joints are hyperflexed (distal interphalangeal joints are sometimes flexed, sometimes hyperextended), thumb is held parallel to palm. The cause in this patient is scarring and skin destruction from a scald of the dorsum of the hands. (See Fig. 39-23.)

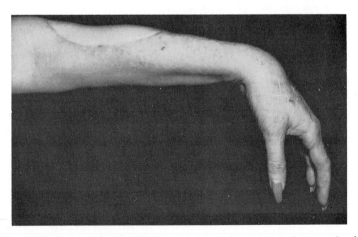

Fig. 39-7. Dropped wrist. Ability to extend the wrist against gravity is lost because of denervation of the extensor-supinator group of muscles from resection of basal cell carcinoma of forearm that invaded the radial nerve.

exaggeration, or disruption of normal arches. Common patterns of pathological postures include claw deformity (intrinsic minus hand) (Fig. 39-6), dropped wrist and hand (Fig. 39-7), and the intrinsic plus hand (Fig. 39-8). Assessing cover implies checking the skin for unstable scars or contractures as well as its color, temperature, and mobility. Mobility must be determined actively and passively. During active motion ask the patient to put his wrist through a full range of motion, to completely extend the wrist and fingers, and then to fully flex all the digits. The normal thumb can describe a cone, oppose, flex and extend, as well as pinch and grasp (Fig. 39-9).

Active and passive motion must be compared and documented quantitatively, and any discrepancies between the two explained. Loss of passive motion is associated with a corresponding loss of active motion, but the converse does not hold. Before active motion can occur, any encumbrances of normal passive mobility such as joint, tendon, and skin contractures or adhesions must be eliminated. Stability requires normal functional integrity of the bones and joints of

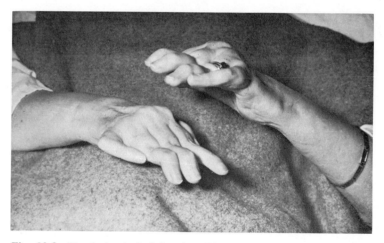

Fig. 39-8. "Intrinsic-plus" deformity. The arches are exaggerated. The metacarpophalangeal joints are flexed, and the interphalangeal joints are in "swan neck" position (proximal interphalangeal joint hyperextended [recurvatum], distal interphalangeal joint locked in flexion). Sometimes both interphalangeal joints are extended (accoucheur's hand). (From Flatt, A. E.: The care of the rheumatoid hand, ed. 3, St. Louis, 1972, The C. V. Mosby Co.)

A

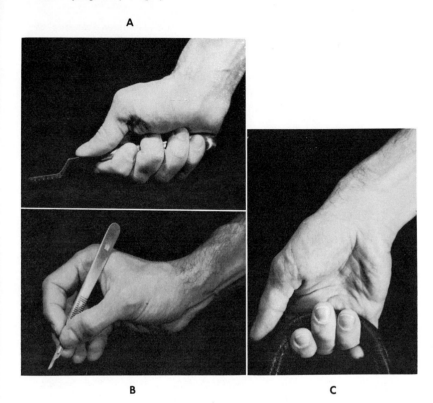

B   **C**

Fig. 39-9. A, Power grip. Object is clamped securely between the flexed fingers and the palm, counterpressure being applied by the thumb. **B,** Precision grip (or "handling"). The object is pinched between the flexor pads of the opposing thumb and fingers. **C,** Hook grip. Only the fingers are used, as a primitive hook.

the hand. Disturbances of this integrity are particularly common after trauma, whether recent or remote, and in rheumatoid arthritis. Sensibility is determined by the usual pin and wisp of cotton, two-point discrimination (Fig. 39-10), a pick-up test (Fig. 39-11), and stereognosis. Normally two points that are as close together as 2 to 4 mm. can be distinguished with the tips and flexor surfaces of the digits, whereas on the dorsal skin two points closer than 10 to 12 mm. are interpreted as one. Viability refers to normal perfusion of the tissues

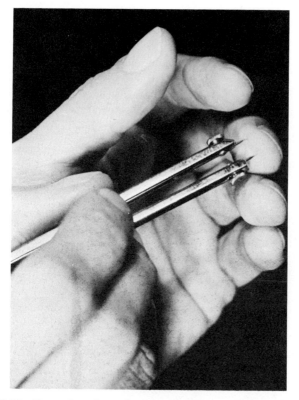

Fig. 39-10. Two-point discrimination. Two points are simultaneously pressed against the skin; the distance between the points is varied to determine the narrowest spread that can be distinguished as two separate points rather than one. The fingertips can usually distinguish two points spread as little as 2 to 4 mm. The proximal dorsal part of the digit can only distinguish two points if the spread is 10 mm. Two-point discrimination is one of the best means of detecting partial nerve injuries and in following nerve repairs.

of the hand. Normal perfusion requires adequacy of arterial supply, the capillary bed, and venous drainage. Loss of any of these three will compromise viability. Aberrations may be focal, as in an unstable scar or crushed skin, or involve the hand as a whole, as in combined radial and ulnar arterial injuries. A hand without adequate circulation will not survive the precipitating trauma; similarly, a hand with marginal circulation comprises a contraindication for reconstructive surgical intervention.

Radiological examination

Radiological examination is an integral part of routine hand assessment. There is no therapeutic benefit conferred by diagnostic radiation. Careful examination will guide inquiry to an appropriate area. For example, the whole hand need not be examined if the terminal phalanx of the thumb has been injured, nor is it diagnostically accurate to assess the scaphoid without special scaphoid views. In short, request appropriate films and reduce needless exposures.

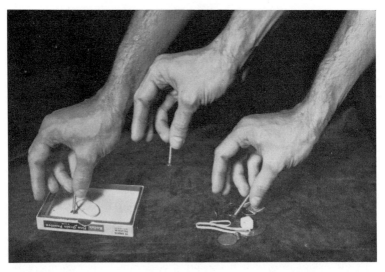

Fig. 39-11. Moberg's "pickup" test. Ask the patient to pick up and place a number of small objects at top speed. This serves to reveal deficiencies in critical sensation and fine coordination that might be missed with cruder tests. Incomplete return of median sensation indicated by patient's preference of ulnar-innervated ring finger.

PRINCIPLES OF MANAGEMENT OF HAND PROBLEMS

Restoration of grasp (both power and precision), fine tactile sense, dexterity, and normal appearance are the sometimes elusive goals of surgery of the hand. These are achieved by restoring cover and stability, mobility, sensibility, and viability to the hand. Skin grafts and pedicles restore missing or contracted skin cover. Fracture fixation, bone grafts, and joint fusions may be required for bone and joint stability. Tendon repairs, grafts, or transfers restore transmission of power for active mobility. Loss of passive mobility is best managed conservatively. Motor nerve deficits may be corrected by nerve repairs, nerve grafts, or tendon transfers. Repairs or grafts of sensory nerves (or occasionally transferring sensory island flaps) (see Chapter 24) may provide some restoration of functional sensibility. Finally, vascular repair may be essential to provide fundamental requirements of viability.

Immobilization is the necessary element in managing trauma, accidental or surgical. The hand reacts badly to prolonged immobilization, worse to swelling, and worst of all to both. Elevation and earliest feasible motion are immutable priorities.

The *intelligent minimum* surgically yields results with the least complications and greatest benefits.

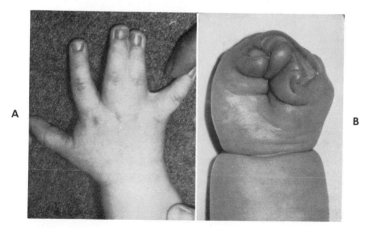

Fig. 39-12. Syndactyly. **A,** Simple syndactyly of ring and long fingers. **B,** Complex syndactyly causing a mittenlike hand in a patient with acrocephalosyndactyly or Apert's syndrome.

Congenital deformities

Congenital deformities of the hand are relatively common and present such a diverse array and range of disorders that they mock attempts at sorting them into an orderly pattern. Polydactyly or excessive number of digits is the most common, occurring in 0.5% of live births. It is frequently bilateral and commonly the extra digit is the ulnarmost or radialmost of the hand.

Syndactyly (Fig. 39-12), failure of digits to separate from one another, is the second most common hand anomaly, occurring in 0.2%

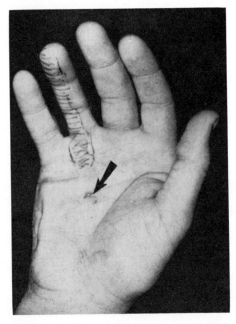

Fig. 39-13. "Tidy" injury of hand. This clean, penetrating wound of the palm was caused by a broken thermometer. Despite its innocuous appearance, examination revealed an area of anesthesia (crosshatches in ink on ring finger), inability to abduct-adduct the fingers, and a positive Froment's sign (Fig. 39-20, *B*). Transection of the motor branch of the ulnar nerve, transection of part of a sensory branch of the ulnar nerve, transection of the deep palmar arterial arch, and partial transection of the flexor digitorum profundus tendon to the ring finger were found at operation.

Table 39-1. Common injuries of the integument and digits

Injury	Treatment
1. Laceration	Cleansing, irrigation, and simple surgical closure
2. Flaplike laceration	1. Suture into place if viable
	2. If not viable, remove skin and close defect directly or with skin graft
3. Amputated skin	1. Defat the skin and replace as a skin graft, or
	2. Take grafts from elsewhere
4. Digital pulp	Cross finger flap, palmar flap, triangular island flaps, or skin graft
5. Degloving injury (skin peeled back from digit as if it were a glove, e.g., ring caught in machinery)	1. Amputate ring finger or unimportant digit, or
	2. Remove degloved skin and cover digit with pedicle (particularly if thumb is injured)
6. Partial amputation	1. Replace severed part if circulation appears adequate
	2. Repair vessels microsurgically if possible, survival without vascular repairs more likely
	If circumstances ideal, replantation by experienced microvascular surgeon
7. Complete amputation	Closure with preservation of all possible length
8. Crushed fingertip	Meticulous reassembly using magnification
9. Avulsion of nail or nail bed	1. Trim nail and replace as a splint to wound; carefully repair nail bed
	2. Replace any missing areas of nail bed with split-skin graft
10. Subungual hematoma	Perforate overlying nail with heated paper clip or needle and evacuate hematoma

of live births. The long and ring fingers are the most commonly adherent, often bilaterally. Syndactyly ranges in complexity from a single slight obliterated web space, to complete fusion of all the digits into a tight mitten.

Brachydactyly (shortened fingers), symphalangy (end-to-end fusion of phalangeal bones), ectrodactyly (absence of a part of one or more digits), and clinodactyly (lateral deviation of the fingers) are some of the less common congenital disorders.

In most instances the safest guiding principle is early referral to a surgeon with special interest in this field. Early operative treatment is mandatory if there is any distortion of growth or progression of deformity.

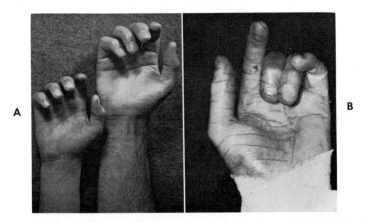

Fig. 39-14. Position of rest. **A,** Normal position of rest. With the hand lying palm upward on a flat surface, muscle tone of the flexors causes slight flexion of the thumb and an orderly gradation of flexion of the fingers, which increases from the index to the little finger. **B,** Loss of position of rest. A razor slash of the flexor compartment of the wrist has caused loss of the position of rest of the thumb and index finger because of complete severance of the associated flexor tendons; a small strand of intact profundus tendon prevents the complete loss of the position of rest in the little finger; all the sublimis tendons were divided, as was the median nerve and the radial artery; areas of sensory loss from transection of median nerve are crosshatched with inked lines; note that much of the damage to the wrist is readily assessed without removing the dressings. (**A,** From Flatt, A. E.: The care of minor hand injuries, ed. 3, St. Louis, 1972, The C. V. Mosby Co.)

Acquired disorders

Traumatic (See Table 39-1.)

Laceration. Skin lacerations or wounds may be tidy or untidy. The tidy wound presents with clean incised margins that heal promptly after simple cleansing and closure. It is, however, essential to maintain a high index of suspicion of hidden problems. Severed tendons, nerves, arteries, and buried splinters of glass or metal can be present in the most innocent appearing wounds (Fig. 39-13). Untidy wounds are ragged, crushed, or torn at the margins and are more widely damaged in the depths. Missing or nonviable skin must be replaced. Dirt, foreign material, and devitalized tissue must be debrided. Complica-

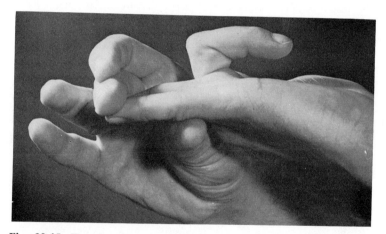

Fig. 39-15. Test for flexor sublimis action. The flexor digitorum profundus muscles and tendons form a more or less solid sheet in the forearm, dividing only quite distally into separate tendons that have little or no independence of action, i.e., the 4 tendons tend to act as one unit. Therefore, if 3 of the 4 digits are forcefully held in extension, the flexor digitorum profundus to the remaining digit is carried into extended position with its fellows and is unable to act as a flexor. However, the flexor digitorum sublimis, which has a distinct and independent muscle belly for each of the four tendons, can still act as a flexor; flexion takes place only at the proximal interphalangeal joint, not at the distal interphalangeal joint. The flexor digitorum sublimis to the middle finger shows normal function in the photograph. (From Flatt, A. E.: The care of minor hand injuries, ed. 3, St. Louis, 1972, The C. V. Mosby Co.)

tions of infection, excessive swelling, and necrosis are more likely to occur in an untidy wound.

No wound, tidy or untidy, should ever be considered for closure until the full extent of the injury is identified. If any uncertainty exists, formal exploration is mandatory.

Tendon—flexor. The diagnosis of digital flexor tendon severance is confirmed by loss of the position of rest (Fig. 39-14) and the inability to perform the test for sublimis action (Fig. 39-15) or the test for profundus action (Fig. 39-16). If these tests are negative but provoke pain, partial division may be indicated.

The level of severance determines the therapeutic approach. Tendons divided distal to "no man's land" (Fig. 39-17) (near bony insertion) may have their proximal end advanced and sutured into the distal phalanx. Tendons severed proximally to "no man's land" are anastomosed immediately with nonabsorbable suture material.

Flexor tendon injuries in "no man's land" (where the flexor digitorum profundus and sublimis cross through the fibrous digital sheath) yield notoriously poor results in anything but optimal circum-

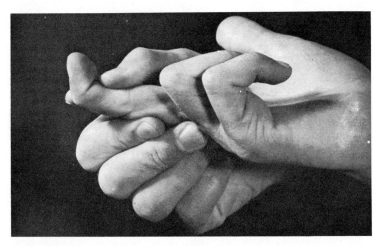

Fig. 39-16. Test for flexor digitorum profundus action. The finger is held forcefully in passive extension at the metacarpophalangeal and the proximal interphalangeal joints. Ability to flex the distal interphalangeal joint indicates normal action of the flexor digitorum profundus. (From Flatt, A. E.: The care of minor hand injuries, ed. 3, St. Louis, 1972, The C. V. Mosby Co.)

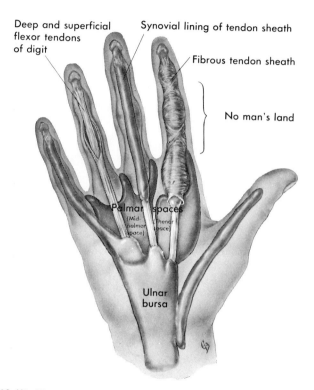

Deep and superficial
flexor tendons
of digit

Synovial lining of tendon sheath

Fibrous tendon sheath

No man's land

Palmar spaces
(Mid-palmar space)

(Thenar space)

Ulnar
bursa

Fig. 39-17. *No man's land:* here the two flexor tendons of each finger of the right hand are tightly enclosed in a synovium-lined fibrous sheath made up of unyielding cruciate and annular ligaments; tendon anastomoses in this region tend to fail because of massive adherence to surrounding structures. *Palmar spaces:* these two fascial clefts are located behind the digital flexor tendons; the midpalmar space is separated from the thenar space by a septum that connects the bursa of the flexor tendons (ulnar bursa) to the third metacarpal bone.

814 Synopsis of surgery

Table 39-2. Extensor tendon injuries

Entity	Mechanisms and level of severance	Treatment
1. *"Drop finger"* (Fig. 39-18, *D*); (injury at level C, Fig. 39-5)	Laceration or rupture of extensor tendon on dorsum of hand or wrist or at metacarpophalangeal joint	Direct suture
2. *"Boutonnière deformity* (develops several weeks after injury (Fig. 39-18, *B-C*); (injury at level B, Fig. 39-5)	Laceration, rupture, or erosion of extensor tendon at proximal phalanx or proximal interphalangeal joint	Immobilization in extension with cast extending to forearm for 3 weeks; if chip fracture present, direct suture; late treatment requires complex operation
3. *"Mallet finger"* (or baseball finger) (Fig. 39-18, *A*); (injury at level A, Fig. 39-5)	Avulsion or laceration of insertion of tendon into distal phalanx (fragment of distal phalanx frequently avulsed with tendon insertion)	Immobilize in plaster with D.I.P. joint in hyperextension and P.I.P. joint in flexion; if wound is open, suture tendon ends and place intramedullary wire through D.I.P. joint

stances. Two large tendons are crowded into a narrow unyielding fibrous tunnel. If divided tendons are sutured primarily, the exuberant fibroblastic outgrowth causes dense adherence between the tendon and sheath and function is lost. The best course of action for the primary physician is to clean the wound, close the skin, and send the patient promptly to an experienced hand surgeon. The surgeon may choose to perform immediate repair of one of the two lacerated tendons, discarding the remaining tendon and removing all of the fibrous sheaths except for two or three 5 mm. pulleys. If the circumstances are less than ideal the surgeon will postpone surgery and instruct the patient in exercises to maintain joint suppleness. When reaction to the initial injury has subsided sufficiently (weeks or months later) elective tendon grafting can be carried out.

In flexor tendon injuries of the wrist (Fig. 39-14, *B*) it is best to assume injuries to major nerves and arteries. If this is confirmed clinically hemorrhage should be controlled by pressure and the patient should be transported to a surgeon competent to perform multiple nerve, arterial, and tendon repairs. Circumstances such as obligatory transfer over great distances sometimes demand exploration with ligation of bleeders, irrigation of the wound, and sterile dressings or closure of the skin.

Tendon—extensor. The extensor tendons are flat, fine structures that are interwoven with tendons of the intrinsic muscles forming the intricate extensor aponeuroses. They do not hold sutures well and surgical restoration is frequently difficult. Diagnostically, the most frequent error is overlooking closed injuries to this extensor apparatus. The most common closed extensor injuries (cited in Table 39-2) must be excluded when assessing a "sprained finger."

The boutonnière deformity (Fig. 39-18, *B*) is caused by loss of restraint of the lateral bands of the extensor mechanism. After the central slip has been divided, these lateral bands become attenuated and migrate volarward, allowing the proximal interphalangeal joint to protrude dorsally as if through a buttonhole. Extensor tendons are prone to attrition injuries. Drop finger (Fig. 39-18, *D*) is seen in rheumatoid arthritis when slips of the extensor digitorum communis rupture because of tendon disease or erosion from a rough bony prominence at the level of the distal radius and ulna. Drummer's palsy or drop thumb is caused by rupture secondary to avascular necrosis of the extensor pollicis longus near the lower end of the radius. Open disruption of an extensor tendon is treated by direct suture unless delay, contamination, or other circumstances contraindicate primary repair. Immobilization for 4 or 5 weeks is customary after suture of extensor tendons, whether open or closed.

Nerve injuries

Compulsive care must be taken to rule out nerve injuries in hand lacerations. For example, children falling with outstretched hand onto broken glass must be assumed to have significant nerve injury. This assumption is essential because of the difficult and frustrating task of attempting accurate clinical assessment of a frightened, agitated child.

If the median nerve is divided (Fig. 39-14, *B*) the hand is blinded from loss of critical sensibility in the most important parts of the thumb and index, long, and ring fingers, while motor power is lost in the thenar muscles. Ulnar nerve transection cripples the greater part of the intrinsic musculature, depriving the hand of dexterity; it also numbs sensation to the ulnar side of the fourth and the entire fifth digit. Accurate testing of the motor and sensory branches of these nerves is mandatory in any hand injury. Even an inconspicuous nick can mark the entry point of glass or steel slivers that may have selectively divided a significant sensory or motor branch (Fig. 39-13).

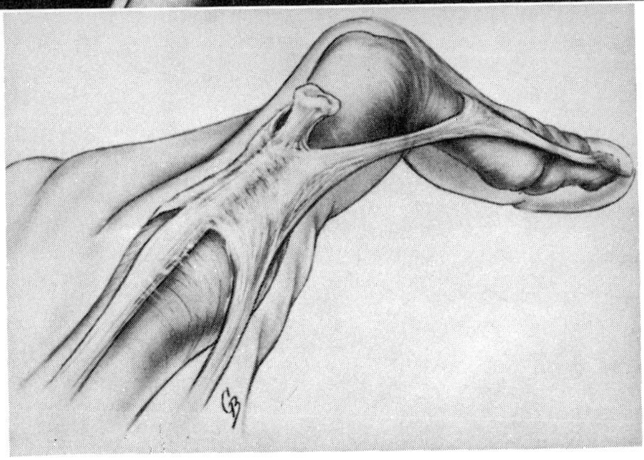

Fig. 39-18. A, *Mallet finger* (baseball finger): disruption of the insertion of the extensor tendon at the distal phalanx. (Injury near level **A,** Fig. 39-5.) **B** and **C,** *Boutonnière* deformity: after disruption of the central slip of the extensor tendon where it inserts on the middle phalanx, the lateral bands of the extensor apparatus tend to migrate in a palmar direction causing flexion of the proximal interphalangeal joint and extension of the distal interphalangeal joint. (Injury near level **B,** Fig. 39-5.) **D,** *Drop finger:* long, ring, and little fingers cannot be extended against gravity (note level **C** of Fig. 39-5) because of tendon rupture at wrist; patient has rheumatoid disease and attrition of the tendons on a bony projection. (Injury proximal to level **C,** Fig. 39-5.)

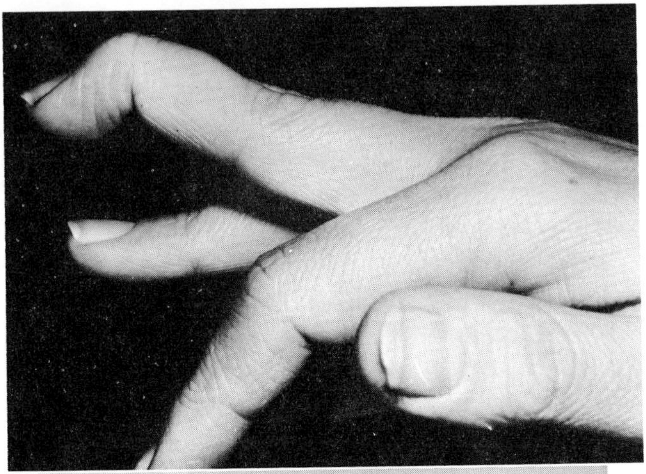

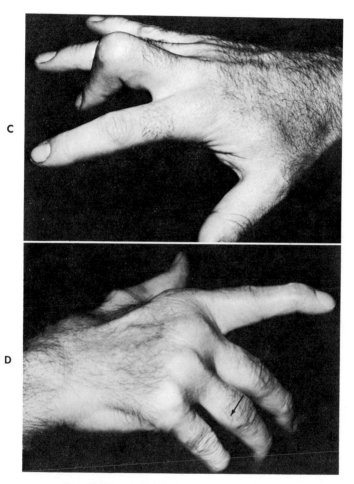

Fig. 39-18, cont'd. For legend see opposite page.

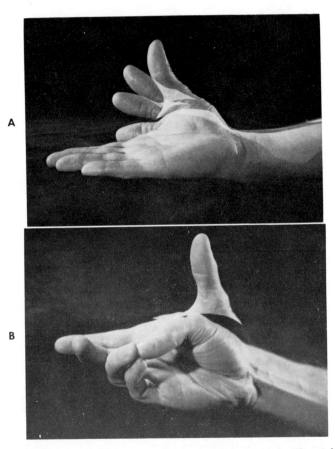

Fig. 39-19. Tests for motor function of median nerve. **A,** The abductor pollicis brevis raises the thumb forward, perpendicular to the plane of the palm; the ability to perform this movement against resistance is the best single test of median nerve function. **B,** The opponens pollicis sweeps the abducted thumb across the palm so that the flexor pad of the thumb meets the flexor pad of the ring or little finger face-to-face and parallel.

In addition to the baseline assessment outlined earlier, the characteristic silky, dry texture of denervated skin should be sought. This texture is caused by disrupted sympathetic fibers which accompany sensory nerve injury. The most reliable tests for isolated motor function of the median nerve in the hand are the abductor pollicis brevis and the opponens pollicis test (Fig. 39-19). For motor function of the ulnar nerve (Fig. 39-20, *A*) the most reliable test is adduction and abduction of the long finger. Froment's sign (Fig. 39-20, *B*) is useful in detecting paralysis of the adductor pollicis.

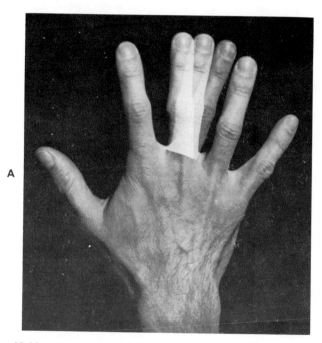

A

Fig. 39-20. Tests for motor function of ulnar nerve. **A,** Independent adduction-abduction of fingers, against resistance, and adduction of thumb with the hand extended on a flat surface demonstrates action of interossei and adductor-pollicis muscles, which are supplied by the ulnar nerve; each muscle should be tested separately for localization of nerve damage.

Continued.

Fig. 39-20, cont'd. B, Froment's sign. The patient pinches a piece of paper forcefully; the examiner then pulls the paper away, or the patient pulls the paper taut with both hands as if to tear it; to prevent the paper from slipping away from the weak adductor pollicis, the patient must bring the flexor pollicis longus into play causing flexion of the interphalangeal joint of the thumb; the patient's right thumb shows Froment's sign because of transection of the motor branch of the ulnar nerve (same patient as shown in Fig. 39-13).

Distal nerve transections, transections of pure motor or sensory nerves, and nerve transections in children have the best prognoses after surgical repair. Immediate repair of cleanly cut nerve ends gives superior results to delayed repair. If a branch 1 mm. or smaller in diameter is divided it can be anastamosed accurately by use of magnification supplied by a high-powered loop or an operating microscope.

Vessel injuries

The hand can usually survive with only one of its two major arteries intact and occasionally with neither. However, arterial anastamosis or grafts should be carried out if blood supply is in question. Clinically, the Allen test (Fig. 39-21) is useful in determining patency of the radial or ulnar arteries. Operatively, viability is best assessed by bright red bleeding occurring at freshly cut edges of muscle or skin. If a tourniquet is used viability may be assessed by the "blush test," i.e., noting the color that develops in the questionable area after the tourniquet is released.

Recently success has been achieved in replanting amputated digits. The key to success is early anastamosis of at least two veins and one artery of the affected digit. This can be accomplished only by a specialty team using appropriate magnification.

Fractures and dislocations

Fractures of the phalanges and metacarpals are the most common of all fractures. If accompanied by no deformity or displacement, they heal quickly with simple immobilization.

Deformity occurs when the fracture creates a disruption in the normal linkage system of the hand. The long bones of the hand constitute a delicate system of levers linked by mobile joints and controlled in space by the balanced pull of the flexor and extensor tendons. With disruption of a long bone a new "joint" is introduced into the system. Since no further controls have been added, the system buckles.

Deformity is tolerated very poorly in the hand, more particularly in the proximal and middle phalanges and least of all in the joints. Rotational deformity must always be looked for and is confirmed if the nail beds are not parallel or if the fingers tend to overlap in flexion (Fig. 39-22).

In treating deformity caused by fresh fractures one must be sure that reduction is obtained and maintained. If any uncertainty exists open reduction and internal fixation are warranted.

Immobilization should be continued until there is clinical and radiological evidence of union. For simple fractures 3 weeks often suffices; however, transverse fractures of phalangeal or metacarpal shafts often require 5 or 6 weeks. There is no justification for including the arm and shoulder in the immobilization. The patient must faithfully exercise the remainder of the upper limb to prevent disuse atrophy.

Carpus. The most common carpal fracture is of the navicular or scaphoid. Classically a fall on the outstretched hand with tenderness in the anatomical snuffbox alerts the examiner to this injury. Even if roentgenographic findings are negative (including scaphoid views), immobilization is mandatory for at least 2 weeks and may be discontinued only if repeat radiological and clinical examination are negative at that time. It is essential to look very closely for evidence of displacement of scaphoid fractures, which may indicate concomitant soft tissue injury and the necessity for open reduction and internal fixation. Furthermore, the possibility of avascular necrosis of the proximal pole of the scaphoid should be considered. It is wise to forewarn the patient of this possibility at the commencement of treatment.

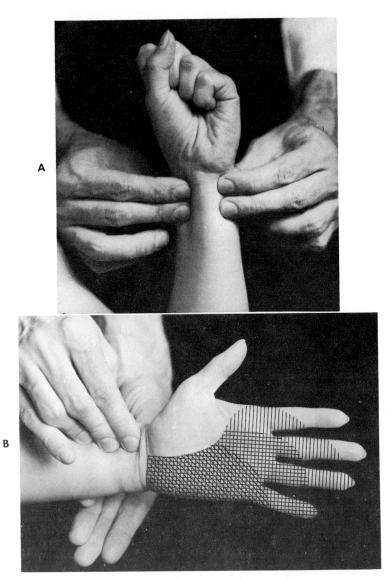

Fig. 39-21. For legend see opposite page.

At times the scaphoid can be very slow in healing and occasionally many months of immobilization are required to gain satisfactory union and function.

The lunate is the most commonly dislocated carpal bone. It usually dislocates in a volar direction and may compress the median nerve in that position. Reduction can usually be accomplished by closed means but there is a risk of subsequent avascular necrosis. Follow-up radiographs are necessary to rule out this complication.

Metacarpus. Bennett's fracture-dislocation is a dislocation of the thumb carpometacarpal joint secondary to a fracture of the metacarpal base extending into the joint, with resultant subluxation or dislocation. Skeletal fixation is generally required to maintain reduction.

The most common fracture of the remaining metacarpals is the "boxer's fracture" of the fifth metacarpal, commonly resulting from a fist fight. Fractures of the shaft of the long and ring metacarpals tend to be more stable than those of the border digits. The usual general principles of reduction and immobilization apply here.

As a rule, dislocations of the metacarpophalangeal joints are easily reduced and maintained unless a phalangeal or metacarpal head is trapped in a "buttonhole" rent in the joint capsule. In the latter circumstance, open reduction of the dislocation is required.

Phalanges. Displaced fractures of the proximal and middle phalanges of an articular surface often require open reduction and internal fixation. Displaced fractures of the distal phalanx are usually caused by crushing injury and are adequately managed by simple immobilization after appropriate soft tissue management. The fingernail should not be thoughtlessly discarded in these crush injuries, for it often serves as an excellent biological splint.

In a patient who presents with a history of trauma and a swollen, tender digit but without any fracture on radiographs, exclusion of

---

Fig. 39-21. Allen's test for patency of major arteries to the hand. **A,** The examiner occludes both the radial and ulnar arteries with his fingertips while the patient holds his hand aloft and milks out any residual blood by repeatedly flexing the digits into a tight fist and extending them; the hand is then lowered to a dependent position, with the arteries still occluded by digital pressure and the digits extended. **B,** The artery in question is then released; a rapid, bright, pink blush beginning near the point of release signifies a patent artery; slow or absent blush denotes occlusion or absence of the artery. If a blush does not occur after releasing one artery, the remaining artery is released after a pause of 1 to 2 minutes; patency of the second artery is demonstrated by a blush.

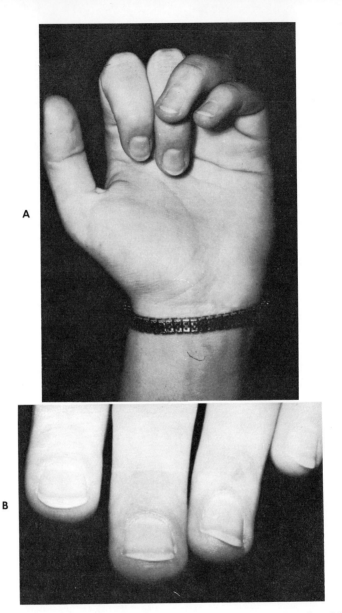

Fig. 39-22. "Scissoring" of fingers. A, Fingers overlap when flexed because of poor alignment and rotational malunion from fractures of index and ring proximal phalanges. B, Clue to malalignment is nonparallel fingernails.

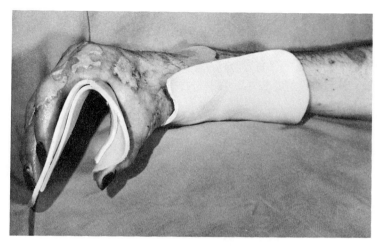

Fig. 39-23. "Anti-claw" splint placed on burned hand when at rest, to prevent claw deformity (see Fig. 39-6). (From Furnas, D. W.: A bedside outline for the treatment of burns, Springfield, Ill., 1969, Charles C Thomas, Publisher.)

significant soft tissue injury is essential. The extensor apparatus and the collateral ligaments of either the interphalangeal or the metacarpal phalangeal joints of the thumb are particularly prone to traumatic disruption.

Burns of the hand

Burns of the exposed and vulnerable dorsum of the hand most commonly result from open flames in adults or scalds in children. Suppleness and extensibility of the dorsal skin are destroyed by edema and inflammation and result in troublesome scar tissue formation in deep second-degree and third-degree burns. The resultant claw deformity (Fig. 39-6) is extremely disabling. Therefore in burns of this depth, begin assiduous physical therapy as soon as possible. The joints should move through a full range of motion many times daily. Between exercise periods, plaster or dynamic splints will prevent clawing (Fig. 39-23). If the above methods fail or are likely to, internal splinting with K-wires immobilizing the P.I.P. joints in slight flexion may be necessary.

Burns of the palmar surface are most often seen in children who have grasped hot objects. For deep second- and third-degree burns skin grafts may be required to prevent flexion deformities.

Electrical burns of the hand usually result from contact of the

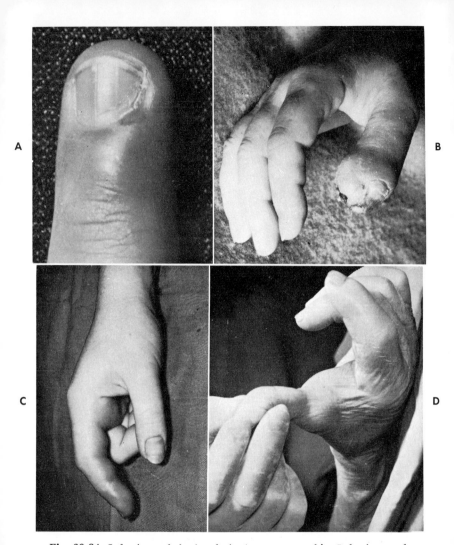

Fig. 39-24. Infections of the hand. **A,** Acute paronychia. Infection tends to run around the nail in the surrounding subcuticular tissue; it may also tunnel beneath the nail, forming a subungual abscess. **B,** Felon. Pus is localized and tightly compressed within the flexor pad or pulp space of the tip of the thumb. **C,** Tenosynovitis. Finger is (1) uniformly swollen, (2) slightly flexed, and (3) tender along tendon sheath, and (4) passive extension causes exquisite tenderness. **D,** Palmar space infection. Thenar space is swollen, tender, and distended with pus. (See Fig. 39-17.)

Table 39-3. Infections originating on the volar surface or around the nail

Entity	Findings	Cause	Site for incision for drainage of pus	Complications
1. *Paronychia* (Fig. 39-24, *A*)	Inflammation of soft tissues around nail that tend to "run around" nail margin	Infection of torn hangnail or cuticle	Directly into pus collection	Subungual abscess
2. *Subungual abscess*	Pus collection under nail	Extension from other infections	Excision of proximal portion of nail	
3. *Felon* (Fig. 39-24, *B*)	Red, tensely swollen, extremely painful throbbing pulp space of distal phalanx; keeps patient awake	Minor puncture wound of fingertip	Lateral aspect of distal phalanx, cutting through fibrous septa	Necrosis and osteomyelitis of phalangeal bone caused by compression of arteries
4. *Tendon sheath infection* (Fig. 39-24, *C*)	1. Uniform swelling of finger; 2. position of slight flexion of finger; 3. exquisite pain on passive extension; 4. maximum tenderness over tendon sheath area	Puncture wound or extension from other sites	Midlateral line of finger	Necrosis of flexor tendon; spread to palmar spaces or other bursae
5. *Palmar space infections* (Fig. 39-24, *D*; Fig. 39-17)	Tenderness and swelling of central and ulnar aspect of palm (*midpalmar space*) or of radial and thenar aspect of palm (*thenar space*)	Extension from tendon sheath infection; direct puncture wound	Skin crease incisions over most prominent area of swelling	Extensive damage to soft tissue of hand; extension to other spaces

hand with a high-voltage conductor. Ongoing deep coagulation necrosis imposes an onerous and frustrating therapeutic burden and frequently necessitates amputation. Arterial hemorrhage and gas gangrene are occasional complications.

Inflammatory conditions

Septic (Fig. 39-24). The dorsum of the hand with hair follicles and sweat and sebaceous glands acquires the same staphylococcal in-

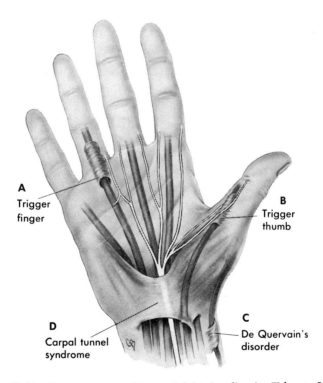

Fig. 39-25. Entrapment syndromes (right hand). **A,** Trigger finger caused by entrapment of digital flexor tendons in proximal portion of fibrous tendon sheath. **B,** Trigger thumb caused by entrapment of long flexor tendon to thumb. **C,** De Quervain's disorders or compression of the abductor pollicis longus and the extensor pollicis brevis tendon near the radial styloid process. **D,** Carpal tunnel syndrome or compression of median nerve by transverse carpal ligament.

fections seen in the skin elsewhere on the body (folliculitis, carbuncles, furuncles, and subcutaneous abscesses). Simple streptococcal infections of either the dorsal or volar aspect of the hand may lead to lymphangitis or lymphadenitis, which respond promptly to appropriate antibiotics and local wound care. Mixed infections with anaerobic streptococcus, bacteroides, or spirochetes (see Chapter 6) may be very destructive and demand aggressive systemic therapy (I.V. antibiotics) with complete and thorough debridement of the wound. A common source of these dangerous infections is the human bite, resulting from the collision of a closed fist with an open mouth.

Infections originating on the palmar surface or around the nail have distinct characteristics, which are listed in Table 39-3. When these infections are seen quite early in their course they may be aborted by antibiotics, bed rest, elevation, and warm moist dressings to the hand. If the infection is not aborted, pus will collect and drainage is required.

In recent years the most common cause of hematogenous septic arthritis in the hand in patients under 40 is *Neisseria gonococcus*. Culture of this organism is extremely difficult and swabs should be

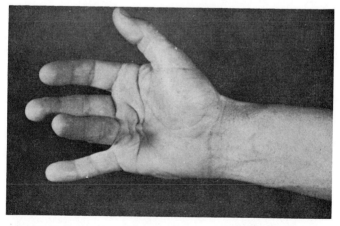

Fig. 39-26. Dupuytren's contracture. Band of hypertrophied and contracted superficial palmar fascia projects distally from nodule in palm; proximal interphalangeal joint of ring finger is forced into permanent flexion.

taken routinely from the oral pharnyx, cervix or urethral meatus, anus, blood, and, if possible, the local site.

Nonseptic. Aseptic tenosynovitis is relatively common in the hand and wrist. DeQuervain's disorder (Fig. 39-25) is caused by compression of the long abductor and short extensor tendons of the thumb in the fibrous sheath near the radial styloid process. It causes severe pain, particularly if adduction of the thumb is carried out while the wrist is held in ulnar deviation. Trigger finger or thumb results from stenosing tenosynovitis in the proximal portion of the fibrous flexor sheath and from nodule formation in the flexor tendon because of

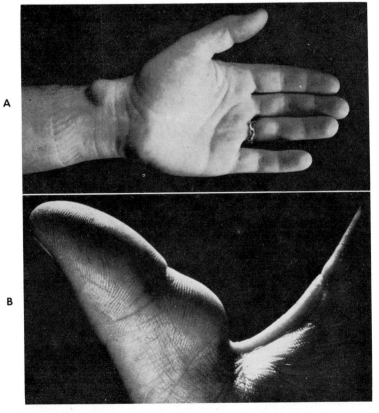

Fig. 39-27. Tumors of the hand. **A,** Ganglia. **B,** Epidermal cyst.

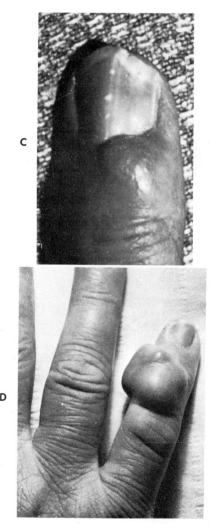

Fig. 39-27, cont'd. C, Mucous cyst. **D,** Xanthoma.
Continued.

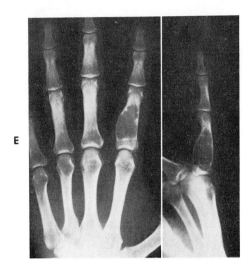

E

Fig. 39-27, cont'd. E, Enchondroma.

injury or rheumatoid disease. The tendon is trapped momentarily as it passes through the mouth of the sheath and then suddenly releases. Either flexion or extension may be blocked.

Treatment of these "ensheathment syndromes" that fail to settle conservatively is surgical decompression by incising the roof of the offending fibrous sheath.

Rheumatoid arthritis commonly presents as an acute arthritis in the wrist or fingers. Multiple symmetrical small joint involvement, fluctuating clinical course, and appropriate lab studies serve to differentiate it from other forms of arthritis.

Degenerative changes

Heberden's nodes are the most common form of involvement of the hand. These are present at the distal interphalangeal joint and reflect a local process of degenerative arthritis.

The carpometacarpal joint of the thumb is also commonly involved by degenerative processes and, as with Heberden's nodes, may reflect a systemic proclivity for osteoarthritis.

Carpal tunnel syndrome

The carpal tunnel syndrome, caused by compression of the median nerve in the flexor compartment of the wrist by the transverse carpal

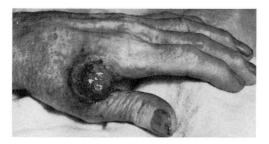

Fig. 39-28. Squamous carcinoma.

ligament, may occur as the result of diminution in the size of the canal (as with Colles' fracture) or of increase in the size of the contents (as with rheumatoid synovitis). Characteristically it results in pain in the hand and forearm, hypesthesia and paresthesia of the radial three digits, and weakness and atrophy of the thenar muscles. Quite commonly the pain is appreciated as far proximally as the shoulder. It is most common in middle-aged women and is frequently bilateral. Surgical decompression of the transverse metacarpal ligament (Fig. 39-25) usually gives results that are gratifying to the surgeon and patient alike.

TUMORS AND TUMORLIKE CONDITIONS
Dupuytren's contracture

Dupuytren's contracture (Fig. 39-26) is a fibrous metaplasia (often bilateral) of the superficial palmar fascia that causes a characteristic flexion contracture located in the subcutaneous layer of the palm. A hypertrophic fibrous nodule appears in the palm or finger (most commonly the ring finger) and is followed by the formation of thick, fibrous bands that may extend distally. These bands slowly shorten until extension of the metacarpophalangeal and the proximal interphalangeal joints is prevented. The contracture is corrected by excision of the offending metaplastic tissue.

Benign tumors

Ganglia, epidermal cysts, mucous cysts, xanthomas, lipomas, enchondromas, glomus tumors, and neurilemomas are benign tumors characteristically found in the hand (Fig. 39-27, *A* through *E*). These are discussed in Table 39-4.

Table 39-4. Benign tumors of the hand

Entity	Description	Comment	Treatment
1. *Ganglia* (Fig. 39-27, *A*)	Multilocular cyst growing from capsule of carpal joint (dorsum of wrist, snuffbox, or just proximal to thenar eminence) or volar aspect of metacarpophalangeal joint	Most common tumor of hand (approximately one-third of tumors of the hand)	Excision using equipment for major hand surgery (aspiration of cyst, injection of cortisone occasionally effective); recurrences are seen after any type of treatment
2. *Epidermal cyst* or implantation cyst, inclusion cyst (Fig. 39-27, *B*)	Subcutaneous cyst filled with epithelial debris located on flexor surface of proximal phalanges or distal palm	Caused by bits of epidermis, stabbed into subcutaneous site by tools or sharp objects	Excision
3. *Mucous cyst* (myxomatous cyst, myxoid cyst, or synovial cyst, Fig. 39-27, *C*)	Translucent cyst embedded in thick, reddish skin just proximal to nail fold; frequently *groove of nail* in direct line with cyst	Filled with synovial fluid; communicates with distal interphalangeal joint usually	Excision of cyst and communication; avoid injury to extensor tendon
4. *Xanthoma* (benign giant cell tumor of tendon sheath; benign synovioma) (Fig. 39-27, *D*)	Firm, irregular, yellowish tumor growing from fibrous flexor tendon sheath	Multinucleated giant cells, synovial clefts, hemosiderin, foam cells seen on microscopic examination	Excision with equipment for major hand surgery

5. *Lipoma*	Soft, multinodular, fatty mass	Frequently grow forward from middle palmar or thenar space displacing tendons and presenting as mass in palm	Excision with equipment for major hand surgery
6. *Enchondroma* (Fig. 39-27, E)	Cartilaginous pocket within bone or proximal phalanx (or other phalanges or metacarpal heads)	Usually asymptomatic, incidental finding on roentgen-ray examination	None, unless symptoms of pathological fracture; then curettage and packing with bone chips
7. *Glomus tumors* (glomangioma or angioneuromyoma)	Tiny, very painful, reddish-purple nodules frequently visible under fingernail, also seen in other sites	Growth of neuromyoarterial glomus, a heat-regulating arterial shunt	Excision
8. *Neurilemoma and neuroma*	Painful, tender nodule along course of previously injured nerve; Tinel's sign (distal paresthesias elicited by percussion at site of neurilemoma)	Most common in a digital nerve of thumb or index finger	If nerve is not functioning, excise neuroma and anastomose the nerve, or excise neuroma and bury stump of nerve in a recess where it will not be stimulated

Malignant tumors

Squamous cell or epidermoid carcinoma (Fig. 39-28) is the most common malignant tumor of the hand. It usually develops from premalignant keratoses on the dorsum of the hand decades after chronic exposure to sunlight, ionizing radiation, or organic hydrocarbons or after long-standing chronic dermatological disorders. Ingestion of arsenicals is associated with keratoses and carcinomas of the palmar surface of the hand. Growth is slow, malignancy is low grade, lymph node metastases occur in only about 5% to 15% of cases, and mortality is proportionately low. Wide excision of the lesion and repair of the defect by skin grafts or pedicles is the usual treatment. In far-advanced cases, amputation, axillary lymphadenectomy, and perfusion of the limb with chemotherapeutic agents must be considered. *Basal cell carcinoma* is rare in the hand.

Malignant melanoma of the hand behaves essentially as malignant melanoma elsewhere on the body surface. Wide excision or amputation with or without regional lymphadenectomy and/or perfusion of chemotherapeutic agents is the usual treatment.

CHAPTER 40

Neurosurgery

HIRO NISHIOKA

Neurosurgery and other surgical specialties constitute areas of limited but essential fields of knowledge for the student. Although details of operative techniques and the complications of surgery are of concern principally to the practitioners of the specialties, the ability to recognize the need for surgical intervention, especially under emergency conditions, remains an indispensable part of every physician's armamentarium. A decision to perform an emergency operation may have to be based upon history and clinical picture only, with little or no confirmatory support from radiographs and other ancillary studies. Therefore, the ability to perform and interpret a neurological examination with proficiency is a prime requisite.

In considering neurosurgical problems, some basic working principles should be borne in mind. The specialized neurons of the central nervous system, once destroyed, are incapable of replacement. Furthermore, the pathways by which neurons are interconnected cannot be reestablished once severed or interrupted. A cell or its connections may be damaged by pressure, penetration by foreign objects, inflammation, invasion by neoplasm, or biochemical processes. Of these, pressure is the only factor that can be relieved surgically. Reparative surgery in the central nervous system is prophylactic only and is utilized to prevent any additional damage by infection, hemorrhage, or trauma.

The degree of cellular or tract damage by pressure is proportional to the amount of pressure, the rapidity of pressure rise, and its duration. The most severe and permanent damage is produced by the sudden application of pressure, e.g., in acute trauma. Pressure of lesser degrees can be tolerated without permanent damage if its rate of increase is slow, e.g., neoplasm. If surgical decompression is to be worthwhile, it must be performed before irreversible damage has

Table 40-1. Common diagnostic studies utilized

Diagnostic test	Procedure	Information obtained
Lumbar puncture	Insertion of needle into lumbar subarachnoid space and withdrawal of fluid	Presence of abnormal amounts of cells, and alterations in chemical content of CSF
Echoencephalography	Transmission of ultrasonic waves coronally through brain and recording of echo at brain-fluid and brain-bone interfaces	Lateral shift of normally midline structures (third ventricle) by mass lesions
Electroencephalography	Application of electrodes to scalp and recording of cortical electrical activity	Abnormal wave forms and seizure discharges from areas irritated or compressed
Isotope scanning (Fig. 40-1)	Parenteral injection of a radioactive isotope and counting of radioactivity transmitted through to scalp	Neoplasms, vascular malformations, and abnormal brain tissue taking up more than normal amounts of isotope
Computerized axial tomography (Fig. 40-2)	Tomograms of head with computer-derived image of structures of different densities	Transverse outlines of ventricular system, fluid and semi-fluid cavities
Pneumoencephalography (Fig. 40-3)	Lumbar puncture and injection of air into subarachnoid space	Outline of subarachnoid cisterns and ventricular system that may be distorted or shifted by mass lesions
Angiography (Fig. 40-4)	Insertion of needle into the carotid or vertebral artery in the neck and injection of contrast medium	Opacification of cerebral blood vessels to show vascular anomalies, or neovascularity and displacement by mass lesion
Myelography (Fig. 40-5)	Lumbar or cisternal puncture and injection of positive contrast medium or air	Outline of spinal subarachnoid space that may be distorted or blocked by mass lesions in the spinal canal
Discography (Fig. 40-6)	Injection of contrast medium into intervertebral disc	Abnormal configuration of disc and leakage of contrast through ruptured annulus fibrosus

Possible complications	Lesions best demonstrated
Herniation of temporal uncus or cerebellar tonsils with compression of brainstem	Meningitis, subarachnoid hemorrhage
None	Lateralized tumors of cerebral hemispheres, subdural and epidural hematoma
None	Brain abscess, seizure focus
Allergic reaction to isotope or its carrier	Meningioma, arteriovenous malformations, highly vascular malignant neoplasms
Allergic reaction to enhancing drugs, if used	Hydrocephalus, neoplasms, cysts, hematomas, infarcts
Herniation of temporal uncus or cerebellar tonsils with compression of brainstem	Tumors in chiasmic cistern, floor of third ventricle, aqueductal obstructions
Thromboembolism with cerebral infarction, local hemorrhage with tracheal compression, allergic reaction to contrast media	Vascular anomalies (aneurysm, arteriovenous malformation), subdural and epidural hematoma, vascular neoplasms, especially meningioma
Spinal arachnoiditis—inflammatory reaction to contrast medium or contaminant	Tumors in the spinal canal, herniated intervertebral disc, avulsion of nerve roots
Extravasation of contrast into subarachnoid space	Degenerated or ruptured intervertebral disc

occurred and it must be sufficiently extensive. The surgeon must occasionally sacrifice nervous tissue that appears grossly nonviable or even normal in the interests of preserving useful functioning tissue that appears capable of recovery.

In contrast to the foregoing, the neurosurgical armamentarium contains procedures for the planned focal destruction of tracts and nuclear elements. These operations are utilized for the relief of intractable pain, involuntary movements, and abnormal states of muscle tonus.

The emphasis of this chapter will be directed toward the management of pressure-producing lesions. Descriptions of infrequently used or highly specialized techniques are omitted, so that the reader may concentrate upon the commonly encountered neurosurgical problems.

SPECIAL DIAGNOSTIC STUDIES

Neurological examination alone is not often sufficiently accurate in localizing intracranial lesions to proceed with operative treatment. In acute trauma, emergency explorations for life-threatening hematomas may be undertaken on clinical grounds alone. In elective situations, however, accurate delineation of the extent and location of the lesion prior to operation is desirable and requires the use of special investigative procedures.

Table 40-1 lists the common diagnostic studies utilized. Whenever possible, the specific tests that give the best chances of demonstrating a lesion should be chosen, based upon the clinical impression of the location and type of pathology expected. Although any test might be abnormal in the presence of a mass lesion, some may provide specific information as to the nature of the pathology; e.g., in the differential diagnosis of extracerebral versus intracerebral mass, an angiogram usually provides a definite distinction, whereas an air study in such a circumstance may show only the site and location of the mass without clearly defining the border between brain and mass. The routine use of a "battery" of tests is to be deplored. All such tests are costly, and some carry significant risks of complications and even death. Therefore, careful neurological evaluation is essential to the efficient and safe investigation of the patient. General screening tests are, of course, never to be overlooked. Blood count, urinalysis, chest radiograph, and any other appropriate tests should be completed prior to special investigations.

Electroencephalography, echoencephalography, and *radioisotope scans* are useful as screening tests since they can be performed without significant risk or discomfort to the patient. *Transverse axial tomography,* in which differential x-ray absorption by the brain and ventricular fluid allows computer derivation of a tomographic picture of the ventricular system, is a promising new radiological technique. By this method, ventricular shifts by mass lesions can be diagnosed without the need for injecting contrast media. As yet, it is a costly and complex technique, and not available as a routine screening test. The final preoperative assessment usually depends on contrast radiological studies *(pneumography, angiography,* etc.). The measurement of heat radiation from the scalp *(thermography)* and the recording of sounds created by abnormal blood flow patterns *(phonoencephalography)* are of occasional value, but they are not part of the essential diagnostic armamentarium.

Considerable confusion exists in the minds of most students regarding the indications for *lumbar puncture.* Whenever intraspinal pathology is suspected, lumbar puncture with the Queckenstedt test

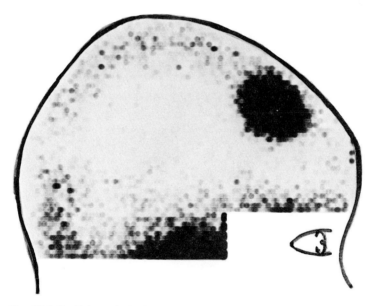

Fig. 40-1. Radioisotopic brain scan. The venous sinuses take up relatively heavy concentrations of isotope, whereas normal brain tissue does not. In this right lateral projection, an area of dense uptake is seen high in the frontal area. The rounded outline suggests a neoplasm. In this case, the lesion proved to be a meningioma.

842 *Synopsis of surgery*

(compression of the jugular veins) is indicated. The complete lack of any change in pressure with the Queckenstedt maneuver indicates the presence of advanced compression within the spinal canal above the site of the needle. In such circumstances, whenever feasible, radiopaque material for myelographic screening, e.g., Pantopaque, should be instilled immediately, for it may be difficult to repeat the spinal puncture at a later time. Lesser degrees of compression are manifested by abnormally slow rates of rise and/or fall of fluid pressure during jugular compression and release. These abnormal pressure changes along with the characteristics of the fluid (xanthochromia, increased protein) serve to differentiate the surgical from the medical neurological problems. It is therefore most important to *measure and record* them accurately.

In the presence of a pressure-producing intracranial pathological

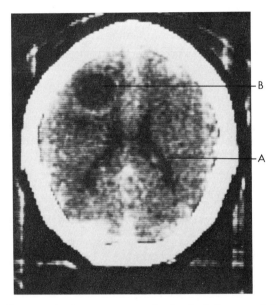

Fig. 40-2. Computerized tomogram at the level of the top of the ears. The skull appears as a dense opaque outline; the semisolid brain tissue as an intermediate density, while the fluid in the lateral ventricles *(A)* appears to be the least dense. A cystic cavity containing fluid *(B)* is clearly demarcated without the need for injecting contrast material into the body.

condition, lumbar puncture is potentially hazardous to the life of the patient. The withdrawal of spinal fluid from below, and particularly the leakage of fluid into the spinal epidural space after the needle has been removed, encourages herniation of the cerebellar tonsils and temporal lobe uncus, with resultant brainstem compression. Therefore, lumbar puncture should be performed for specific indications only. Increased intracranial pressure is usually associated with clinically recognizable symptoms and signs such as vomiting and papilledema. There is no advantage in measuring the exact degree of abnormal pressure in the presence of such signs. The diagnosis of infections (menin-

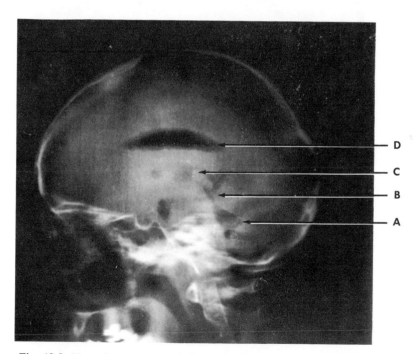

Fig. 40-3. Normal pneumoencephalogram. Air has been injected into the lumbar subarachnoid space, with the patient sitting upright in a special chair. The air enters the cerebral ventricular system via the foramina of Magendie and Luschka and then fills successively the fourth ventricle (**A**), the aquaduct of Sylvius (**B**), the third ventricle (**C**), and finally the lateral ventricles (**D**).

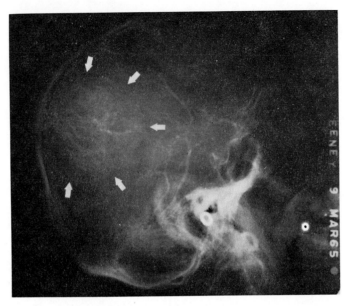

Fig. 40-4. Angiogram showing meningioma. The tumor (outlined by arrows) contains many neovascular channels that, when filled with contrast medium, produce a stain or blush in the angiogram. Malignant gliomas may also show vascular stains, and the differentiation is not always possible.

gitis, encephalitis) and of subarachnoid hemorrhage depends on the finding of the appropriate cells in the cerebrospinal fluid. Lumbar puncture is therefore indicated in all patients suspected of harboring the preceding, based upon the clinical finding of *nuchal rigidity*. That these same conditions are likely to be associated with increased intracranial pressure is apparent, but the possible risks of the procedure are outweighed by the necessity for deriving information that may be vital to the selection of proper treatment. In brain tumors, the information obtained from lumbar puncture is usually not worth the hazards; in subdural hematoma, the fluid may be entirely normal, misleading the clinician into a false sense of security. The Queckenstedt, test, for all practical purposes, should *never* be performed when intracranial pathology is suspected, for the potential hazards of uncal or tonsillar herniation are acutely increased by compressing the jugular veins.

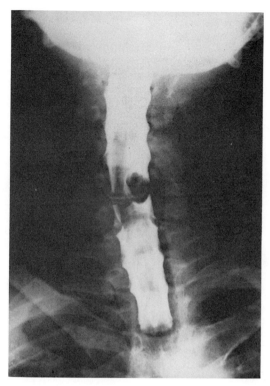

Fig. 40-5. Myelogram showing intradural extramedullary tumor. The sharp outline of the tumor mass is diagnostic of a lesion inside the dura but extrinsic to the spinal cord. Neurofibroma and meningioma are the usual lesions.

INCREASED INTRACRANIAL PRESSURE
Clinicopathological correlations

The addition of fluid, blood, or neoplastic tissue to the normal contents of any body cavity may result in (1) increase in the volume of that cavity, (2) increase in the pressure within the cavity, or (3) both. Adding to the contents of the cranial cavity results in an increase in the size of the head only in infants when the cranial sutures are still open, but even then the increase can occur only slowly.

846 *Synopsis of surgery*

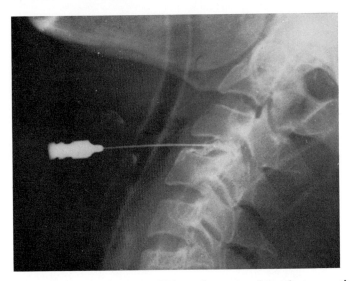

Fig. 40-6. Cervical discogram. This study was performed at operation for anterior interbody fusion in a patient with a reduced but unstable dislocation at C3-C4. Contrast medium has been injected into the disc space. The outline is ragged, and some of the medium has passed posterior to the vertebral body, indicating rupture of the annulus fibrosis.

For practical purposes the cranial cavity may be regarded as a rigid box divided into two compartments, one above and one below the tentorium. Each has one principal outlet, the tentorial hiatus and the foramen magnum, respectively. Every increase in volume within these compartments is accompanied by a tendency for brain tissue to herniate through their outlets. The herniating tissue directly compresses and distorts the brainstem and is the primary cause of death from increased intracranial pressure.

Institution of treatment before irreversible damage has occurred depends on the recognition of danger signs indicating beginning or advancing herniation. The patient's responses to common environmental stimuli are the most reliable indicators of his intracranial pressure. As pressure increases, the responses are progressively impaired in speed, accuracy, and propriety. Pupillary dilatation is always late in onset, occurring only in the presence of dangerous herniations. The "classic" alterations of vital signs (increasing blood pressure with slow-

Table 40-2. Clinical changes with progressive brainstem compression

Stage	Response to:			Pupils	
	Addressing patient by name	Patting or shaking patient's shoulder	Pinching tendon of pectoralis major	Relative size	Reaction to light
Normal	Looks at examiner, remains attentive	Looks at examiner, remains attentive	Removes pinching hand quickly and effectively, moves body away	Equal	Reactive
I	Opens eyes but tends to fall asleep while being spoken to	Opens eyes and remains awake as long as stimulus is applied	Removes stimulus and moves away, but not as quickly as in "normal"	Equal	Reactive
II	No response	Little or no response	Sluggish and ineffectual attempts to remove stimulus, shrugs shoulders	Dilated on side of lesion*	Sluggish or no reaction
III	No response	No response	Extensor thrust (decerebrate posture) on side opposite the lesion*	Widely dilated on side of lesion	No reaction
IV	No response	No response or bilateral extensor thrusts	Bilateral extensor thrusts	Widely dilated bilaterally	No reaction
V	No response	No response	No response	Moderately dilated	No reaction

*Dilatation of the pupil and the appearance of extensor posturing occasionally occur first on the side opposite that listed in this table. For the anatomic explanation for this phenomenon refer to text and to Fig. 40-7.

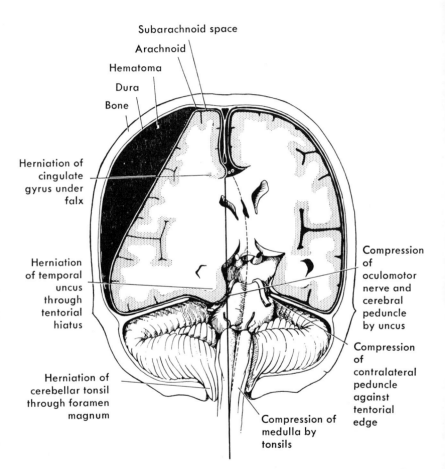

Subarachnoid space

Arachnoid

Hematoma

Dura

Bone

Herniation of
cingulate
gyrus under
falx

Herniation
of temporal
uncus
through
tentorial
hiatus

Herniation of
cerebellar tonsil
through foramen
magnum

Compression
of
oculomotor
nerve and
cerebral
peduncle
by uncus

Compression
of
contralateral
peduncle
against
tentorial
edge

Compression of
medulla by
tonsils

Fig. 40-7. Subdural hematoma. Although the hematoma displaces and distorts the surface of the cerebral hemisphere, the more serious and life-threatening changes are occurring in deeper structures at some distance from the hematoma itself. These changes result in displacement and compression of vital centers within the brainstem.

ing of the heart rate) may not occur until it is too late for effective treatment, if they occur at all.

Table 40-2 lists the progression of observable responses as intracranial pressure increases. Note that the categorized responses for each stage are not absolute; these are general guidelines and are subject to some variation. Fig. 40-7 shows how a subdural hematoma distorts the brain and produces the neurological signs of herniation. Dilatation of a pupil signifies herniation of the temporal uncus with compression of the oculomotor nerve. The nerve adjacent to the herniated uncus is usually affected first, resulting in dilatation of the pupil on the side of the lesion. Occasionally, however, the midbrain is shifted to the extent that the opposite oculomotor nerve is compressed against the edge of the tentorium, resulting in pupillary dilatation on the side opposite the lesion.

Compression of the cerebral peduncle either directly by the herniating uncus or indirectly by shifting against the opposite tentorial edge results first in a *paresis* on the side opposite the primary lesion (since these fibers cross in the medulla at the decussation of the pyramids), commonly followed by a change in response to *extensor thrust* (decerebration). At this stage, vasomotor and respiratory centers are easily compromised, so that cessation of respirations may occur at any moment.

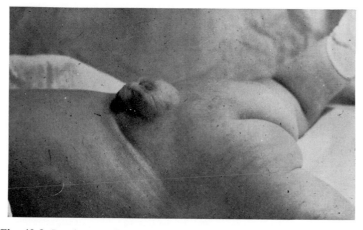

Fig. 40-8. Lumbar meningomyelocele. The lesion usually has a wide base, so that closure of the skin after excision of the sac often requires extensive undermining and rotation of flaps.

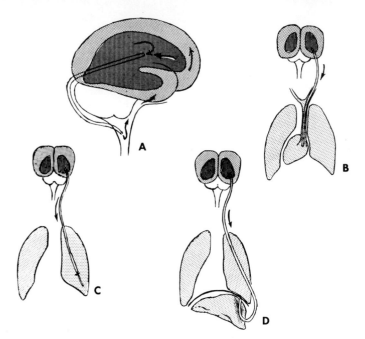

Fig. 40-9. Shunt procedures used in the treatment of hydrocephalus.
A, Ventriculocisternal shunt. Fluid is shunted into the cisterna magna to
circulate upward over the cerebral hemispheres and be absorbed in the
normal manner. B, Ventriculocaval shunt. Fluid is shunted directly into
the bloodstream via a catheter inserted into the jugular vein and passed
downward so that its tip lies in the superior vena cava; a one-way valve
within the system prevents reflux of blood upward from the vena cava
and also controls the pressure under which fluid leaves the ventricles.
C, Ventriculopleural shunt. Fluid is drained into the pleural cavity where
it is absorbed; failure to absorb the fluid quickly enough may result in
accumulation and compression of the lung. D, D₁, D₂, Ventriculoperi-
toneal shunts: D, into suprahepatic space; D₁, into the pelvic cavity
utilizing the fimbriated end of a fallopian tube; and D₂, into the left para-
colic gutter. Fluid is shunted into the peritoneal cavity to be absorbed;
the area into which the fluid is directed frequently becomes walled off
or covered with omentum so that the shunt ceases to function; the variations (D and D₁) are designed to avoid omental obstruction. E, Ven-
triculoureteral shunt. One kidney is removed and the fluid is drained
into its ureter; ventricular fluid and its electrolytes are lost from body
fluids and must be replaced carefully. F, Lumbar peritoneal and ureteral
shunts. These procedures can be used only in communicating hydrocephalus, i.e., when the ventricular system communicates with the spinal
subarachnoid space.

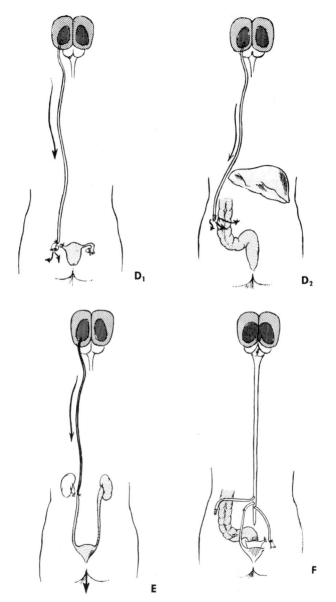

Fig. 40-9, cont'd. For legend see opposite page.

The stage-by-stage progression to total decerebration and finally to complete flaccidity with no response to any stimulus may occur gradually over a period of hours, or suddenly within a few seconds. Thus, there is no margin of safety after the onset of signs indicating midbrain compression.

CONGENITAL MALFORMATIONS

Three conditions merit the attention of the student. These are meningomyelocele, hydrocephalus, and craniosynostosis.

Meningomyelocele (Fig. 40-8) occurs most frequently in the lumbar region but can occur at any point in the midline of the neuraxis, including the vault of the skull. Lumbar meningomyeloceles are variable in their content of neural tissue; they almost always contain some nervous elements and are frequently associated with varying degrees of paraparesis. If no neural elements are present, the lesion is called a meningocele. Surgical repair of the sac is performed to prevent rupture with its attendant danger of meningitis, but little can be done to improve the neurological deficit.

Meningomyeloceles, regardless of location, are very often associated with the *Arnold-Chiari malformation,* a caudal displacement of the medulla and cerebellar tissue through the foramen magnum into the cervical canal. For reasons that have never been explained adequately, repair of the meningomyelocele is frequently followed by rapid enlargement of the head from *obstructive hydrocephalus.* Numerous methods of shunting the accumulated fluid out of the ventricular system (Fig. 40-9) have met with limited success and many complications. At present, the most satisfactory shunting procedure is the ventriculovenous shunt using a one-way check valve to prevent the reflux of blood from vein to cerebral ventricle (Fig. 40-9, *B*). The successful long-term control of pressure may result in useful survivals— children at least capable of being educated. On the other hand, inadequate control of pressure results in a child with very limited potential for mental development, with a monstrously large head.

Craniosynostosis, or premature closure of the cranial sutures, is a curious condition that affects males six times more frequently than females. The abnormal shape of the head depends on the suture(s) prematurely fused. In most cases, early treatment is indicated to prevent mental retardation, blindness, and permanent disfigurement. Operation consists of cutting out an artificial suture (linear craniectomy) and preventing early reclosure.

CRANIOCEREBRAL TRAUMA

The high incidence of head injuries in the general civilian population makes an adequate working knowledge of the problem essential to every physician. The pathological condition that may result from trauma is dependent on the mechanism of injury so that this must be considered carefully in each patient. In this section, the pathogenesis is considered along with the diagnosis and management of the various types of patients.

The management of the patient may be divided into four phases, which are discussed in the following paragraphs.

Phase I
Assessment of the type and severity of injury

The history of the traumatic event may provide valuable clues to the nature and areas injured. Unfortunately, patients are usually unable to provide this history because they are unconscious, or because of the amnesia generally associated with the injury. Therefore, fragments of information from relatives, spectators, and police officers may have to be pieced together. Since head injury occurs frequently in conjunction with injuries to other parts of the body, the physician must learn to evaluate quickly the relative severity of each and to determine which deserves priority in the order of treatment. The force of a blow to the head is always transmitted in some degree to the cervical spine, so that one must be aware constantly of the possibility of a fracture and/or dislocation of the cervical spine in association with every head injury. Respiratory and cardiovascular distress always take precedence over neurological injury, for they are immediately life threatening, and the resultant hypoxia enhances any damage to other tissues including those of the nervous system. (See Chapter 35.)

The type of injury may be classified according to the mechanism of trauma. It may be kinetic or static, nonpenetrating or penetrating. The kinetic injury results from the differential rates of motion between skull and brain tissues. Nonpenetrating kinetic injuries are by far the most common in civilian life. The stationary head may be struck, resulting in sudden movement of the cranium (acceleration), or the head in motion may strike a stationary object such that motion of the cranium is suddenly arrested (deceleration). The latter is more common and produces a more severe lesion. When movement is in a forward direction (Fig. 40-10, *A*), the major lesion is usually directly under the point of impact; when movement is in the lateral plane (Fig. 40-10, *C*), there is greater tendency for the maximal damage to occur on the side of the brain opposite the point of impact (contrecoup). Penetrating injuries are primarily static. In civilian life they are not uncommonly seen after a kick by a horse, or after direct blows with small objects such as balls or hammers.

The *key* to the initial and subsequent neurological evaluation of the head-injured patient is the assessment of the *level of responsiveness or*

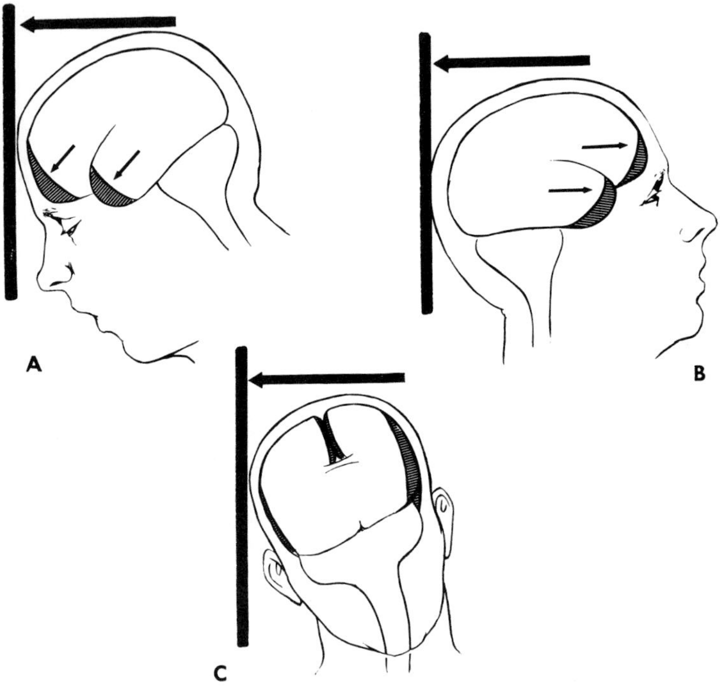

Fig. 40-10. Cortical contusion with relation to the direction of head movement. **A,** Head moving forward and striking stationary surface— major injury found at the tips of the frontal and temporal poles. **B,** Head moving backward and striking stationary surface—major injury found in the frontal and temporal lobes (contrecoup). **C,** Head moving laterally and striking stationary surface—major injury found on the side opposite that which strikes the surface (contrecoup); the medial surfaces of the hemispheres are also injured by impingement on the relatively rigid falx.

"*consciousness.*" This point cannot be overemphasized. Instability of the vital signs is common immediately after head trauma, whereas localizing neurological deficits may not become manifest until complications are far advanced. The rapidity, propriety, and accuracy of a patient's responses to verbal commands or to noxious stimulation wherever necessary must be observed carefully and recorded. The patient should be evaluated according to the *brain* injury as diagnosed by neurological examination, and the *bony* injury as diagnosed by physical and radiological examinations.

Brain { Concussion, Contusion, Laceration } Hemispheres, brainstem, or both

Bone { Closed fracture, Open fracture } Linear, Comminuted with or without depression of fragments

The severity of the brain injury does not correlate with the degree of skull damage. Therefore, each component should be described, e.g., cerebral concussion with closed linear fracture, or cerebral laceration from open comminuted fracture with depression of fragments.

Concussion implies that the trauma has been sufficient to impair cerebral function temporarily, that there is no immediate structural damage, and hence that recovery may be expected. *Contusion* denotes a more severe injury, producing bruises or petechial hemorrhages in brain substance. Complete neurological recovery can occur, but severe contusion may progress to infarction with permanent deficits or even death of the patient. *Laceration* denotes a break in the anatomic continuity of brain substance. It is usually associated with penetrating wounds, e.g., depressed fracture, bullet wounds, but can occur in nonpenetrating injuries.

By far the most common type of head injury seen in practice is concussion with or without skull fracture. A blow to the head sends the victim into a state of unresponsiveness from which he cannot be aroused. Within seconds or minutes, he begins to move his extremities, and then to open his eyes. He may be confused and disorientated for minutes or hours. During the first 6 to 12 hours, there may be lethargy, nausea, and vomiting. Within 24 to 48 hours, he is lucid and orientated, with no neurological deficit except for amnesia for the events just prior to and/or after the injury. Headache and giddiness are common when ambulation is begun, except in young children, who complain very little of symptoms after 24 hours.

Since skull fractures without gross displacement will heal without specific treatment, they are not of therapeutic importance except in two instances. Fractures of the base of the skull with dural and arachnoid tearing resulting in *leakage of cerebrospinal fluid* (mixed with blood) from the ear or nostril call for prophylaxis against meningitis. Ampicillin is most satisfactory for this purpose. Fractures of the petrous temporal bone frequently cannot be seen in skull radiographs, so that *diagnosis is based entirely upon the finding of bloody spinal fluid otorrhea*. Fortunately this leakage from the ear will almost invariably cease spontaneously. Cerebrospinal fluid rhinorrhea, however, often persists, with its attendant threat of meningitis. In such cases, intracranial repair of the meningeal laceration is necessary. *Depression of bone fragments* of such magnitude or in an area where functional cortex is compressed calls for immediate surgical elevation. In most instances, the blow that produces such depression of bone also lacerates the scalp, so that there is danger of infection in sequestrated bone fragments.

Performance of ancillary emergency procedures

Establishment and maintenance of an unobstructed airway is the first and most important consideration. Wherever indicated, *tracheostomy* should be performed without delay. It is desirable whenever deeply unresponsive patients must be transported to a neurosurgical facility several hours away. Where shorter periods of transport are involved, temporary intubation with an endotracheal tube is preferable. *Replacement of blood loss* from scalp lacerations is not often necessary except in infants and children where the blood loss may become sufficient to result in shock. Bleeding from the scalp edges can be controlled for short periods by tamponing, but if there is an extensive underlying fracture, then bleeding from the *bone edges* may continue despite the application of pressure to the scalp. *Debridement* and *suture* of lacerations should be performed with adequate shaving and cleansing of the lacerated area and under good operating conditions. Too often, scalp lacerations are roughly sutured under the premise that the scar will be hidden by hair. Patients who may be expected to remain unresponsive for prolonged periods should have an *indwelling catheter* in the bladder. This will not only facilitate nursing care but will also allow accurate measurement of the urinary output.

Summary of phase I:

1. General examination—define areas and extent of injuries and perform necessary emergency measures
2. Record cerebral functional status:
   a. Level of responsiveness
   b. Memory and mentation
   c. Motor power in face and extremities
   d. Pupillary size and reactions
   e. Vital signs

3. Examine skull radiographs for:
   a. Type and location of fractures, especially with relation to sinuses and middle meningeal grooves
   b. Position of the pineal gland if calcified
   c. Any other related or unrelated skull abnormality

Phase II
Observation of clinical progress

The clinical course is observed to detect the development of complications. What are these complications, and what are their symptoms and signs? Four types are under consideration at all times: *increased intracranial pressure, hemorrhage, infection,* and *convulsive seizures.* Increased intracranial pressure after head injury may result from reactive cerebral edema or from the development of a localized hematoma in the epidural or subdural spaces, or within brain substance. Lethargy, vomiting, and dulling of responses are common to all cases regardless of the underlying pathology, and localizing neurological deficits are inconstant except in patients with intracerebral hematoma.

Cerebral edema begins immediately after injury and may continue to increase for 48 to 72 hours before commencing to subside. In relatively minor injuries, it diminishes after 6 to 12 hours and requires no treatment. After severe cerebral contusions, edema and generalized infarction may convert the white matter into a pulpy mass.

Subdural hematoma is by far the most common of the complicating hematomas. The acute hematoma, which produces signs within 48 hours of injury, is usually caused by bleeding from a vein bridging between the superficial middle cerebral vein and the sphenoparietal sinus. Hence, these hematomas are maximal in the *temporal region.* The clot may become organized and liquefy so that it becomes converted into a cystic cavity limited by a capsule and containing fluid having a much higher osmotic pressure than that of the adjacent cerebrospinal fluid. By osmosis through this semipermeable capsule or membrane, cerebrospinal fluid is imbibed, resulting in gradual expansion of the cavity. Symptoms may then appear after a delay of several weeks or months after injury (chronic subdural hematoma). Small subdural collections may occur that cause no symptoms and require no treatment; they may resolve into thin scars and sometimes become calcified. An intermediate entity, the subacute hematoma, is recognized. Its definition is arbitrary, but generally it applies to hematomas that become clinically manifest between the third and fourteenth day after injury. An alternative explanation for the formation of chronic hematoma is that there is tearing of the Pacchionian granulations from their dural attachment, resulting in the immediate leakage of cerebrospinal fluid and blood into the subdural space. This lesion is therefore maximal

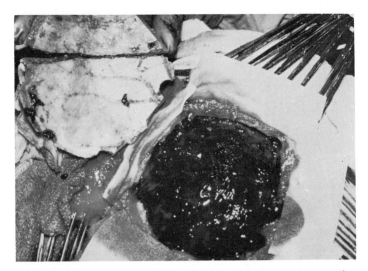

Fig. 40-11. Epidural hematoma. The reflected skull flap shows a linear fracture crossing the grooves formed by the middle meningeal artery. The underlying hematoma is an entirely solid clot, so that it could not have been drained through burr holes only.

over the *convexity of the hemisphere.* After a lapse of about 3 months from the time of injury, the possibility of a clinically significant subdural hematoma is so small that for practical purposes it need not be entertained seriously in the differential diagnosis.

Epidural hematoma (Fig. 40-11) usually results from laceration of branches of the middle meningeal artery. Often a fracture line can be seen radiologically in the temporal region, crossing the grooves formed in the inner table of the skull by the artery. Because bleeding is arterial, the symptoms are rapid both in onset and in progression. This lesion is less common in the elderly because the dura becomes so adherent to the inner table with advancing age that the artery is tamponed effectively.

Intracerebral and intracerebellar hematomas of sufficient magnitude to require evacuation are relatively rare. Bleeding occurs into softened and bruised brain tissue, so that the "hematoma" is usually a mixture of blood and necrotic white matter.

The appearance of signs of increased intracranial pressure varies with the lesion producing the pressure. Signs develop within the first

24 to 48 hours from cerebral contusion and edema and from epidural hematoma, whereas they tend to appear slightly later with intracerebral hematomas. Evidence of subdural hematoma may appear early or up to 3 months later, by which time the causative traumatic episode may have been forgotten. Since every head injury of any consequence is followed by some degree of increased pressure from reactive edema, one must establish a critical level at which point specific investigation and treatment are indicated. This level is generally reached *when the patient is no longer able to respond appropriately to verbal or nonnoxious tactile stimuli.* If the patient has been incapable of such a response from the time of injury, it is appropriate, in the absence of localizing neurological deficits, to await signs of progression.

The presence of hemiparesis is inconstant and unpredictable in patients with traumatic hematoma. Hemiparesis present immediately after injury is likely caused by cerebral contusion rather than by a compressing hematoma. The slow development of a mild hemiparesis is consistent with the presence of an extracerebral hematoma (epidural or subdural), whereas a dense hemiplegia, especially in an alert patient, is rarely produced by such a lesion. Subdural hematoma may arise with no paresis, or with hemiparesis contralateral or ipsilateral to the hematoma. Hence, the *neurological picture of subdural hematoma is often confusing and nonspecific.*

Frequent recording of the vital signs—pulse, respirations, blood pressure, and temperature—is an integral part of the observation routine. Unfortunately, the so-called classic alterations in the vital signs described under the section on increased intracranial pressure are so *frequently absent* in patients with proved intracranial hematomas that they cannot be relied upon to occur. Intracranial pressure may not be assumed to be normal because the vital signs are stable. Shock is never produced by increased intracranial pressure, except in the terminal stages. The development of shock demands a search for an extracranial source of blood loss. (See Chapter 35.)

Hemorrhage from the gastrointestinal tract not uncommonly accompanies severe head injuries, particularly with brainstem damage. The pathophysiology of this phenomenon is presumably the same as stress ulcers associated with burns and other major traumatic incidents. Bleeding may occur from a single acute ulcer or from multiple superficial erosions, and it may cause death by exsanguination. Whenever shock occurs during the clinical course of an unresponsive patient, gastrointestinal hemorrhage should be suspected. Subgaleal bleeding (cephalohematoma) in infants can be of sufficient magnitude to produce shock. In adults, it is impossible to lose a sufficient quantity of blood intracranially or into the subgaleal space to produce shock from volume loss alone.

Infections involving the pulmonary and urinary tracts are frequently encountered in patients who remain unresponsive for prolonged periods of time. Tracheostomy is often indicated for adequate removal of tracheobronchial secretions. Prophylactic antibiotic therapy should be given in certain circumstances, particularly in the elderly. *Meningitis* is a threat when an open fracture allows the leakage of cerebrospinal fluid outside the cranial cavity. Whenever there is bleeding from the ears, nose, mouth, or scalp, the blood should be examined for spinal fluid content. Blood containing cerebrospinal fluid is usually watery, forms a pale outer ring when dripped onto a gauze sponge, and does not clot. High fever and nuchal rigidity call for diagnostic lumbar puncture. Abscess formation produces pressure symptomatology similar to that of hematoma, except that seizures and localizing paresis are much more common.

Convulsive seizures occur infrequently after head injury. They are much more likely to occur in infants and children under the age of 10 years. The seizures may be focal or generalized (grand mal) and usually denote cerebral contusion. Except in infants, subdural hematoma is rarely associated with seizures prior to treatment.

Supportive medical care

Vomiting is common during the first 8 hours after head injury, so that oral intake should be withheld during that period. Clear fluids may be given thereafter if the patient desires it, and solid food after 24 to 48 hours depending on the severity of the injury. If parenteral fluids are required, the volume administered during the first 48 hours should be somewhat less than the normal daily requirement—1,500 to 2,000 ml. for an average adult. Overhydration enhances cerebral edema. Feeding by nasogastric tube should be instituted if the patient is unable to swallow after 3 days.

Seizures must be vigorously treated with anticonvulsant drugs. Respiratory embarrassment accompanying convulsive seizures adds the insult of hypoxia to an already injured brain. Intravenous diphenylhydantoin (Dilantin) should be tried first. Barbiturates produce sedation that interferes with the assessment of the level of responsiveness. Therefore, they should be given only after maximum doses of Dilantin have proved ineffective in controlling seizures. Repeated seizures progressing toward status epilepticus are most effectively stopped by the direct intravenous injection of diazepam. Sedation should be avoided whenever possible, but the extremely restless, struggling, and vociferous patient should be quieted with small doses of chlorpromazine or other tranquilizing drugs rather than by the simple application of restraining bonds.

Attention to the care of the eyes, oropharynx, and respiratory and urinary tracts is essential to the prevention of ulcerative and infectious complications. The program for such supportive care is the same as that required after any major operation or trauma.

Phase III
Performance of special diagnostic tests

Table 40-1 showed that *echoencephalography, computerized tomography,* and *cerebral angiography* are the most useful tests for detecting traumatic hematomas. Since echoencephalography involves no risk to

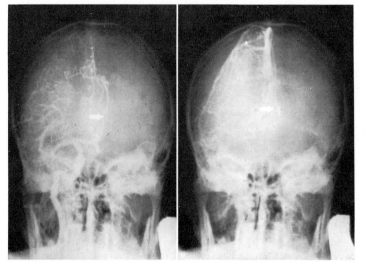

Fig. 40-12. Carotid angiogram demonstrating an extracerebral hematoma. The arterial phase, **A,** shows the surface arterioles to be displaced inward from the inner surface of the skull, leaving a large avascular area. The anterior cerebral artery *(arrow)* is shifted to the left of midline. The venous phase, **B,** shows the same avascular area, and a shift to the left of the internal cerebral vein *(arrow)*. If the middle meningeal artery is visualized, a subdural hematoma can be differentiated from an epidural hematoma; in the former, the artery lies in its normal position, whereas in the latter, it is displaced inward along with vessels on the surface of the brain. The artery is not visible in these photographs.

the patient, it may be utilized routinely. The position of midline structures can be checked easily and repeatedly during the period of critical observation. When performed accurately, a diagnostic echo can be recorded from the interface between cortex and hematoma.

Cerebral angiography is indicated, but not necessarily essential, in any patient whose level of responsiveness has dropped to the critical level previously discussed, in those who develop progressive neurological deficit, and in those who fail to show clinical improvement. Precise angiographic localization is desirable before operation (Fig. 40-12), but discretion must be used in each case. The patient in extremis with brainstem compression may suffer irreversible damage during periods of nonessential delays. Therefore, when the patient's condition demands immediate exploration and decompression, all diagnostic tests should be bypassed.

Lumbar puncture is of no value except in the diagnosis of meningitis or gross subarachnoid hemorrhage. Subdural taps can be performed on infants, but only liquefied (chronic) hematomas can be aspirated through the small-bore needles used for such taps.

Phase IV
Nonsurgical treatment

The goal of definitive treatment is to alleviate increased intracranial pressure. Although the removal of a significant hematoma is mandatory, that alone may be insufficient to accomplish this goal if there is severe cerebral swelling. Nonsurgical decompressive aids may then be necessary if the patient is to derive practical benefit from the removal of the primary lesion. These aids are to be used only if angiography or exploration has ruled out the presence of a major hematoma; their indiscriminate use prior to definitive diagnostic tests can mask the signs of a lesion that demands surgical removal.

Three nonsurgical agents are applicable: the infusion of dehydrating agents, the administration of adrenocorticosteroids, and hypothermia. Intravenously administered *urea* or *mannitol* produces dramatic and profound reductions of intracranial pressure. The effects generally do not last more than 6 to 10 hours. After that, the intracranial pressure tends to rise to a level even higher than before the substance was given (rebound phenomenon). Subsequent infusions are much less effective, so that their use is, for practical purposes, limited to a maximum of two doses. High-potency adrenocorticosteroids *(dexamethasone)* and the *reduction of body temperatures* to the range of 30 to 33° C. theoretically reduce the degree of cerebral edema, but their effectiveness in reducing the morbidity and mortality of head injuries has not been proved.

Surgical treatment

Surgical management comprises the evacuation of hematomas, debridement of necrotic nonfunctional brain tissue, and extracerebral decompressive procedures. Liquid hematomas can be drained through simple burr holes, whereas solid clots and necrotic brain require larger openings for effective removal. This may be provided by rongeuring the bone (craniectomy) or by removing a full bone flap. Additional decompression may be accomplished by the complete removal of large bone flaps and by sectioning the tentorium to relieve direct pressure on the brainstem. The use of the latter procedures has largely been supplanted by the application of the nonsurgical adjuvants discussed previously.

The following general rules are useful in the surgical intervention for *acute subdural* or *epidural hematoma:*

1. Exploratory openings should be made low in the temporal region.
   Reason: The source of bleeding is usually a vessel located in that region.
2. Exploration should be bilateral unless prior angiography has ruled out a hematoma on one side.
   Reason: a. Contrecoup lesions are common.
   b. Bilateral subdural hematomas are common.
   c. Localizing signs may occur on either side regardless of the side of the hematoma
3. Provision should be made for proceeding with a major craniotomy.
   Reason: a. Acute hematomas usually consist of solid clot that cannot be evacuated adequately through a small burr hole.
   b. Sources of persistent bleeding cannot be located through a burr hole.
4. An adequate quantity of blood should be available for transfusion.
   Reason: Bleeding from the original source may be persistent and difficult to locate.

Of special interest in the postoperative care of patients with subacute and chronic subdural hematomas is the high incidence of convulsive seizures. The risk is sufficiently great as to warrant routine use of anticonvulsant medications for 3 to 6 months after operation.

Prognosis after head injury

Although the threat of serious or fatal complications attends every head injury, no matter how trivial, some general prognostications may be applied to the majority of patients, depending on their neurological findings immediately after injury. The capacity for neurological recovery is profoundly influenced by the age of the patient. An infant or child suffering a concussion with loss of consciousness for not more than a few minutes will usually be asymptomatic within 48 hours. The young and middle-aged adult often complains of postural headache and giddiness for perhaps a week, whereas the elderly patient is often mentally confused for days and complains of symptoms for weeks. Severe brainstem injury with decerebrate responses may be completely reversible in the child and young adult, although several months are required for recovery. Such an injury is quite likely to be fatal in the middle-aged, and even more so in the elderly.

If epidural hematoma is diagnosed and treated in time, complete recovery usually occurs. However, the younger age group sustaining this complication contributes to the low mortality and morbidity. Acute subdural hematoma is fatal in the great majority of cases, even with immediate operation. Gross cerebral contusion that accompanies most of these hematomas contributes to the high mortality. Chronic subdural hematomas can usually be satisfactorily treated, but the incidence of postoperative complications remains high.

SPINAL TRAUMA

Management of the spine-injured patient may be considered in the same four phases as described for craniocerebral injuries. It is directed toward achieving the following goals:

1. Relief of compression on the spinal cord or nerve roots.
2. Prevention of additional trauma to neural elements until bony healing has taken place.
3. Provision of conditions such that bony healing will result in permanent stability and satisfactory alignment.

Phase I

Assessment of the type and severity of injury

The mechanism of injury, resultant neurological disability, and prognosis differ greatly depending on the level of injury. Table 40-3 lists the types of deficits with relation to the vertebral segments injured. Fracture-dislocations of the cervical spine (Fig. 40-13) usually result from acute hyperextension, e.g., a blow to the forehead or chin driving the head backward. Thus there may be significant craniocerebral injury associated with any cervical spine injury, and, conversely, any *injury to the head may be accompanied by damage to the cervical spine.* The thoracic and lumbar spines are more often damaged by hyperflexion (Fig. 40-14).

Table 40-3. Clinical picture after injury to the spinal cord and cauda equina

Vertebral segment	Neurological segment	Paralysis resulting from physiological transection	
		Partial transection	Complete transection
C1–C4	Spinal cord, cervical plexus level	Quadriparesis, becoming spastic*; Brown-Séquard syndrome	Instant or early death from respiratory failure
C5–T1	Spinal cord, brachial plexus level	Quadriparesis, becoming spastic; Brown-Séquard syndrome	Quadriplegia, becoming spastic
T2–T10	Dorsal spinal cord	Paraparesis, becoming spastic; Brown-Séquard syndrome	Paraplegia, becoming spastic
T11–L1	Conus medullaris	Flaccid or spastic paraparesis	Flaccid or spastic paraplegia
L2–S1	Cauda equina	Flaccid paraparesis	Flaccid paraplegia
Sacrococcygeal	Filum terminale	No deficit	No deficit

*Paresis or paralysis is always flaccid in the acute phase.

As in craniocerebral trauma, the spinal injury is considered from two aspects, the neurological and the vertebral:

Neurological Concussion
                Contusion   Spinal cord
                Compression Nerve roots
                Hematomyelia

Vertebral   Compression   Vertebral body

                           Laminal arch   With dislocation
              Linear fracture Spinous process Without dislocation
                           Pedicle

             Dislocation without fracture

Description of the injury should include the level of the injury, assessment of major motor and sensory functions, and the bony lesion, e.g., complete paraplegia with motor and sensory loss to T6 dermatome, fracture of pedicles of T5, with anterior dislocation of T5 on T6.

Concussion and contusion denote the same gross pathological changes as in the brain. Hemorrhage into the substance of the cord may be petechial or localized into a hematoma (hematomyelia). Sub-

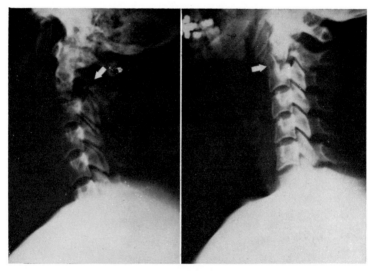

Fig. 40-13. Fracture-dislocation of C2 anteriorly on C3. The body of C2 is displaced anteriorly, and the pedicles are fractured *(arrow)*. In the right half of the photograph, the dislocation has been reduced by traction, and anterior interbody fusion is performed with the insertion of a bone dowel *(arrow)*.

dural and epidural hematomas sufficient to produce significant compression are so rare in the spinal canal that they are not of practical importance.

Unfortunately, the most frequent presenting neurological picture is that of complete bilateral cord transection. There is usually a band of hyperesthesia at the dermatomal level of injury, with complete loss of all motor power and sensation, autonomic function (anhydrosis and paralytic ileus), and reflexes below this level. This is the picture of *spinal shock*. Autonomic activity returns in 48 to 72 hours, and reflexes in 1 to 5 weeks. Paralysis of voluntary movement is permanent, but hyperactivity of reflexes often leads to severe spasms in paralyzed

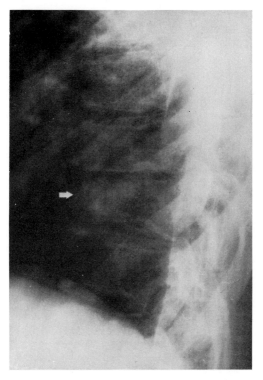

Fig. 40-14. Compression fracture of a thoracic vertebral body. The vertebra *(arrow)* has become squeezed into a wedge shape. In this instance there is no dislocation.

Table 40-4. Clinical syndromes of partial spinal cord damage

Portion of cord involved	Neurological picture
Central core	Severe paresis at level of injury only, with relatively intact motor and sensory functions below that level
Anterior half	Bilateral paresis and loss of pain and temperature sensation, with relative preservation of touch, position, vibration senses below level of injury
Lateral half	Ipsilateral paresis with contralateral loss of pain and temperature sensations below level of injury (Brown-Séquard syndrome)
Whole cord	Partial loss of all motor and sensory functions to approximately equal degree below level of injury

muscles. Lesser degrees of functional deficits are shown in Table 40-4.

Compression fractures of the vertebral body and linear fractures of laminae and spinous processes are generally not associated with neurological deficit. Fractures of the pedicle are usually accompanied by dislocation and frequently result in neural damage, depending on the extent to which the spinal canal is narrowed. Gross dislocations of the vertebral bodies are still compatible with cord function if fractured laminal arches separate from the bodies so that the spinal cord is not acutely squeezed. Occasionally, severe deficits are present in the absence of any visible bony abnormality. In such cases, acute herniation of the intervertebral disc may cause compression of the cord.

In assessing the bony damage radiologically, the patient should be moved as little as possible. In cervical spine injuries, the *neck must be protected* against movement at all times until the vertebral alignment has been defined. This is accomplished best by placing heavy sandbags on each side of the head. If the patient must be moved from the transporting stretcher, his head should be *supported in a neutral position,* preferably with slight *traction.*

Performance of emergency procedures

Any dislocation of cervical vertebrae, with or without associated neurological deficit, requires the immediate application of skull tongs (Crutchfield, Vinke, or similar type) or wires for skeletal traction (Fig. 40-15). *Halter traction is unsatisfactory and dangerous to life in any patient with upper limb paresis.* The halter may asphyxiate, and the patient with paresis may not have sufficient strength to adjust or remove it. In most instances, proper alignment can be restored with traction alone. Traction is begun with 10 to 15 pounds, and weight

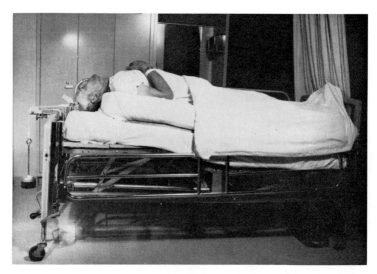

Fig. 40-15. Skeletal traction for dislocation of cervical spine. Crutchfield tongs *(white arrow)* have been inserted into the patient's skull, and traction has been applied by suspending weights on a pulley at the head of the bed. The position of the head required to maintain vertebral alignment varies with the individual features of the dislocation. The patient is lying on an automatic alternating-pressure mattress, controlled by a motor located at the foot of the bed.

successively added as indicated by progress radiographs until reduction has been accomplished. Progress radiological examinations and the addition of weights should follow within minutes of each other. Realignment usually occurs with 25 to 35 pounds' traction, and can be maintained with 10 to 15 pounds during the period required for bone healing.

Cervical dislocations above C6 associated with gross neurological deficit may produce respiratory insufficiency from paresis of intercostal muscles and diaphragm. Tracheostomy plus the assistance of a mechanical respirator may be necessary.

Little can be done to restore the alignment after fracture dislocation in the thoracic and lumbar vertebrae. Since most of these fractures are the result of hyperflexion, the patient should be placed in bed on soft supports such that the spine tends to be slightly extended. Pelvic traction is of no value.

If the patient is unable to urinate without leaving a significant residual, an indwelling catheter should be placed and drainage established.

Phase II
Observation of progress and supportive medical care

The development of secondary compressive hematomas is so rare after spinal trauma that it is not the major consideration that it is after head injury. However, lack of neurological improvement and certainly any progressive deterioration of function may be indications for surgical exploration and decompression.

Paralytic ileus constantly accompanies paralysis of the limbs, so that oral intake should be withheld until there is evidence of return of good bowel activity. The normal daily requirement of fluids should be given parenterally.

Care of the skin is a major nursing problem in patients who are unable to change position in bed. Decubiti rapidly develop over the sacrum and heels. Use of revolving frame beds, e.g., oscillator, Foster, Stryker, etc., and of the alternating pressure mattress aid in the frequent redistribution of pressure on different areas of skin.

Phase III
Special diagnostic procedures

Evaluation of the degree of pressure on the spinal cord or nerve roots is difficult and inaccurate. After reduction of a dislocation, there may be persistent compression by cord swelling or by hernated disc. Myelography involves considerable manipulations and changes in position that the acutely injured patient tolerates very poorly. Neither myelography nor the Queckenstedt maneuver can measure the amount of pressure exerted by any lesion. Therefore, the presence of a surgically significant compression is a diagnosis based primarily upon clinical impressions rather than upon objective measurements.

Phase IV
Nonsurgical treatment

Contusion and laceration of the spinal cord are accompanied by reactive edema as in brain injuries. Dexamethasone to reduce the reaction has gained increasing usage, although its efficacy in reducing the ultimate neurological deficit has yet to be scientifically proven.

The unstable fractured spine requires approximately 6 weeks of immobilization before the patient may be ambulated. For unstable cervical fractures, skeletal traction must be maintained during that period. An external cervical support such as a Thomas collar or a metallic brace can be fitted, and the patient can be ambulated progressively after removal of the traction tongs. Periodic radiological checks should be made to detect any subsequent dislocation. Lateral roentgenograms taken with the neck in flexion and then in extension are used to determine the degree of stability or instability. Prolonged immobilization is hazardous to the elderly because of the rapid development of pulmonary complications. Thoracic and lumbar injuries may be mobilized in a body cast or braces. These protective devices are worn for an additional 6 weeks to 3 months.

Surgical treatment

Internal decompression of neural elements is accomplished initially by realigning dislocated vertebrae. Posterior decompression by removal of the laminal arches may also be necessary, particularly when a dislocation is not correctable, e.g., thoracic and lumbar regions. Therefore, injuries below T1 associated with neurological deficits and a manometric block on Queckenstedt maneuver are usually treated by decompressive laminectomy, even though the chances for functional recovery may be small. Local hypothermia applied directly to the injured segment of spinal cord has been shown to be markedly beneficial in the experimental animal, but its efficacy in humans has not yet been proved.

Operative interbody fusion in cervical fracture-dislocations accomplishes (1) the removal of a possibly herniated and compressing intervertebral disc, (2) much earlier mobilization and discharge from the hospital, and (3) a guarantee, barring complications, of achieving a permanently stable spine. The procedure may be undertaken as soon as the patient has recovered from the immediate constitutional effects of trauma, and ambulation may be begun within 2 weeks of operation. Anterior interbody fusion is applicable to all dislocations between C2 and T1. It is frequently necessary when there has been marked subluxation without major fracturing, for while a fracture reunites with strong new bone formation, interspinous ligamentous tears heal poorly and chronic instability is a common result. Odontoid fractures and chronically unstable thoracic and lumbar fracture-dislocations can be fused by use of interlaminar or interpedicular struts.

Prognosis for recovery after spinal injuries

The prognosis for neurological recovery varies with the neurological segment injured and the severity of the initial deficit. If there is immediate loss of all motor and sensory function below the level of injury, the chances for functional recovery are extremely small regardless of the promptness and type of treatment. Any preservation of neurological function alters the prognosis from one of almost complete hopelessness to one of possible, if partial, recovery. Complete recovery is rare with spinal cord injuries but occurs not infrequently when the cauda equina is the only area damaged. Death may ensue early or late as the result of pulmonary or urinary tract infection, especially after cervical cord transection.

The permanently paraplegic patient can usually be rehabilitated to an economically useful life. For some, crutch walking can be accomplished with external bracing of the legs, but for most, the wheelchair is the only method of locomotion. The complete quadriplegic is usually a permanent invalid, incapable of gainful employment despite the availability of prosthetic aids.

PERIPHERAL NERVE INJURIES

In contrast to the central nervous system pathways, the peripheral nerves are always capable of regrowth and reestablishing neural connections after they have been traumatized or severed. The goal of surgical treatment is to provide the best possible conditions for the transected nerve to reestablish its connections with muscles and skin. Without the most optimum conditions, neuronal regrowth may be blocked, retarded, or disorganized, and may result in incomplete or ineffective reinnervation.

Pathological changes after injury

Trauma to a peripheral nerve sufficient to produce clinically recognizable denervation may be accompanied by pathological changes both proximal and distal to the site of injury. *Proximally,* there is central chromatolysis *(axonal reaction)* in the cells of origin in the central nervous system; this is a temporary change and is reversible. *Distally,* there is *Wallerian degeneration,* which, once begun, is irreversible and continues until all axonal debris is removed. Within 4 to 6 days after the onset of Wallerian degeneration, the nerve can no longer be made to conduct an electrical stimulus, so that direct stimulation of the nerve trunk through a needle electrode results in no contraction of the muscles that nerve normally innervates.

Axonal regrowth begins within 48 hours. If a proper pathway is available, regrowth proceeds at a rate of 1 to 1.5 mm. per day until the target (muscle or skin) has been reached. If such a pathway is blocked, the axons curl back upon themselves, forming a heaped-up tangle of fibers called a *neuroma.* Although no recognizable degenerative changes occur in denervated skin, loss of tonus and fiber size occur in denervated muscle. The latter is most noticeable in the first 6 weeks after injury. If denervation is prolonged, the muscle becomes progressively replaced with fibrous tissue until it can no longer contract effectively even when stimulated directly. Thus, if effective reinnervation is to occur, the nerve must make contact with its muscle before too much fibrosis has occurred.

Using the foregoing principles, one can calculate the potential for effective treatment of most nerve injuries. Given a minimum neuronal regrowth rate of *1 mm. per day or 1 inch per month,* and considering that a muscle remaining denervated for more than *1 year* may be extensively fibrosed, then if a nerve is severed more than 1 foot proximal to its muscles, the potential for good functional motor recovery is poor. Furthermore, if, for example, a nerve is severed 9 inches proximal to its muscles but the lesion is neglected or goes undiagnosed for 6 months, a late anastomosis may not restore good function. Thus, although it may be prudent to delay exploration in cases in which the anatomic continuity of a nerve is thought to be preserved, *too long a delay may result in missing the opportunity for functional reinnervation.* There are, of course, exceptions to these mathematic calculations, so that they may not be used as absolute criteria to determine whether surgery is indicated.

Management

The management of peripheral nerve injuries will be considered according to the three types of lesions encountered: stretching, compression and contusion, and laceration.

Stretch injuries affect principally the brachial plexus and, to a lesser extent, the sciatic nerve. A downward blow on the shoulder, or falling and landing on the shoulder such that it is forced downward, puts sudden tension on the roots and trunks of the brachial plexus. Axis cylinders may be ruptured, and the roots may be avulsed from the spinal cord. The result almost invariably is permanent loss of function. Management consists only of placing the limb in a position such that there will be minimal tension on the plexus, i.e., arm abducted 90 degrees and supported by an airplane splint. Myelography may be performed as soon as the patient can tolerate the maneuvers required without undue discomfort; extravasation of contrast medium at the site of an avulsed root is diagnostic. The lesion is untreatable (Fig. 40-16). Posterior *dislocation of the hip* may result in stretching of the sciatic nerve over the head of the femur; other nerves may occasionally be stretched over the fractured ends of long bones. Surgical treatment of the stretch injury is most unsatisfactory because it is impossible to determine by gross inspection how long a segment of nerve has been damaged. Furthermore, such injuries in the brachial plexus and sciatic

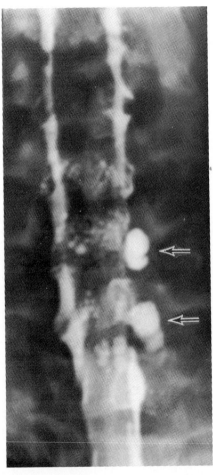

Fig. 40-16. Cervical myelogram showing extravasation of contrast media at the site of the avulsed C7 and C8 nerve roots *(arrows)*.

nerve at the hip are located so far proximal to denervated muscles that even if regeneration occurs, it cannot reinnervate muscles before extensive fibrosis has occurred.

Compression and contusion most commonly affect nerves that are relatively superficial and not protected by thick layers of muscle. The ulnar nerve at the elbow and the superficial peroneal nerve at the neck of the fibula are such examples. Severe crushing trauma may injure any nerve trunk. There are three possible pathological courses after peripheral nerve compression and contusion:

1. No Wallerian degeneration—functional recovery within 2 to 6 weeks regardless of the distance from site of injury to denervated muscle or skin.
2. Wallerian degeneration without significant internal fibrosis—regeneration and functional recovery after a delay consistent with the distance as calculated by distance from injury to muscle or skin ÷ rate of regrowth.
3. Wallerian degeneration followed by significant internal fibrosis—formation of a neuroma-in-continuity (Fig. 40-17), partial reinnervation only, regardless of length of time elapsed.

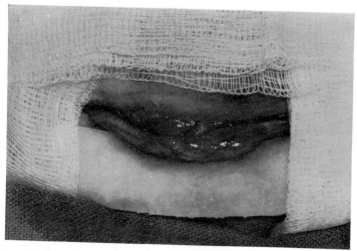

Fig. 40-17. Neuroma-in-continuity. Ulnar nerve in a patient who fell on her elbow 6 months prior to operation and developed a partial paralysis of the interossei with preservation of all other ulnar nerve functions. The nerve is expanded to double its normal diameter by the neuroma.

When there is no reason to suspect that a nerve has been severed (no penetrating wound, no fractured bone ends that might lacerate nerve), management entails following the patient's course with frequent neurological examination to determine whether regeneration is occurring. Paresthesias referred to the peripheral distribution of a nerve when the nerve is lightly percussed *(Tinel's sign)* indicate the most distal end of the regenerating nerve. If the sign can be elicited more than 2 inches beyond the point of injury, recovery will be likely to occur without surgical intervention. Electromyography is useful in detecting early reinnervation. If, after 6 weeks, there is no evidence of reinnervation or regeneration, exploration is indicated. If a significant neuroma is present with no electrical conduction distal to it, resection and anastomosis should be performed.

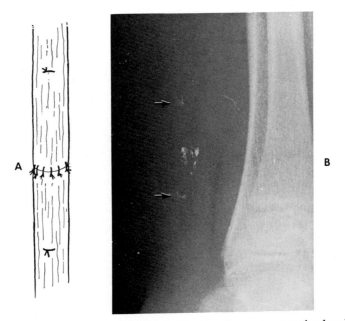

Fig. 40-18. Peripheral nerve anastomosis. A radiopaque suture is placed through the epineurium on each side of the line of anastomosis. Postoperative radiograph, **B**, reveals these marking sutures to be approximately equidistant from the anastomosis. Separation of the nerve ends is diagnosed if the marking sutures become separated.

Laceration or transection of a peripheral nerve may be produced by penetrating foreign bodies or internally by the jagged ends of fractured long bones. Whenever such an injury occurs, neurological function must be evaluated accurately, and any deficit pointed out to the patient. The importance of the latter lies in the fact that surgical treatment of some kind is usually necessary in the treatment of associated injuries to bones, muscles, and tendons, so that a neurological deficit that is not pointed out prior to such surgery may be blamed on the surgical procedure rather than on the injury. A clean field free of potential infection is a strict requirement for the anastomosis of a transected nerve. The great majority of open wounds do not fulfill this requirement, and, therefore, emergency nerve repair is seldom indicated. Apposition of the lacerated ends with one or two sutures prevents their retraction and also facilitates identification at the time of definitive anastomosis. Such wounds should be debrided thoroughly and closed, and anastomosis should be delayed until clean healing has occurred. However, though it is prudent to wait whenever the sterility of a wound is in doubt, there is *equal disadvantage in waiting too long,* particularly when the site of transection is nearly a foot proximal to denervated muscles, for reasons stated previously. Anastomosis can be performed by use of suture or various adhesives. Fresh cuts are made until healthy nerve ends are bared; the nerve trunk proximally and distally may be mobilized with its mesoneurium and/or transplanted in order to bring the ends together without tension. Marking the ends with radiopaque sutures through the epineurium provides a useful method of checking to see that they have not separated postoperatively (Fig. 40-18).

INTRACRANIAL NEOPLASMS

The morbidity and mortality potentials of an intracranial neoplasm differ from those of tumors elsewhere in the body. Local compression and invasion are as important to the prognosis as the histological picture. Therefore, the anatomic localization of a tumor is all-important in the clinical diagnosis. A histologically benign tumor may inevitably be fatal if it is so located that surgical removal cannot be undertaken without undue risk of operative death or the production of an incapacitating neurological deficit. The histologically malignant neoplasms spread infrequently within the subarachnoid space and very rarely outside the central nervous system. They cause death by invading or compressing vital centers.

The symptoms of intracranial neoplasms are of three types:
1. Increased intracranial pressure—headache, lethargy, vomiting
2. Local or neighboring compression and invasion—paralysis and sensory loss
3. Local irritation—convulsive seizures

Persistent headache, often accompanied by subtle changes in mental behavior and by vomiting, indicates abnormal pressure rather than common migraine or nervous tension headaches. The progressive onset of neurological deficit distinguishes neoplasm from cerebrovascular accident with its sudden ictus. Convulsions, especially focal or Jacksonian, beginning in adult life suggest neoplasm rather than idiopathic epilepsy.

Objective neurological findings depend on the size, location, and rapidity of growth of the tumor. A slowly growing neoplasm, located at some distance from the sensorimotor cortex, may attain great size before producing recognizable neurological signs other than those of generalized increased intracranial pressure. Conversely, a small irritative lesion growing within the sensorimotor cortex may produce localized seizures and paresis long before there are any symptoms or signs of increased intracranial pressure.

Any of the foregoing symptoms coupled with any objective neurological abnormality is sufficient to warrant investigation for brain tumor. In certain situations, such investigations may be called for in the absence of any recognizable deficit. In general, investigations begin with tests that carry no risk to the patient. An elective order of preference is as follows:

1. Complete blood count, sedimentation rate, urinalysis
2. Posteroanterior and lateral chest radiographs; lateral, anteroposterior, Towne, and submental views of skull
3. Electroencephalography
4. Isotopic brain scan
5. Computerized axial tomography of head
6. Contrast-injected radiologic studies—angiography, pneumoencephalography, and ventriculography

One or several intermediate tests may be omitted as indicated by clinical examination.

Table 40-5 gives a classification of more commonly encountered neoplasms. For a detailed classification and description of all tumors, the reader is referred to textbooks of neuropathology. Only the clinical aspects of the common tumor are discussed here.

The age of the patient and the anatomic location of the lesion are of considerable importance in predicting the type of neoplasm. Infants and children under the age of 2 years rarely develop intracranial neoplasms. Up to the age of 15 years, tumors most often arise in the *cerebellum.* Of these, medulloblastoma and cystic astrocytoma comprise the vast majority. The highly malignant *medulloblastoma* occurs in the cerebellar vermis (disequilibrium) and blocks the outlets of the fourth ventricle (headache, vomiting from obstructive hydrocephalus). Removal of sufficient tissue to unblock the ventricular

Table 40-5. Primary intracranial neoplasms*

Neuroepithelial	*Ectodermal*
Astrocytoma, grades I, II, III, and IV	Craniopharyngioma
Ependymomas	Pituitary adenomas
Oligodendrogliomas	
Medulloblastoma	*Congenital*
Pinealoma	Epidermoid
Papilloma of choroid plexus	Dermoid
Paraphyseal (colloid) cyst	
Neurilemoma	
Mesodermal	
Meningiomas	
Hemangioblastoma	
Chordoma	

*Neoplasms occurring with extreme rarity have been omitted from this classification; those tumors listed in the *plural* term occur with varying histological types and grades of differentiation.

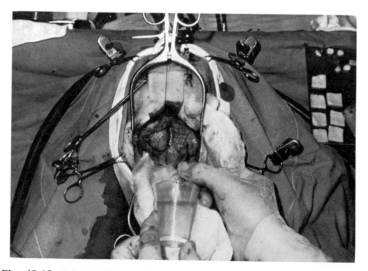

Fig. 40-19. Suboccipital craniectomy for cystic tumor of the right cerebellar hemisphere. The cerebellar hemispheres are exposed, and their tonsils are seen herniated downward into the cervical canal, the right tonsil being larger than the left. A cannula has been introduced into the right hemisphere, and about 25 ml. of fluid is drained off, resulting in collapse of the hemisphere. The fluid is usually xanthochromic and often will clot on standing.

system followed by radiation therapy is the usual method of treatment. Total surgical removal is impossible because of the infiltrative propensity of the tumor, and although the neoplasm is highly radiosensitive, complete eradication cannot be achieved. It frequently spreads in the subarachnoid space, producing secondary impants along the spinal neuraxis. Survival ranges from 1 to 15 years. The *cystic astrocytoma* occurs in the cerebellar hemisphere (limb ataxia) and later obstructs the fourth ventricle (headache, vomiting). The tumor consists of a large cyst containing xanthochromic fluid (Fig. 40-19) and a small nubbin of solid neoplasm. If this nubbin is resected completely, as it frequently can be, permanent cure results. Tumors of the cerebral hemisphere are less frequent in children, but when they occur, are likely to be *ependymomas*. These tumors are moderately radiosensitive; therefore, as much of the mass as possible is resected, followed by radiation therapy. Recurrence and death within 2 to 3 years is to be expected.

Of the remaining supratentorial tumors of children, *craniopharyngioma* deserves mention. This tumor, rising above the optic chiasm,

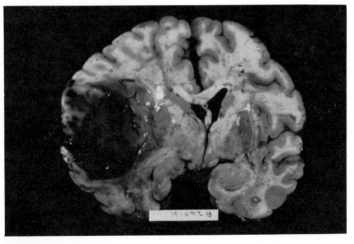

Fig. 40-20. Astrocytoma grade IV (glioblastoma multiforme). The tumor is often hemorrhagic. Its gross demarcation from surrounding brain tissue may appear fairly distinct at times, but microscopic examination will show invasion. Therefore, curative resection is not possible.

is very often partially calcified, so that the combination of visual field defect, optic atrophy, and suprasellar calcium deposits almost provides a definitive diagnosis. Complete resection and cures have been reported, but temporary relief by decompression and radiation is frequently all that can be accomplished.

The 30- to 60-year age group produces the largest group of primary neoplasms, the great majority of which are cerebral hemisphere malignancies with survival prognoses of less than 5 years. The *astrocytomas,* particularly the most malignant *glioblastoma* (Fig. 40-20), are the most frequently found lesions. They occur anywhere in the hemispheres, so that the signs and symptoms are dependent on the anatomic location. If located at the pole of a hemisphere, radical resection with lobectomy may be accomplished, where as if located close to or in the sensorimotor cortex, only a limited excision and external decompression are possible. The neoplasms may infiltrate extensively (Fig. 40-21) and, when located near the midline, tend to cross to the opposite hemisphere via the corpus callosum; therefore, recurrence and eventual death of the patient are invariable, even with the most

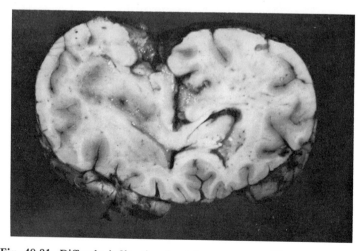

Fig. 40-21. Diffusely infiltrating frontal astrocytoma. The tumor blends imperceptibly with the surrounding brain tissue and microscopically infiltrates the brain. At operation, it is impossible to determine the extent of the tumor tissue by gross inspection.

radical resections. The effects of radiotherapy are, at best, moderately palliative; noticeable clinical improvement directly attributable to radiation is seen only infrequently.

The most common benign tumor in adulthood is the *meningioma* (Figs. 40-22 and 40-23). A majority of meningiomas occur close to the midline, over the vault, or along the sphenoid wing. In the former position they are closely related to the superior longitudinal sinus and the falx cerebri, and they may invade the sinus or produce hyperostosis of the overlying bone. Focal or Jacksonian seizures of months' or years' duration with a slowly developing paresis are hallmarks of this tumor. Total removal can usually be accomplished, but there is still a significantly high postoperative morbidity and mortality.

A neoplasm presenting primarily with visual loss in the adult is likely to be a *pituitary adenoma*. Characteristically, the visual deficit is a *bitemporal hemianopsia* because the tumor compresses the optic chiasm, damaging the crossing temporal field fibers (Fig. 40-24). Skull radiographs show enlargement of the sella turcica. The tumor is usually

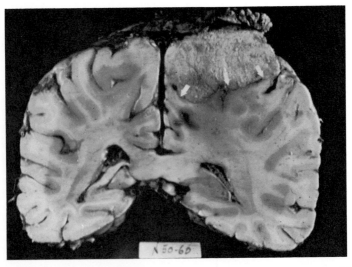

Fig. 40-22. Parasagittal meningioma. The tumor may arise from the falx or from the convexity and may invade the superior longitudinal sinus. It does not invade brain tissue but slowly compresses it inferolaterally *(arrows).*

treated satisfactorily by radiation. However, when compression is severe enough to compromise visual acuity, surgical removal of tumor with decompression of the chiasm is the treatment of choice.

The *acoustic neurilemoma* arises from the intracranial portion of the eighth cranial nerve and produces tinnitus, loss of hearing, and ataxia of the limbs. This symptom-complex, called the *cerebellopontine angle* syndrome, may include impairment of adjacent cranial nerves (fifth and seventh). Complete removal is difficult, except in small tumors, and may result in paralysis of the facial nerve that is intimately associated with the tumor capsule.

Above the age of 50, the possibility of *metastatic carcinoma* must always be considered in the differential diagnosis of any intracranial expanding lesion. The metastases are frequently multiple (Fig. 40-25). In the male, the most common source is the lung; in the female, the breast is the usual source. A metastasis may become evident months or even years after the primary lesion has been removed; it may be solitary, particularly with hypernephroma, and surgical removal may

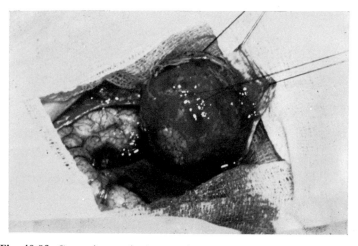

Fig. 40-23. Convexity meningioma. When the tumor arises from the convexity and has a wide base, it can be removed from its bed in one piece, with it attached to the dural flap. Since the dura is invaded, the flap to which tumor is attached is excised widely. The brain may then be covered with a graft of tissue such as pericranium, or the bone may simply be replaced over the cortex.

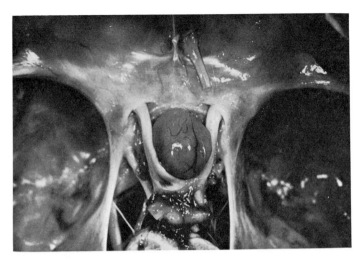

Fig. 40-24. Pituitary adenoma. Having ruptured through the diaphragma sellae, the tumor balloons upward between the optic nerves, stretching them as well as the optic chiasm to produce the characteristic bitemporal hemianopsia.

extend the life expectancy and has even resulted in apparent cures. Despite the ominous prognosis of metastatic carcinoma in the brain, one should not abandon hopes for worthwhile palliation. Surgical removal of any solitary intracranial metastasis may be worthwhile in selected cases, provided, of course, that there are no other known secondaries elsewhere in the body. In most instances a metastatic lesion excites considerable edema in the surrounding white matter. This edema can be overcome with high doses of dexamethasone and may result in dramatic symptomatic improvement. Hormone-dependent carcinomas of the breast, and bowel carcinoma, that have previously responded to chemotherapy, may produce metastases that are sensitive to a combination of hormonal agents and cytotoxic chemicals. With a proper selection of modes of treatments, these unfortunate patients can be offered several months or even years of additional comfortable life. Therefore, they should not be abandoned to die untreated simply because of the known presence of metastatic or recurrent malignant disease.

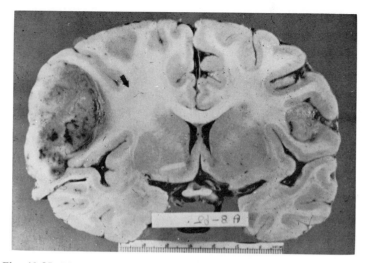

Fig. 40-25. Bilateral metastatic neoplasms. The multiplicity of metastases is an unfortunate common characteristic. The lesions are grossly quite well demarcated in most instances. They often produce marked swelling of the white matter *(arrow)*. This patient had a bronchogenic carcinoma.

INTRASPINAL NEOPLASMS

Neoplasms, within the spinal canal produce symptoms and signs by compression of the adjacent spinal cord and/or nerve roots, and by obstruction of the blood supply to the cord. The patient complains of progressive weakness, clumsiness, or numbness of the extremities below the lesion. If a nerve root is involved, there may be pain radiating out into the dermatomal distribution of that root. In these respects, the symptomatology mimics that of vertebral spondylosis and herniated intervertebral disc. Spinal cord compression per se produces no pain, and loss of specific sensations is often not noticed by the patient.

Tumors involving the spinal cord almost invariably produce recognizable neurological signs *bilaterally* by the time the patient is aware of any deficit. The small diameter of the cord makes it practically impossible for any mass lesion to produce compressive damage to one side only. Therefore, when the findings on examination are strictly unilateral, cord tumor is an unlikely diagnosis. The exact level of compression cannot be established reliably by clinical examination, for paresis and sensory loss do not necessarily extend up to the level of the tumor; e.g., a tumor at C5 may produce paresis and sensory loss only to the T4 dermatomal segment. Only in the later stages when function has been greatly impaired does the neurological level correlate with the anatomic site of the lesion.

Lumbar puncture with Queckenstedt maneuver is indicated in all

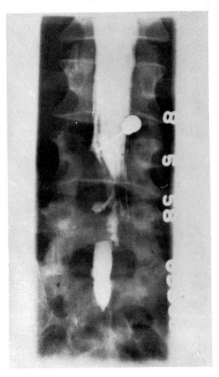

Fig. 40-26. Myelogram showing extradural mass. The irregular, ragged appearance of the lower end of the dye column is usually characteristic of an extradural mass. This patient's lesion was an extruded intervertebral disc; the myelographic picture of extradural neoplasm is the same except that it may not be centered over an intervertebral space.

cases, preferably with facilities for immediate myelographic study. Whenever possible, puncture should be performed below and as far away from the lesion as possible. When the needle is inserted below the lesion, varying degree of block may be shown on jugular compression, and the spinal fluid protein is usually elevated. The color of the spinal fluid should be noted carefully; slight xanthochromia is frequently present, and pellicle formation may occur when there has been long-standing obstruction.

Definitive diagnosis is established by myelography (Figs. 40-5, 40-26, and 40-27). Clinical differentiation between the various types of tumors is difficult and not of practical value to the student. Early recognition of the presence of an intraspinal mass is important, for the sooner the mass is removed, the more rapid and complete will be the neurological recovery. Operation performed after the patient has lost all cord function below the lesion stands little chance of producing worthwhile, if any, neurological recovery.

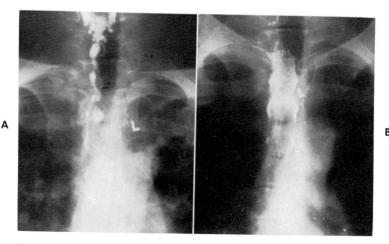

A　　　　　　　　　　　　　　　　　　　　　　　　　　**B**

Fig. 40-27. Myelogram showing a primary tumor of the spinal cord. This lesion is intradural and intramedullary, i.e., within the substance of the cord. The dye column gently thins out at the level of the tumor, and the spinal cord shadow expands to fill the subarachnoid space. The lower limit of the tumor, **A,** is about T6; the upper limit, **B,** is about T2.

The common types of tumors are classified as follows:

Intradural
  Intramedullary
    Ependymoma
    Astrocytoma
  Extramedullary
    Primary
      Meningioma
      Neurofibroma
    Secondary
      Medulloblastoma (seeding from cerebellar tumor)
Extradural
  Primary
    Bone tumors
  Secondary
    Carcinomas (from prostate, lung, breast, gastrointestinal tract)
    Lymphoma
    Myeloma

Neoplasms within the cord substance (intramedullary) can sometimes be removed by splitting the cord in the midline posteriorly. However, decompressive laminectomy followed by radiation is often the only treatment possible. The meningioma and neurofibroma can almost always be totally excised, with excellent neurological result. Metastatic extradural neoplasms are seen more commonly than the aforementioned primary neoplasms. The history is usually short, with progession from apparently normal neurological status to complete loss of all cord function within a few days. Such rapid progression indicates impairment of blood supply to the cord rather than compression as the principal feature and explains the overall lack of success of emergency decompressions. Laminectomy with partial removal of tumor followed by radiation is offered in the hope of at least delaying progression to total paralysis.

INTRACRANIAL INFECTIONS

Infections within the central nervous system are generally chemotherapeutic rather than surgical problems. Two possibilities for surgical treatment exist, namely, the evacuation of an abscess and the prevention of reinfection. The abscesses are most frequently intracerebral, arising within the white matter by hematogenous spread from the lung, or by contiguous spread via a tract from a paranasal sinus or the middle ear. The symptoms may be acute or chronic, characterized by headache, lethargy, vomiting, and paresis depending on the location of the lesion. Fever is often absent. Abscesses are a common complication of *cyanotic heart disease.* Subdural abscess or empyema is next in frequency, arising almost invariably from a paranasal sinus or middle ear. Symptoms are acute and dramatic, with severe headache, convulsive seizures, and dense neurological deficits. Epidural abscess also arises by direct extension from sinus or bone but presents less dramatically with pressure signs.

The presence of a focus of infection raises the possibility of abscess in the differential diagnosis of any mass intracranial lesion. It is obviously to the surgeon's advantage to be prepared for the finding of an abscess before undertaking intracranial surgery. Subdural and epidural abscesses can usually be drained effectively through burr holes. Intracerebral abscesses, whenever encapsulated, are preferably resected completely. Postoperatively, the patient is treated with the same dosages of antibiotics as are used for active meningitis.

After management of the abscess problem, any possible primary source for reinfection should be investigated. Meningitis without abscess formation also deserves such consideration if the responsible organism is other than *Meningococcus* or *Haemophilus influenzae.*

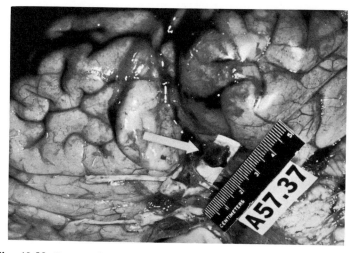

Fig. 40-28. Ruptured aneurysm, internal carotid artery. The aneurysm has ruptured at its neck *(arrow),* producing fatal subarachnoid hemorrhage. The great majority of aneurysmal ruptures occur at the dome rather than at the neck of the sac.

SPONTANEOUS INTRACRANIAL HEMORRHAGE

Intracranial bleeding in the absence of trauma may occur primarily into the brain substance (cerebral hemisphere, brainstem, or cerebellum) or into the subarachnoid space.

Intracerebral and intrapontine hemorrhages are most commonly seen in *hypertensives* in the 50- to 70-year age group. They are catastrophic in onset, with initial loss of consciousness and a severe lateralized neurological deficit, e.g., hemiplegia. The hemorrhage usually occurs deep in the cerebral hemisphere near or in the internal capsule in the distribution of the lenticulostriate branches of the middle cerebral artery. The immediate mortality is very high. Surgical treatment is directed toward preserving viable functioning tissue by

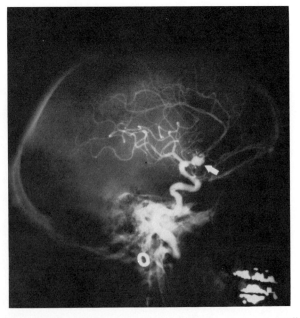

Fig. 40-29. Angiogram showing aneurysm of the circle of Willis. The aneurysm *(arrow)* arises from the anterior communicating artery. It is associated with local spasm of the anterior cerebral artery and is irregular in outline with a small nubbin protruding from the superior surface. These two features indicate that the aneurysm has recently ruptured.

evacuating hematomas and debriding swollen and necrotic brain. However, because of the deep location of the hemorrhage and the extensive destruction of tissue, operation is not worthwhile in the majority of cases.

Subarachnoid hemorrhage is most often caused by a ruptured aneurysm of the circle of Willis (Figs. 40-28 and 40-29) and occurs maximally in the 40- to 60-year age group. In over 20%, more than one aneurysm is present, but rarely does more than one aneurysm rupture at any given time. About 7 to 15% die as a direct result of the initial hemorrhage, and recurrent hemorrhages, particularly within the first 2 weeks, result in an aggregate mortality of 40 to 45%. Recurrent hemorrhage may be prevented by various surgical procedures, each of which adds its own potential risk of death or complications to the natural risk. Aneurysms of the internal carotid artery frequently shrink or disappear angiographically after ligation of the carotid artery in the neck, but the procedure itself carries a 33% risk of producing a

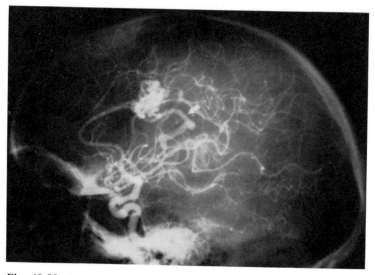

Fig. 40-30. Angiogram showing arteriovenous malformation. The lesion is fed principally by the pericallosal artery. Rapid passage of contrast medium through the malformation into the venous system *(arrow)* is characteristic. The principal feeding and draining vessels are dependent on the location of the malformation.

hemiparesis or hemiplegia, and a lesser but significant risk of death from cerebral ischemia and infarction. Intracranial procedures have been performed to ligate the neck of the sac, to invest the sac with muscle, gauze, or plastic coatings, or more recently to induce thrombosis within the aneurysms by electrocoagulation, piloinjection, and the injection of iron particles. No single mode of treatment has proved to be optimum for every case, and extensive studies are still being performed to find methods that will lower the overall mortality from the lesion that is prevalent in a relatively young, productive age group.

Subarachnoid and/or intraparenchymal hemorrhages occurring in the young (under 30) normotensive patient may result from an *arteriovenous malformation* (Fig. 40-30). The mortality from hemorrhage from this lesion is low, but recurrent hemorrhages are likely to occur over many years or decades. Total extirpation of all abnormal vessels is the goal of surgical treatment but is feasible only in those malformations that are so located that operation does not carry a great risk of producing a disabling neurological deficit.

PROTRUSION OF INTERVERTEBRAL DISCS AND VERTEBRAL SPONDYLOSIS

Herniation of an intervertebral disc into the spinal canal or hypertrophic changes in the vertebral bodies resulting in spur formation (spondylosis) may result in compression and irritation of nerve roots and/or spinal cord. The former is a common condition affecting principally the 30- to 60-year age group, whereas symptomatic spondylosis is seen somewhat later in life (45 to 70 years). Though any vertebral segment may be involved, there are definite sites of predilection. The fourth and fifth lumbar and the fifth and sixth cervical disc are the most frequently herniated; herniation of discs at other levels is distinctly rare. Spondylosis sufficient to produce *neurological* symptoms occurs most commonly in the lower three cervical vertebrae (Fig. 40-31). Spondylotic spurs on the lumbar vertebrae may produce the symptoms and signs of nerve root compression; in the thoracic segments, neurological involvement is rare.

The symptoms of the two types of pathology are clinically indistinguishable from each other. When nerve roots are involved, pain is the principal symptom, accompanied by variable degrees of sensory and motor impairment. The characteristics of the pain are the following:

1. It is referred to the dermatomal distribution of the compressed nerve.
2. It is aggravated by any maneuver that increases intraspinal cerebrospinal fluid pressure such as (a) coughing, sneezing, (b) strain-

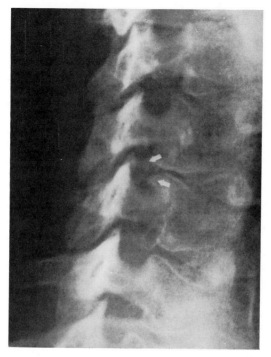

Fig. 40-31. Cervical spondylosis. Oblique view of the cervical spine shows the presence of osteophytic spurs *(arrows)* encroaching on an intervertebral foramen. The remainder of the foramina are normal.

ing at stool, and (c) compression of jugular veins (Naffziger's test).

3. Cervical root pain is usually aggravated by extension or flexion of the neck.

4. Lumbar and sacral root pain is aggravated by straight leg raising, which may be accentuated by forced dorsiflexion of the foot; occasionally, raising the contralateral leg may produce pain referred to the ipsilateral side.

Spinal cord symptoms may be produced either by direct compression of the cord or compression of the incoming radicular arterial supply. The clinical picture is one of progressive spastic quadriparesis (or paraparesis in rare thoracic disc herniations).

Distribution of symptoms and signs depends on the nerve roots compressed, as shown in Table 40-6. Because of individual variations in segmental innervation, the sensory pattern is much less reliable in the upper extremity than in the lower. In contrast, the motor pattern is less reliable in the lower extremity than in the upper.

Management depends on the severity of symptoms and signs. Conservative measures, consisting of bed rest, traction (for cervical root pain), or immobilization, can be tried in all cases in which there is no disabling neurological deficit. If symptoms are relieved satisfactorily, continued support of the involved area with a collar or brace may be the only treatment required. The presence of a definite neurological deficit, particularly muscle weakness and atrophy, usually indicates surgical removal of the compressing lesion. Interference with bladder function by acute disc herniations requires immediate surgical treatment.

Diagnosis is confirmed by myelography (Figs. 40-32 and 40-33). Myelography is necessary in cervical lesions because of the inaccuracy of clinical localization, but is optional in lumbar disc herniations in which the typical history and physical findings leave little doubt about the nature and location of the lesion. Lateral disc herniations in the lumbar or cervical regions can be removed through small hemilaminot-

Table 40-6. Neurological manifestations of vertebral spondylosis and herniated intervertebral disc

Inter-vertebral level	Nerve root involved	Distribution of pain and sensory loss	Principal motor deficit	Reflex dimi-nution
C5–C6	C6	Neck, shoulder, arm, radial side of hand, thumb, index finger	Biceps	Biceps
C6–C7	C7	Neck, shoulder, arm, middle of hand, index and middle fingers	Triceps	Triceps
L4–L5	L5	Lower back, posterior thigh and calf, medial side of foot, medial two or three toes	Anterior tibial group	None
L5–S1	S1	Lower back, posterior thigh and calf, lateral side of foot, lateral two or three toes	Gastroso-leus group	Achilles

omies posteriorly. In cervical spondylosis, however, the bony spurs are better removed from an anterior approach. In this procedure, interbody fusion is accomplished at the same time by use of bone graft from the hip.

SURGICAL RELIEF OF PAIN AND DYSKINESIAS

Intractable pain for which the causative lesion cannot be treated directly may be satisfactorily alleviated only by interrupting the pathways by which painful sensations are perceived. Carcinomas of the

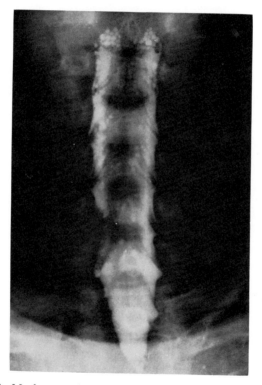

Fig. 40-32. Myelogram showing herniated cervical disc. The cervical canal is outlined by the dye column, and the nerve roots are seen exiting at each interspace. At the C6-C7 interspace, the dye column is indented from the right and the root shadow obliterated. At times the differentiation between disc and tumor is difficult to make myelographically.

cervix, bladder, prostate, and lower bowel frequently produce severe and continuous pain, both in the abdomen from local invasion and in the leg from involvement of the lumbosacral plexus. Advanced carcinomas of the breast and lung may similarly produce pain in the chest and arm, the latter from nodal or rib involvement in the region of the brachial plexus. Analgesics provide only partial and short-lived relief, and the prolonged use of narcotics may result in addiction. Therefore, although every attempt should be made to obtain relief

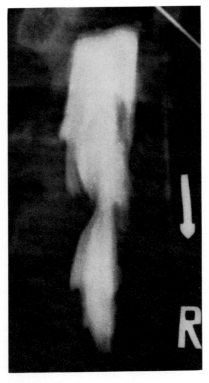

Fig. 40-33. Myelogram showing herniated lumbar disc. The arrow indicates that the patient is standing upright so that the dye column sinks to the caudal end of the subarachnoid space. The patient has then been turned obliquely to demonstrate the large mass indenting the canal and distorting the outline of a nerve root as it descends to a lower segment.

of symptoms by treating the causative lesion, the use of neurosurgical procedures should not be withheld unduly in patients with malignant disease.

Table 40-7 shows the two most common procedures in use: *cordotomy* and *rhizotomy*. Spinal rhizotomy is of limited value in the trunk and extremities for two reasons: (1) the extensive overlapping of dermatomal segments necessitates the sectioning of many more roots adjacent to the area of pain, and (2) extensive deafferentation of an extremity renders it *functionally useless* from loss of proprioception, regardless of the integrity of motor innervation. Cerebral destructive procedures, e.g., *prefrontal lobotomy* and *cingulumotomy*, designed to alter the patient's interpretation of pain, are useful only in certain specific situations. Malignancies of the oropharynx and paranasal sinuses frequently produce extreme pain and suffering that cannot be satisfactorily alleviated by sensory denervation, unless that denerva-

Table 40-7. Surgical procedures for the relief of intractable pain

	*Ventrolateral cordotomy**	*Posterior rhizotomy*
Pathway interrupted	Lateral spinothalamic tract	Posterior root proximal to its ganglion
Sensations lost	Pain and temperature	All sensory modalities
Distribution of sensory loss	Up to a level of 1 to 2 segments below operation, on the side of the body opposite cordotomy	In the dermatomal distribution of the sectioned root(s) only
Level of operation*	C2	Fifth and ninth cranial nerves
	T2	Any spinal nerve root
Indications	C2—Chest and arm pain, e.g., carcinoma of lung	Fifth cranial—trigeminal neuralgia
	T2—Abdomen and leg pain, e.g., carcinoma of cervix, prostate	Ninth cranial—glosso-pharyngeal neuralgia
		Fifth, ninth, C2, C3—oropharyngeal pain, e.g., carcinoma of tongue
Complications	Paralysis from trauma to adjacent lateral corticospinal tract	Same complications as any intracranial operation when fifth and ninth nerves are sectioned

*Cordotomy may be performed percutaneously rather than by open operation; the lesion is produced by a radiofrequency generator via a percutaneously inserted needle.

tion is very extensive. In these conditions, a simple procedure such as cingulumotomy performed through burr holes under local anesthesia may produce gratifying alleviation of the patient's suffering. *Hypophysectomy* in patients with hormone-dependent breast carcinoma often provides dramatic relief from the bone pain of widespread metastases and may temporarily arrest the metastatic process. Section of anterior spinal roots *(anterior rhizotomy)* is a procedure reserved for the permanently paraplegic or quadriplegic in whom mass flexor reflexes result in painful spasms of the paralyzed extremities.

Trigeminal neuralgia (tic douloureux) is a relatively common condition characterized by lightninglike stabs of pain in the distribution of one or more branches of the trigeminal nerve. Occasionally the pain may follow the distribution of the glossopharyngeal nerve (glossopharyngeal neuralgia). The condition occurs predominantly in the elderly and affects females more frequently than males. Attacks of pain can often be precipitated by touching or rubbing the area of skin involved ("trigger point"). In most instances no causative pathological condition can be demonstrated, so that treatment is symptomatic. Analgesics are of no value, for the pain is transitory. Diphenylhydantoin (Dilantin) may decrease the frequency of attacks. Carbamazepine is a highly specific and effective drug for trigeminal neuralgia, but untoward reactions occur frequently so that the drug must be discontinued in a significant proportion of patients. Alcohol injection of peripheral branches usually provides satisfactory relief, but the sensory loss obtained is not permanent so that pain returns as the nerve regenerates. "Decompression" of the Gasserian ganglion usually stops the pain, but late recurrences are frequent. Destruction of the ganglion by radiofrequency current is also effective, but the late recurrence rate is unknown. Section of preganglionic fibers subserving the area of pain affords permanent relief, but at the cost of a permanent area of facial numbness.

From the foregoing descriptions of various techniques, it is apparent that practically any painful area in the body can be rendered analgesic by neurosurgical deafferentation. These procedures are intended primarily for clearly defined painful syndromes such as occur with incurable malignancies. They are not generally recommended for the variety of common pain problems that have no provable etiology. Once nerve pathways have been purposely destroyed, they can never be reestablished; the resulting sensory loss is permanent. Trigeminal root section performed for nonmalignant facial pain that is not typically trigeminal neuralgia will leave the patient with a permanently anaesthetic face while the original pain for which the operation was performed may persist or recur in spite of the sensory loss.

Rhizotomies, cordotomies, or other procedures performed for post-herpetic neuralgia or for phantom limb pain fail too frequently to provide lasting relief of symptoms. Denervation should be resorted to only after all reasonable attempts to control the cause of pain have failed. If the patient remains disabled by pain, an operation having permanent con‑equences may be justified.

Stereotactically placed destructive lesions in the ventrolateral nucleus of the thalamus have, in selected cases, been effective in abolishing or reducing the tremor of Parkinson's disease. Patients under the age of 60 with unilateral tremor and without bradykinesia or pseudobulbar manifestations are the best candidates for the operation. The physiological mechanism by which the tremor is stopped is unknown. The procedure has been tried with little success in the treatment of other disorders characterized by abnormal states of muscle tone and movement (dyskinesias).

CHAPTER 41

Urology

JOSEPH D. SCHMIDT
†RUBIN H. FLOCKS

Urology is that branch of medicine and surgery devoted to the study, diagnosis, and treatment of diseases and abnormalities of the urogenital tract of the male and the urinary tract of the female.

Urologists must work in close association with members of all other branches of medicine, but particularly with internists and surgeons in the study and care of diseases of the adrenal gland, of so-called medical diseases of the kidney, and of abdominal masses of all types.

The kidney is the most important organ of excretion. A clear understanding of the status of the urinary tract of every patient is essential to a complete evaluation of the patient's condition. Only by a complete history and general examination of the patient, analysis of the urine, estimation of renal function, and radiological visualization of the urinary tract can the physician obtain an accurate knowledge of his patient's urological status. Cystoscopy is occasionally necessary to complete the urinary tract evaluation.

ANATOMY AND PHYSIOLOGY

The kidney has some endocrine functions that are related to the maintenance of blood pressure, but the kidney's main function is to form urine. This is the main pathway by which water, salts, nitrogenous wastes, and other products are excreted from the body, thereby helping to maintain the internal balance of these substances. The urine that is formed then travels down through the calyces, renal pelves,

---

†Deceased.

and ureters to the bladder. When about 400 ml. have collected, the desire to urinate triggers contraction of bladder muscle, emptying the urine through the urethra. The kidneys, calyces, pelves, and ureters are normally duplicated, but there is normally only one bladder and urethra.

PATHOLOGY AND SYMPTOMATOLOGY

Diseases of the genitourinary tract conveniently fall into the following general classes: congenital anomalies, injuries, inflammations, neoplasms, and certain miscellaneous diseases. Since its excretory function links the genitourinary tract anatomically and physiologically to other organ systems of the body, lesions involving the urinary tract may give rise to symptoms suggestive of lesions in organs and tissues outside the urinary tract. Moreover, since there is a direct communication and interrelationship between the functions of the various portions of the urinary tract, lesions in one portion may in turn produce disturbances of function in another portion of the urinary tract. These two facts are extremely important to the understanding of urinary tract disease.

Thus, disorders of this system may not only be multiple in distribution in the tract itself, but they also may be secondary to, or influenced or mimicked by, lesions arising primarily in other organ systems. This is particularly true in *children* with congenital anomalies of the genitourinary tract. If an early diagnosis is to be made, a complete urological survey must be made of all children with any unexplained symptoms or signs.

One should not infer from the preceding remarks that every individual with a genitourinary disease should be subjected at the first visit to all the procedures necessary to evaluate his entire genitourinary system. This is not only unnecessary, but in many instances may also be distinctly harmful; e.g., in the presence of an acute inflammation of the urethra, prostate, or bladder, the instrumentation necessary to examine the bladder, ureters, or kidney may be contraindicated. Only those examinations are necessary that establish accurately the location and nature of the disease needing active and immediate treatment. The more complicated diagnostic manipulations are deferred until the acute inflammatory findings subside, or until the progress of the disease makes these examinations imperative.

Since *obstruction* and *infection* are complications common to most urinary tract lesions, the physician must determine whether they are primary or secondary.

THERAPY

Therapy, in general, consists of two phases, after an accurate diagnosis has been established. The first, or palliative phase, is designed to relieve pain, dysuria, and increased frequency or signs of infection. The *sine qua non* is the *relief of obstruction* anywhere in the urinary tract, performed in the simplest way possible. In addition, antibiotics are given to control infection. With even this temporary relief of obstructive signs and symptoms, the patient's general condition will improve rapidly, and then one may proceed with the definitive phase of therapy.

The definitive phase is designed to cure, correct, or eradicate the causative lesion. This is done in such a way as not to disturb function but rather to restore it to as near physiological as possible. Here again, adequate urine drainage is of paramount concern. All therapeutic efforts are aimed at restoring or maintaining normal renal function and urinary transport.

EXAMINATION OF THE PATIENT
Approach

Urological patients may be shy with regard to their complaints because of taboos connected with the genitourinary tract, and it is especially important for the physician and nurse to assume a correct professional attitude toward them. Sympathy must be expressed and embarrassment avoided. They must be made to feel at ease. Deep human understanding and an intense feeling of responsibility on the part of the physician and nurse are highly desirable qualities.

Remarks

The patient's history and chief complaints are important because (1) they may point directly to some portion of the genitourinary tract, and (2) they may indicate lesions elsewhere, but these extra–urinary tract disturbances of function may be caused by impaired renal function caused by primary disease of the genitourinary tract. There may be no symptoms, and only a complete examination of the urinary tract will show the asymptomatic abnormalities.

History

Patients usually present themselves with one or more of the following situations:

1. Trauma-urinary extravasation
2. Abnormalities of the urine:
   a. Pyuria
   b. Hematuria
   c. Chyluria
   d. Pneumaturia
3. Abnormality in voiding:
   a. Incontinence
      (1) Ordinary
      (2) Paradoxic
   f. Small stream
   g. Difficulty or retention

  (3) Dribbling between
    normal urination
 b. Frequency
 c. Dysuria
 d. Oliguria
 e. Polyuria

h. Dribbling (Is it incontinence or is it associated with apparently normal voiding? The latter is almost pathognomonic of ectopic ureteral meatus.)

 4. Tumors or swellings in urogenital area:
  a. Scrotum:
   (1) Painful
   (2) Tender
   (3) Associated redness

  b. Abdominal masses:
   (1) In the flank
   (2) Suprapubically
   (3) In the groin

 5. Pain and tenderness in region of genitourinary tract:
  a. Infection
  b. Stone

  c. Trauma
  d. Congenital or acquired obstruction

6. Uremia: A blanket term used to designate the syndrome that results from renal insufficiency of any type. It may be characterized by nausea, vomiting, stupor, coma, azotemia, night anuria and oliguria, etc. The signs and symptoms vary with the myriads of variations in pathophysiology associated with renal insufficiency.

7. Azotemia may be part of the picture of renal insufficiency (uremia) but may be present with no renal insufficiency (dehydration, severe gastrointestinal tract hemorrhage).

8. Chills or fever may mean infection of the urinary tract.

9. Loss of weight may indicate urogenital malignant neoplasm or uremia.

10. Evidences of metastatic lesions to the bones: (a) osteogenic lesions to the bones of the pelvis usually are metastases from carcinoma of the prostate in the male; (b) hypernephroma frequently metastasizes to the lungs, as does tumor of the testis; (c) pulsating bone tumors, osteolytic in nature, usually are metastases from hypernephroma.

11. Poor growth in children may be an indication of renal insufficiency, related to congenital urinary tract obstruction.

12. Sexual dysfunction: Impotence, total or partial, is a common symptom and is based on psychological (nonorganic) problems in 80 to 90% of cases. Premature ejaculation likewise is unrelated to organic disease, whereas retrograde ejaculation usually results from anatomic disturbances of either the lumbar sympathetic ganglia or bladder neck (internal sphincter).

Examination
General appearance

The general appearance of the patient frequently suggests urinary tract disease. However, many serious diseases of the urinary tract produce no external changes, even in their late stages. In children, abnormalities of growth, particularly dwarfism, suggest disease of the urinary tract with associated renal insufficiency. In all ages, edema, sallow complexion, shortness of breath, and anemia or dehydration may herald serious genitourinary tract disease.

Findings

General findings that often justify careful diagnostic evaluation of the urinary tract are discussed in the following paragraphs.

Fever. Fever may be an indication of primary or secondary urinary tract infection; it is usually high, erratic, and frequently associated with chills.

Hypertension. Hypertension is frequently associated with glomerular disease of the kidneys, late stages of chronic pyelonephritis, congenital polycystic disease of the kidney, and decreased perfusion of one or both kidneys or even a segment of one kidney.

Edema. Edema associated with urinary tract disease is of two types. It may be peripheral to venous and lymphatic obstruction caused by primary or metastatic urinary tract neoplasm, or it may be generalized and associated with renal insufficiency or hypoproteinemia.

Abnormalities of growth. Abnormalities of growth in children may be associated with changes in the adrenal function or severe renal insufficiency.

Secondary anemia. Secondary anemia is frequently seen with renal insufficiency and urinary tract neoplasm from bleeding and bone marrow involvement.

Evidence of metastasis. Neoplasms of the prostate, kidney, and testes frequently metastasize to the lungs, the brain, and the bones of the torso.

Neurological findings. Diseases of the spinal cord frequently produce abnormalities in function of the bladder and the upper urinary tract, especially infection, stone formation, and residual urine in the bladder and kidney pelves. Early urological work-up is particularly important, since damage to the urinary tract caused by spinal cord disease may be so insidious that very marked change may occur before symptoms arise.

Loss of weight, dehydration. Loss of weight and dehydration are concomitants of renal insufficiency and other urinary tract diseases.

Abnormal breathing. Abnormal breathing may herald acidosis accompanying renal insufficiency.

Abdominal masses. Abdominal masses require complete urinary tract investigation, including roentgenography. A suprapubic mass may simply be a full bladder caused by obstruction of the bladder neck. Pelvic or abdominal masses may be ectopic kidneys that should not be removed.

Local examination and findings

Careful examination in the region of the kidneys and ureters should be a part of every physical examination. The skin should be inspected for enlarged, dilated veins that indicate collateral circulation. Palpation of the costovertebral angle for muscle spasm and tenderness should be carefully carried out.

Suprapubic dullness and masses should be noted.

The inguinal canal should be palpated for an undescended testis and hernia.

The scrotum should be carefully studied. The vas deferens, the epididymis, and the testis should be examined separately and abnormalities noted in their size, consistency, and form. Any mass in the scrotum should be transilluminated. A varicocele on the left side is not of great significance, but may signal a mass in the retroperitoneal area if present on the right side. The patient should be examined in the standing position to allow filling of any varicocele or hernia.

The perineum, urethra, and penis should be palpated carefully and inspected for swelling, tenderness, and urethral discharge.

The rectal examination includes the following:

1. The anal sphincter tone should be noted; if lax, it may be an indication of neurological cord disease.
2. Hemorrhoids may be caused by urinary or genital tract neoplasm producing vascular obstruction.
3. The prostate and seminal vesicles should be palpated carefully. The prostate normally is triangular with its apex caudad, each side measuring one inch, and its consistency is firm and rubbery. Hard areas should be noted; they may be caused by chronic inflammation (such as tuberculosis) but are more likely composed of prostatic neoplasms or calculi. The seminal vesicles are not normally palpable; if palpable, this may be evidence of inflammation (tuberculosis) or neoplastic invasion.
4. The prostatic secretion should be examined microscopically; it is obtained by digitally milking the prostate after the patient has urinated, so that as the prostatic secretion is discharged per urethra it will not be contaminated with urethral secretion. Normally, 5 to 10 pus cells or less are visible in each high-powered field. Tumor cells or large numbers of pus cells indicate prostatic neoplasm or infection, respectively. If bacterial prostatitis is suspected, the secretions should be cultured.

LABORATORY EXAMINATION—THE URINE

Urinalysis is an integral part of the examination of any patient. However, important urinary tract abnormalities may occur with relatively normal urine.

Under normal conditions the urine is formed by a process of physical filtration of the blood plasma through the glomeruli, followed by selective or vital reabsorption of a large part of the filtrate by the renal tubules. What is left, plus a few substances (like phenol red) that are excreted by the tubules, is the urine.

Abnormalities of the urine may be classified in three separate categories: (1) physical changes, (2) chemical changes, and (3) microscopic changes.

Physical changes
Volume

The amount of urine excreted is of great importance, particularly in relation to the intake. One of the most important single duties of the nurse in charge of a patient who has a urological condition is to measure accurately the intake and output, especially the urinary output. Normally, the adult excretes anywhere between 1 and 2.5 liters of urine in 24 hours, depending on his intake. Children excrete about three times as much as adults, per kilogram of body weight. About two-thirds of the urine is excreted during the daytime.

Anuria. *Anuria* is the failure to excrete urine. Anuria from renal failure must be differentiated from acute *retention* of urine, in which the kidneys secrete a normal amount of urine that cannot be voided because of obstruction somewhere in the drainage system. Bladder outlet obstruction is most common and may readily be determined by urethral catheterization. Occasionally, anuria is caused by bilateral obstruction of the ureters. This is *not* relieved by bladder catheterization.

Oliguria. When the adult secretes less than 400 to 500 ml. of urine in a 24-hour period, the condition is called *oliguria*. It is definitely pathological; the physician must ascertain its cause. It is *rarely* caused by an obstructive lesion in the urinary passageway.

Polyuria. Polyuria is a condition in which an excess amount of urine is secreted. Diabetes mellitus and insipidus and simply a large intake of fluids are the most common causes. Frequency of urination may occur, which must be distinguished from the much more common frequency of urination secondary to bladder outlet obstruction with overflow. Accurate measurement of the total amount of urine excreted per 24 hours will distinguish these two causes for frequency of urination. True polyuria is characterized by urine of a low specific gravity.

Turbidity

Normally the urine is clear. The clarity of urine may be disturbed by phosphates, fat, chyle, and pus. Most urine gets cloudy on standing because of the action of bacteria, and, therefore, turbidity must be studied on the fresh specimen. Phosphaturia will clear when the urine is acidified.

Color

Urine is normally light amber in color. Occasionally it changes because of the administration of drugs, like methylene blue. With hematuria, it may be smoky, red, or brown, depending on the amount, duration, and age of the blood in the urine. When the urine is brown and turns black on standing after alkalinization, it may be caused by alkaptonuria caused by homogentisic acid, or it may be caused by melanin.

Odor

Urine has a characteristic odor. Urea-splitting organisms in the urine give it a distinct ammoniacal smell. These organisms produce severe urinary tract infections and predispose to phosphate stones, and therefore an ammoniacal odor to the urine requires investigation of the urinary tract. Some commonly prescribed drugs such as ampicillin impart a characteristic odor to the urine.

Reaction

Normally urine has a pH of about 6.2 but may range from 4.5 to 8.0. Renal tuberculosis produces an acid urine, but most other types of urinary tract infections are associated with an alkaline urine. Urine pH is important in the work-up of patients with urolithiasis, since certain types of stones (e.g., cystine, uric acid) tend to occur when the urine is acid, and others (e.g., calcium phosphate, calcium ammonium magnesium phosphate) when the urine is alkaline. Testing a fresh specimen with Nitrazine paper is the most practical way to study the urine pH. Urine pH often reflects the acid-base balance status of body fluids. Many of the newer paper-strip indicators (Combistix, Hema-Combistix, and Labstix) afford the patient and the physician an opportunity to rather accurately detect glycosuria, proteinuria, pH, and other urinary changes simultaneously. Similarly, frequent pH testing can monitor a patient's response to therapy for infection or urolithiasis.

Specific gravity

The specific gravity of the urine varies from 1.001 to 1.030, according to the percentage of solids in the urine. It is usually reduced in chronic nephritis, with a tendency to fixation at 1.010. Inability to concentrate after dehydration is a valuable clinical renal function test.

Chemical changes

The following chemical changes in the urine are important: albuminuria, glycosuria, hemoglobinuria, and abnormalities in the excretion of chloride, phosphates, and calcium. Albuminuria may be orthostatic in type and transitory because of changes in position that interfere with the circulation through the kidney. It may be renal in origin because of chronic disease of the kidney, or even extrarenal (Tables 41-1 and 41-2).

Microscopic examination. Careful microscopic examination of the urine for casts, red cells, leukocytes, epithelial cells, and other organized substances is of great value. Special stains allow study of urinary tract cytology, and occasionally transitional cell tumors or renal cell tumors may be diagnosed by this means.

The microscopic examination should always include a thorough search for urinary organisms. Grossly, this is possible in the freshly voided, unstained specimen, but if more positive information is de-

Table 41-1. Diagnostic measures in hematuria*

1. General examination (including eye grounds, B.P., cuff test, studies of bleeding and clotting mechanisms, etc.)	Nephritis, hemorrhagic diathesis, Dicumarol
2. Urinalysis†	Verifies presence of blood
3. Plain x-ray (K.U.B.)	Stone, enlarged kidney
4. Excretory urogram	Tumor, tuberculosis, stone
5. Cystoscopy (preferably during bleeding)	Source of blood (vesical tumor, stone, renal origin)
6. Retrograde pyeloureterogram	On side of bleeding; on both sides if not localized to side
7. Abdominal aortogram and renal arteriogram	Renal neoplasm, vascular malformation
8. Renal biopsy (open, percutaneous)	Glomerular, interstitial disease
9. Repeated studies at intervals	To discover lesion at first overlooked

*Hematuria must be regarded as serious until unquestionably proved otherwise.
†Red urine does not necessarily contain red blood cells; so this point must be settled by microscopic examination unless clots are present. Other causes of red urine include hemoglobin (March and cold hemoglobinuria), porphyria, and ingestion of certain azo dyes or of large quantities of beets. Malingerers may add blood to the urine; this practice may be difficult to prove if the patient is clever.

sired, the sediment should be stained with Gram stain. *Staphylococcus, Streptococcus, Gonococcus* or gram-negative bacilli may be distinguished in this manner. Cultures of the urine are confirmatory and help one select the proper antibiotic. In cases of "sterile pyuria," particularly in an acid urine, guinea pig inoculations for tubercle bacilli should be done (Table 41-3).

ESTIMATION OF RENAL FUNCTION

Evaluation of renal function is an extremely important part of examination of any patient, but particularly so in the patient with urological disease. Moreover, the renal function is variable from one time to another, justifying serial evaluations in many patients.

Table 41-2. Origin of hematuria in 2,400 cases

Cause		Site	
Neoplasm	800	Vesical	860
Inflammation	500	Renal	840
Miscellaneous (systemic, indeterminate, etc.)	400	Prostatic	300
		Ureteral	250
Stone	425	Urethral	60
Tuberculosis	275	Systemic	20
		Unidentified	70
	2,400		2,400

Table 41-3. Diagnostic measures in chronic pyuria

Test	What it measures
1. Two-glass test	Exclusion of urethritis
2. Culture, Gram stain	Selection of antiseptic or antibiotic
3. Acid-fast stain, culture, and guinea pig inoculation	Tuberculosis (Mantoux, chest radiograph)
4. Residual urine	Prostatism, neurogenic dysfunction, stricture of urethra
5. Plain x-ray (K.U.B.)	Stones, perinephritic abscess
6. Excretory urogram	Stasis, anomalies, tuberculosis, impaired function
7. Cystourethroscopy	Dilated prostatic ducts, diverticula, etc.
8. Ureteral catheterization	Source of pyuria, divided cultures
9. Retrograde pyelogram	When excretory urogram fails
10. Foci of infection	Prostate, cervix, Skene's glands

The most common ways by which renal function is estimated are the following: (1) history of loss of appetite or nausea and vomiting, (2) edema or marked dehydration—"uremic snow," (3) urinary output—quantity, specific gravity, (4) specific renal function tests—the most important of these are the following:

1. Mosenthal specific gravity test
2. Phenolsulfonphthalein test
3. Blood urea nitrogen and creatinine (blood nonprotein nitrogen and creatinine)
4. Urea clearance test
5. Inulin, Diodrast, and phenol red clearance tests
6. Excretory urography
7. Differential renal function test during cystoscopy
8. Endogenous creatinine clearance

Mosenthal specific gravity test

In progressive renal damage, one of the earliest changes is impairment of the concentrating power of the kidney. Fluids are omitted after 6:00 P.M., and the first urinary specimen passed in the morning is tested for specific gravity. Normally the urine will be concentrated to 1.028. This test may be unreliable during diuresis.

Phenolsulfonphthalein (P.S.P.) test

The P.S.P. test is one primarily of the renal tubular excretion capacity. It shows change relatively early in the course of progressive renal damage and is reduced to zero before much change is found in the blood urea, nonprotein nitrogen (N.P.N.), or creatinine.

Procedure. The patient, who should be in bed, drinks two glasses of water. Then, 6 mg. of P.S.P. in 1 ml. of sterile water are injected intravenously. The patient voids every 30 minutes, and four specimens are collected during the next 2 hours. Each specimen is compared colorimetrically with standards to estimate the patient's excretion of the dye.

In a normal individual, the dye appears in about 3 minutes. About 60% is excreted in the first hour and about 20% in the second hour. The amounts are decreased and sometimes reversed in patients with renal disease. Residual urine in the bladder will make the test less accurate; catheterization prior to the test is required.

Blood urea nitrogen and creatinine

Normally, the blood urea nitrogen is 10 to 20 mg.% and the creatinine 0.6 to 1.5 mg.%. Both values are elevated with marked renal damage or obstructive disease causing impairment of function.

Urea clearance test

The term "clearance" is defined as the volume of blood in milliliters "cleared" by the kidneys in 1 minute. To carry out the test, one must collect the urine for a 2-hour period and obtain a blood urea determination at the end of the first hour.

Procedure. In the morning after breakfast the patient drinks at least 1 liter of water to ensure maximum diuresis; the bladder is emptied and the specimen is discarded. The next 2-hour urine is the one that is studied. Normally about 75 ml. of blood is cleared of urea per minute.

Inulin, Diodrast, and phenol red clearance tests

These clearance tests are restricted to the few occasions when information is desired of renal blood flow or separate glomerular and tubular function. The inulin clearance measures glomerular filtration rate, and the other two substances precisely evaluate renal tubular function.

Excretory urography

Excretory urography is the most *important single test of renal function* available today. It not only gives an estimation of total renal function, but it also differentiates each kidney and gives information about the urinary passageways. With renal impairment, the time of the appearance is delayed, excretion is prolonged, and there is a less dense shadow cast on the radiograph. On the contrary, with incomplete obstruction the shadow may be more dense than normal. Known sensitivity to iodinated contrast media is the main contraindication.

Differential renal function tests during cystoscopy

The urine emerging from the ureters at the time of cystoscopic examination may be observed after the intravenous injection of 5 ml. of indigo carmine. Normally, the dye appears in 3 minutes and concentrates to a deep blue.

Another method is to insert ureteral catheters up to each kidney and collect the urines separately; 6 mg. of P.S.P. are injected intravenously, and the appearance time and the total excretion in 15 minutes of the dye are studied.

Endogenous creatinine clearance

This test measures a patient's ability to clear the plasma of circulating creatinine. A 24-hour urine collection is made, and a serum creatinine concentration is drawn midway during the collection. The clearance is calculated using the formula $Cl_{cr} = \dfrac{U \times V}{P}$ where U represents the urine creatinine concentration, P the serum creatinine concentration, and V the 24-hour urine volume expressed in ml./1,440 minutes. Correction for body surface area variation should be made for children and large or small adults. The normal range of creatinine clearance is 70 to 130 ml. per minute.

INSTRUMENTAL EXAMINATION OF THE URETHRA

Besides examining the urethra by palpation, the urethra may be examined by means of a catheter, a bougie, a urethroscope, or urethrography. Urethral obstruction will prevent passage of a catheter into the bladder, its precise cause (stricture, foreign body, or tumor) requiring further work-up with urethroscopy and cystourethrography. Spasm of the external bladder sphincter must be differentiated carefully from organic obstruction.

Residual urine in the bladder may be determined as follows: The patient is asked to void, and the character of the stream is noted. A good strong stream that voids from 100 to 300 ml. of urine usually eliminates the possibility of residual urine in the bladder. The patient is then placed on his back (unclothed) on the examining table. Suprapubic percussion and palpation are carried out. Any lower abdominal mass, even if it is not in the midline, should be suspected of being a full bladder, or an undrained diverticulum of the bladder. Aseptic catheterization should then be performed; more than 30 to 75 ml. of urine in the bladder indicates significant residual urine. The cause of this should be ascertained.

Technique for catheterization in the male. The patient should lie on his back with the thighs slightly separated and moderately flexed. The penis, scrotum, and pubic area are cleaned thoroughly with soap and rinsed with sterile water. In the average adult a No. 18 French rubber catheter is used. A sterile tube of lubricant jelly is removed from the antiseptic solution in which it is stored, and the first teaspoonful or so is discarded. Then the nozzle of the tube is inserted into the urethral meatus, and with steady pressure the entire urethra is filled with jelly.

The operator stands at the right side of the patient, grasps the shaft of the penis between the third and fourth fingers and the glans penis at each side of the meatus with the thumb and index finger of the left hand, so as to open the meatal lips widely enough to admit the tip of the catheter. The penis is drawn gently forward and upward from the body so as to stretch it slightly and thus straighten the anterior urethra. When using soft rubber or woven catheters, the penis is kept in the midline and the catheter is advanced to the bladder; the penile shaft is lowered as the catheter tip passes the external sphincter and enters the bladder. If the catheter does not enter the bladder easily, the tip is probably caught in the side part of the bulb, or is held by the contracted external sphincter. In the former instance the catheter is withdrawn a little and advanced again drawing the penis over it with the left hand, much as a glove is drawn over a finger, at the same time depressing the penile shaft to between the thighs. In case the external sphincter is in spasm, the tip of the catheter is held against it with gentle but continuous pressure for several minutes. The contraction generally relaxes partially, and the catheter enters the bladder. Larger instruments overcome the spasm of the sphincter more easily than small ones. Irrigation is then carried out since the lubricating jelly may have closed off the lumen of the catheter.

Technique for catheterization in the female. Follow the same general principles as in the male. Since the urethra is short, once the meatus is located, the catheterization is easily carried out.

Cystourethroscopic examination. The modern cystoscope is used to visualize the urinary bladder and urethra for diagnostic purposes. It allows operative procedures to be carried out under vision, without making an incision into the bladder or urethra.

Cystoscopy and urethroscopy may be carried out with ease in patients of all ages, including infants. Ordinarily in the adult female patient, no anesthesia is necessary. In children and adult males, however, or with severe inflammatory lesions, it may be necessary to carry out the procedure under either general or regional anesthesia. When operative procedures are to be performed, anesthesia is, practically speaking, always necessary.

Technique of cystoscopy. Asepsis is observed and then the instrument is introduced in much the same manner as a stiff catheter is introduced. After careful observation of the bladder neck, trigone, ureteral orifices, fundus, anterior and lateral walls of the bladder, and the urethra, any indicated operative procedure may be carried out.

ROENTGENOLOGICAL EXAMINATION OF THE URINARY TRACT

Roentgenological examination of the urinary tract is just as important as a chest radiograph in general evaluation of a patient. No other single technique so clearly evaluates renal function or diagnoses urinary tract disease. Early diagnosis is essential to avoid severe and irreparable damage to the urinary tract.

Examination of the urinary tract is carried out by a plain film, by cystograms, urethrograms, intravenous pyelography, and retrograde pyelography. Retrograde pyelography is carried out after cystoscopic examination and the passage of ureteral catheters up to the kidney pelvis.

For the best results in interpreting the films, it is wise to establish a definite routine for each type of examination and follow that pattern. This may seem tedious, but it produces the best results. The routine that we recommend is presented in the outline that follows:

I. The plain film (K.U.B.)
    A. Procedure: The patient lies flat on his back, and the film is taken to include the area from the lower ribs to the pubis.
    B. Bone survey
        1. Look for bony changes in the ribs, spine, sacrum, pelvis, and femurs.
        2. Metastatic lesions of carcinoma are particularly important:
            a. Osteoblastic bone lesions: carcinoma of the prostate.
            b. Osteolytic bone lesions: carcinoma of the kidney, breast, thyroid, lung, and urinary bladder.
            c. Bone tumors such as multiple myeloma, sarcoma, etc.
        3. Other bony changes such as arthritis, Paget's disease, bone cysts, syphilis, and fractures.
    C. Soft tissue survey
        1. Kidney outline:
            a. Size, shape, and position.
            b. Frequently not seen because of gas or poor detail.
        2. Psoas shadow outline:
            a. Are the outlines bilaterally the same?
            b. Note if the outline is sharp and distinct.
            c. Frequently is not seen because of gas or poor detail.
        3. Other tissue masses:
            a. Such as liver, spleen, tumors.
    D. Foreign bodies, stones
        1. Show up as opaque shadows.
        2. A phlebolith can be differentiated from a stone by its typical hollow center and ectopic location with respect to the ureter or kidney pelvis or bladder.
    E. Intestinal gas pattern
II. Excretory urography (I.V.P.)
    A. Procedure: Check for sensitivity to iodine. If possible, the patient is prepared previously by being dehydrated—no fluid or food for 12 to 18 hours prior to the films. (An important exception to the dehydration preparation is the patient with multiple myeloma involving the kidneys. These patients should not be dehydrated so that renal failure may be avoided.) First, a plain film (K.U.B.) is taken. Then, 20 to 60 ml. of radiopaque contrast material (Hypaque, Renografin, Renovist, Conray) are injected slowly intra-

venously. If injected too rapidly, it may cause flushing, abdominal distress, nausea, and vomiting. Exposures covering the same area as the K.U.B. are usually made at 5, 10, and 25 minutes. A fifth film, the excretory cystogram, is taken over the bladder region alone.

Visualization of the urinary tract is improved by the technique of infusion urography. Here, the patient need not be dehydrated in advance. An infusion consisting of 1 ml. of contrast per pound of body weight added to an equal volume of 5% dextrose in water is administered intravenously over 15 or 20 minutes. Appropriate films are taken after the infusion is completed. This study is more expensive but results in improved filling of the collecting systems.

B. Value of the intravenous pyelogram
   1. It is useful when retrograde pyelograms would be difficult or dangerous to do such as in children, urethral or ureteral strictures, impassable stones, suspected rupture of the kidney, suspected anomalies, and poor-risk patients.
   2. It is a quick, simple, safe screening test to help rule out urinary tract pathological conditions.
   3. It is a good indicator of kidney function. A normal kidney is visualized well; a nonfunctioning kidney will not be visualized.

C. The size, shape, and position of the drainage pathways of the tract are established.

D. Iodinated contrast medium may be given intramuscularly or subcutaneously if a vein cannot be entered, such as in children. The amount of contrast medium varies from 5 to 20 ml., depending on the age of the child. An infant should take about 5 to 8 ml. and a child over 10 years of age, 15 ml. The contrast medium can be mixed with an equal volume of saline, divided in half, and each portion injected intramuscularly into one buttock. The addition of 1 ml. of hyaluronidase (Wydase) improves absorption of the contrast medium. The first film is exposed in about 10 minutes. The next film is taken about 5 minutes later and the third in another 5 to 10 minutes. If the contrast medium is injected intravenously into children, three roentgen-ray exposures are taken 5 minutes apart. We have used this technique in newborns as young as 1 day of age.

III. Cystography: The patient's bladder is entirely emptied by means of a urethral catheter. Any iodinated contrast medium can be used, depending on the effect desired, and there are times when air is used as the contrast medium. The cystogram may be taken in many different positions, depending on the nature of the lesion to be studied. An emptying cystogram is made by having the patient void while the film is exposed.

IV. Opaque cystogram

    A. Procedure: The patient lies flat on his back and an iodinated contrast solution is instilled into the bladder per catheter until the patient complains of a feeling of fullness. This amount is usually less than 400 ml. of solution. Anteroposterior and oblique exposures are taken.

    B. Size, shape, and location of the bladder

        1. The normal bladder configuration is a rounded shadow, centrally placed, about the size of a grapefruit.

        2. Chronic cystitis is characterized by an extremely small, spastic bladder, atony by an extremely large, flaccid bladder.

        3. Pelvic tumors displace the bladder from the midline.

    C. Character of the bladder wall

        1. Normally it is slightly rough or irregular to smooth.

        2. Long-standing obstruction causes a hypertrophied and markedly roughened bladder wall with many coarse trabeculations.

    D. Diverticula

        1. A diverticulum is a herniation of mucosa through the hypertrophied muscle fibers. This outpouching most commonly results from long-standing obstruction. The normal bladder has no diverticula.

        2. Sometimes the diverticulum may be larger than the bladder itself, or there may be many diverticula, creating a problem of identifying the true bladder. Distinguishing features of the diverticulum are the following:

            a. It has a smooth outline, whereas the bladder is normally slightly roughened.

            b. It is usually eccentrically located.

            c. The urethral catheter usually does not enter it.

        3. Emptying: Does the diverticulum empty, or does urine stagnate? This may be distinguished by the position of the diverticulum, or by a postevacuation film.

    E. Reflux up the ureters

        1. It is not normal to have the contrast solution pass up the ureters.

        2. Ureteral reflux is due to incompetence of the ureterovesical valve, caused by infection, long-standing obstruction, congenital anomalies, surgery, or neurogenic disease.

    F. Rupture of the bladder: The contrast extravasates from the bladder.

    G. Bladder contents: The contrast cystogram may outline tumors or foreign bodies within the bladder, but this is better done with the air cystogram.

V. Air cystogram
   A. Procedure: The bladder is emptied of the contrast and washed out. The patient is placed in the right oblique (semilateral) position. The bladder is filled with air, by catheter, until the patient complains of a feeling of fullness.
   B. The air acts as a lucent contrast medium and will help to visualize:
      1. Intravesical position of the prostate.
      2. Bladder tumors.
      3. Foreign bodies, especially stones.
VI. Urethrography
   A. Procedure: Urethrography is of great value in the study of trauma, strictures, contractures, congenital deformities at the bladder neck, and deformities of the prostatic urethra associated with prostatism. A urethrogram is made after the technique of Flocks by emptying the bladder of fluid, filling it with air with the patient in the oblique position, and then filling the urethra with a mixture of iodinated contrast and sterile lubricating jelly. During the exposure of the film, 50 ml. of this mixture is injected into the urethra. This gives a simultaneous air cystogram and opaque urethrogram and is particularly valuable for outlining the posterior urethra to evaluate the adequacy of prostatectomy. At times a voiding urethrogram is helpful. This is usually done by filling the bladder with contrast and exposing the film during micturition.
   B. The following landmarks should be noted:
      1. The pendulous urethra.
      2. The bulbous urethra—the usual seat of inflammatory strictures.
      3. The external sphincter and the internal sphincter.
      4. The prostatic urethra: elongation, widening, and anterior angulation are indicative of benign prostatic enlargement:
         a. Are there prostatic calculi?
         b. Are there periurethral abscesses?
VII. Retrograde pyelography
   A. Retrograde pyelography is the most exact method of visualizing the upper urinary tract. Its purpose is fourfold.
      1. Accurate visualization of the anatomic structure of the upper urinary tract.
      2. Procurement of segregated specimens of urine from each kidney for culture, cytology, and microscopy.
      3. When the ureteral catheters are in place, the differential function of each kidney is determined accurately by the intravenous injection of phenolsulfonphthalein.
      4. Relief of ureteral obstruction.
   B. Procedure: A cystoscope is introduced into the bladder, and after cystoscopy has been completed, the ureteral orifices

are catheterized with ureteral catheters that are advanced gently into each renal pelvis. Specimens of urine are then obtained from each renal pelvis for the examinations mentioned previously.

After this, plain films are taken to mark the course of the ureters and to locate any radiopaque density, such as stones. Either air or an iodinated contrast is injected into the kidney pelvis, and radiographs are made to visualize the renal calyces accurately.

If visualization of the ureters is desirable, the catheters are withdrawn to the lower portion of the ureter and contrast is injected for a ureteropyelogram. Air is used instead of contrast to show nonopaque calculi or other relatively nondense filling defects of the ureter. Retrograde pyelography is not an innocuous procedure. Reflex anurias and pyelonephritis are rare complications of retrograde pyelography.

The vast majority of cystoscopies and retrograde pyelograms are done without any anesthesia whatsoever, and the patients experience no undue discomfort. All in all, retrograde pyelograms are probably one of the most accurate and definitive diagnostic procedures in medicine.

VIII. Special roentgenographic studies

There are many special types of studies that have limited use:

A. Perirenal air and gas injections: These are used to outline the kidneys and possible adrenal tumors. This is not an innocuous procedure but does, at times, give sufficient additional information to justify its risk.

B. Gastric air injections: Air introduced into the stomach may aid in demonstrating a renal mass, especially in children.

C. Air cystograms for diagnosis of possible placenta previa: The bladder is filled with 120 ml. of air, and exposures are made in the anterior, posterior, and lateral positions. The relation of the fetal head to the air-containing bladder helps determine if a placenta previa exists.

D. Nephrotomography: Very valuable particularly to outline masses in the renal area.

E. Abdominal aortography: Contrast media injected into the aorta outlines the renal arterial system. Uses:

1. The main advantage of aortography is to differentiate malignant lesions of the kidney from benign cysts. Contrast fills the vascular spaces within a neoplasm but outlines only the periphery of a cyst.

2. The nephrogram demonstrates certain parenchymal lesions before they are large enough to encroach on the calyces or pelvis, or produce detectable reduction of renal function. This is particularly true in early tuberculous and neoplastic renal lesions.

   3. Visualization of the renal artery may help diagnose renovascular hypertension (some obstructive mechanism of the arterial supply to the kidney). Massive arterial renal infarct may also be detected by this procedure.
   4. The question of renal ptosis versus ectopia is clearly settled, but these usually can be distinguished by retrograde pyelograms.
   5. Aberrant vessels that obstruct the ureteropelvic junction in congenital hydronephrosis may be documented by aortography. This may be demonstrated better if one does a retrograde pyelogram immediately preceding the arteriogram, superimposing one on the other.
   F. Selective renal angiography: Very useful for visualizing renal artery lesions and renal tumors and has in many instances supplemented aortography.

OTHER SPECIAL DIAGNOSTIC STUDIES

Other special diagnostic studies are the following:

1. Radioactive renography
2. Renal scanning
3. Needle biopsy
4. Cinefluorography
5. Urodynamic studies: ureters, kidney pelvis, and bladder
6. Endocrine function studies
7. Chromatin test for somatic sex
8. Skeletal scanning
9. Ultrasound scanning

THE KIDNEY
Renal anomalies

The congenital anomalies of the renal parenchyma may be classified as follows: abnormalities of number, position, form, structure, and vascularization.

Anomaly of number

The most common anomaly is that of number and usually is asymptomatic. Obviously, if both kidneys are absent, life is impossible. Congenital *solitary kidney* does occur. This means that whenever nephrectomy is to be considered, the possibility that the other kidney may be absent or hypoplastic makes preoperative study mandatory. Occasionally a true *supernumerary kidney* may be present. The most common type of abnormality of number is *duplication* of the pelvis and ureter. Many of them are associated with ectopic ureteral openings, usually of the ureter draining the upper kidney pelvis, which are the source of the presenting symptoms. (See discussion on congenital anomalies of the ureter, p. 940.) Many are also associated with anomalies of vascularization that produce partial urinary obstruction as the presenting symptom and sign.

Anomaly of position

Anomaly of position occurs when the embryological process of ascent and rotation of the kidney is interfered with at any point. Usually failure of rotation is associated with compression of the pelvis and/or ureter by renal vessels, producing obstruction. The *ectopic kidney* can easily be recognized by its short ureter and anterior position of its pelvis. Sometimes *crossed ectopia* with fusion occurs, which resembles a large tumor mass. This may actually be all the renal parenchyma the patient has, and removal of such a fused kidney would be lethal.

Anomaly of form

Anomalies of form occur during embryological migration of the kidneys upward. Their lower poles may fuse to form a *horseshoe kidney*. After fusion one kidney may ascend and pull the other to the opposite side *(crossed ectopia with fusion)*. The anterior surface of one may be fused to the posterior surface of the other, and they remain in the pelvis (so-called disc kidney). These anomalies frequently are confused with other masses, or are associated with obstruction to the outflow of urine from their pelves, because of the necessity of renal vessels crossing the pelvis and ureter to get to the kidney. Treatment is tailored to the exact difficulties each produces.

Anomaly of structure

Anomalies of structure may be unilateral or bilateral and are characterized by *hypoplasia* or *cystic formations*. If hypoplasia is unilateral, no symptoms may occur. If hypoplasia is bilateral, renal insufficiency will result. Cystic formations may be asymptomatic, but massive replacement of remaining renal tissue will produce renal insufficiency (Fig. 41-1). Multicystic kidney is usually associated with an atretic ureter.

Congenital polycystic disease. Congenital polycystic disease is one of the important congenital anomalies of the kidney. It is usually *bilateral, familial,* and seems to be caused by a lack of fusion of most of the renal elements with the excretory elements of the tubules. This produces a large number of varying-sized cysts in each kidney that grow slowly, destroy renal substance, and produce gradual renal insufficiency. Bilateral palpable masses usually result. The cysts distort the kidney outlines and the kidney pelves, to produce a characteristic radiographic appearance.

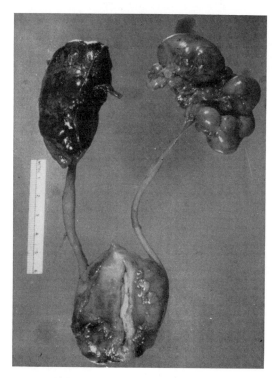

Fig. 41-1. Multicystic kidney, left.

If polycystic disease is unilateral, it cannot be differentiated from hypernephroma.

When bilateral, the diagnosis is usually easily made. Hypertension with red and white cells and casts in the urine herald the gradual onset of renal insufficiency. The treatment is symptomatic and operative. *Symptomatic treatment* consists essentially of avoiding trauma and infection to the kidneys, since massive hemorrhage may result. *Surgical treatment* consists of relocating each kidney into the subcutaneous area, and at intervals aspirating as many of the cysts as possible to reduce the pressure upon the normal-functioning renal substance. This, of course, is purely palliative. The prognosis varies with the rapidity with which renal insufficiency and hypertension develop, which in turn probably depends on the extent of the renal involvement. Some patients live only a few years, most die in middle age, and a few live out their normal span. In a small percentage of cases this is associated with cystic disease of the liver and lungs and cerebral artery aneurysms. Hemodialysis and renal transplantation have been effective in the treatment of the chronic renal insufficiency related to polycystic kidney disease. Bilateral nephrectomy is indicated to make room for the renal graft or for relief of hypertension.

Anomaly of vascularization

Anomalies of vascularization may occur in otherwise normal kidneys. They are hazards during operative procedures upon the kidney, or they may produce obstruction at the ureteropelvic junction that requires correction (Fig. 41-2).

• • •

Abdominal masses, renal insufficiency, abdominal pain, or urinary symptoms may indicate a congenital anomaly of the kidney. This is true, no matter what the age of the patient.

Congenital anomalies of the renal pelvis are essentially *obstructive* from bands, high insertion of the ureter, or stricture at the ureteropelvic junction. They may produce enormous hydronephrotic sacs with renal atrophy. They are bilateral in over 50% of the cases and need to be differentiated from renal cysts, renal neoplasms, and obstructive uropathy originating lower in the urinary tract. They may be silent, or produce an ache or pain in the side or evidence of severe infection. They may produce a large abdominal mass. The treatment is surgical— removal or plastic repair—with the surgeon always keeping in mind that the condition is frequently bilateral. The pathognomonic findings are demonstrated readily with intravenous and retrograde pyelography.

Urolithiasis

Stones in the urinary tract are common disorders with marked geographic variations in incidence (Fig. 41-3). So-called stone belts occur in various parts of the world, in which certain types of stone predominate; e.g., in the southern part of the United States, calcium oxalate stones are common. In this country as a whole, about 75 to 80% are calcium oxalate, calcium phosphate, or magnesium ammonium phosphate stones. Of the remaining, four-fifths are uric acid stones, and the others are cystine stones. Magnesium ammonium phosphate stones commonly occur after infection in the urinary tract with urea-splitting organisms (Fig. 41-4).

Stones in the urinary tract are the end result of a series of predisposing factors. Elucidation of these factors is necessary for correct

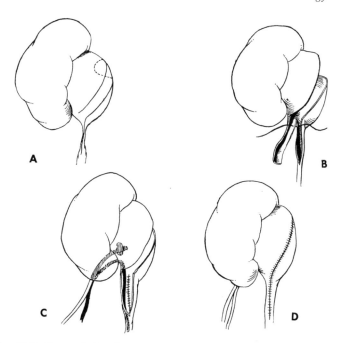

Fig. 41-2. Congenital stricture of ureteropelvic junction and its surgical correction. **A,** Incision is outlined that crosses stricture and raises a flap from the kidney pelvis. **B,** Flap swung down to widen the strictured area. **C,** Nephrostomy tube and ureteral catheter splint inserted. **D,** End result.

therapy (Table 41-4). In some instances a matrix, or nucleus, acts as a template for further precipitation of crystalloids. However, in certain types of recumbency calculi, such a matrix is obviously not necessary. Some factors are important in the formation of a nucleus, and others facilitate precipitation of the various stone-forming crystalloids.

We want to emphasize some of the factors that are precursors of certain types of stone. Any *foreign body* in the urinary tract favors the formation of calcium phosphate and ammonium magnesium phosphate stones. Nonabsorbable suture material used in operation upon the bladder or renal pelvis will act as a nucleus around which precipitation of the supersaturated calcium salts occurs. Ulcerating lesions and retained blood clots in the urinary tract act similarly.

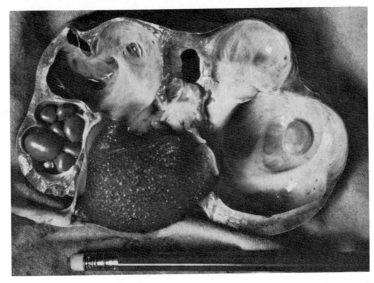

Fig. 41-3. Urolithiasis. Multiple large stones (cystine) have obstructed and totally destroyed the kidney.

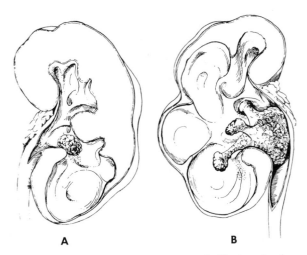

A   B

Fig. 41-4. A, Single calculus obstructing and dilating the lower renal calyx. **B,** "Staghorn" calculus obstructing and dilating all the renal calyces.

Table 41-4. Stones in the urinary tract

Renal stone is a symptom of one or more of the following:
1. Vitamin A deficiency
2. Focal infection
3. Urinary tract infection
4. Urinary tract stasis
5. Foreign body in urinary tract
6. Increased crystalloid excretion (cystinuria, hyper-parathyroidism, etc.)
7. Changes in the urine that lessen the solubility of the crystalloids in the urine

In man, the relationship of *vitamin A deficiency* to urinary calculi is debatable, but in animals it may produce urinary stones in several ways: (1) by producing ulceration of the epithelium of the urinary tract, (2) by causing desquamation of the epithelium (the desquamated epithelium acts as a nucleus), and (3) by predisposing the urinary tract to infection that may change the precipitability of the stone-forming crystalloids.

Urinary tract infection is believed to be the most important single cause of urolithiasis. It may produce a stone by creating a nucleus in a manner similar to vitamin A deficiency, by changing the pH of the urine, or by altering the protective colloids of the urine.

Urinary stasis from acquired or congenital obstruction of the urinary passageway is an important predisposing cause of urolithiasis. In a series of 60 patients with obstruction at the ureteropelvic junction without infection who were studied at the University of Iowa Hospitals, the incidence of urolithiasis was 10 times higher than it was in a series of patients without such obstruction. If other causes for urolithiasis exist and a tiny stone forms, it may pass without becoming clinically manifest if obstruction is not present. If recurrent urolithiasis is to be prevented, urinary stasis must be corrected.

Metabolic disturbances

Certain metabolic disturbances produce qualitative and quantitative changes in the urinary crystalloids that predispose to the formation of calculi, particularly if a nucleus has formed, if urinary stasis and infection occur, or if changes in the urine aid in the precipitation of such crystalloids. The most frequent of these metabolic changes are cystinuria and alterations of calcium metabolism.

Cystinuria is a familial abnormality of the amino acid cystine metabolism characterized by the excretion of a large amount of cystine in the urine. Normally, 10 to 100 mg. of cystine is excreted in the urine in 24 hours. With abnormal cystine metabolism, 300 to 1,500 mg. may be excreted in 24 hours. At present, no method for altering this abnormality is known. The following measures are helpful: forced administration of fluids, correction and avoidance of all factors that lead to the formation of a nucleus, correction of urinary stasis if present, and alteration of the hydrogen-ion concentration of the urine so that it will be continuously alkaline (cystine is insoluble in acid urine and highly soluble in alkaline urine). The urine usually is made alkaline by administering sodium bicarbonate and sodium citrate and by the use of an alkali-ash diet. The chelating agent D-penicillamine (Cuprimine) is also indicated in cystinuria. The drug forms a complex with cystine that is more soluble than the cystine alone. Large cystine calculi have been dissolved by such therapy.

Metabolic conditions that predispose to an increased excretion of *calcium phosphate* are very common. The most important of these is recumbency. If other factors that predispose to the formation of urinary calculi can be avoided by a proper regimen, the precipitated calcium salts can be washed out readily before irreparable renal damage occurs. Tiny stones can be demonstrated on roentgenograms of the kidneys every month during the first year of a period of recumbency.

Hyperparathyroidism from adenoma or hyperplasia of the parathyroid glands may be the underlying cause of urolithiasis. Up to 50% of patients with hyperparathyroidism will have renal stones. Hyperparathyroidism is characterized by localized or generalized osteoporosis, urinary calculi, and a high serum calcium and low serum phosphorus in the early stage of the disease before renal insufficiency develops. The serum alkaline phosphatase usually is increased. In most cases, treatment of the hyperparathyroidism should precede treatment of the urinary calculi. Exceptions to this are cases in which acute urinary obstruction or infection is present.

Other metabolic diseases may be important in the formation of urinary calculi. Uric acid stones are seen with hypersecretion of uric acid associated with a disturbance of purine metabolism. The medical management and prevention of these calculi are very similar to those utilized in cases of cystinuria, i.e., an alkaline reaction of the urine and a low purine diet. The xanthine oxidase inhibitor allopurinol (Zyloprim) is useful in that it decreases both serum and urine uric acid concentrations. With improved chemotherapy for various malignancies, more cancer patients are at risk for the hyperuricemia and subsequent hyperuricosuria related to increased cell destruction and release of nucleic acids.

Changes in the urine predisposing to crystalloid precipitation

At the time a urinary stone is formed, the hydrogen ion concentration of the urine is the final factor that determines the chemical composition of the stone. Infection of the urinary tract plays an important role since urea-splitting organisms alkalinize the urine to favor the precipitation of calcium oxalate. Treatment includes control of urinary infection and acidification of the urine by the administration of sodium acid phosphate. In addition, this drug decreases the urinary excretion of calcium by as much as 50%. Ascorbic acid (vitamin C) is also useful to acidify the urine.

Other etiological factors

In some cases, a primary renal defect may be associated with hyperexcretion of oxalates and calcium phosphate. In such cases, diets relatively low in oxalates and phosphorus may be useful.

Stress influences the formation of stones in animals, although its role in humans is obscure. It is thought to be a factor in the production of uric acid and oxalate calculi. Avoidance of stress should be a part of the treatment of patients with these calculi.

The prolonged administration of ACTH and corticosteroids produces osteoporosis and an accompanying hypercalciuria. Hypercalciuria should be considered in any case in which either of these drugs in administered for a long time.

Ureteral stones

Ureteral stones essentially are renal stones that have passed down into the ureter. They rarely arise in the ureter itself, except when a foreign body, such as a ureteral suture, acts as a nucleus for precipitation of calcium and magnesium ammonium phosphate salts.

In general, stones under 1 cm. pass spontaneously. Those over 1 cm. in diameter usually must be removed, whether they are causing symptoms or not. Uric acid calculi are nonopaque on radiographic examination and show up as filling defects in the pyeloureterogram; they must be differentiated from blood clots and tumors of the ureter.

Vesical stones

Vesical stones are common. They are associated with infection and obstruction at the bladder neck, or with ulcerating lesions or foreign bodies in the bladder itself. Vesical calculi, therefore, are commonly found in the bladder itself, although many of them are actually stones that have passed down from the kidney and have been retained in the bladder because of bladder neck obstruction. They may be removed suprapubically or transurethrally by cystolitholapaxy or cystolithotripsy, depending on their size, consistency, and the condition of

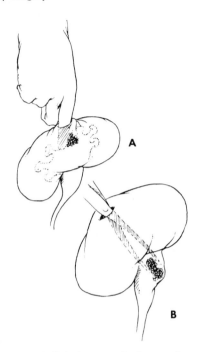

Fig. 41-5. **A,** Transrenal digital removal of stone from calyx. **B,** Transrenal removal of stone from kidney pelvis by instrument.

the bladder itself. Calculi may form in bladder diverticula because of increased stasis. Here treatment must be directed against the underlying cause of the diverticulum as well as removal of the stone.

Nonopaque uric acid stones require differentiation from bladder tumors, large subcervical prostatic lobes, or blood clots. Opaque calculi are readily recognized on the radiograph. Since many of them are secondary to ulcerative lesions of the bladder or bladder neck obstruction, these accessory or predisposing conditions must be treated simultaneously. Surgical treatment is shown in Figs. 41-5 and 41-6.

Renal neoplasms

Neoplasms of the kidney are common and are generally malignant. Benign tumors are clinical curiosities. The best clinical classification

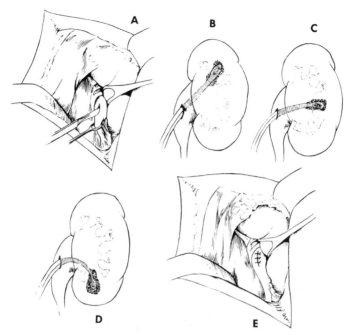

Fig. 41-6. Removal of stones through renal pelvis. **A,** Incision into renal pelvis. **B** to **D,** Extraction of stones from various locations in renal calyces by stone forceps. **E,** Closure of incision in renal pelvis.

is related to age. All tumors in children under the age of 8 are so-called Wilms' tumors, or nephroblastomas. Generally, few malignant tumors occur between the ages of 8 and about 25 or 30 years. About 95% of renal tumors in adults are highly malignant neoplasms of the renal parenchyma, the so-called hypernephroma (renal cell carcinoma) and cystadenocarcinoma. The other 5% are tumors of the renal pelvis: squamous cell, transitional cell, or adenocarcinoma.

The general trend in the treatment of malignant renal neoplasms favors more radical surgery. Preoperative or postoperative deep roentgen-ray therapy is debatable, although the current consensus strongly endorses irradiation as part of the therapy for Wilms' tumor. In the adult, irradiation alone is not of great help, either in hypernephromas or tumors arising primarily from the urothelium.

Kidney neoplasms of childhood

Renal neoplasms of childhood are mixed mesenchymal tumors, the so-called Wilms' tumors. They appear very early in life and constitute one of the most frequent malignant tumors of childhood, closely followed in incidence by neuroblastoma, which frequently invades the kidney and resembles Wilms' tumor. Wilms' tumors grow rapidly and metastasize early through the bloodstream and lymphatics, with the lungs being frequently involved. Over 30% of patients have metastases when first seen: The most common presenting sign is a large abdominal mass. The urine is often normal, and there are generally no urinary symptoms. Gastrointestinal disturbances and pain are frequent because of the weight and bulk of the tumor. Metastatic lesions produce a variety of symptoms and signs. The diagnosis is usually readily made by means of pyelography; intravenous pyelograms show a mass deformity or no function from the involved kidney, and retrograde pyelograms show a distorted and deformed pelvis. Wilms' tumors must always be differentiated from congenital hydronephrosis and cystic disease of the kidney, which are frequently bilateral and in which removal of a kidney might be contraindicated. A differential diagnosis between neuroblastoma and Wilms' tumor should also be

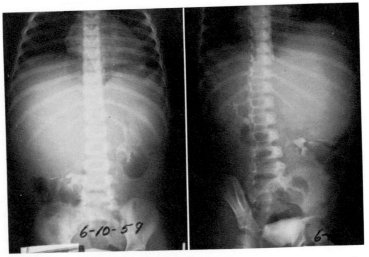

Fig. 41-7. Mass above right kidney in child, depressing and distorting the kidney. Oblique view on right. Neuroblastoma.

made, since therapy is different: a very fine stippled calcification is seen in the neuroblastoma, which involves the kidney only indirectly (by pushing it down and involving the cortex or a portion of the cortex so that the intravenous pyelogram shows good function in a portion of the kidney) (Fig. 41-7). On the other hand, Wilms' tumor usually involves the entire kidney and usually has no calcification.

Treatment. The treatment of Wilms' tumor consists of three modalities: (1) surgical removal of the primary tumor, (2) irradiation therapy, and (3) chemotherapy. For Wilms' tumors, actinomycin D seems to be almost specific. Treatment must be carried out over a long period of time so that metastatic lesions are destroyed. Results have been steadily improving, so that in patients who do not have obvious metastases, an 80% 5-year survival can be expected. Vincristine sulfate is also useful in chemotherapy for Wilms' tumor.

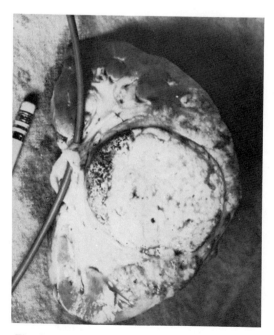

Fig. 41-8. Carcinoma of the kidney parenchyma.

Neoplasms of the adult kidney substance (Fig. 41-8)

A. General
    1. All neoplasms are malignant, with rare exceptions.
    2. There is no definite agreement on the pathological classification of these tumors, but for practical purposes we can call them all hypernephromas (renal cell carcinoma, clear cell carcinoma, adenocarcinoma).
    3. Treatment is the same.

B. Metastasis
    1. Most frequent to the lung and roentgen-ray evidence is characteristic (snowball lesion).
    2. Almost as frequent to bone (pulsating osteolytic lesion).
    3. 30% have metastases when first seen.

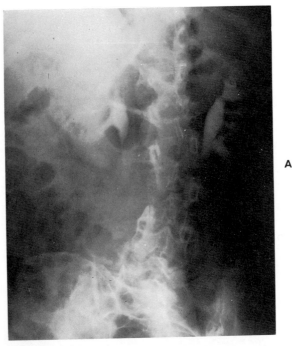

A

Fig. 41-9. Carcinoma of right kidney in a 52-year-old female shown on, A, intravenous pyelogram, B, retrograde pyelogram, and, C, selective renal arteriogram. Note metastasis to third lumbar vertebra.

C. Cardinal signs and symptoms
  1. Pain
  2. Mass—unilateral
  3. Hematuria
D. Diagnosis
  1. Suspicion is aroused by:
     a. Any of the preceding cardinal signs or symptoms
     b. Unexplained fever
     c. Unexplained weight loss
     d. Unexplained anemia
  2. However, diagnosis at the stage when these signs and symptoms appear is usually too late for curative therapy.
  3. Cytological studies of the urine show promise of aiding early diagnosis in those tumors developing close to the urothelium.

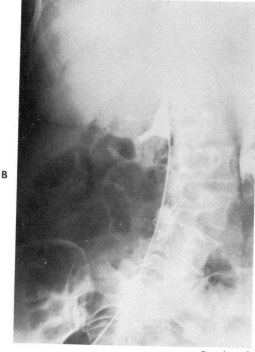

Continued.
Fig. 41-9, cont'd. For legend see opposite page.

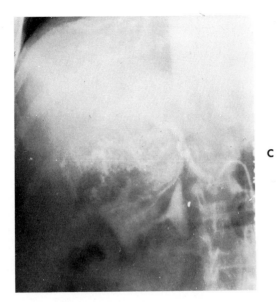

C

Fig. 41-9, cont'd. For legend see p. 932.

4. Roentgen-ray diagnosis:
   a. Characteristic pyelogram (Fig. 41-9):
      (1) Quite characteristic splaying or spiderlike deformity of calyces
      (2) Asymmetric enlargement of kidney substance on film
      (3) Obscuring of the renal outline
      (4) Irregular calcifications
   b. Pulmonary metastasis
   c. Bone metastasis
E. Differential diagnosis
   1. Congenital lesions:
      a. Cysts
         (1) Polycystic—usually bilateral
         (2) Solitary—cannot tell by radiographic examination, calcification less frequent, radiolucent center, smooth wall
         (3) Multiple solitary—same as for solitary
   2. Trauma: Hematoma—history, blood clot is not smooth in outline, clot is generally movable in the pelvis and will gradually disappear.
   3. Infection:
      a. Renal carbuncle—tenderness, renal mass, chills and fever, W.B.C. count elevated, history of diabetes mellitus

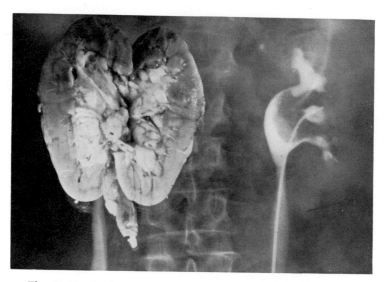

Fig. 41-10. Carcinoma of renal pelvis: pyelogram and specimen.

    b. Tuberculosis—history of contact and above
    c. Parasites—unlikely from environment
4. Stone—smooth, movable, does not disappear, roentgen-ray evidence, blood chemistry studies.

Treatment. Surgical removal (in some cases with external radiotherapy) has improved results. A 40 to 50% 5-year survival is expected if there are no metastases when the diagnosis is made.

Neoplasms of the urothelium

Tumors arising from the urothelium are relatively uncommon but present a serious diagnostic problem (Fig. 41-10). The most common symptoms are gross hematuria and pain that simulates a renal calculus. Retrograde pyelography shows filling defects or distortions of the calyces that are quite characteristic but need to be distinguished from nonopaque stone and blood clot. They frequently metastasize along the ureter or into the bladder, and sometimes this presents a problem in differential diagnosis in that the tumor blocks the ureter, presents itself in the bladder, and appears to be a carcinoma of the bladder that is blocking off the outflow of urine from the kidney.

Separate bladder tumors are seen in about half the patients with renal pelvic or ureteral tumors.

The treatment is surgical. At times cytology of the urine from the ureters is helpful in differential diagnosis.

Renal injuries

Renal injuries may be divided into two types: *penetrating* and *blunt*. The former are caused by bullet or knife wounds, and the latter are caused by indirect injury. With regard to the latter type, a kidney that is already the seat of a pathological lesion is more easily injured because (1) inflamed or tumor tissue is more friable and (2) the increased size of the diseased kidney makes it more accessible to the forces producing the injury. Renal injuries may also be classified according to the extent of the injury: (1) a sight tear or

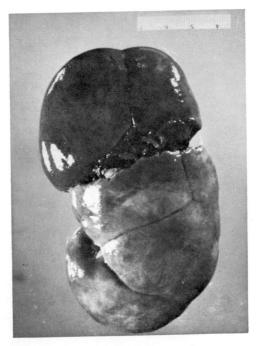

Fig. 41-11. Total rupture of kidney from trauma.

contusion, (2) a marked tear of the renal substance, (3) a tear of the kidney substance involving the renal pelvis, (4) a hematoma about the kidney, and (5) the vessels or ureter may be torn off.

The ensuing symptoms, signs, and pathological changes depend on the nature and extent of the lesion. Extravasation of urine into the kidney substance may occur, producing necrosis and subsequent infection. Massive hemorrhage or massive renal infarction may result. Serious late sequelae to kidney trauma can occur, including scarring and caliectasis with poor drainage from portions of the kidney, leading to hypertension, stone formation, and renal infection.

Symptoms and diagnosis. After the history of injury, pain, hematuria, a mass on the injured side, marked muscle spasm, and tenderness with shock may appear. Physical, urine, blood, and radiographic examinations should be done immediately. The findings are varying degrees of shock, hemorrhage, a mass with tenderness in the area of the renal injury, and abdominal distension. Hematuria is variable, depending on whether the blood has access to the ureter. Intravenous and retrograde pyelograms confirm the diagnosis, although intravenous pyelograms are useless if the patient is in shock. Abdominal aortography plus renal arteriography and even celiac axis injection are most helpful in identifying the site and character of vascular injuries. Pyelography may be required in the operating room. Careful consideration of both kidneys and all the renal substance involved is necessary. The best surgical approach is transabdominal to allow evaluation of all other intra-abdominal organs as well as both renal arteries and both kidneys. The surgical procedure is tailored to the precise injury, from simple suture to nephrectomy (Fig. 41-11).

Postinjury checkup examinations should be done every 2 months for at least a year (with intravenous pyelography) to evaluate possible permanent damage to the kidney.

One other form of injury associated with trauma, called the *crush syndrome,* must be considered. Massive amounts of crushed tissue can cause severe oliguria and acute tubular necrosis. Fluids must be managed carefully. (See Chapter 3.) In severe cases peritoneal or hemodialysis may be required.

Renal tuberculosis

Renal tuberculosis is decreasing in incidence with more effective general control of the disease by public health measures and antituberculous drugs, since it is part and parcel of hematogenous dissemination from a primary focus in the lung or gastrointestinal tract. The primary focus produces a temporary bacteremia of tubercle bacilli, which are filtered out in the cortex of both kidneys and produce lesions that

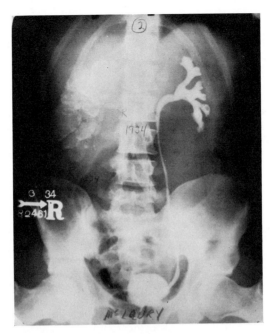

Fig. 41-12. Pyelogram showing tuberculosis of right kidney ("putty kidney").

usually go on to repair themselves. Occasionally, however, they progress and involve the collecting system to produce an open renal tuberculosis. Prior to the advent of specific chemotherapy, this condition became bilateral in nearly 100% of the cases and required prolonged sanitarium care. With gross unilateral involvement, nephrectomy was the treatment of choice. At the present time, with the use of INH, ethambutol, and rifampin, most of these cases can be controlled if massive lesions can be removed surgically.

Hematuria or pyuria is present with no evidence of pyogenic organisms, but with tubercle bacilli in the urine detected by guinea pig inoculation and cultures. Any patient with marked pyuria, with no obvious organisms on smear or ordinary culture, should be suspected of having renal tuberculosis. This is particularly true if there is a history of pulmonary tuberculosis, even though inactive and completely repaired. Pyelography usually shows the typical lesion: scarring and obliteration of some of the infundibula of the calyces and distortion and irregularity of several of the calyces in a kidney (Fig. 41-12). Tuberculous lesions frequently calcify. In fact, renal tuberculosis can present in so many different ways that it might be called "the great masquerader" and is similar to generalized syphilis in this regard. If there is no marked destruction of renal tissue or abscess formation, the treatment should be conservative and medical. If surgery is contemplated, chemotherapy prior to and after the surgical procedure is indicated.

Nontuberculous infections of the urinary tract

Renal infections are common and may arise as primary lesions, with entrance of the organisms into the kidney from a *hematogenous* source, much as we have just described in renal tuberculosis. On the other hand, they may be associated with *ascending infection,* starting with lesions primarily in the urethra, the prostate in the male, the urethra in the female, and the bladder in both. They may also arise from *infections outside the urinary tract,* producing lesions that allow the entrance of organisms into the perirenal lymphatics and periureteral lymphatics. If the ureterovesical junctions are incompetent, because of bladder infection, congenital anomaly, or neurogenic involvement of the bladder, renal infection is almost sure to ensue because of reflux of the infected urine into the renal pelvis.

Symptoms and signs. Urinary tract infection may manifest itself in many different ways. It may be discovered in an asymptomatic patient whose urinalysis shows bacteriuria or pyuria. It may produce disturbances of urination or pain over the region of the bladder or kidney. It may be associated with chills, fever, and leukocytosis, indicative of a general reaction. The history is important to rule out previous infections elsewhere in the body that might have acted as a primary source or some other pathological lesion in the urinary transport system. Thus intravenous pyelography, cystography (to evaluate ureteral reflux), careful examination and culture of the urine, and cystourethroscopy may all be necessary for complete evaluation.

General supportive therapy, specific antibiotics for the organism that is cultured, and correction of urinary tract obstruction or other lesions that predispose to infection are keystones of treatment. An ulcerated bladder tumor, stones, bladder neck obstruction, benign prostatic hypertrophy in the adult male, or urethral stenosis in the elderly female produce obstruction that sustains the infection. These lesions *must* be corrected if the infection is to be eliminated. Pyuria or bacteriuria does not mean pyelonephritis. It means simply that an infection exists somewhere in the urinary passageway or the kidney. Intelligent management demands a thorough quest for contributory anatomic deformities. The eventual sequelae of uncontrolled urinary tract infection are loss of renal function (renal failure) and destruction of the urinary transport system.

THE URETER
Congenital anomalies

Anomalies of the ureter are frequently associated with anomalies of the kidney, which have been discussed previously. They include duplications, fused ureters, and aberrant course.

Ureterocele is a cystic dilatation of the vesical end of the ureter caused by a congenital narrowing of the ureteral orifice (Fig. 41-13). It is symptomless until obstruction leads to hydronephrosis, stone formation, and infection. Diagnosis is made by cystoscopic examination and pyelograms. Cystoscopy reveals a thin-walled cystic body that intermittently fills and balloons with urine, then collapses as the urine is discharged from the tiny orifice. Pyelograms may show the cystic

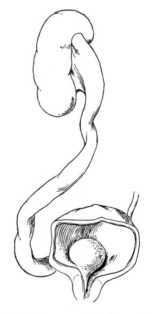

Fig. 41-13. Diagram of right ureterocele.

mass in the bladder and the secondary damage to ureter and kidneys. Treatment consists of removal of the ureterocele with ureteral reimplantation.

Megaloureter is a tremendously atonic and dilated ureter (Fig. 41-14). The etiology is obscure, although a functional disturbance of the neuromuscular mechanism of the ureter is the most likely cause. The condition is symptomless until hydronephrosis, infection, and stone formation occur.

Diagnosis is made by cystoscopy and pyelograms. On cystoscopy one sees the classical "golf ball" ureteral openings. Pyelograms reveal a dilated and tortuous ureter. The essence of treatment is to secure good drainage and relieve stasis, which may require ureterovesical implantation or cutaneous ureterostomy.

Ectopic ureteral orifices are often associated with other congenital anomalies of the genitourinary passageways. In the female, the aberrant opening of the ureteric orifice may be found in the vesical trigone, urethra, vagina, or even uterus. In the male the ectopic ureter usually opens proximal to the external sphincter. The symptoms affecting micturition vary greatly. In the female sphincter control of the ectopic ureter is absent, and urinary incontinence is always present.

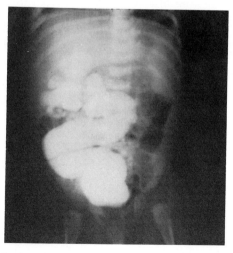

Fig. 41-14. Pyelogram showing right-sided megaloureter and hydronephrosis.

Diagnosis is made by history, urography, and cystoscopy. If the abnormality is discovered before renal damage is serious, the ureter may be implanted into the bladder, but if discovered after hydronephrotic atrophy and infection have occurred, nephrectomy is indicated if adequate renal function remains on the other side.

Other relatively rare congenital anomalies of the ureter include diverticulum, postcaval ureter, and stricture. Postcaval ureter is actually an anomaly of the vascular system, for the vena cava forms in front of, instead of behind, the ureter. The ureter is compressed by this overlying vena cava, causing a hydronephrosis that may later become infected. True congenital strictures are very rare; they result in hydroureter and hydronephrosis.

Injuries to the ureter

Injuries from external violence are relatively infrequent because of musculoskeletal protection and relative mobility of the ureter. When injury does occur, it is accompanied by other injuries of great severity, such as shattered pelvis, and generally involves complete division of the lower ureter.

Injuries from instrumentation are most frequently perforations made while attempting to extract a stone or to pass a catheter.

Injuries from surgery, particularly gynecological pelvic surgery, are the most common cause of ureteral injury. Normally the uterine artery and ureter are only 2.5 cm. apart, but neoplastic or inflammatory disease distorts this relationship and makes identification difficult. Injuries include incision, complete transection, occlusion, and necrosis from interference with blood supply.

Symptoms with unilateral injury include urinary fistula, progressive silent hydronephrosis, or pyonephrosis after infection. Symptoms with bilateral injury include anuria, uremia, and death.

Diagnosis. Indications of ureteral injury are the following:

1. Urinary fistula exists without bladder injury.
2. If methylene blue solution is introduced into the bladder and no dye appears through the fistula, but does appear through the fistula when methylene blue is given intravenously, ureteral fistula must be suspected.
3. Further confirmation is obtained by cystoscopy and pyelographic studies.

Treatment. Treatment varies with the extent of injury to the ureter and the location of the lesion. Small incisions or minor damage to the ureteral wall may require no repair. Large incisions or transections should be repaired over a ureteral catheter, if possible, and the catheter left in place for 8 to 10 days. Other procedures include ureterovesical anastomosis, ureterointestinal anastomosis, cutaneous ureterostomy, transureteroureterostomy, or even nephrectomy.

Ureteral calculus

Etiology. A ureteral calculus is usually a small stone that has passed down from the kidney pelvis. It rarely starts in the ureter, although an impacted fragment may grow larger there. The majority are composed of uric acid or calcium oxalate, since the phosphatic and cystine stones rapidly grow too large to pass down the ureter. The etiological factors responsible for stones in the kidney pelvis are also responsible for ureteral stones, particularly those of stasis associated with strictures and congenital hydroureter.

Symptoms. The types of symptoms produced by ureteral calculi are the same as those produced by a stone in the kidney. However, pain, hematuria, evidences of obstruction, infection, and renal insufficiency are more common with ureteral stones than they are with renal stones. Rarely ureteral calculi may be present for long periods of time without producing symptoms. They may produce gradual destruction of the urinary tract above because of obstruction.

Diagnosis. History, particularly of the known predisposing factors, chemical examination of the blood and urine, and dramatic relief of pain when the ureteral catheter is passed (beyond the obstruction) are important in diagnosis. Radiographic examination is important, particularly oblique films that will show the relationship of the stone to the course of the ureter.

Differential diagnosis. Calcified lymph nodes, phleboliths, pills, gas in the bowel, and skin moles must be distinguished radiographically from ureteral calculi. Of course, all other causes of acute abdominal disease must be ruled out.

Treatment. Surgically remove all stones over 1 cm. in diameter anywhere in the ureter, whether they are causing symptoms or not.

Stones under 1 cm. in diameter may pass spontaneously. Antispasmodics and morphine are given as needed, and fluids are forced. If the stone does not pass, a ureteral catheter is inserted above the stone for 48 hours. The catheter is then removed for another trial at passing the stone. If the stone is already down in the lower one-third of the ureter, an extractor is used to attempt to remove it under general or spinal anesthesia, after having dilated the ureter with an indwelling ureteral catheter for 2 to 3 days. Attempted basket extraction of calculi in the upper or middle third of the ureter is associated with a significantly increased complication rate. Ureterolithotomy is usually a safer procedure.

Carcinoma of the ureter

Carcinoma of the ureter may be either primary, arising from the urothelium, or secondary, arising from such organs as the ovary or the gastrointestinal tract. The reported age incidence varies from 22 to 89 years. There seems to be no sex difference or preference for either side. The lower third of the ureter is the most common site of primary carcinoma.

Pathology. The most striking characteristics of ureteral tumors are their ability to seed elsewhere on the urothelium (Fig. 41-15). The primary growth may be in the renal pelvis, and the secondary "seedlings" may appear in the ureter, the bladder, or even the urethra. Some investigators believe that a virus is the cause of these new growths.

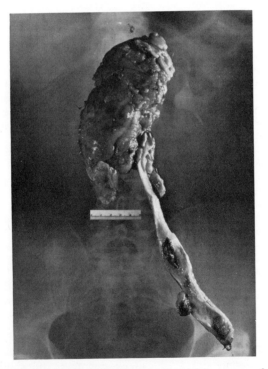

Fig. 41-15. Pyelogram and specimen of multiple tumors of ureter.

Ureteral tumors characteristically are slow growing and confined to the urinary tract. Two general types of tumor are recognized: *papillary transitional cell carcinoma,* which may either be pedunculated or have a base as large as the tumor mass itself, and the *squamous cell* type, which is nonpapillary, more solid, less cellular, and tends to be invasive. Metastases occur in the areas drained by the lymphatics of the ureter.

Symptoms. Hematuria is the initial symptom in 70% of patients with ureteral neoplasms; renal colic or a mass in the flank area are less common heralding complaints. The hematuria is usually painless and may be accompanied by fishworm clots. Pain may be colicky because of obstruction of the ureter but is more commonly dull and aching in character. The mass usually is a hydronephrotic kidney and not the tumor itself. Weight loss, easy fatigue, and a general rundown feeling are late symptoms of ureteral tumors.

Diagnosis. The urine consistently contains red blood cells, either grossly or microscopically. The significance of hematuria is that it tells you *where* the pathological condition is, not *what* the pathological condition is. Cystoscopy is indicated to locate the source of the bleeding: bleeding from ureteral tumor is usually continuous, not episodic, and the tumor may protrude from the meatus at each efflux of the urine. The drip from the ureteral catheter may be bloody initially, and then suddenly clear as the catheter rises above the source of the bleeding. On the other hand, vigorous hemorrhage may be provoked by the passage of a ureteral catheter. All of these signs point toward a tumor of the ureter.

The intravenous urograms may show nonfunction or hydronephrosis on the involved side. The retrograde pyelograms may indicate hydronephrosis and hydroureter, but the most reliable sign of ureteral tumor is a constant filling defect in the ureter.

Nonopaque stones or a blood clot must be distinguished from ureteral tumors. The nonopaque stone is usually sharp in outline, its position may move from time to time as progressive roentgen-ray studies are made, and it may scratch a waxed catheter bulb. A blood clot may also change position or disappear, indicating that the lesion is not constant.

One of the more recent and reliable methods of differentiating a ureteral tumor from a nonopaque stone or blood clot is the examination of the urinary sediment for abnormal cells, i.e., "cytology studies." Characteristically, the neoplastic cells have an increased nuclear:cytoplasmic ratio, a thickened nuclear membrane, and prominent and bizarre nucleoles, and often the cells are tadpole-like, indicating their origin from transitional cell epithelium. Cytological detection of abnormal cells in the urine is a useful adjunct but does not replace any standard diagnostic procedures.

Treatment. The treatment of ureteral neoplasia is early nephroureterectomy, with extirpation of the entire upper urinary tract, including a cuff of the bladder at the ureterovesical junction. (Remember that these tumors tend to seed themselves on the urothelium.) A single-stage procedure is usually employed.

An attractive alternative treatment is local resection of the neoplasm and adjacent ureter with end-to-end ureteroureterostomy. This therapy obviously conserves renal function in a disease that tends to be bilateral and recurrent. Follow-up includes interval urine cytology, excretory urography, and cystoscopy.

Prognosis. The prognosis of ureteral tumor is good in the papillary type, especially if the tumor is small, if the pathological sections show noninvasive characteristics, and if the involved ureter is completely removed with the accompanying kidney. The squamous cell type has a poor prognosis; invasion and metastases occur early.

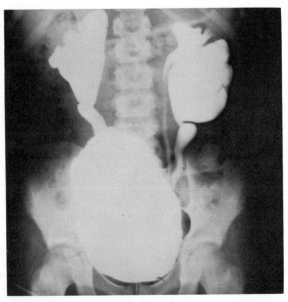

Fig. 41-16. Cystogram showing congenital bladder neck stricture with dilated bladder, bilateral ureteral reflux, and hydronephrosis.

Ureteral reflux

Ureteral reflux (Figs. 41-16 and 41-17) has recently captured the interest of urologists and internists. Although the relationship of ureteral reflux to chronic bladder infection has been known for many years, the common occurrence of ureteral reflux in many other conditions was not generally recognized until the past decades. Ureteral reflux plays a major role in renal infection and gradual renal deterioration in patients with neurogenic bladder and in children (particularly female) with bladder infections from urethral stenosis or bladder neck contracture. Renal failure may result from neglected bilateral reflux.

In some instances, ureteral reflux is associated with a congenital patulous state of the ureteral orifice with failure of the ureterovesical valvelike mechanism to prevent ureteral reflux. Urinary tract obstruction or infection may well predispose to ureteral reflux. Many operative procedures have been devised for its correction, the most common being the "tunneling procedure." This is usually successful in patients

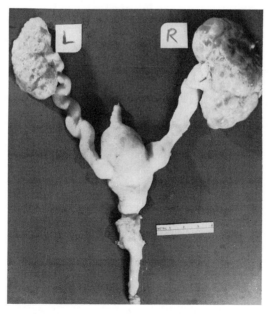

Fig. 41-17. Specimen of congenital bladder neck stricture.

who do not have markedly dilated ureters and in whom infection can be controlled satisfactorily. Ureteral reflux is usually readily demonstrated by delayed cystography or by cystourethrography.

THE URINARY BLADDER

The function of the bladder is twofold: to store urine and to remove it from the body. Any pathological condition changing these functions will usually be accompanied by frequent, difficult, and painful urination, nocturia, hematuria, and pyuria. These symptoms will be discussed thoroughly under the primary pathological conditions responsible for producing them.

A markedly or moderately distended bladder is percussible or palpable on abdominal examination. A midline suprapubic tumor should always make one consider the possibility of a distended bladder, which may also be palpated per rectum as a fullness above the prostate. Evaluation of the size of the prostate by rectal examination is hindered by a distended bladder.

Bladder function may be accurately assessed by simple tests. Catheterization will yield a great deal of information. *Residual urine,* the amount of urine remaining in the bladder after voiding, is diagnostically important. Residual urine in the bladder in any amount is significant of abnormal bladder function.

Roentgenography of the bladder may reveal valuable information. Stones and radiopaque foreign bodies will be seen on the plain film. The injection of radiopaque medium through a catheter into the bladder (cystography) outlines the size and shape of the bladder, trabeculation, diverticula, and ureteral reflux. Extravasation of radiopaque medium indicates bladder rupture. Micturition cystograms (roentgenray photographs of the bladder taken after the patient voids after instillation of radiopaque media into the bladder) pinpoint the presence and location of residual urine (which may reside in a diverticulum). Air cystograms best demonstrate filling defects from tumors, nonradiopaque stones, and foreign bodies.

Examination of the interior of the bladder by cystoscopy allows precise evaluation of the mucosa for inflammation, trabeculation, stones, ulcers, tumors, scars, and fistulous tracts. Cystoscopy is also valuable in determining the source of hematuria, i.e., whether it is coming from the bladder or the right or left ureteral orifice.

Cystometry is useful in determining the neuromuscular function of the bladder.

Congenital anomalies of the bladder

Complete aplasia of the bladder is rare and is usually diagnosed at autopsy. *Double bladder* is also rare; it may be complete or incomplete, transverse or sagittal. An hourglass bladder with a constricting fibrous band in the midportion has also been described. *Exstrophy of the bladder* occurs about once every 50,000 births. Complete exstrophy of the bladder is characterized by a lack of the anterior bladder wall with a fascial-muscular defect in the anterior abdominal wall. The posterior wall of the bladder and the trigone occupy this defect. Exstrophy in the male is usually accompanied by complete epispadias, undescended testes, and a bifid scrotum. In the female the clitoris is bifid, the labia are separated, and the urethra is epispadic. In both sexes the symphysis is absent, with a wide separation of the pubic bones. This creates the characteristic waddling gait of these children. Incomplete exstrophy of the bladder presents only a defect in the upper or lower portion of the anterior bladder wall. About 90% of exstrophies occur in males. The existing bladder wall is basically defective and often is associated with hydroureteronephrosis or even reflux.

Clinical picture. The diagnosis of exstrophy of the bladder is easy. The exstrophied bladder presents as a red outpouching of mucous membrane on the anterior abdominal wall in which the ureteral orifices and the interureteric ridge are clearly visible. The patient is constantly urine soaked and is physically and socially miserable.

The anomaly is not compatible with long life (50% are dead by the age of 10 years) because of upper urinary tract damage leading to renal failure. Another complication of exstrophy of the bladder is malignant change of the epithelium of the exstrophied bladder, which is said to occur in about 5% of the cases. An adenocarcinoma is the most common malignancy developing in an exstrophied bladder.

The management of bladder exstrophy consists of diversion of the urinary stream and resection of the exstrophied bladder. Attempts to close and reconstruct the bladder have been generally unsatisfactory. Diversion of the urinary stream is carried out either into the sigmoid colon, or into a rectal bladder from which feces have been diverted. This is a very successful operation if the anal and rectal sphincters are functioning. Otherwise an ileal conduit urinary diversion is indicated.

Results of treatment by this method are uniformly good and offer the patient comfort, social acceptability, and a good prognosis. At a later time the associated epispadias and undescended testes are surgically corrected. In all cases of the female and in some cases of the male, adequate sexual relationships and procreation can be achieved.

The *urachus* may give rise to anomalies that create definite clinical entities. Patent urachus is characterized by a fistula draining urine at the umbilicus, or in the midline between the symphysis and the umbilicus. The urachus may obliterate at the upper end only, forming a pouch off the bladder that may harbor stones and infection. Both ends of the urachus may obliterate, leaving a blind pouch in which calculi may also form. Adenocarcinoma and sarcoma in these urachal cysts have also been reported. Diagnosis of these lesions is confirmed by (1) cystography and (2) cystoscopy and endoscopic examination of the lower urinary tract. The treatment consists of surgical removal of such lesions.

Hernias of the bladder are uncommon. They are usually found in "sliding" direct inguinal or femoral hernias.

Traumatic injuries of the bladder

Traumatic perforations of the urinary bladder result in two different pathological entities: intraperitoneal or extraperitoneal urinary extravasation. Rupture of the bladder is caused by a variety of agents: instrumentation, penetrating wounds, and direct or indirect blows. The most common causes of ruptured bladder are comminuted fracture of the bony pelvis and operative damage incurred during transurethral manipulation or open pelvic operations. Penetrating wounds of the bladder are commonly associated with damage to other abdominal viscera. Sudden changes in directional force when the bladder is full may cause rupture of the urethra at the junction of the prostatic and membranous portion.

Diagnosis. The diagnosis of bladder or urethral rupture is not always simple. A history of trauma followed by hematuria and pain suprapubically with voiding abnormalities suggests a ruptured bladder. Extraperitoneal extravasation of urine may produce only moderate tenderness and rigidity of the lower abdomen, although later a mass becomes apparent on the anterior abdominal wall that may extend upward to the umbilicus and laterally to the inguinal ligament, or may be felt as a mass above the prostate on rectal examination. By this time the patient is extremely ill with fever, chills, nausea, and vomiting. Urinalysis reveals gross or microscopic hematuria. Leukocytosis is also present.

If the rupture is intraperitoneal, the patient will have generalized abdominal tenderness and rigidity, paralytic ileus, shock, and the other well-known signs of generalized peritonitis.

Final diagnosis rests on visualization of the bladder extravasation by cystography with radiopaque media. Differentiation between rupture of the bladder and the prostatic urethra is important; if a catheter passes easily into the bladder it is presumptive evidence that the urethra is intact.

Treatment. The treatment of a ruptured bladder (or urethra) is prompt surgical closure of the rent with perivesical drainage. The bladder itself is drained with an indwelling urethral or suprapubic catheter. Supportive treatment and large doses of antibiotics are vitally important. To temporize by catheter drainage alone in a suspected rupture of the bladder invites disaster.

Foreign bodies

Foreign bodies arrive in the bladder in a number of different ways. They may come through the bladder wall, through the urethra, or through fistulous openings into the bladder from some other viscera. The variety and number of foreign bodies introduced into the bladder through the urethra by children and adults is amazing: e.g., paraffin, chewing gum, hairpins, matches, insects, worms, snakes, rubber tubing, and balloons.

The clinical features are those of marked bladder irritation: frequency, dysuria, tenesmus, hematuria, and pyuria are prominent. The diagnosis of foreign bodies rests upon demonstration by radiographic and cystoscopic studies.

Treatment is removal either transurethrally with an instrument or through a suprapubic cystotomy.

Inflammatory disease of the bladder

Inflammatory disease of the bladder is very common. This is true in women of all ages, but particularly in young girls and elderly women. It is associated with frequency, dysuria, aching in the suprapubic area, and bacteria and pus cells in the urine in abnormal quantities.

Extravesical sources for the infection must be ruled out, as well as vesical tumor, vesical stones, and obstructions.

Ureteral reflux is evaluated by delayed cystography. Cystoscopy will distinguish a vesical infection from some other underlying lesion such as a diverticulum, a neurogenic bladder, a stone or a tumor, or a bladder neck contracture. The urethra must be calibrated to rule out urethral stenosis. Careful study of the bladder neck is indicated to rule out congenital bladder neck contracture, valves at the bladder neck, or some other bladder neck obstruction. Prostatitis in the male is a common cause. When these conditions are eliminated, the diagnosis of primary bladder infection is made. The treatment is straightforward. Culture and sensitivity tests indicate the proper antibiotic to be used, generally one with a broad spectrum of effect because colon bacilli of various kinds are almost invariably responsible. Vaginal infections and cervical infections must be treated, because the short female urethra allows reinfection from these adjacent areas. Topical application of 1:1,000 or 1:750 silver nitrate solution or 1:6 nitrofurazone (Furacin) solution helps in the treatment of the local infection.

Interstitial cystitis or *Hunner's ulcer* is a peculiar type of cystitis,

Table 41-5. The neurogenic bladder

Type	Voluntary control	Condition of bladder; muscle tone	Bladder capacity	Micturition
Sensory atonic	Absent	Flaccid and distended; myogenic tone decreased	Considerably increased	Early stage—incomplete emptying Late stage—overflow incontinence; dribbling
Motor atonic	Absent	Flaccid and distended; myogenic tone decreased	Considerably increased	Early stage—incomplete emptying; sense of distension Late stage—overflow incontinence; dribbling
Autonomous	Absent	Myogenic tone preserved	Variable—may be increased or somewhat reduced	Early stage—inability to void; distended bladder Late stage—dribbling and straining
Reflex (automatic)	Absent	Variable—may be below normal, normal, or above normal	Variable—may be reduced or increased	Early stage—inability to void Late stage—reflex and precipitous urination
Uninhibited	Maintained by external sphincter but often insufficient to preserve continence	Normal	Decreased	Precipitous and frequent

Residual urine	Infection	Etiology	Responsible conditions	Comment
Large volume	Common	Loss of sensory supply to bladder, as in lesions of posterior roots and columns	Acute (shock) stage of spinal injury; tabes dorsalis; diabetic radiculitis; subacute combined sclerosis	With the subsidence of spinal shock this type will merge into the reflex bladder unless severe myogenic disturbance has occurred through overdistension
Large volume	Common	Loss of motor supply to bladder, as in lesions of anterior horns and roots of sacral segments 3 and 4	May be part of the picture of spinal shock or occur in acute poliomyelitis	This type of bladder disturbance is also susceptible to myogenic disturbance, as above, but usually not to such severe degree
Present, usually in small or moderate amounts	Generally present	Complete interruption of reflex arc when both the sensory and motor components are destroyed	Traumatic lesions of sacral cord or conus; spina bifida manifesta; traumatic lesions of nervi erigentes	Patient may be able to express some urine by straining or manual compression
Present in variable amounts, depending on muscle tone of bladder	Often present	Complete interruption of upper motor neuron control; spinal arc present	Traumatic lesions of spinal cord above sacral level (after period of shock); spinal cord tumor; multiple sclerosis	Patient may discover "trigger areas" for induction of micturition
None	Absent	Loss of cerebral inhibitory control	Cerebral arteriosclerosis; brain tumor; brain injury; incomplete lesions of spinal cord; delayed development of cerebral inhibitory mechanism	This type shows least variance from normal bladder activity

much more frequently found in women than in men. It is characterized by sterile, clear urine, without inflammatory cells but with painful and frequent urination. Cystoscopic examination reveals areas of hemorrhage and cracking of the vesical mucosa, usually in the fundus, when the bladder is distended. This lesion responds best to increasing strength of silver nitrate solution instilled into the bladder, starting with 1:1,000 and going up to about 1:500. Etiology of this lesion is unknown.

Other treatments include anticholinergic drugs plus hydraulic dilatation performed under anesthesia. An unfortunate sequel of interstitial cystitis is the small-capacity, contracted fibrotic bladder. In situ carcinoma may masquerade as interstitial cystitis.

Enuresis

All patients age 5 or older with enuresis should be studied radiologically and endoscopically to rule out an underlying lesion. Ectopic ureteral orifices, urethral diverticulum, foreign body in the bladder, congenital obstructions to the outflow of urine, and other bladder lesions are often the cause of enuresis. If a search for anatomic abnormality is unrewarding, therapy consists of anticholinergic agents and general psychological support for both child and parents. Many children with enuresis have delayed maturation of their central nervous systems, resulting in persistent infantile, small-capacity bladders.

Neurogenic bladder

In the adult, function of the normal bladder is controlled by conditioned reflexes, the highest center of which is in the cortex; any break in the pathway or derangement affecting the cortical center produces some type of neurogenic vesical dysfunction.

In infancy the bladder is controlled by a simple reflex arc synapsing in the sacral cord. Sensory stimulation from distension of the bladder is carried to this sacral center, triggering motor impulses over the afferent limb that cause the detrusor muscle to undergo a series of contractions of increasing amplitude until a massive contraction occurs and the bladder evacuates its contents. This pattern is influenced by training and environment until, in a normal child, the bladder is completely controlled by the conditioned reflex mechanism arising in the cortex. The contractions occurring in an infant bladder may be termed uninhibited contractions and do not occur in the normal adult bladder.

The bladder may be evaluated neurologically much as any other portion of the nervous system, for perception of temperature, pain, touch, contraction, and filling. The motor function of the bladder is examined by cystometry. Table 41-5 lists the types and summarizes the features of neurogenic bladders.

Diverticulum of the bladder

Diverticulum and trabeculation of the bladder are produced by obstruction to the outflow of urine from the bladder itself. Urethral stricture, bladder neck contracture, benign prostatic hypertrophy, urethral stenosis, and congenital valves are the most common causes. Diverticula of the bladder may occur at any age, and the large ones should be removed surgically and their cause eliminated. They occur in at least 10% of the patients with benign prostatic hypertrophy.

Carcinoma of the bladder

Carcinoma of the bladder accounts for approximately 10% of all admissions to the Urologic Service at the University of Iowa, numbering over 100 new patients each year. The majority of these cancers occur near the trigone and ureteral orifices, suggesting the action of a carcinogenic agent in the urine acting on the bladder mucous membrane. No proof of this thesis exists, except in patients who are exposed to hydrocarbons, as in the dye industry. The carcinogenic agent is beta-naphthylamine. Chronic irritation, vesical calculi, and chronic cystitis

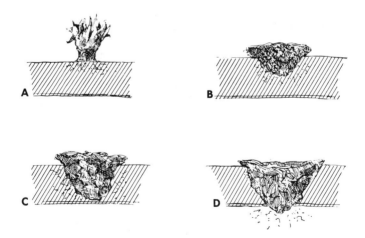

Fig. 41-18. Bladder tumors. **A,** Papillary, noninvasive. **B,** Partially invading bladder wall. **C,** Invading the bladder wall completely. **D,** Invading perivesical tissue, generally with metastases.

are not present in any sizable portion of the cases. Studies are being carried out to see if tryptophan derivatives may be related to vesical cancer.

Fig. 41-18 shows the four classifications (degree of invasion) of bladder tumors. Group A tumors are potentially 100% curable; Group C tumors are 23% curable.

Signs and symptoms. Although painless hematuria is the cardinal sign of carcinoma of the bladder, many patients do not manifest hematuria at all or only in the latter stages. Any disturbance of micturition or change in the urine may be a manifestation of carcinoma of the bladder. In our series, patients have been referred to the hospital with a mistaken diagnosis of chronic prostatitis or cystitis. Therefore, any patient over the age of 20 who has any disturbance of micturition should have a cystoscopic examination to rule out carcinoma of the bladder. Early diagnosis makes a tremendous difference in the type of therapy recommended and in the result of treatment. In our series of 540 patients, the average time interval between the occurrence of the first symptom and the diagnosis was 1½ years.

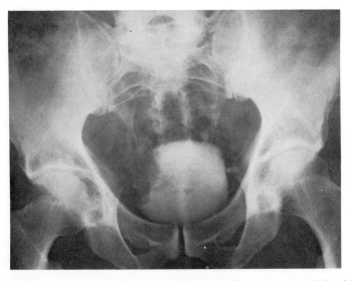

Fig. 41-19. Cystogram of tumor producing "filling defect" in right side of bladder.

Diagnosis. Absolute diagnosis is based upon cystoscopic examination with biopsy of suspicious tissue. The lateral air cystogram and the intravenous pyelogram may visualize a bladder tumor, particularly if it is large and papillary or if it obstructs a ureter (Fig. 41-19).

Cytology studies of the bladder urine may reveal suspicious cells; this line of investigation is still in its infancy.

The differential diagnosis between transitional cell carcinoma of the bladder and adenocarcinoma of the dome of the bladder (urachal rest tumor), carcinoma of an adjacent organ invading the bladder (sigmoid colon, prostate, cervix, uterus), and intense chronic cystitis may be difficult even after microscopic study of sections of the tumor. All these lesions require thorough investigation.

Treatment. The surgical treatment of carcinoma of the bladder is summarized as follows:

1. Destruction by means of electrocoagulation, either through the resectoscope transurethrally or through an open cystostomy.
2. Removal by open surgical procedure (partial cystectomy or total cystectomy with diversion of the urinary stream) to include the removal of the regional lymph nodes.
3. Palliative treatment: transurethral resection, high-energy roentgen-ray therapy, or diversion of the urinary stream.

In recent years surgical treatment has been greatly aided by the ileal conduit (ureteroileal cutaneous anastomosis) for supravesical diversion. This has proved to be superior to ureterosigmoid anastomosis, particularly in patients treated with irradiation. Several forms of irradiation (cobalt, electron beams, and intravesical radioactive gold solution) are valuable therapeutic aids. Systemic chemotherapy needs to be more thoroughly studied. Local application of thiotepa for recurrent superficial tumors appears promising.

THE PROSTATE
Congenital anomalies

Congenital anomalies of the prostate are extremely rare and then only in association with other anomalies of the genitourinary tract, such as hypospadias. Congenital cysts of Müllerian duct remnants arise between the lobes of a normal prostate. They may be felt on bimanual (rectal and abdominal) examination. They are treated by complete excision.

Inflammatory lesions

Inflammatory lesions of the prostate are quite common, particularly during middle life. They are caused by enteric bacteria, by gonorrhea, or by tuberculosis. They may be acute or chronic and can produce abscesses. The signs and symptoms vary, depending on the organism, the stage of the infection, and whether an abscess has formed. Acute prostatitis is marked by dysuria (frequency, burning, smarting) and retention of urine if a large abscess or an acutely swollen gland compresses the urethra. On the other hand, a dull, aching sensation in the perineum may be the only symptom of chronic prostatitis.

Treatment consists of general supportive care, prostatic massage, drainage (if an abscess is present), and appropriate chemotherapy after the organisms have been cultured. Tuberculous prostatitis justifies a search for a primary tuberculous focus elsewhere in the body, and appropriate antituberculous therapy.

Prostatic calculi may be an underlying cause for chronic prostatitis, and they need to be removed, either transurethrally or by open prostatectomy.

Frequently prostatitis is associated with impotence and with infertility. Both of these problems improve once the infection has been cleared.

Benign prostatic hypertrophy

Etiology. Benign prostatic hypertrophy is a common disease, probably the second most common disease of the aged male (Fig. 41-20) (generalized arteriosclerosis is first). It is of tremendous importance in geriatric practice; 75% of all males over the age of 60 years have

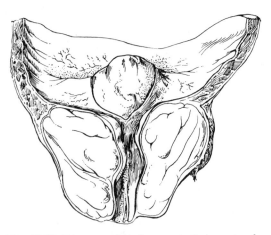

Fig. 41-20. Diagram of benign prostatic hypertrophy.

benign prostatic hypertrophy which causes complete bladder outlet obstruction in 50% of these (i.e., 38% of the total).

The prostate is a compound racemose structure composed of 100 or more outer (paraurethral) glands and 100 or more inner (periurethral) glands. Between these inner and outer glands is a thin line of compressed tissue known as the false capsule. A true capsule surrounds the entire gland, known as Denonvilliers' fascia. In benign prostatic hypertrophy the inner glands hypertrophy as nodules of fibroadenomatous tissue. These nodules push inward to distort the prostatic urethra, and outward to compress the tissue between the inner and outer glands. Thus the outer (paraurethral) glands are not involved in benign prostatic hypertrophy. The hyperplasia so distorts the urethra as to cause a ball-valve effect leading to urinary retention. The disease begins as small spheroids of hypertrophy beneath the mucosa of the prostatic urethra and interferes with urination, not by constricting the urethra but by acting as a valve.

With long-standing obstruction in the prostatic urethra, the bladder muscle hypertophies and the bladder wall becomes trabeculated. Later, small herniations of vesical mucosa are pushed outward between these hypertrophied muscle bundles, forming diverticula. Stagnation of urine, infection, and sometimes stone formation occur in these diverticula.

Eventually, the bladder can no longer compensate by hypertrophy, and the bladder wall becomes stretched and atonic. The ureterovesical valve becomes impaired by constant back pressure; reflux, hydroureter, hydronephrosis, destruction of kidney tissue, uremia, and death result. *The most common cause of a lower abdominal mass in males over 50 years of age is a full bladder obstructed by benign prostatic hypertrophy.*

Symptoms and signs. Urinary obstruction from prostatic hypertrophy has many clinical manifestations, including frequency, nocturia, hesitancy, urgency, inability to empty the bladder completely, episodes of complete retention, hematuria, pyuria, dysuria, episodes of chills and fever, back pain, renal colic, and a progressive history of slowing of the stream and diminution in its caliber. Oddly enough, hematuria is more common in benign prostatic hypertrophy than in carcinoma of the prostate, with about 25% of patients complaining of initial or terminal hematuria.

Long-standing bladder obstruction with renal damage also produces nonspecific complaints of poor appetite, anemia, general weakness, and at times excessive thirst and spells of disorientation.

The residual urine that remains after the patient attempts to empty his bladder is the most conspicuous sign of urinary obstruction. True, rectal examination can estimate the size of the prostate, but it cannot tell the degree of obstruction. Frequently, a huge gland will cause no obstruction, whereas a tiny nodule, strategically located, can cause complete retention.

Differential diagnosis of obstructive uropathy of the bladder

Many conditions, outlined below, produce obstruction to the outflow of urine from the bladder. In adult males, benign hypertrophy is the most common.

A. Conditions of prostate that cause obstruction
    1. Acute prostatitis
    2. Prostatic abscess
    3. Tuberculous prostatitis
    4. Prostatic cyst
    5. Prostatic calculi
    6. Benign hypertrophy
    7. Carcinoma of the prostate
    8. Sarcoma of the prostate

B. Conditions about the prostatic urethra that cause obstruction
    1. Perirectal abscess
    2. Carcinoma or sarcoma adjacent to the urethra

C. Conditions of prostatic urethra that cause obstruction
    1. Congenital conditions
        a. Enlargement of verumontanum
        b. Urethral valve
        c. Congenital stricture
    2. Urethral stone
    3. Traumatic stricture of prostatic urethra

D. Conditions in bladder that cause obstruction
    1. Congenital folds
    2. Hypertrophy of trigone
    3. Vesical stone
    4. Ureterocele
    5. Bladder neck contracture

E. Conditions of bladder that cause obstruction
    1. Disturbances of position—prolapse
    2. Diverticulum
    3. Neurogenic
        a. Upper motor neuron
        b. Lower motor neuron
        c. Sensory disturbances
    4. Spasm of the sphincters
    5. Myogenic atony
    6. Carcinoma of the bladder

F. Conditions outside the bladder that cause obstruction
    1. Abscess in pelvis
    2. Carcinoma of the cervix
    3. Diverticulitis of sigmoid colon
    4. Carcinoma of sigmoid colon

Disturbances of urination are the chief symptoms of diseases that involve any portion of the urinary tract, and not just those originating in the bladder or prostate. Thus the characteristic symptoms of obstructive uropathy must be regarded merely as evidence of nonspecific urogenital disease, until definite abnormality of the bladder or prostate is proved. Only complete urological investigation will differentiate among these many conditions that produce obstruction to the outflow of urine from these conditions that give symptoms of bladder dysfunction without obstruction.

Diagnosis

The following are necessary procedures for diagnosis.

Rectal examination. The prostate is smooth, usually symmetric, elastic, and mobile. We usually grade it from 1+ to 4+, 1+ being a gland of small size and 4+ being one so large the examining finger cannot go over it.

Residual urine. After voiding, the patient is catheterized and the amount of urine remaining in the bladder is measured. The normal bladder is able to empty itself to less than 1 ml. of urine. But on practical clinical grounds residual urine volumes of less than 50 to 75 ml. are not considered "significant" unless complications such as infection, calculi, or severe voiding difficulty supervene. The urine obtained in this manner should be examined for pH, specific gravity, blood, pus, sugar, and microscopic elements.

Cystourethrograms, cystoscopy, pyelography, renal function tests. Use these tests as indicated.

General physical examination, particularly cardiac status. The patient must be evaluated as a whole to determine whether he will benefit from surgical relief of his bladder neck obstruction.

Treatment

Treatment includes nonsurgical treatment, treatment of acute retention, and surgical treatment.

Nonsurgical treatment. In mild cases with an acute episode of retention, conservative measures are often successful for a time. Prostatic massage, hot sitz baths, urinary antiseptics, antibiotics, bed rest, and catheter drainage may take the patient through an acute episode and avoid surgery. Progestational drugs to "shrink" the prostate are still being investigated.

Treatment of acute retention. The essence of treatment of acute retention is to drain the bladder slowly enough so as to prevent hemorrhage and bladder spasm, yet rapidly enough to draw off more urine than is being formed. Should the patient develop bladder spasms or hemorrhage, fluid is immediately replaced into the bladder and the patient is watched carefully. Once equilibrium has been achieved, surgical treatment is carried out.

Surgical treatment. The four surgical approaches to the prostate for the cure of benign prostatic hypertrophy are (1) *transurethral,* (2) *suprapubic,* (3) *perineal,* and (4) *retropubic* prostatectomy. Although called "prostatectomy," they are truly only an adenectomy, or a partial prostatectomy. The end result of each approach is identical—removal of the adenoma to the plane of cleavage at the false capsule, with the outer prostatic glands left undisturbed. In none of these methods is the entire prostate removed. The operation called the radical total prostatectomy is not performed for benign prostatic hypertrophy and is discussed under cancer of the prostate, p. 964.

Transurethral resection (TUR). The resectoscope is introduced into the urethra and under direct vision the adenomatous tissue is cut away with a high-frequency current until the plane of the false capsule is reached (Fig. 41-21). *Advantages* are (1) low mortality and morbidity with short and mild convalescence, (2) average postoperative hospital stay is 6 days, (3) the disadvantages of open surgery are avoided, and (4) damage to the rectum or external sphincter is avoided. *Disadvantages* are that (1) the procedure is technically difficult and hard to learn and (2) hemolytic reactions, urethral trauma, and stricture sometimes occur.

Suprapubic (transvesical) prostatectomy. The bladder is opened extraperitoneally through a transverse incision above the pubis, and

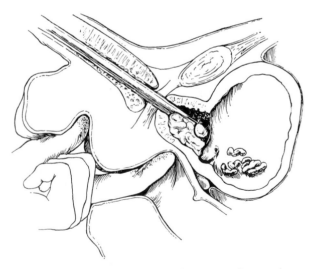

Fig. 41-21. Diagram of transurethral prostatic resection.

the adenoma is enucleated with the finger. *Advantages* are that (1) this is an easy operative technique, best suited for the surgeon who infrequently does prostatic surgery and (2) it avoids the rectum and external sphincter. *Disadvantages* are (1) relatively high mortality and morbidity and (2) delayed healing with urinary fistula and long hospitalization (up to 3 to 4 weeks).

Perineal prostatectomy. Enter through the perineum (Fig. 41-22). The prostate is detached from the rectum by cutting the rectourethralis muscle. The plane of cleavage is established, and the adenoma is

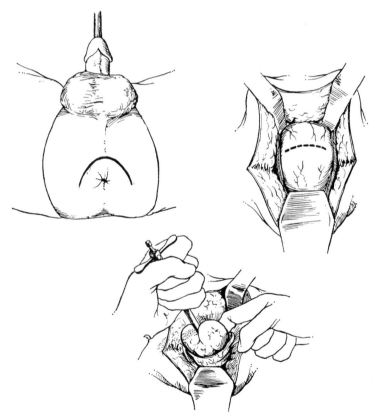

Fig. 41-22. Diagram of perineal prostatectomy.

enucleated. *Advantages* are (1) low mortality and morbidity and a mild convalescence second only to transurethral resection and (2) dependent drainage. The *disadvantage* is that it is technically difficult and occasionally damages the rectum and external sphincter.

Retropubic prostatectomy. A transverse incision is made just above the symphysis. The prostate is exposed in the prevesical space beneath the pubic arch. The plane of cleavage is established below the level of the internal sphincter, and the adenoma is enucleated via an incision in the anterior prostatic capsule. *Advantages* are (1) relatively low mortality and morbidity and a relatively short hospital stay and (2) a simple anatomic approach that avoids the rectum and external sphincter. *Disadvantages* are that hemorrhage from the prostatic venous plexus is not infrequent, and osteitis pubis may (rarely) complicate the convalescence.

Vasectomy. Many clinics precede a prostatectomy by vasectomy in hopes of preventing epididymitis. We have found approximately the same incidence of epididymitis with or without vasectomy. Probably bilateral vasectomy has its greatest place in preventing postprostatectomy epididymitis when it is performed *prior* to any urethral instrumentation. The scrotal route is most often employed, but an intrapelvic vasectomy can be achieved at the time of open prostatectomy.

Prognosis and results

The overall mortality in recent years for all types of prostatic resection in this country is less than 1%. Patients void well after resection, and only a small percentage suffer from incontinence or sufficient regrowth to cause prostatic obstruction.

Cancer of the prostate

Cancer of the prostate is the most common malignant growth in aged males, and, next to carcinoma of the lung, it is the most frequent cause of death from cancer in the male in this country. It is relatively rare below the age of 40 but occurs in 20% of all Caucasian males over the age of 50. About 40% of all elderly males suffer from urinary obstruction, and one-fifth of these cases are attributed to carcinoma of the prostate. There is no causal relationship between prostatic carcinoma and other lesions of the gland such as benign prostatic hypertrophy or chronic inflammatory disease. The etiology is unknown.

Unlike benign prostatic hypertrophy, carcinoma arises in the periphery of the prostate (in the outer glands). Thus, rectal examination may detect a carcinomatous nodule before it gives symptoms of obstruction and frequently before metastases have occurred, if rectal examination is carried out routinely. The neoplasm may remain limited to the gland itself for a relatively long period of time; then by direct invasion it involves the inner glands, the seminal vesicle area, and the vas deferens. Later it breaks through the capsule to involve the urethra and bladder, rectum, periurethral tissues, the lymph nodes along the rectum, the internal and external iliac vessels, and the seminal vesicles. Blood-borne metastases carry the malignancy to the bones, primarily the spine and pelvis, and to the lungs. In advanced cases, metastases occur to any other portion of the body.

Grossly, carcinoma of the prostate is a firm, white-yellow, irregular mass. It is an adenocarcinoma, histologically, which characteristically produces an increase in the serum acid phosphatase when it has disseminated. Bony metastases are usually osteoblastic and associated with an elevation of the serum alkaline phosphatase as well.

Signs, symptoms, and diagnosis. Carcinoma of the prostate produces no symptoms until there is a spread to the urethra or until the bones are involved, causing pain. Urethral involvement produces dysuria, hematuria, and difficulty in urination. Detection of a hard prostatic nodule palpable on rectal examination requires confirmatory biopsy of the nodule. Chronic inflammatory disease of the prostate and prostatic calculi may mimic prostatic carcinoma. Fig. 41-23 lists efficacy of various tests for carcinoma of the prostate.

Treatment. The treatment for prostatic carcinoma depends on the stage. If the lesion is localized completely to the prostatic area, a

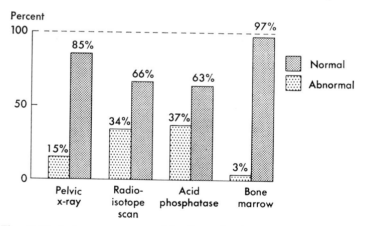

Fig. 41-23. Laboratory tests used in diagnosis of carcinoma of the prostate.

total prostatectomy can be carried out with a high incidence of cure. On the other hand, once the lesion has invaded the capsule, the base of the bladder, or the area around the seminal vesicles, there is a 50% chance that the regional lymph nodes are involved and a 10 to 15% chance of vascular metastases. Partial prostatectomy is often followed by local recurrence unless adjunctive therapy is carried out. Radical prostatectomy with instillation of radioactive gold may be helpful in cutting down local recurrence and bringing about cures in those patients who do not have dissemination beyond the local area. External irradiation (cobalt teletherapy, linear accelerator, and betatron treatment) has also been used as adjunctive therapy for this type of patient. If dissemination has occurred, local therapy to relieve obstructive symptoms must be supplemented by systemic treatment. The local therapy usually consists of transurethral prostatic resection.

Palliative systemic therapy of disseminated prostatic cancer consists essentially of altering the hormonal environment of the lesion by orchiectomy and the administration of estrogens. Progesterone-like agents and alkylating agents have some effect on disseminated prostatic carcinoma. Controlled clinical trials to evaluate the efficacy of chemotherapeutic agents in this disease are now being conducted at several institutions. Recently open cryosurgical destruction of the malignant prostate has been utilized to destroy the large local lesion and alleviate pain from bony metastases. As yet there is no good objective evidence of regression of metastases or of an enhanced immunological defense mechanism.

THE URETHRA
Congenital anomalies
Male urethra

Congenital valves of the posterior urethra may obstruct the passage of urine and, if not detected early, will produce marked back pressure with hydroureter, hydronephrosis, and ultimately renal insufficiency. Treatment consists of destruction of the valve leaflets, either by open surgery or through the resectoscope, to relieve the obstruction. Plastic procedures upon the bladder, the ureters, and the kidney pelvis may be required to correct the effects of long-standing back pressure on the urinary transport system.

Hypospadias. The urethra opens on the ventral surface of the penis in hypospadias, the distal urethra not having been formed. In addition, there is a marked ventral curvature, or *chordee,* of the penis. The corrective operations must first straighten the penis by removal of the fibrous band causing the chordee; then, a tube is fashioned of skin leading from the intact urethra to the glans penis. The untreated patient must urinate in the sitting position and is sterile, even if the chordee is mild enough to permit coitus, since ejaculation occurs outside of the vagina.

Epispadias. The urethra opens dorsally on the penis, appearing as a flat strip of mucous membrane on the upper surface of the penis between the separated corpora cavernosa. The severe forms involve the sphincters, causing incontinence of urine and often are associated with exstrophy of the bladder. Treatment consists of closure of the urethral groove by plastic operation.

Diverticulum of the urethra. Urethral diverticulum is rare and should be excised.

Female urethra

The female urethra is homologous with the posterior urethra in the male. Congenital anomalies are associated with defective development of the bladder, as in exstrophy and epispadias. In epispadias the urethra appears as a trough in the mons veneris.

Urethral stenosis. Congenital urethral stenosis is a possible cause of urinary obstruction in the female. It may be associated with urethral valves. The obstruction must be corrected surgically, usually by dilatation.

Infections

Infections of the urethra are common. They may produce prostatitis in the male and stricture formation in both the male and the female, with back pressure effects on the urinary transport system. They are the result of various types of organisms, pyogenic, *Trichomonas vaginalis,* pleuropneumonia-like organisms, and tuberculosis.

Treatment centers around identifying the specific organism and administering appropriate antibiotics. Obstruction to urine drainage must be relieved.

Gonococcal urethritis, caused by venereally transmitted *Neisseria gonorrhoeae,* continues to be the most common specific urethral infection. Symptoms in the male are an intense dysuria and a yellow-green purulent urethral discharge, whereas the female is usually asymptomatic. Diagnosis can be made in addition by identification of gram-negative intracellular diplococci on a Gram stained urethral discharge or via new culture techniques. Treatment in nonallergic individuals consists of high-dose parenteral penicillin G (4.8 to 7.2 million units) plus oral probenecid to increase further tissue drug levels. A combination of oral ampicillin and probenecid is an alternative. Patients allergic to penicillin can be given either intramuscular spectinomycin or an oral tetracycline. Treatment of sexual contacts as well will reduce the reinfection rate.

Stricture of the urethra

Stricture of the urethra narrows the urethral channel and is generally caused by cicatrix from old inflammation. It is seen in both sexes but is more common in the male. It gradually develops months or years after the initial episode of urethritis.

The urethral stricture is evaluated by radiographs or cystourethroscopy, with its length noted and the size of the lumen calibrated. Minor strictures may respond to dilatations, but severe ones require surgical resection to restore the natural size of the lumen. Unless this is done, there is gradual persistent damage to the proximal portion of the urinary transport system. Periurethral abscess, urinary fistulas, and infertility are other complications of urethral stricture.

Injuries of the urethra

Simple contusion may be caused by forcible instrumentation, false passage, or acts of sexual violence. There is slight to moderate bleed-

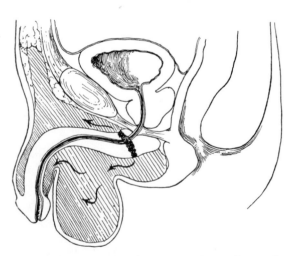

Fig. 41-24. Diagram of traumatic rupture of anterior urethra; shaded areas indicate routes of extravasation. Treatment consists of catheter splinting and drainage.

ing. Treatment generally consists of splinting the area of injury by an indwelling catheter, or suture of the area if accessible.

If *severe trauma* occurs, one must differentiate among ruptures of the anterior urethra, posterior urethra, and bladder.

Rupture of the anterior urethra is most frequently caused by forcible use of urethral instruments or lacerating wounds (Fig. 41-24). Injuries to the bulbous urethra are generally caused by straddle injuries or direct blows to the perineum. In both of these injuries there is a continuous drip of blood from the urethral meatus. A hematoma may form under Buck's fascia. The patient has no desire to urinate and later develops lower abdominal pain. He may have difficulty in urinating, and urine may extravasate into the scrotum. Treatment consists of antibiotic administration, immediate drainage of the area of extravasation, and splinting of the urethra by an indwelling catheter.

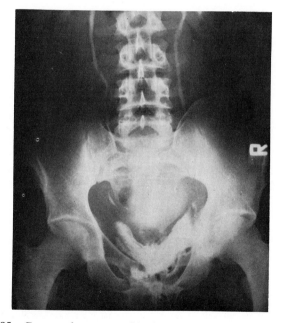

Fig. 41-25. Cystourethrogram with intravenous pyelogram showing rupture of posterior (prostatic) urethra with fractured pelvis. Note extravasation of contrast medium about base of bladder, which has been displaced upward.

Rupture of the posterior prostatic urethra is usually associated with fractures of the pelvis, severe physical trauma, and occasionally instrument perforations during transurethral resection. The patient becomes just as ill and "toxic" as in rupture of the anterior urethra, but there is no dripping of blood from the urethra, no hematoma under Buck's fascia, and no scrotal swelling, and the urine extravasates posteriorly into the ischiorectal fossa or anteriorly into the suprapubic area. The urethral catheter passes easily but may go through the false passageway rather than into the bladder (Fig. 41-25). Injection of contrast through the catheter determines if the catheter is really in the bladder. The patient will not void spontaneously even though

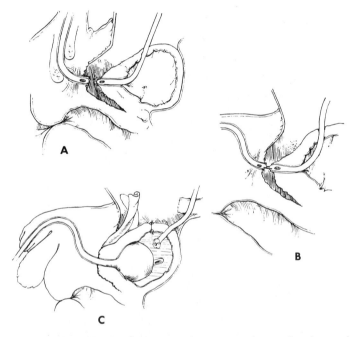

Fig. 41-26. Diagram showing traumatic rupture of posterior (prostatic) urethra and its repair. **A,** Catheters passed from urethra and bladder to meet at point of rupture. **B,** Catheter ends joined, and urethral catheter pulled on into bladder. **C,** Urethral catheter bag inflated and pulled down to splint the urethra; perivesical space drained, suprapubic catheter placed.

the bladder is distended with urine, because of spasm. Many of these patients die of shock or sepsis, if treatment is neglected.

Treatment of rupture of the posterior urethra consists of a suprapubic cystostomy, with possible retrograde catheterization of the urethra if the splinting urethral catheter passed from below does not enter the bladder. Later, plastic procedures may be necessary if fibrosis and scarring produce urethral stricture leading to chronic infection and calculi formation (Fig. 41-26). Long-term complications of posterior urethral injuries include impotence, urinary incontinence, and stricture.

Rupture of the bladder occurs from severe external trauma, usually with associated fracture of the pelvis, or from operative trauma. There is no immediate suprapubic extravasation or scrotal swelling, and frequently the patient is able to void. Diagnosis is suspected when saline injected into the bladder by catheter is not returned, and it is readily confirmed by cystography. Treatment consists of immediate suprapubic drainage with surgical repair of the wound.

Neoplasms of the urethra
Benign neoplasms

Benign neoplasms of the urethra occur rarely in both sexes. They are usually caruncles, papillomas, or adenomatous polyps. Initial hematuria is the most frequent entering complaint. Treatment consists of electrocoagulation through the panendoscope or direct excision.

Malignant neoplasms

Etiology. Primary carcinoma of the urethra is a very rare disease that, unlike carcinoma of the penis, occurs in both circumcised and uncircumcised individuals. A history of chronic urethral stricture is common.

Pathology. This neoplasm is usually an epidermoid carcinoma, but may be an adenocarcinoma; it is a relatively slow-growing neoplasm that arises with equal frequency in the anterior and posterior urethra. Urethral carcinoma spreads to the inguinal, external iliac, hypogastric, and common iliac nodes. One should suspect spread to the pelvic nodes if there is marked local extension into the corpora, or metastases to the inguinal nodes.

Symptoms. The symptoms result from progressive narrowing of the urethra and associated infection: diminution in size and caliber of the stream, dysuria, pyuria, and hematuria.

Diagnosis. Diagnosis is made by palpation of an indurated urethral mass and confirmed by panendoscope.

Treatment. If there are no pelvic node metastases, we advocate preoperative and postoperative deep roentgen-ray therapy and wide surgical excision. Palliative treatment consists of providing a free passageway for urine and amputation of the penis for cosmetic purposes in neglected cases.

THE PENIS
Anomalies

The most comon anomalies of the penis are associated with hypospadias and epispadias (discussed on p. 966). Anomalies of absence or multiplicity are extremely rare, as are micropenis and macropenis.

Phimosis may be either congenital or acquired and consists of a long, narrow prepuce with a minute orifice that limits the urinary flow and causes local irritation and inflammation. Treatment consists of circumcision.

Paraphimosis results from the retraction of the prepuce behind the glands. The prepuce becomes so edematous that replacement becomes difficult, and local ulceration or gangrene may result. Again the treatment consists of reduction and circumcision. A dorsal slit may be required if manual reduction is unsuccessful.

Inflammatory lesions of the penis

Inflammatory lesions of the penis are relatively common. They consist essentially of balanitis, chancre, granuloma inguinale, chancroidal infection, and lymphogranuloma venereum. These are all venereal in nature and yield to cleanliness, accurate diagnosis, and proper chemotherapy. Dark-field examination may be necessary to rule out syphilis. Yeast or fungal infections may not respond completely to anti-infective agents until circumcision is performed. Condylomata accuminata can be eradicated by topical podophyllin or by excision. Herpes progenitalis, caused by the herpes simplex virus, as yet has no specific therapy but is usually self-limited with proper hygiene and prevention of secondary bacterial infection.

Neoplasms of the penis

Neoplasms of the penis are not uncommon. Venereal warts are probably caused by a viral infection and are associated with poor hygiene and a redundant foreskin. They are readily treated by circumcision, coagulation of the papillomatous areas, cleanliness. They may be precursors to carcinoma and should be cleared up at all costs.

Carcinoma of the penis is very rare in patients who have been circumcised in childhood or adolescence. Uncircumcised people living in a hot, humid climate and who have poor genital hygiene are predisposed to carcinoma of the penis. It is a slow-growing, painless, fungating epidermoid carcinoma that usually begins as a small pimple

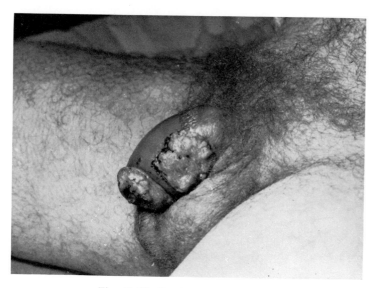

Fig. 41-27. Carcinoma of the penis.

or wart on the glans, prepuce, or shaft of the penis (Fig. 41-27). Diagnosis is readily made by biopsy; certain types of chronic inflammatory lesions (chancre and chancroid) need to be differentiated. The treatment consists of surgical removal of the penis and regional lymph nodes. The prognosis is good if the regional lymph nodes are not involved.

THE SCROTUM AND SCROTAL CONTENTS
Anomalies

Anomalies of the scrotum are rare and have little significance. A bifid scrotum usually is seen with congenital anomalies of the urethra such as epispadias, severe hypospadias, and intersex conditions. Congenital deformities of the scrotum are of importance only for cosmetic reasons.

Diseases

Carcinoma of the scrotum is seen occasionally as a soft, warty growth that soon becomes ulcerated. *Sebaceous cysts* of the scrotum are common; they are yellowish, rounded, firm, and may grow to the size of a marble. The cysts are asymptomatic unless secondarily infected; then they should be removed.

THE TESTIS
Anomalies

Anomalies of position of the testis are common, but anomalies of number are very rare. There as two types of anomalies of position: failure of descent (cryptorchism) and abnormal location (ectopia).

Cryptorchism is usually unilateral, but may be bilateral; it occurs approximately in 1 out of every 25 boys and is commonly associated with an inguinal hernia. The etiology of undescended testis is not completely understood, but it is probably related to maldevelopment of the structural route along which the testis must descend, or to atrophy of the gubernaculum testis. Cryptorchism is frequently associated with atrophy and alteration in the composition of the testis itself; degenerative changes of the seminiferous tubules are progressive after puberty, with sterility unless the testis is surgically brought into the scrotum (orchidopexy).

Failure of the testis to enter the scrotum is not abnormal until after the first year of life; after this, orchidopexy should be seriously considered, and in all cases should be carried out before the age of 5. The use of gonadotropic hormones from the anterior lobe of the pituitary gland has many advocates, particularly in bilateral cryptorchism. However, we believe it is better to bring the testis down surgically rather than depend on hormones or wait until the onset of puberty.

Inflammation of the testis and epididymis
Orchitis

Orchitis may be either acute or chronic. Chronic orchitis is usually secondary to tuberculous epididymitis, and it will be discussed later. Acute orchitis, too, may be secondary to infection of the epididymis, vas deferens, and seminal vesicles, or it may be primary and not involve the cord structures. Primary orchitis is seen most commonly in adults who develop mumps and other contagious diseases more characteristic of childhood. The diagnosis is made by palpation of an acutely tender, swollen testicle with or without involvement of the epididymis and vas defgerens.

Mild cases of orchitis are treated conservatively and symptomatically; bed rest, analgesics, elevation of the scrotum, and application of heat. However, severe orchitis is treated surgically by incision and drainage of the tunica vaginalis and albuginea; this will prevent the severe testicular atrophy that otherwise might occur. Corticosteroid therapy is indicated in postpubertal mumps orchitis to prevent post-inflammatory fibrosis and subsequent sterility.

Acute epididymitis

Etiology. Acute epididymitis may be gonorrheal or nonspecific in origin. In either case, the pathogenesis and treatment are generally the same. Usually epididymitis is secondary to infection of the lower urinary tract from prostatitis, urethral manipulation, or too vigorous prostatic massage. The infection travels by a direct route from these structures up the seminal vesicles, the vas deferens, and to the tail of the epididymis.

Diagnosis. The diagnosis is made by palpation of a markedly inflamed, hot, tender, and swollen epididymis, with or without involvement of the testis. Usually, the epididymis can be palpated separately from the testis. Accompanying these findings are systemic reactions with chills, fever, and leukocytosis.

Treatment. The treatment of acute epididymitis is medical, be it gonorrheal or nonspecific. The use of large doses of antibiotics, elevation of the part, bed rest and local heat will usually arrest the process within a few days. However, it may be a matter of months before the swelling and induration have completely subsided. One should eradicate the focus of infection in the lower urinary tract to prevent the opposite epididymis from subsequently becoming involved.

Complications. The principal complication of acute epididymitis is sterility, caused by obliteration of the epididymal canals and lumen of the vas deferens. Complete aspermia is commonly found after bilateral epididymitis even though testicular biopsy reveals entirely normal testicular tissue.

Chronic epididymitis—tuberculosis

Etiology. Chronic epididymitis is usually tuberculous in origin and should be considered such until proved otherwise. Whether epididymal tuberculosis is primary or secondary is in dispute. Many feel that it arises from the prostate and seminal vesicles as does acute epididymitis, traveling to the epididymis via the vas deferens. Others feel it arrives in the epididymis via embolic metastases and spreads down along the genital tract into the testis.

Signs and symptoms. Tuberculous epididymitis begins in the globus minor as a painless mass and may reach an advanced stage before the patient is aware of its presence. Palpation reveals a hard, irregular, and commonly fixed mass involving a part or all of the epididymis; the vas deferens is often irregular and beaded, and there may be a secondary hydrocele. Chronic epididymitis may be bilateral and associated with one or many draining scrotal sinuses.

Diagnosis. The diagnosis is often difficult. A history of pulmonary tuberculosis (usually arrested) is helpful. Careful palpation of the vas deferens and rectal examination may disclose tuberculous involvement of other genital organs. One must rule out testicular tumor, the Aschheim-Zondek test being of some differential value. A spermatocele will frequently cause confusion, but spermatoceles usually transilluminate. Tumors of the epididymis are rare and seldom confusing.

Treatment. The treatment of tuberculous epididymitis continues to be surgical. The prompt removal as soon as the diagnosis is made frequently prevents testicular involvement by direct extension. It may also prevent involvement of the other side. Simple epididymectomy usually suffices.

Chemotherapy has not yet proved itself capable of curing any but the superficial tuberculous lesions, but is helpful as an adjunct in the treatment of genitourinary tuberculosis. Treatment for 2 years is indicated.

Torsion of the testis

Etiology. Torsion of the testis is caused by a sudden twisting of the spermatic cord producing an acute partial or total obliteration of the vascular supply to the part. Torsion may occur in a normal testis, but it is more frequently seen in the cryptorchid. It frequently follows minor trauma and may be confused with an acute epididymitis. The immediate and mechanical cause of the torsion is thought to be a spastic contraction of the cremasteric muscle. The combination of an abnormal attachment of the testis, a deficiency in the gubernaculum, or an unusually large tunica vaginalis more frequently leads to a partial or complete rotation with subsequent vascular obstruction.

Diagnosis. Sudden pain usually occurs, followed by swelling, induration, and tenderness. It may be extremely difficult to differentiate from an acute epididymitis but usually careful history will assist in clinching the diagnosis. Elevation of the testis relieves the pain of acute epididymitis but does not help in testicular torsion. The testis undergoing torsion may assume a more horizontal axis and superior position because of shortening of the spermatic cord.

Treatment. The treatment of torsion of the testis is a serious, distinct emergency, and, if relief is not prompt, sterility and subsequent atrophy will ocur. The scrotum should be explored as soon as the diagnosis is even suspected. If, after straightening the cord, the testis regains its normal color, it may be fixed securely in the scrotum. Unfortunately, by the time the diagnosis is made, the part is often gangrenous, and the only recourse is surgical extirpation. In either event the contralateral scrotum should be explored and orchiopexy carried out since the tendency to testicular torsion is often bilateral.

Neoplasm of the testis

Incidence. In general, all tumors of the testis are malignant and should be removed if the diagnosis is suspected. Tumors of the testis constitute about 1 to 2% of all the malignant tumors in the male. Although uncommon, the significance of these tumors lies in the age group (20 to 40 years) affected.

In descending order of frequency, malignant tumors of the testis are as follows: seminoma, embryonal carcinoma, teratocarcinoma, adult teratoma, and the least common is chorioepithelioma or chorio-carcinoma.

Etiology. Although the etiology of testicular tumors is unknown, the undescended testis is distinctly a predisposing factor. All cryptorchid testes should be either removed or brought down into the scrotum as prophylaxis against testicular tumor development.

Pathology. There is no unanimity in the pathological classification of testicular tumors. From a practical viewpoint, they are probably best understood by classifying them according to cells. They may develop from any cell type found in the testicular tissue but usually from the germ cells.

The adult *teratomas* are thought to arise from isolated blastomeres. They are a mixed cell type, relatively benign, and uncommon. They cause no gonadotropic hormone to be excreted in the urine; grossly they may be solid or cystic. They are encapsulated. The cysts contain sebaceous and mucoid material. Microscopically they are characterized by a variety of well-differentiated and often unrecognizable structures.

The *seminoma* closely resembles the cells of the seminiferous tubules. Seminomas are believed to be derived from the primordial and primitive sex cells. They usually are unicellular tumors and are the most common of the testicular tumors. They are definitely malignant. Their gonadotropic hormone production is usually nil.

The *embryonal carcinoma* is a more highly malignant tumor and elaborates gonadotropic hormone in the urine but to a lesser degree than chorioepitheliomas. Embryonal carcinomas are rapidly growing and metastasize readily. Grossly they are soft, often necrotic appearing, and hemorrhagic in the cut specimen. They may be unicellular, in which case they are difficult to differentiate from the seminomas. Usually they are multicellular and may appear either papillary or adenomatous. These tumors are therefore often spoken of as either embryonal *adenocarcinoma* or embryonal *papillary adenocarcinoma*.

The *teratocarcinoma* is a mixture of fairly well-defferentiated teratoid structures. This tumor is definitely malignant, unlike the adult teratoma. The teratoid structures are seen intermingling with masses of malignant cells recognized as embryonal carcinoma, seminoma, or chorioepithelioma. Grossly, they are solid and contain many cystic areas. The solid areas contain the malignant tissue.

The most malignant and fortunately the most rare of the testicular tumors is the *chorioepithelioma*. These tumors elaborate large quantities of gonadotropic hormone. Grossly, the primary lesion may be small and often hidden until postmortem examination, at which time there may be metastases throughout the body. The tumors are soft, extremely hemorrhagic, and necrotic, because of the tumor's propensity to outgrow its own blood supply. Microscopically it is distinguished by Langhans' and syncytial cells.

Metastases. The mode of metastases is primarily lymphatic, passing up along the cord to be regional nodes: the para-aortic, the mediastinal, and the supraclavicular nodes. These tumors may, in addition, metastasize by the bloodstream, and lung metastases have occasionally been excised with apparent cure with no systemic treatment.

Signs and symptoms. Testicular tumors arise insidiously. The initial symptoms are usually a painless swelling of the testis and a sensation of increased weight. Because of the tumor's insidious onset, minor trauma to the part frequently directs attention to the mass. The mass slowly enlarges and continues to be painless. However, all too frequently the testicular mass goes unnoted until widespread metastases have developed with weight loss, abdominal mass, abdominal or back pain, edema of the lower extremities, or pulmonary complaints. This is especially true of chorioepitheliomas.

Diagnosis. Testicular tumors must be differentiated from hydroceles. Differentiation is often very difficult since a hydrocele frequently accompanies the tumor. Usually the mass will not transilluminate, but if any doubt remains, the scrotum should be explored from an inguinal approach. Hematocele may be ruled out by palpation. Chronic or acute epididymitis is frequently confused with testicular tumors.

The Aschheim-Zondek test for pregnancy was first applied to the diagnosis of testicular tumors in 1929. It should always be included in any investigation to rule in or out the possible diagnosis of testicular tumor. A positive test will clinch the diagnosis. Serial A-Z tests are useful in following patients with hormonally active testicular tumors. If after orchiectomy and irradiation the test remains negative, the possibility of metastases is remote. On the other hand, if it continues high after adequate therapy, the prognosis becomes much more grave. Some workers use the original height of the gonadotropic hormone excretion as an index for prognosis: the higher the gonadotropic hormone excretion, the higher the degree of malignancy. This is especially true in chorioepithelioma. Also, the lower the gonadotropic excretion, the less malignant and extensive the lesion is thought to be.

Prognosis. The prognosis of testicular tumors largely depends on the type of tumor and the time elapsing between its onset and adequate treatment. In this clinic, the average survival rate for all tumors is 5 years.

Treatment. The treatment of seminoma of the testis is high inguinal orchiectomy followed by irradiation therapy over the common routes of metastasis. In all other types of malignant testicular neoplasms, high inguinal orchiectomy plus complete node dissection of the inguinal, iliac, and the para-aortic nodes up to the renal arteries is indicated. Irradiation therapy is not as helpful for lesions other than seminoma. Chemotherapy is the treatment of choice in disseminated testicular tumors, and the effective agents are methotrexate, chlorambucil, and actinomycin D or the combination of vinblastine sulfate and bleomycin.

VARICOCELE

Etiology. Varicocele is the name given to varicosities of the pampiniform venous plexus. The veins become distended, elongated, and tortuous; 97% of varicoceles are found on the left side, and 5% are bilateral. Although etiology is unknown, the high incidence of left-sided varicocele suggests that the 90 degree angle by which the left spermatic vein enters the renal vein is, in some way, causative. On the right side, the spermatic vein empties into the inferior vena cava at an oblique angle. Since obstruction of the inferior vena cava may produce a varicocele on the right side, all right-sided varicoceles must be thoroughly investigated to rule out this cause. Defective valves in the spermatic venous system may also cause varicocele.

Varicoceles are usually seen between the ages of 15 and 30 years. Frequently they are asymptomatic. Some patients complain of a dragging sensation or neuralgia of the testis.

Diagnosis. The diagnosis of a varicocele is simple. The involved testis hangs distinctly lower than its mate, and its cord has a "bag of worms" sensation to palpation. The distended veins empty when the scrotum is elevated, and the "bag of worms" sensation disappears only to return when the patient stands. If the varicocele does not disappear with scrotal elevation, an intra-abdominal tumor or vena caval obstruction must be suspected.

Treatment. The treatment of varicocele is nearly always nonsurgical. In most instances surgical treatment is both unwarranted and unwise since varicoceles tend to disappear spontaneously with time. Furthermore, surgical ligation of the involved veins rarely relieves the neuralgia and commonly is followed by atrophy of the testicle, hydrocele, hemorrhage, thrombosis, and epididymitis, leaving the patient worse off than before surgery. Therefore, we recommend a scrotal support as the only treatment of simple varicocele. Infertility associated with varicocele may respond to ligation of the spermatic veins. Improvement in sperm count, motility, and morphology with subsequent pregnancy has been reported in up to 50% of men so treated. Although this surgery can be performed at the scrotal or inguinal levels, we prefer the retroperitoneal route to expose the internal spermatic veins superior to the internal inguinal ring.

SPERMATOCELE

Etiology. Spermatoceles are retention cysts of the vasa efferentia, epididymis, or appendix testis, and they contain spermatozoa. Most spermatoceles are thought to arise from scarring and deformity of the epididymis because of inflammatory obliteration of the lumen of the vasa efferentia, although some are traumatic in origin.

Signs and symptoms. Spermatoceles are manifest as slowly enlarging cystic masses of the scrotum in young and old men, and generally they produce only mild local discomfort.

Diagnosis. A spermatocele is palpable as a cystic mass separate and distinct from the testis, usually arising from the globus major. It transilluminates as well as a hydrocele, the fluid contents being gray-white in color and containing inactive spermatozoa.

Treatment. Spermatoceles usually require no treatment. When they become large they may be aspirated or excised.

HYDROCELE

Etiology. Hydrocele is an accumulation of fluid within the serous sac of the scrotum lying between the tunica vaginalis and the tunica albuginea. Hydroceles are classified as idiopathic or congenital, acute or chronic, and may involve the testis or the cord.

By far the most common hydrocele is the idiopathic variety, which may occur at any age. Congenital hydrocele occurs in the infant with an imperfect closure of the processus vaginalis; it may be associated with a congenital type of inguinal hernia, depending on the size of the opening into the peritoneal cavity.

Hydrocele of the cord may also be congenital. In this case there is obliteration of the funicular process proximally and distally, leaving an intervening lumen in which fluid accumulates. Hydrocele of the cord presents as a cystic mass along the cord, which transilluminates and is separate from both the testis and the epididymis.

Diagnosis. Diagnosis of hydrocele is established by palpation and transillumination, which will usually rule out a hernia and hematocele. It must then be differentiated from spermatocele. In a hydrocele, the testis is either not felt or is palpated within the hydrocele sac. The spermatocele is felt as a mass distinct from the testis.

Treatment. The treatment of hydrocele may be either medical or surgical. The hydrocele may be aspirated from time to time, with infection being the most likely complication of this conservative form of treatment. Surgical treatment consists of excision of the redundant portion of the hydrocele sac, with inversion of the remainder about the testis, or any other procedure that enhances reabsorption of fluid produced by the tunica vaginalis testis.

DISEASES OF THE VAS DEFERENS

The vas deferens is afflicted by the same diseases as the epididymis. Deferentitis may be of gonorrheal or nonspecific origin, as well as tuberculous. The acute pyogenic infections cause pain, swelling, and tenderness to deep palpation over the vas deferens and the lower quadrants of the abdomen. Systemic manifestations are nausea, vomiting, fever, and leukocytosis.

The treatment of vasitis is the same as for epididymitis: bedrest, heat applications, and antibiotics. The prognosis is usually good, with infection subsiding in approximately a week to 10 days. However, obliteration of the lumen is a distinct possibility, leading to sterility.

Chronic infection of the vas is usually tuberculous in origin and has been discussed in the section on tuberculous epididymitis.

DISEASES OF THE SEMINAL VESICLES

Seminal vesiculitis may be of gonorrheal, nonspecific, or tuberculous origin. In gonorrheal and nonspecific vesiculitis, it is often associated with prostatitis, epididymitis, and seminal vesiculitis and is simply a part of a general infection of the genital tract. The posterior urethra is the most frequent source of infection, which involves the vesicles by direct extension.

The acute phase of seminal vesiculitis begins with marked engorgement of the vesicles, which may progress to suppuration and abscess formation if the process fails to resolve. Later, a chronic stage develops with thickening and induration of the vesicles. This accounts for the ease with which they are palpated on rectal examination in the chronic stage of seminal vesiculitis.

Acute seminal vesiculitis may begin with systemic manifestations of chills and fever with or without urinary disturbances. Pain is variable; when present it is referred to the suprapubic and inguinal regions, but rarely as high as the kidney. In nongonorrheal seminal vesiculitis the onset is more insidious, with few systemic manifestations and little discomfort. Chronic vesiculitis is frequently asymptomatic except for pain the perineum, hip, and low back area. As it is frequently associated with prostatitis, there may be increased urinary frequency, dysuria, and the symptoms of prostatitis.

On examination one finds tenderness, induration, and thickening of the vesicles, in addition to epididymitis and vasitis. Seminal vesiculitis will frequently be followed by aspermia, oligospermia, or even a complete lack of ejaculate.

Treatment of acute seminal vesiculitis consists of massive doses of antibiotics, bed rest, and sedation. Chronic vesiculitis is treated with antibiotics and massage or stripping of the vesicles. No treatment is needed if the patient is asymptomatic. Hematospermia is a common symptom.

STERILITY IN THE MALE

Etiology. Fertility in the male requires (1) normal, actively motile spermatozoa formed within the testis, (2) free transport of the spermatozoa through the epididymis, vas deferens, and ultimately out the urethra, and (3) deposition of the sperm into the vaginal fornix.

There are a multitude of causes for sterility. *Impotence* may produce a relative state of sterility because of the inability to deliver spermatozoa into the vaginal vault. Impotence may be either neurological or psychogenic in origin. If the lesion is psychogenic, the prognosis is good with proper psychiatric care, but if it is neurological, the prognosis is usually poor.

Hypospadias frequently results in sterility on the same basis as impotence, the chordee and foreshortened urethra precluding delivery of the ejaculated specimen into the vaginal vault.

Stricture of the urethra will produce aspermia or oligospermia if the lumen is so narrow as to prohibit the extremely viscid semen from passing.

Prostatitis and seminal vesiculitis are thought by many to be a cause of sterility by altering the pH of the prostatic secretions to decrease seriously the motility and longevity of otherwise healthy spermatozoa.

The most common cause of sterility in the male is bilateral *epididymitis*. It may be acute, gonorrheal, or nonspecific, perhaps resulting from a prostatitis. In any case, after the acute inflammatory reaction, scarring of the tubules results with either total or partial obliteration of their lumen.

Orchitis is another common cause of sterility. Orchitis of mumps usually occurs during or after puberty and may result in extreme atrophy of the seminiferous tubules.

Patients with cryptorchism after the age of puberty are sterile on the involved side, and complete aspermia is the usual finding if bilateral. Secondary sex characteristics will develop normally, since the testicular atrophy does not involve the interstitial cells of Leydig.

Diagnosis. The examination for sterility should include a careful history of past or present prostatitis, seminal vesiculitis, epididymitis, or orchitis.

The testes, epididymes, vasa deferentia, seminal vesicles, prostate, and urethra are examined carefully, as a pathological condition anywhere along the genital tract may eventuate in either partial or complete sterility.

Examination of the semen. After a complete history and physical examination, the semen is examined. It must be obtained after at least 5 days of sexual abstinence, so that the sperm count can return to its optimal level. This clinic obtains the semen specimen by masturbation, and it is extremely rare that the patient complains of this method. There are other less satisfactory methods of obtaining semen specimens. Coitus interruptus may result in a partial loss of the fluid, making the count unreliable. The semen may be obtained from the vaginal vault of the female partner, but this, too, is an unsatisfactory method, since it is impossible to obtain the total volume of ejaculate. The use of a condom to collect the ejaculate is wholeheartedly condemned since the latex rubber is impregnated with solutions and powders designed to act as spermicides.

The semen is first checked grossly. Normal semen is milky in appearance, of a thick consistency, and has a high viscosity. The volume averages 3 to 4 ml.; the pH varies from 7.7 to 8.5. Any marked alteration from these norms should be noted; a low pH will result in decreased motility and longevity of the spermatozoa. A positive fructose test indicates the presence of seminal vesicle fluid; this function is extremely sensitive to even low concentrations of plasma testosterone.

The specimen is studied best microscopically about 30 minutes after delivery. By this time it has lost its high viscosity and can be diluted easily for an accurate count; little change in the motility of the sperm occurs during this interval of time. Normally, 80% or more of the sperm are actively motile; any decrease of the motility percentage lowers fertility.

A cell count of the semen is next done, which normally averages 50 to 150 million spermatozoa per milliliter. The specimen is diluted in a white blood cell pipette in the same manner as for a white blood cell count, using a diluent composed of 1% formalin and 5% sodium bicarbonate in water. This immediately kills the sperm cells. Two large squares are counted, as for a white blood cell count, and the result is multiplied by 100,000 (i.e., add 5 zeros to the total count). This will give the spermatozoa count per milliliter.

Although great reliance is placed on the total sperm count, it has little practical significance inasmuch as only the actively motile spermatozoa can impregnate the ova. Many clinics classify their degree of fertility on the actively motile count, obtained by this formula: % motility × sperm count per milliliter × volume of specimen in milliliters. At least three seminograms are required.

Medical treatment of sterility in the male. Thyroid extract, vitamin E, gonadogens, and gonadotropins have been found on careful experimentation to produce no significant increase in sperm count. Parenteral testosterone therapy predictably results in a decreased sperm count. Some authors have described a subsequent "rebound" phenomenon to justify the treatment, but our studies do not bear this out. Furthermore, and more importantly, since the entire process of spermatogenesis requires 75 to 90 days, any attempt to assess the efficacy of a treatment modality on the seminogram should be postponed until at least 3 months following the completion of the therapy.

Surgical treatment of sterility. The surgical treatment of male sterility is equally disappointing. The surgery may be divided into prophylactic and therapeutic. Prophylactic surgery is of vital importance: undescended testes should be brought into the scrotum before puberty, and severe orchitis associated with mumps may be saved from sterility by prompt opening and draining of the tunica vaginalis and tunica albuginea or by corticosteroid therapy. Urethral strictures should be dilated, and hypospadias with chordee should be corrected by appropriate plastic surgery.

Surgery has little to offer aspermic patients. Epididymis–vas deferens anastomosis has been attempted in patients with sterility secondary to old epididymitis with little success. Catheterization of the ejaculatory duct and injection of the vas deferens are mentioned only in condemnation. Vasovasostomy is successful in at least 50% of patients previously rendered sterile by bilateral vasectomy.

In this clinic, bilateral testicular biopsy is recommended for patients with oligospermia or aspermia. This procedure may be done under local anesthesia. The biopsy specimen is fixed in Bouin's solution, stained, and studied microscopically to determine the degree of spermatogenesis and to lend some insight into the etiology of the sterility. Biopsy allows a more accurate prognosis of fertility.

Treatment of low-fertility patients. Discouraging as are the medical and surgical approaches to male sterility, definite progress is being made in the management of low-fertility males. The date of ovulation must be determined accurately to allow the maximum number of spermatozoa to be ejaculated at the most opportune time. Spermatozoa are rarely viable for more than 48 hours in the uterus. The date of ovulation may be estimated by a sharp drop in the daily basal temperatures, taken just after awakening. This method will usually localize the time of ovulation to within 48 hours. It has proved a definite boon to the subfertile males, even though its accuracy is limited. Recent tests may be accurate to within 6 to 12 hours of ovulation.

Instructions to the low-fertility groups. After determining the exact time of ovulation, we are able to suggest the following course: sexual abstinence for a week prior to the date of ovulation; then, coitus should be undertaken the day before, twice during the 8-hour period of ovulation, and daily for the next 3 days. By this method the husband will be able to concentrate the maximum number of spermatozoa at the most crucial period. Strict adherence to this routine has produced very encouraging results in subfertile couples.

Men with documented high-volume ejaculates (6 to 10 ml.) usually have their spermatozoa concentrated in the first portion of the ejaculate, whereas the overall sperm count may be normal or low. Instruction about the technique of coitus interruptus at the time of expected ovulation to deliver the undiluted active spermatozoa has resulted in pregnancies in this select group of subfertile couples.

Artificial insemination. The initial successes with artificial insemination occurred at this clinic. Two general types are now practiced: artificial insemination by husband (A.I.H.) and artificial insemination by donor (A.I.D.). The former is indicated when physical abnormalities make normal sexual intercourse impossible or in the use of split ejaculates when coitus interruptus is unsuccessful. Unidentified donor insemination (A.I.D.) has many medicolegal ramifications, and the exact status of this technique may vary from state to state. Presumably its use would benefit those couples in which the husband is sterile, the wife is fertile, and adoption is considered less attractive. The concept of sperm banks has recently received much publicity, especially in the lay press, but the unclarified medical and moral issues involved make the use of sperm banks highly controversial and thus not recommended at this time.

CHAPTER 42

Head and neck surgery

CHARLES J. KRAUSE
BRIAN F. McCABE

A clear understanding of otolaryngological and head and neck diseases is important for the general physician, since somewhere between 20 and 40% of all the illnesses he treats will center above the clavicles. Upper respiratory tract infections (nasal, sinal, aural, and pharyngeal) are by far the most common sources of infection. A knowledge of these diseases is important for the specialist as well, because the number of general practitioners is diminishing in this country. Even the specialist must occasionally practice some general medicine. Furthermore, the specialist must not neglect disease in another organ system while treating that disease for which he is primarily trained. We must continuously dedicate ourselves to the welfare of the whole patient.

This section deals primarily with identification of otolaryngological disease by pointing out the *nature* of the process. Principles of diagnosis are stressed, and treatment methods are described only so far as they are pertinent. The student is cautioned that treatment methods in this field change very rapidly.

CONGENITAL ANOMALIES
Congenital anomalies with respiratory obstruction

Congenital abnormalities of the head and neck are important because they may affect vital processes such as respiration, deglutition, and nourishment. Some anomalies in this region impair the important modalities of communication. Of no small import are the cosmetic defects imposed by congenital abnormalities of the head and neck. Function is the most important consideration, but appearance is also of concern. Here we do not speak of the gross abnormalities, such as anencephaly or cyclops deformity, and the other monstrous deformities that are for the most part incompatible with life. The minor abnormalities, such as hawk nose, outstanding ears, cleft lip, and hypognathia, although not necessarily compromising function, are major concerns to the patient as a person. The good physician bears in mind that in one's physiognomy dwells the entity that a person calls "himself."

In this section we will consider chiefly those entities that alter function and that therefore demand early recognition and treatment.

Respiration obstruction in the newborn is a problem of prime importance, and a thorough knowledge of its differential diagnosis is essential. The following is a list of some of the important causes:

1. Secretory obstruction (mucus or amniotic fluid)
2. Choanal atresia
3. Tracheoesophageal fistulas
4. Congenital vascular ring
5. Laryngeal cysts and webs
6. Congenital laryngeal stridor
7. Pierre-Robin syndrome
8. Treacher-Collins syndrome
9. Rhinomeningoceles or encephaloceles
10. Laryngomalacia and tracheomalacia
11. Laryngeal paralysis
12. Diaphragmatic hernia
13. Bronchial or pulmonary agenesis
14. Brain damage and/or agenesis

Choanal atresia is obstruction of the posterior nares attributed to retention of the embryonic plate that separates the nasal chambers from the nasopharynx. The atresia may be unilateral or bilateral. Neonates afflicted with this abnormality do not breathe normally because *mouth breathing is not normal to the infant within the first 2 weeks of life.* Careful observation of the infant with bilateral choanal atresia reveals the following sequence of events: cyclic episodes of upper airway obstruction when the mouth is closed, associated with cyanosis and labored respiratory efforts that are dramatically relieved when he cries. Air is freely exchanged when the infant cries, he becomes pink and quiet, closes his mouth, and the cycle is then repeated. The infant cannot rest, and feedings are often aspirated because of the airway obstruction that this provokes. There exists a true respiratory emergency. The diagnosis is made by inability to pass a catheter through the nasal chamber into the oropharynx. Radiocontrast studies confirm the diagnosis: lateral skull films show complete retention of dye instilled into the nasal chambers while the infant is supine. Treatment consists of tiding the infant over the 2-week period required for mouth breathing to be learned. Feedings are given by orogastric tube. A patent airway is obtained by whatever means proves most satisfactory: decubitus position, frequent suction, oropharyngeal airway, and rarely tracheotomy. The nasopharyngeal plate may be perforated with a blunt instrument, but extreme care must be taken to avoid passing the instrument through the fragile and largely cartilaginous cervical vertebrae into the brainstem. Definitive operation for removal of the atresia plate transpalatally can be carried out as early as 1 year of age.

Tracheoesophageal fistulas are discussed in Chapter 28.

Congenital vascular ring is discussed in Chapter 31.

Laryngeal cysts and webs produce respiratory obstruction of the larynx and usually result in hoarseness. In the infant, this is manifested as a husky or nonclear cry. Cysts arise anywhere within the endolarynx or hypopharynx and are caused by malformations of mucus glands. Web formation occurs through incomplete separation of the true vocal cords. The cords are joined at the anterior commissure, much as fingers are connected in syndactylism. The laryngeal web is of minor consequence if it involves only the anterior commissure but is serious if it is nearly total, with a small breathing hole at the posterior commissure. *Subglottic stenosis* is a less common condition of congenital narrowing of the airway at the level of the cricoid cartilage. Diagnosis is made by direct laryngoscopy. The treatment includes tracheotomy and removal or repair of the lesion endoscopically, or by splitting the larynx. An indwelling stent for a period of several months is frequently necessary.

Congenital laryngeal stridor produces a clear, sharp inspiratory stridor upon crying or straining. When the infant is breathing normally and quietly, the stridor is not present. Mild cyanosis is seen occasionally, but unconsciousness by hypoxia does not occur. The lesion is caused by immaturity of the epiglottis ("infantile" or omega-shaped epiglottis), so that on sharp inspiration the aryepiglottic folds are drawn down into the glottic aperture, with consequent stridor. The stridor occurs *only on inspiration*. The condition is self-limited, but the parents require strong reassurance. The child usually outgrows his symptoms during the second year of life, as the epiglottis gains maturity.

Pierre-Robin syndrome is one of the family of mandibulofacial dysplasias produced by anomalies of the first and second branchial arches. Respiratory obstruction of the oropharynx is immediate and alarming with the baby supine, but is relieved in the prone position. The syndrome is recognizable at birth by simple observation of hypognathia, glossoptosis, cleft palate, and usually a cleft lip. The descriptive term *micrognathia* is used if there is no cleft palate. There is not room for the relatively large tongue in the patient's oropharynx because of the failure of anterior growth of the mandible. This must be differentiated from cretinism, in which the tongue is abnormally large and cannot be accommodated by the oral cavity of normal size. On inspection, the bulging floor of the mouth may resemble the tongue, but on pushing this down, the tip of the tongue can be seen pointing up toward the hard palate, well back in the mouth. Although feeding may be difficult, airway obstruction is the most acute threat to life. Careful positioning of the baby in the lateral decubitus or prone position is necessary for gravity to prolapse the dependent tongue away from the posterior pharyngeal wall to disobstruct the airway. An anterior tongue-tie, attaching the undersurface of the tip of the tongue to the lower lip, may also hold the tongue forward to keep the airway clear. Tracheotomy may be necessary. Tube feedings are often required. Curiously enough, the airway problems improve with time. Other congenital anomalies are frequently present. The fatality rate of this syndrome is high, exceeding 20% in most series.

Treacher-Collins syndrome, another of the mandibulofacial dysplasias, is a striking developmental defect of the first and second branchial arches and the first branchial groove (Fig. 42-1). Hypognathia and glossoptosis are present, as in the Pierre-Robin syndrome. In addition, there is an underformed maxilla producing the appearance of an abnormally prominent nose, outward and downward slanted eyes (sometimes called "antimongoloid"), a notched lower lid, bony atresia of both external auditory canals with severe deafness, and small, low-

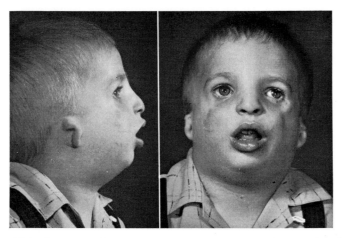

Fig. 42-1. Treacher-Collins syndrome, one of the congenital craniofacial dysplasias. The "bird shape" to the face and the eye and ear anomalies are striking. It is extremely important to place a bone conduction hearing aid on such a patient by age 1 or 2, so that normal speech and intellectual development may occur.

set, and deformed ears. The palate and the lip are usually intact. Early in life, the respiratory problem requires attention, but past infancy the mandible grows enough for adequate respiratory exchange without obstruction or stridor. In the second and third years of life, deafness is the greatest problem; the child needs a bone conduction hearing aid to develop speech and learn at an adequate rate. The external auditory canal atresia is corrected surgically to improve hearing at about the time the child enters school; this should take precedence over cosmetic improvement of the external ears. These patients have such a characteristic appearance that they are sometimes called "bird people" (Fig. 42-1).

In *rhinomeningoceles* or *encephaloceles* cerebral contents herniate through an unformed cribriform plate or other portions of the floor of the anterior cranial fossa to produce masses in the nasal chamber of the newborn that may obstruct the airway. The appearance externally may be normal, or paranasal masses may pulsate. Rhinomeningoceles or encephaloceles are smooth, pale, and pulsate on close inspection. Biopsy is disastrous, of course, and must be avoided by awareness of this diagnostic possibility. Rhinomeningoceles are approached by anterior craniotomy, and the mass is retracted back into the cranial cavity with repair of the defect.

Laryngomalacia and *tracheomalacia* are congenital defects in the ground substance of the airway cartilage, which cannot retain its shape on inspiration. The walls of the airway collapse proportionate to the degree of negative pressure created during inspiration. The only treatment is tracheotomy. Congenital laryngeal stridor may be misdiagnosed as laryngomalacia and wrongly treated by tracheotomy.

Laryngeal paralysis may be unilateral or bilateral. If unilateral, the condition is asymptomatic, but if bilateral, severe inspiratory stridor is present at birth, and tracheotomy is mandatory. Bilateral laryngeal paralysis seldom occurs without associated neurological disturbances, such as cerebral palsy. The diagnosis is made by direct laryngoscopy; the cords stay at or near the midline and do not abduct upon inspiration.

Diaphragmatic hernia is discussed in Chapter 27, pulmonary agenesis in Chapter 30, and central nervous system disturbances in Chapter 40.

Congenital anomalies not associated with respiratory obstruction

Branchial and *thyroglossal remnants* are discussed in Chapter 28.

A *cleft lip* or *cleft palate* (Fig. 42-2, *A*) is always alarming to the parents of the afflicted newborn, and they need reassurance that the

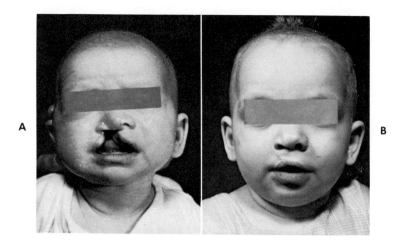

A   B

Fig. 42-2. Cleft palate and lip. **A**, Preoperative. **B**, Postoperative.

child can develop almost normally in function and appearance with medical care that is properly timed and carried out. The appearance of the cleft lip or cleft palate is so varied as to defy description. It ranges all the way from a minor notch or slight alteration of the vermillion portion of the upper lip to complete clefts of both sides of the upper lip that extend into the floor of the nostrils and nasal chambers, completely back through the hard and soft palate. Restoration of the intact palate is as important for function as repair of the lip is for cosmetic appearance (Fig. 42-2, *B*). Multiple operations, properly timed, are needed to avoid interference with proper growth of the middle third of the face. Dental anomalies, sometimes gross and bizarre, are invariably present. Speech and nourishment are difficult and require special help; cleft palate adds vexing ear problems, such as repeated acute infections and chronic serous otitis media. Thus the modern care of cleft palate patients is a multidisciplinary effort of a highly specialized team. The cleft palate team includes an otolaryngologist, a plastic surgeon, an orthodontist, a prosthodontist, a speech therapist, a pediatrician, a pedodontist, an audiologist, a social worker, and a psychologist.

Lingual thyroid, a prominent mass overlain by normal mucosa (Fig. 42-3), is located at the junction of the middle and posterior thirds of the tongue. It is diagnosed by biopsy or scintiscan. Lingual thyroid

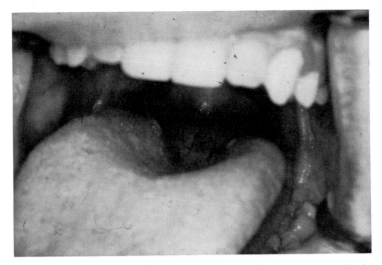

Fig. 42-3. Lingual thyroid, occurring at the foramen cecum of the tongue. Note the intact, unulcerated covering. Such lesions may be biopsied for diagnosis but should not be removed as a tumor, for this may be the only thyroid tissue the patient has. An ^{131}I scintiscan is a simpler method of diagnosis.

A 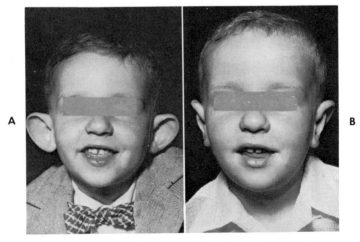 B

Fig. 42-4. Lop ears. **A,** Preoperative. **B,** Postoperative.

should not be removed until it is proved that other thyroid tissue is present, unless thyroid extract replacement is given.

Outstanding ears (lop-ears) result from failure of development of the anthelix of the auricle, so that the rim of the ear stands outward from the skull (Fig. 42-4, *A*). The ear is often cup shaped. Otoplasty will restore good contour if the patient is sensitive of the cosmetic deformity (Fig. 42-4, *B*).

Pretragal cysts or granulomas appear just anterior to the tragus of the ear and are caused by entrapped skin below the surface, from the developing hillocks of cartilage that form the outer ear. Incision and drainage is inadequate treatment; the entire skin-lined tract must be removed to effect a cure.

Floor-of-the-mouth cysts and tumors may be of many varieties. The *ranula* is the most common (Fig. 42-5). The *pseudoranula* is merely a blocked minor salivary gland in the floor of the mouth and is submucosal. The *true ranula* is an embryological deformity of the sublingual glands and perhaps other glands, with fingerlike ramifications into the substance of the genioglossus muscles. Simple intraoral excision

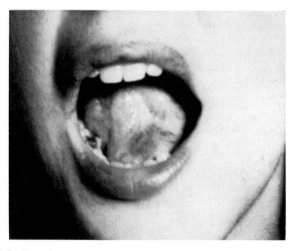

Fig. 42-5. Ranula. Note the intact epithelium over it. It is soft and cystic. Such lesions may be superficial in the floor of the mouth ("pseudo-ranula") or have deep extensions into the diaphragm of the floor of the mouth and genioglossus muscles ("true" ranula).

of the pseudoranula suffices. The true ranula generally requires an external approach for complete excision, although it may be managed satisfactorily by creating a fistula of the ranula into the mouth. *Dermoid* and *epidermoid cysts* cannot be distinguished clinically. They are fusion fault cysts, in which epithelial tissue is trapped between the joining mandibular arches. Differential diagnosis includes *minor salivary gland tumors, salivary gland calculi,* and *desmoid* or *desmoplastic tumors.*

INFECTIONS

Certain principles in diagnosis and treatment of head and neck infections are important. Infections in this region are very common and may constitute as much as 20% of the family doctor's office practice. Despite the proliferation of the antibiotic drugs, infection, like the poor, will always be with us.

Despite their frequency, head and neck infections should not be taken lightly or dismissed with a superficial evaluation. The complications may be serious and life threatening, e.g., extension to bone or metastatic spread to other organ systems such as the kidney, heart, or joints. On the other hand, they hold no mystery to the alert physician who understands the specialized structures involved.

In the treatment of acute infections, full-dosage antibiotic therapy must be instituted early and maintained for several days after symptoms have subsided. Whenever possible, cultures should be obtained prior to instituting antibiotic therapy. Selection of a specific antibiotic will rest upon what organism is suspected, a history of drug allergy, and route of administration desired. The antibiotic may later need to be changed when culture and sensitivity results are available. Acute abscesses, whether in the middle ear, neck, or another part of the body, must be afforded the time-honored principle of incision and drainage. Supportive measures are necessary, including aspirin for pain and fever, local wet or dry heat, bed rest, and increased fluid intake.

Chronic infections in this region are seldom amenable to antibiotic therapy alone, especially chronic sinusitis, mastoiditis (Fig. 42-6), and tonsilitis. The treatment of chronic infections in this region is surgical. When bone is infected acutely, it is usually amenable to antibiotic therapy, but when chronic infection is present, the bone must be removed. This can usually be done without significant alteration of function or cosmetic deformity.

Viral infections

The *viral nose cold* is the most common infection of man. Little need be said about it except that antibiotics of any kind render the

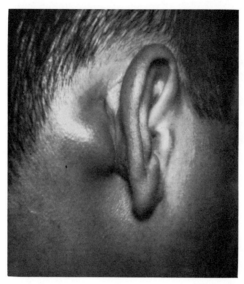

Fig. 42-6. Acute mastoiditis. Swelling with pain and fluctuance in this region is most unlikely to be misdiagnosed. The incidence of acute mastoiditis has been very low in the antibiotic era, but that of chronic mastoiditis is steadily rising. This patient has an acute exacerbation of chronic mastoiditis. The disease chose to perforate the mastoid cortex. If it had chosen rather the middle fossa plate (roof of the mastoid) or inner ear, the results could have been disastrous.

patient a disservice. The symptoms are well known, and the treatment is entirely supportive. The nose cold is generally said to be 3 days coming, 3 days present, and 3 days going. Any nose cold lasting longer than this is probably becoming complicated by suppurative infections of the nose, sinuses, or lower respiratory tract. *APC fever* (adenopharyngoconjunctival fever) is a mildly epidemic viral infection of the nasopharynx that, after several days of sore throat, produces a nonsuppurative conjunctivitis of first one and then the other eye. *Infectious mononucleosis* is also a mildly epidemic disease of young people, often heralded by petechiae of the palate or buccal mucosa. The tonsils are usually involved in the nonsuppurative process. The tonsilitis may on occasion be extreme, with severe sore throat and necrotic slough of the surface of each tonsil. Diagnosis is made when two of the following are present: (1) posterior cervical adenopathy, (2) a significant rise in the number of atypical "foamy" lymphocytes in peripheral blood, and (3) a positive heterophile agglutinin test in rising titer. The treatment is nonspecific but should include prolonged bed rest because of the possible complications of the disease, which include hepatitis and prolonged postinfectious fatigue state.

Bacterial infections
Acute suppurative oropharyngitis, nasopharyngitis, laryngitis, and tonsillitis

As with acute suppurative infections anywhere, acute infections of these organs result in fever, general malaise, pain in the affected organ, and altered function. The diagnosis is made by observing pus over the markedly inflamed tissue. Antibiotic and supportive therapy is the treatment. A mirror is necessary in the diagnosis of all head and neck infections, or one may be led astray; e.g., the oropharynx of a patient with acute suppurative nasopharyngitis may be profusely inflamed but without pus visible on tongue-blade examination, suggesting a viral oropharyngitis. These infections are not communicable, although there are infections of this region that are communicable (diphtheria and Vincent's infection). When the suppuration involves the larynx and/or trachea, modified voice rest must be a part of therapy in order to avoid the complication of speaker's nodule, vocal cord granuloma, or vocal polyp.

Paranasal sinusitis

Clinically, the important forms of sinusitis are acute and chronic suppurative. Other forms of sinusitis exist, e.g., atrophic sinusitis, rhinoscleromatous sinusitis, and tuberculous sinusitis, but they are rare.

Acute suppurative sinusitis is accompanied by the usual signs of acute infection together with facial pain, usually over the involved sinus, and a purulent rhinorrhea (Fig. 42-7). The pain of sphenoiditis is either fronto-occipital or bitemporal. The history is that of change of the watery nasal discharge to a suppurative one at the end of a viral nose cold. The diagnosis is not difficult to make on examination: pus at one of the sinus ostia within the nasal chamber. The edematous nasal mucosa is easily shrunk with a drop or spray of 1 to 3% ephedrine in normal saline solution, or with any of the commercial nose drops. The treatment is similar to that for any acute febrile infection, as described previously. Codeine may be necessary for relief of pain, and some benefit is afforded by antihistamines or similar agents to produce mucosal shrinkage, aid drainage, and diminish the mucoid element of the discharge. The vast majority of acute suppurative sinus in-

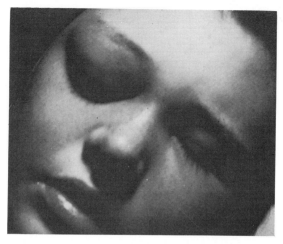

Fig. 42-7. Acute right frontal sinusitis that has perforated the floor of the sinus and produced an orbital abscess. The disease is now surgical. The differential diagnosis includes orbital cellulitis, cavernous sinus thrombosis or fistula, frontal or ethmoid neoplasm, and osteomyelitis.

fections are never seen by the physician, resolving spontaneously after a course of several weeks—but the *complications* of acute sinusitis always bring the patient to the physician. The most common complication is that of chronicity, and this will be discussed later. Perhaps the second most common complication is *acute serous otitis media,* producing a stuffy ear, deafness, tinnitus, and autophony, of which the patient may complain bitterly without mention of the nasal complaint. The sinusitis is then discovered as the cause during routine examination. More serious complications are *acute osteomyelitis, orbital abscess* (Fig. 42-7), *epidural, subdural, and brain abscess, cavernous sinus thrombosis,* and *acute empyema* of the sinus. All of these complications are of major consequence, and each is accompanied by a specific set of symptoms that requires treatment by an appropriate specialist. They all produce external swelling and a marked worsening of the general condition of the patient, which should immediately alert the physician.

Chronic suppurative sinusitis, however, is unaccompanied by facial pain, headache, or any signs of systemic infection, unless complicated.

Let us dispel the widely prevalent notion that frontal (or frontal and occipital) headache plus a stuffy nose is equatable with chronic sinus disease. This set of symptoms generally signals tension headaches plus chronic vasomotor rhinitis. The diagnosis of chronic suppurative sinusitis is untenable if pus is not visible at one of the sinal ostia. This is true almost regardless of the roentgen-ray findings, especially report of a "cloudy sinus." Perhaps the only diagnostic roentgen-ray sign is that of an air-fluid level. The "cloudy sinus" frequently means nothing more than thickening of the lining—testimony of an old healed infection and scarification (Fig. 42-8, *A*).

The treatment of chronic suppurative sinusitis is surgical (the nasoantral window operation, or sinusectomy). Sinusectomy is accomplished transorally (antral region), intranasally (ethmoid or sphenoid sinus), or externally (for the frontal or frontoethmoid sinus). The *complications* of chronic sinusitis are of major importance, including those listed under acute sinusitis, plus one other, mucocele. *Mucocele* arises as a slowly enlarging cyst filled with mucus, or mucopus *(mucopyocele),* from the frontal sinus or a frontal ethmoid cell; it invades the surrounding sinuses and the orbit, often taking several years to produce proptosis and a down-and-outward displacement of the eye (Fig. 42-8, *B*). A cystic mass is felt above the inner canthus of the eye. Treatment is always surgical removal.

The *role of allergy* in suppurative sinus disease deserves mention. There is no question that patients with allergic rhinitis are more predisposed to acute and chronic suppurative sinusitis than nonallergic patients. Identification of the underlying allergy directs treatment beyond that of the infection alone, which will not produce resolution of the basic disease. Allergic hyposensitization is then in order. An allergic component should be suspected whenever suppurative sinusitis fails to respond to the usual measures. Generally there is a family history of extrinsic allergy or a positive history of drug or food allergy in the patient, asthma in childhood, a labile nasal airway, perennial hay fever, or merely prolonged repetitive bouts of sneezing and epiphora. Pale, boggy, or violaceous nasal mucosa is often a clue, and the presence of allergic polyps (which resemble peeled grapes) is usually diagnostic. The treatment of allergic polyps is always surgical, but prior hyposensitization is carried out if allergies are found.

Infections of the ear

External otitis, frequently mistermed otomycosis or "fungus of the ear canal," is a suppurative infection of the skin of the ear canal. In the *acute form* it is extremely painful and produces marked edema of the skin. It does not produce deafness unless the canal is occluded by

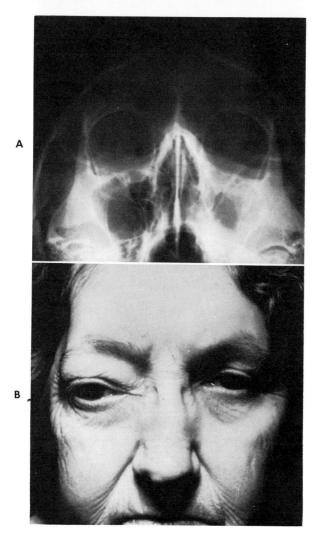

Fig. 42-8. A, Lining thickening of the right maxillary antrum; this is not diagnostic of chronic sinusitis but may represent old healed disease; the only diagnostic radiographic sign of active sinusitis is an air-fluid level; view the radiographs you order; the good physician realizes that if a radiograph is worth ordering, it is worth going to look at. **B,** Frontal mucocele; the right eye is pushed down, out, and forward; a cystic mass is palpable and easily visible above the inner canthus of the eye; this is one of the complications of chronic suppurative sinusitis; surgical intervention is necessary before the eye is ruined.

the edematous skin or exudate. Over half the reported cases are caused by *Pseudomonas aeruginosa,* and the remainder are caused by *strepto-cocci, staphylococci* or *Haemophilus influenzae*. Since it is an acute pyo-derm, the treatment is the administration of wet soaks (not systemic antibiotics). A cotton wick is placed deeply in the ear canal and kept soaked with Burow's solution or an antibiotic-cortisone eardrop. The pain is relieved in 24 to 48 hours if the cotton wick extends the entire length of the ear canal. The wick is left in place for 1 to 3 days, after which drops are continued along with meticulous periodic cleaning of the ear canal until the infection has subsided.

The *chronic form of external otitis* may have a number of causes. The most frequent is atrophy of the cerumen glands resulting in a chronically dry, pruritic canal. Other causes are seborrheic dermatitis, eczematoid dermatitis, and the end result of an untreated acute external otitis. Repeated trauma to the canal is the usual result of the pruritus. Such trauma from a finger, cotton-tipped applicator or pin propagates the infection. Treatment consists of avoidance of all trauma, careful cleaning by a physician, and long-term use of cortisone cream or ointment.

Acute suppurative otitis media is second in incidence to the nose cold. Few children escape it. It is also called *acute otitis media, middle ear abscess, acute ear, red ear,* and *bulging drum*. Signs and symptoms are those of an acute febrile infection with ear pain, which may be severe and protracted. Relief of the pain comes with either spontaneous drainage or the myringotomy knife. In the infant, irritability and diarrhea may be the only symptoms; this has been termed "cholera infantum." The etiology is the ascension of suppurative organisms from the nasopharynx (*streptococci, pneumococci, Haemophilus influenzae, staphylococci,* sometimes other organisms) through the eustachian tube or more probably via peritubal lymphatics. It should be stressed here that not all "red ears" are acute suppurative middle ear infections. Distinction must be made from mere hyperemia of the membrane or tympanum, which can be caused by holding a struggling, crying child for otoscopy. Diagnosis is made by observing a bulging, inflamed tympanic membrane, or pus in the ear canal that has recently perforated the tympanic membrane. Bulging is recognized by a diminished or absent prominence of the short process of the malleus. The eardrum changes may be obscured by the thickening and desquamation that occur in the tympanic membrane in the medial portion of the canal with acute middle ear infection, requiring cleaning of the canal.

Treatment consists of myringotomy (if the drum is bulging) and appropriate antibiotic therapy for at least 10 days. The following complications of an acute suppurative otitis media are probably more important than the disease itself:

Acute mastoiditis	Subperiosteal abscess
Acute osteomyelitis of the temporal bone	Acute suppurative labyrinthitis
	Acute meningitis
Acute petrositis	Sigmoid sinus thrombus
Facial nerve paralysis	Epidural abscess
Chronic nonsuppurative otitis media	Subdural abscess
	Brain abscess (cerebellar or
Chronic suppurative otitis media	temporal lobe)

Each of these complications poses its own diagnostic and treatment problems. The most common complication of acute suppurative otitis media, *chronic nonsuppurative otitis media,* is considered in the following paragraphs.

Chronic nonsuppurative otitis media is the most common cause of deafness in children and is conductive in type. It is of the magnitude of about 30 dB. The precise cause is not completely understood, although it follows eustachian tube obstruction and antibiotic-treated acute suppurative otitis media. Mucus-secreting glands migrate from the eustachian tube ·epithelium into the middle ear mucosa and produce a thick viscid, gluelike substance. The eardrum is gray, lusterless, retracted, and immobile. A synonym for the disease is *glue ear.* Treatment includes adenoidectomy, resolution of any suppurative disease of the upper respiratory tract, eustachian tube inflations by Valsalva maneuver or politzerization (forcible insufflation of the ear into the nasal chambers), elimination of inhalant allergies, antihistaminics, and, in recalcitrant cases, temporary intubation of the tympanic membrane to give the middle ear a rest. In each case, myringotomy and aspiration of the gluelike material should accompany any other treatment.

Chronic nonsuppurative otitis media, with true secretion of mucus into the middle ear, should be differentiated from acute nonsuppurative otitis media, which is a transudation of thin amber fluid into the middle ear after acute eustachian tube obstruction. This is most commonly caused by a viral upper respiratory infection, with edema about the nasopharyngeal end of the tube. However, the physician must be aware that neoplasms of the nasopharynx usually result in a middle ear effusion, and he must carefully examine the nasopharynx of each patient who presents with middle ear effusion.

Chronic suppurative otitis media is another sequela of acute middle ear infection. It is essentially a nonresolution of the acute infection. This is always accompanied by a perforation of the tympanic membrane and chronic, usually fetid, otorrhea. It is incumbent upon the physician to distinguish a *safe* from a *dangerous* chronic suppurating ear. A "safe ear" seldom shortens anyone's life by one day; a "dangerous ear" produces the same complications that may occur after acute suppurative otitis media. The following criteria for this distinction demand careful consideration:

Character of the discharge
Progressive unexplained hearing loss
Site of the perforation
Presence of vascular pyogenic granulation
  tissue growing on bone
Positive reservoir sign
Positive fistula test
Presence of a cholesteatoma
Presence of bone destruction on inspection or
  radiographic examination

The *discharge* suggests dangerous chronic osteomyelitis if it is highly fetid in smell, the result of bone digestion by bacterial enzymes. Simple mucosal infection produces predominantly a mucoid discharge with no odor, or merely a musty odor from stasis and the action of saprophytic organisms.

Marginal perforations, including "attic" perforations or those in the pars flaccida, generally indicate a dangerous ear condition. Central perforations, or those in the pars tensa away from the annula region, generally indicate the nondangerous ear condition.

A *cholesteatoma (skin in the middle ear, where skin does not belong),* is virtually diagnostic of a dangerous ear condition. Once skin enters the middle ear space, it casts off layer upon layer of desquamated epithelium, which is surrounded by the thinned-out matrix. The matrix is the surrounding layer of living skin. The cholesteatoma invades and destroys bone by two processes: enzymatic digestion in the presence of vascular pyogenic granulation tissue, and pressure necrosis by a solid ball of cholesteatoma whose center is filled with desquamated keratin debris or "squame." The cholesteatoma may enlarge slowly over many years with no symptoms except the chronic otorrhea, and perhaps increasing deafness. Then the cholesteatoma invades one of the many vital structures surrounding the middle ear, and catastrophe follows. These vital structures are the cochlea, the vestibular labyrinth, the sigmoid sinus, the jugular bulb, the dura of the cerebellum, the dura of the temporal lobe, and the subarachnoid space. Septic retrograde thrombosis of vessels may also be induced by chronic osteomyelitic bone. The cholesteatoma is recognized by its characteristic cheesy-white, flaky content. *The presence of bone destruction on either*

<u>*visual inspection or on roentgen-ray examination*</u> indicates either a destructive osteomyelitic process or an expanding cholesteatoma. *Vascular pyogenic granulation tissue growing on bone* is diagnostic of chronic osteomyelitis. The *positive reservoir sign* is the re-formation of pus a few minutes after it has been thoroughly wiped away. A *positive fistula test* is conjugate deviation of the eyes to the opposite side on compression of the air in the external auditory canal, diagnostic of a fistula through the bone over a semicircular canal, without actual suppurative invasion of the inner ear. It is then only a matter of a few days to a few weeks before suppurative invasion takes place. When this occurs, sudden irrevocable total deafness follows, together with severe and prolonged vertigo and nystagmus. A labyrinthectomy is then necessary.

Only a few of these criteria may be present in a given patient, and no single test (except the positive fistula test in a chronic draining ear) is absolutely diagnostic of a dangerous ear. Thus it becomes a matter of meticulous observation, careful interpretation, and judgment to establish this. Recognition of the dangerous state is crucial *because the impending complication may be diagnosed in advance and prevented by surgical intervention.* Recognition is the physician's responsibility.

Fascial space abscesses

Peritonsillar abscess (quinsy) is the most common fascial space abscess. The organism is usually a *streptococcus* or a *staphylococcus* and an acute or chronic tonsilitis the etiology. There occurs marked edema of the tonsillar bed with fanning out of the anterior pillar over the swollen mass. The uvula may be pushed across the midline. It is severely painful, causing marked odynophagia and pain on opening the mouth. True trismus may be present. Incision and drainage is the treatment, along with antibiotic therapy. Distinction between peritonsillar abscess and peritonsillar cellulitis may be difficult. The cellulitis precedes abscess formation, which takes at least 48 hours to form.

Retropharyngeal space abscesses are uncommon. They are generally seen in children, in whom an infected retropharyngeal lymph node gives rise to the infection. These nodes are usually absent in the adult. Diagnosis is made by a characteristic spongy or cystic feel to the posterior pharyngeal wall and widening of the retropharyngeal space on the lateral soft-tissue radiograph of the neck. The collection of pus exists between the superior constrictor muscle and the prevertebral fascia. Treatment is incision and drainage.

Pharyngomaxillary space abscess (lateral or parapharyngeal space) is an abscess in the potential space between the fascia of the parotid gland and the internal pterygoid muscle laterally, and the fascia of

the superior constrictor muscle medially. In it are the carotid sheath structures and the styloid process with its muscle group. The abscess is recognized by medial displacement of the tonsil *and* lateral angle of the pharynx and brawny induration of the upper neck just below the angle of the mandible. However, bulging may be present in only one of these places. Trismus is marked. Treatment is external incision and drainage with antibiotic therapy.

A *masticator space abscess,* usually of dental origin, is an abscess under the periosteum of the mandible. Trismus is usually present. Ludwig's angina is a floor of the mouth phlegmon and is also usually of dental origin. The patient frequently is a diabetic. The floor of the mouth is markedly swollen, and the tongue is pushed up and back, endangering the airway. Tracheotomy must be contemplated. Later, all the potential spaces of the floor of the mouth are involved, and the infection may spread down to clavicular level. Wide incision and drainage is frequently necessary, although intensive antibiotic therapy early in the infection may suffice.

TRAUMA

Automobile accidents account for most severe maxillofacial trauma today. Though reduction and fixation of facial bone fractures may be delayed for as much as 14 days, a very careful evaluation of the patient must be carried out at the time of the injury. Other emergent conditions that require immediate attention may be developing such as airway obstruction, cervical vertebra fracture, long bone fracture, progressive intracranial or intra-abdominal injury, or soft tissue lacerations.

Trauma of the nose

The *nasal bone* is the most commonly *fractured* bone in the body. Even relatively minor nasal trauma may result in a fracture. When the patient is evaluated immediately after the trauma has occurred, the diagnosis may be obvious. Mobility of the nasal bones on palpation is diagnostic. Roentgenograms may be misleading when old fractures have healed with scar tissue or when recent fractures are not demonstrated. Within a few hours after trauma the swelling about the nose may be extensive, making a clinical evaluation extremely difficult. In such a case, treatment may be delayed for as much as 7 days to allow the swelling to subside. Because of their intimacy, both nasal bones are usually fractured. After the nose is anesthetized, a blunt instrument may be placed beneath the nasal bone on the concave side and elevated outward. The other nasal bone is then moved medially into its proper position. This position is maintained with external splinting.

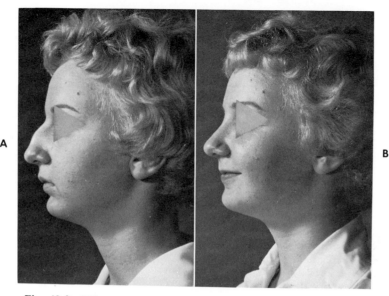

Fig. 42-9. Old nasal fracture. **A,** Unreduced. **B,** After rhinoplasty.

When the nasal fracture is allowed to heal in a deviated position, a rhinoplasty is required later to restore normal nasal contour (Fig. 42-9).

Fracture of the nasal septum sometimes occurs without nasal bone fracture. If the fractured septum is displaced significantly, it produces permanent airway obstruction. Fractures of the nasal septum are often difficult to reduce because the septum becomes dislocated off the palatine crest. If the septum does not go easily back to the midline, submucous resection of the septum (discussed on p. 1006) may be required at the time of the acute fracture.

Another late sequela of untreated septal fracture is *"saddle" type deformity of the nose*. The middle third of the dorsum of the nose is supported by the nasal septum and not by the nasal bones. The support is lost by an inward fracture of the septum that may not be apparent immediately on external examination because a hematoma forms in its place, so that the nose retains roughly its former appearance. The "saddle" deformity then becomes apparent after resolution of the hematoma. Correction of this deformity requires a bone graft and rhinoplasty, a complicated procedure.

Deviation of the nasal septum may also be acquired by differential growth pattern. Nasal septal spurs and bending of the nasal septum with encroachment of one nasal chamber are usually the result of unequal growth of the two sides of the septum. Deflection of the caudal (anteroinferior) edge of the septum into one nasal vestibule is usually traumatic. Septal deflections are important to the degree they produce airway obstruction. Significant obstructions should be treated by *submucous resection of the nasal septum*. In this operation, the mucoperiosteum and mucoperichondrium of each side of the septum are elevated, and the deviated part of the rigid septum is removed. An entire septectomy is never necessary, but the deviated parts of the septum that provide support to the external nose may be removed and replaced in proper position. Such an operation is called a *septal reconstruction*. These operations are relatively minor and often produce gratifying results. Deviated septa do not cause headaches, sinus disease, nervousness, weight loss, or the like. Submucous resection of the nasal septum only cures airway obstruction.

Digital trauma to the nasal septum may eventually cause a septal perforation and today is its most common cause. Years ago, the most common cause was *syphilis*. A perforated nasal septum is not significant unless it produces annoying crusting and bleeding from perichondritis or chondritis at the edge of the perforation. This is treated by cutting the cartilage and bone back well beneath the mucosal covering. Occasionally a septal perforation causes whistling in the airstream, when the perforation is of a critical size relative to the speed of the airstream. This may be resolved by making the perforation larger, or by closing the septal perforation with a special surgical procedure.

Epistaxis (nosebleed)

Epistaxis is an almost invariably benign disease, but frequently a trying one because it is frightening to the patient and difficult for the physician to treat.

The single most common cause of epistaxis in the adult is *hypertension*. The most common season is the late fall, when the home heating plant is turned on and the humidity drops precipitously. This dries out the inspired air, cracking or splitting the delicate respiratory mucosa. In children, *digital trauma* to the anterior nose promotes this cracking, as crusts build up inside the nares. The usual location of the bleeding vessel is at the anteroinferior portion of the nasal septum, where a plexus of submucosal vessels is located (Kiesselbach's plexus) in *Little's area*. The plexus is formed by the confluence of the septal branch of the sphenopalatine artery, the anterior ethmoid artery, and the perforating branch of the anterior palatine artery. Such epistaxes are termed *anterior bleeders;* they account for nine out of ten nose-bleeds.

The management of *posterior epistaxis* is sometimes difficult. In addition, the patients deserve a complete work-up in search of specific causes, such as hypertension, leukemia, neoplasms of the nasal chambers and paranasal sinuses, and hemorrhagic disorders.

The first step in the management of a patient with epistaxis is to locate the bleeding vessel. Important principles are threefold: *spot lighting, spot suction,* and *spot hemostasis.* Spot lighting requires a head mirror or a head light, because overhead operating room lighting or a flashlight is totally inadequate to the task. Spot suctioning apparatus (which will reach 25 mm. Hg negative pressure with a high flow) is available in every hospital emergency room. To this should be added a (Frazier type) suction tip, which has a finger cutoff valve. All clots are aspirated from the nasal chamber with the patient in a sitting or semi-Fowler's position, and free-flowing source of blood is located.

Anterior septal bleeders may be managed as a rule by silver nitrate bead cautery. The silver nitrate bead must be placed directly over the opening in the bleeding vessel and held in position for 10 to 15 seconds. The patient is cautioned against straining and noseblowing for several days. Occasionally petroleum jelly gauze packing is necessary. The use of topical vasoconstrictor agents such as adrenaline on a cotton tampon must be looked upon as a temporary measure in the treatment of epistaxis.

Posterior epistaxis arises from either the ethmoid arteries, part of the internal carotid system, or from the sphenopalatine arteries, a part of the external carotid system. In the former, the bleeding will be from above the level of the middle turbinate, and in the latter from below the level of the middle turbinate. This distinction is of vital importance should all local methods fail and vascular ligation be necessary.

Fractures of the facial bones

Fractures of the middle third of the face involving the maxilla have been conveniently classified by LeFort (Fig. 42-10). Type I is a fracture involving the alveolar ridges or palate, and the bodies of the maxillary bones are intact. Type II involves the medial portion of the middle third of the face, with the fracture line crossing the zygomaticomaxillary suture lines, so that grasping the incisor teeth allows motion of the entire middle third of the face, and not just the palatal portion. Type III is termed a craniofacial separation, with the fracture line on almost a horizontal plane, separating the maxillary and

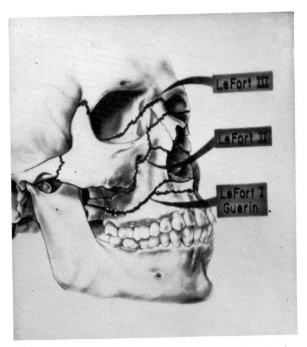

Fig. 42-10. Mid-third (maxillary) fractures of the face tend to occur along certain lines and may be classified. The LeFort classification is pictured here. LeFort III is a craniofacial separation, LeFort II a pyramid-shaped fracture, and LeFort I a palatal separation.

zygomatic bones from the rest of the skull. *Proper treatment is very important because occlusion of the teeth is involved as well as cosmetic appearance.* Improper treatment results in malocclusion of varying types and degrees. If the molar teeth come together before the incisor teeth, biting through food with the front teeth is impossible. Arch bars must be placed across the teeth so that the upper and lower teeth can be brought together with wires in the proper alignment. This stabilizes the upper fragments of broken jaw upon a stable lower jaw. The middle third of the face is stabilized by snugging the arch bars up to the base of the skull with suspension wires circling the arches of the zygoma, or passed subcutaneously through drill holes in the lateral orbital rims.

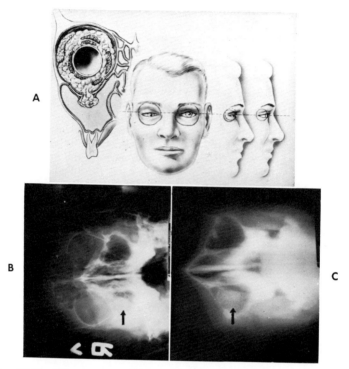

Fig. 42-11. Blowout fracture of the orbit. A sharp blow to the soft tissues of the eye may fracture the thin floor of the orbit and allow orbital contents to drop into the antrum, **A.** The eye is thus dropped, becomes enophthalmic, and upward-following gaze is lost. This is permanent unless recognized and treated. A Water's view of the sinuses can be very helpful, **B,** but sometimes a laminagram, **C,** is necessary.

The supraorbital ridge, being very thick, is fractured only by a heavy blow. The infraorbital rim, however, is formed by thin bone and may be fractured by a relatively minor blow. A blow to the orbit may generate tremendous elevations of intraorbital pressure and result in a "blowing out" of the thin, bony orbital floor with herniation of orbital contents into the maxillary sinus below. Such an injury may result in enophthalmos, a depressed interpupillary line, and limitation of upward gaze in the affected eye (Fig. 42-11). Failure to recognize this fracture may result in permanent enophthalmos and diplopia. Treatment consists of retrieving the herniated tissue and restoration of integrity of the orbital floor.

Fractures of the zygoma occur by a direct blow high over the cheek. A crushing blow may fracture the arch of the zygoma to produce cosmetic deformity. The *tripodal fracture* involves the zygomaticofrontal suture, the zygomaticomaxillary suture, and the arch, resulting in a depression of the malar eminence. This fracture usually requires open reduction and fixation to assure a good cosmetic result.

Mandibular fractures are important for the same reason that maxillary fractures are important: faulty treatment will produce nutritionally crippling malocclusion. The most common types are *subcondylar,* which results in trismus; *ramus,* with displacement of the fracture ends produced by different muscle pulls exerted on the fragments; *body,* usually across the mental foramen; and *symphyseal.* Treatment is by closed reduction, using arch bars to restore normal occlusion, and wiring of the fragments together where indicated. External support with appropriate hardware may be necessary.

Fractures of the frontal sinus are important to recognize to avoid the late sequelae of *cosmetic deformity, obstruction of the nasofrontal duct* (with ultimate production of a mucocele of the frontal sinus), and *cerebrospinal fluid leak* from a fracture tear of the posterior wall to which dura is firmly attached. An unrecognized cerebrospinal fluid leak may result in repeated meningitis, months or years apart. Open reduction is usually necessary.

Fractures of the temporal bone

Temporal bone fractures are the result of severe head injury, with the fracture line extending through the base of the skull, of which the temporal bone is a part. Hemorrhage from the ear canal or cerebrospinal fluid otorrhea is frequent, although not invariable. If there has not been a direct blow to the soft tissue over the mastoid, a bruise in this area is diagnostic (Battle's sign).

Temporal bone fractures are of two types. *Transverse temporal bone fractures* occur across the internal auditory canal and inner ear, producing immediate total deafness, labyrinthine vertigo and nystagmus, and frequently a facial nerve paralysis. *Longitudinal temporal bone fractures* cross the posterosuperior canal wall, middle ear, and eustachian tube, producing conductive deafness. A facial paralysis in this type is less common. Immediate facial nerve paralysis indicates severance of the nerve, which should be repaired as soon as the patient's general condition permits. A delayed facial nerve paralysis usually will resolve spontaneously.

Fractures of the larynx

Laryngeal fractures are extremely important to recognize and treat early to avoid loss of the important faculties of speech and normal breathing. *In any patient with a neck injury, particularly an anterior blow to the neck, the symptoms of hoarseness or dyspnea demand laryngoscopy.* Within a week or 10 days of injury the diameters of the larynx can be reconstituted to restore normal speech and breathing. After this time, consequent scarring may require repeated operations on the larynx before the tracheotomy tube can be removed or may even sentence the patient to a permanent tracheostoma. The preceding points are of extreme importance and should be firmly in the mind of every physician attending an emergency room or treating acutely traumatized patients.

Frostbite

Cold injuries to the head and neck most frequently involve the external ear and the tip of the nose. The old maxim that a frozen member should be rubbed with snow is false. This resutls only in needless trauma to already damaged tissue. Cold, or frostbite, produces its injury by infarction, and through cellular rupture by large ice crystals that form when tissue is slowly cooled below the crystallization point. Some tissue loss is then inevitable, but frequently this need be only the outer layers of the skin.

There is no uniformly successful method of treating frostbite, but it is generally agreed that the frozen tissue should be thawed reasonably rapidly. Further injury to the tissue should be avoided by immobility. Anticoagulation is not widely accepted. The skin should be protected against drying, fissuring, and the development of superficial infection by the application first of petrolatum jelly, and later antibiotic ointments if necessary.

NEOPLASMS
Neoplasms of the face

Basal cell carcinoma (rodent ulcer) is the most common neoplasm of the skin of the face. The lesion begins as a roughened area that ulcerates and fails to heal, classically above a line drawn from the tragus of the ear to the nasal ala. Farmers, because of their high exposure to actinic radiation, are prone to develop this lesion, as well as other skin neoplasms in exposed areas. Basal cell carcinomas do not metastasize but continue to enlarge and destroy anything in their path until properly treated. Treatment is adequate excision, by use of skin lines for the incisions to obtain optimal cosmetic results, especially for small lesions. When large basal cell carcinomas are excised, some type of skin graft is required for coverage. Excellent results are also obtainable by radiation therapy given in cancericidal doses, which usually means at least several weeks of daily treatments. Dermatologists frequently prefer to treat by electrodesiccation and curettage, or cryotherapy.

Epidermoid (squamous cell) carcinoma occurs anywhere on the face, including the lips, nose, lids, and external ear. Classically, the ulcerated lesion has a rolled, pearly border. The indurated border represents infiltration of adjacent normal tissue. In contrast to basal cell carcinoma, epidermoid carcinoma can metastasize. The nodes first involved are the submaxillary or submental nodes, and then the deep cervical nodes, or the deep cervical nodes alone. Treatment is adequate excision of the primary lesion, which must include 1 cm. of normal tissue around its borders. Radiation therapy is also effective, but higher doses are necessary than in the basal cell carcinoma. When lymph nodes are involved, a radical neck dissection is necessary.

Carcinomas of the lids, lips, or external ear pose special problems in treatment and are best treated by a specialist. Where cartilage is immediatley subjacent, as in the ear or nasal ala, special handling is required to prevent chondritis, whether treated surgically or by radiation. Immediate reconstruction is necessary if ear, eye, or nose is removed or is grossly deformed. Eyelid lesions must be managed with special care to avoid entropion, ectropion, and exposed cornea, which may lead to corneal damage and blindness. Lip lesions are treated by wedge resection or vermilionectomy. If the wedge is large, a plastic reconstructive procedure must be performed to supplant the tissue sacrificed so that a tight lip that limits speech and feeding does not ensue.

The *differential diagnosis* of facial skin cancer includes senile keratoses, seborrheic keratoses, nevi, and the keratoacanthoma. The latter is an ulcerating reactive lesion of the skin closely resembling cancer, but that is a self-limited disease.

Neoplasms of the mouth and oropharynx

Epidermoid (squamous cell) carcinoma is by far the most common neoplasm of this region. This lesion occurs most commonly in the tongue, floor of the mouth (Fig. 42-12), buccal mucosa, and tonsil, but may involve the palate, alveolar ridges, mucosa of the jaws, uvula, and oropharyngeal walls. *Treatment* is simple excision to include an area 1 cm. around the periphery or radiation therapy if the lesion is 2 cm. or smaller in size. A wedge resection is performed if the primary lesion involves the tongue. Tonsillar lesions are treated differently because of their propensity for early metastasis; small lesions are treated

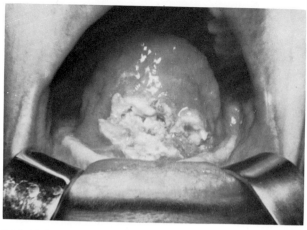

Fig. 42-12. Epidermoid carcinoma of the floor of the mouth. Note its exophytic character and purulent membrane over the entire ulcerated surface. Indurated lesions with ulceration anywhere in the mouth demand biopsy.

by irradiation, but those larger than 2 cm. in size have usually metastasized and require neck dissection for cure. The involved cervical lymph nodes may be impalpable (subclinical metastases). Epidermoid carcinomas of the mouth and oropharynx that are larger than 2 cm. in diameter require a large operation. Combination therapy is frequently used: preoperative radiation therapy in a submaximal dose followed with a radical neck dissection. Excision of the primary lesion usually by definitive operation that combines removal of the primary lesion requires hemimandibulectomy, hemiglossectomy, and resection of the angle of the pharynx if the lesion is oropharyngeal. Reconstruction of the surgical defect is begun immediately to provide early functional and cosmetic rehabilitation. Five-year survival may approach 75% in small lesions located anteriorly in the mouth, whereas large lesions posteriorly with regional lymph node metastasis represent 25% or less 5-year survival.

Adenocarcinomas also occur in the mouth and oropharynx that are identical to those of the major salivary glands, because they arise in one of the many minor salivary glands in the region. They may be of many types. (See discussion on neoplasms of the salivary glands, p. 1021.) Thus mixed salivary gland tumors may occur on the palate, tonsillar pillars, or lateral angle of the pharynx. *Treatment* is always sur-

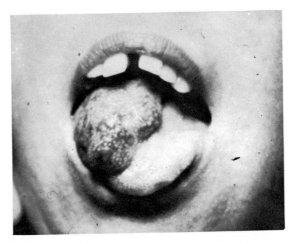

Fig. 42-13. Hemangioma of the tongue. This lesion is common in the upper digestive tract. The lesion is characteristically deep blue and empties and refills slowly on application and release of pressure. Varices on the undersurface of the tongue should be readily distinguishable from them and do not require treatment.

gical because adenocarcinomas generally are not radiosensitive. The prognosis for these lesions is less favorable than for epidermoid carcinomas.

Connective tissue tumors are not unusual in this area. The most common are lymphomas that occur in tonsillar tissue. Connective tissue tumors of the bones of the jaws may occur, such as osteogenic sarcoma, fibrosarcoma, and giant cell tumor of bone. Muscle tumors such as rhabdomyosarcoma occur here, as well as neoplasms of other connective tissue elements, e.g., myxomas, fibromas, lipomas, and hemangiomas (Fig. 42-13).

Tumors of dental origin appear as expansile lesions widening the alveolar ridge or the body of the mandible, or, less commonly, the upper jaw. The only common neoplasm of this type is the adamantinoma (ameloblastoma), a neoplasm of the enamel organ of the developing tooth. This is a benign tumor, cured by adequate simple excision. A dentigerous cyst is not a neoplasm, but it requires simple excision because it can be distinguished from an adamantinoma only by histological examination.

Leukoplakia (white plaque) occurs wherever there is moist, strati-

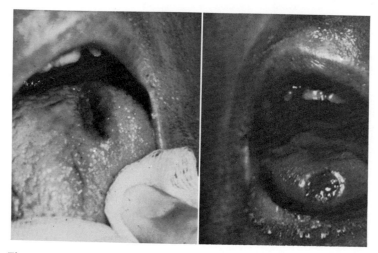

Fig. 42-14. Histoplasmosis of the tongue. Note the sharp margination of the ulceration and lack of exophytic response. This probably occurs by primary inoculation from chronic weed chewing. It is easy to confuse this or any other chronic specific granuloma with malignancy.

fied squamous, nonkeratinizing or respiratory epithelium. It appears as a thin, whitish plaque, most commonly in areas subject to chronic irritation, and can be identified in almost any denture-wearing patient. It is also very common on the buccal mucosa, lips, the mucosa over the ascending ramus of the mandible, floor of the mouth, tongue, and palate. It occasionally takes on a lacy pattern and may resemble lichen planus. Histologically, there may be any degree of abnormality from hyperkeratosis to invasive carcinoma. Not all leukoplakia requires treatment, but it must be observed periodically. If the lesion becomes *palpable,* or assumes an opaque, milky appearance indicating possible premalignant change, or if punctate ulceration occurs, excision must be carried out. If the area of leukoplakia is large, it may be excised in stages, or radiation therapy may be considered. Ordinarily, radiation therapy is not utilized unless there is evidence of malignant change.

The *differential diagnosis* of oral cancer includes the *epulides, chronic specific granulomas,* and *trauma* from ill-fitting dentures or jagged teeth. Giant cell epulis is not a neoplasm but a reactive phenomenon, found most frequently on the alveolar ridges. It is caused by trauma or marked alterations in hormonal levels, such as in pregnancy.

Chronic specific granulomas masquerading as neoplasms include *tuberculosis* (rare), *Vincent's angina, histoplasmosis* (Fig. 42-14), *actinomycosis, syphilis,* and *lethal midline granuloma* perforating the hard palate. The *brown hairy tongue* (Fig. 42-15), a peculiar biological phenomenon that is poorly understood, should not be mistaken for a neoplasm. It is common in the chronically ill patient but also is seen in a healthy individual. Brown hairy tongue is essentially a marked hypertrophy of filiform papillae, with proliferating chromogen bacteria deeply embedded between the papillae. *Treatment* consists of repeatedly trimming the hypertrophied material down with sharp dissection.

Early biopsy of lesions of the mouth and oropharynx is essential to cure. Once the lesion becomes larger than 1 cm., the cure rates drops

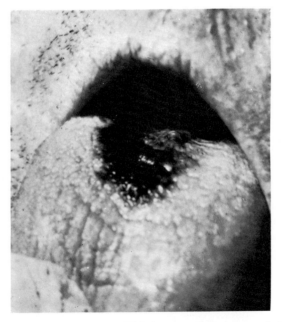

Fig. 42-15. Brown hairy tongue. This is not a disease per se, but is often of great concern to the patient. It is a frequent accompaniment of a chronic disease state. Chromogen bacteria growing between greatly elongated filiform papillae produce the picture. Treatment is by "tongue shave."

precipitously. The prudent physician biopsies any suspicious lesion in this area. Practically no harm can be done, as functional or cosmetic losses from mouth or oropharyngeal biopsy are virtually negligible, but a positive biopsy of a small lesion will yield high dividends for the patient. Retain a high index of suspicion. The physician should never feel chagrined at a negative biopsy.

Neoplasms of the nasopharynx

Cancer of the nasopharynx is common, especially in people of Oriental extraction. *Epidermoid carcinoma* and *lymphoepithelioma* of the nasopharynx are most insidious neoplasms, for in the majority of patients the first symptom is hearing loss from a middle ear effusion. Symptoms that may follow are presence of a firm mass in the neck, odynophagia, epistaxis, or blood-streaking of oral secretions. Any patient who presents with a middle ear effusion or a hard mass in the neck must have a thorough examination of the nasopharynx before treatment is instituted. *Treatment* of the primary nasopharyngeal carcinoma is radiation therapy. Once the primary is controlled, neck dissection is performed if the cervical nodes are involved.

Connective tissue neoplasms of the malignant variety, including reticulum cell sarcoma, lymphosarcoma, and giant follicular lymphoma, may also occur in this area. Liposarcoma and fibrosarcoma are rare neoplasms of the nasopharynx.

Benign tumors of the nasopharynx include the juvenile nasopharyngeal angiofibroma. This is a highly vascular tumor of young boys that is thought to arise in cartilaginous rests of sphenoid ossification centers. Its symptoms are nasal obstruction and epistaxis. The tumor can be diagnosed by mirror examination of the nasopharynx. The tumor contains a great many dilated blood spaces unlined with smooth muscle, and even biopsy may provoke profuse bleeding. Although it does not metastasize, it is "malignant" by position in that, in time, it erodes the base of the skull. *Treatment* is by excision, usually with cryotherapy. The operation is extremely difficult and attended with much blood loss. *Craniopharyngioma* is a tumor arising from the embryonic Rathke's pouch. Most of these neoplasms are intracranial, but if the stalk of Rathke's pouch is persistent and becomes entrapped in the sphenoid bone, a sphenoid or nasopharyngeal tumor will result. This is also a benign tumor that is malignant by position; an aid to diagnosis is calcification of the embryonic notochord. Chordomas occur most frequently in the body of the sphenoid bone and in the sacrum. Contents of the tumors are usually gelatinous; thus the tumor may be thought to be merely a cyst, but unless excision of the entire capsule is accomplished, it will recur.

Differential diagnosis of tumors in this area includes *chronic sphenoiditis, sphenoid mucocele, mucous retention cyst of nasopharyngeal mucosa, Tornwaldt's bursa,* and *chronic adenoiditis.*

Neoplasms of the larynx and hypopharynx

Epidermoid carcinoma of the larynx afflicts men more commonly than women, in a ratio of about 10:1. One classification of neoplasms of the larynx is by location and divides into (1) glottic, including the entire true cord, (2) supraglottic, including the false vocal cord, the aryepiglottic folds, epiglottis, and valleculae, and (3) subglottic, involving the conus elasticus and the upper trachea. Cancer of the true cord has a good prognosis, ranking second only to epidermoid carcinoma of the skin in curability. The overall cure rate of carcinoma of the larynx is about 65%.

Carcinomas of the true cord are highly curable for two reasons: (1) symptoms (hoarseness, excessive throat clearing) annoy the patient enough to prompt an early visit to the physician, and (2) there is a paucity of lymphatics in the true cord so that metastases are rare. The 5-year cure rate of carcinomas of the true cord is between 80 and 90%. Treatment is by radiation therapy if cord mobility is unimpaired and the lesion extends to neither end of the cord; hemilaryngectomy is perferred if the lesion does extend to either end of the true cord. Because lesions of this area are so amenable to cure and because they are so readily visible, *any patient with hoarseness of 2 weeks' duration or longer must have examination of his larynx.*

Larger glottic or supraglottic lesions without vocal cord fixation may be treated with a partial laryngectomy. These patients retain a serviceable voice with survival rates equal to those with total laryngectomy. Even larger lesions require total laryngectomy and radical neck dissection. The patient must learn esophageal speech to gain full speech rehabilitation. Five-year survival is approximately 65%.

Epidermoid carcinoma of the laryngopharynx involves the lateral pharyngeal wall, posterior pharyngeal wall, or piriform sinus. Carcinomas that arise in the introitus of the esophagus are referred to as postcricoid lesions. These lesions are more common in women than in men, dysphagia is the first symptom, and loss of laryngeal crepitus is the most outstanding finding on examination. Laryngeal crepitus is that crackling sensation obtained by pushing the larynx side to side over the cervical vertebrae. Barium swallow is indicated, and esophagoscopy confirms the diagnosis. *Treatment* consists of preoperative cobalt therapy followed by partial or total laryngopharyngectomy and radical neck dissection.

Adenocarcinomas of the larynx and hypopharynx are uncommon but do occur.

Differential diagnosis. *Leukoplakia* occurs on the true vocal cords and may be indistinguishable from carcinoma in situ or early invasive carcinoma. *Speaker's nodules* occur at the junction of the anterior and middle thirds of the vocal cords in patients who use their voices excessively. The nodules may be pinhead in size, or polypoid and ulcerated, resembling a neoplasm. *Laryngocele* is a progressive enlargement of a noncommunicating portion of the laryngeal ventricle, producing a laryngeal cyst. Initially the laryngocele is internal, encroaching on the airway, and then dissects up over the thyroid cartilage and presents as a neck mass as it becomes external. Laminagrams of the larynx are helpful in diagnosis of laryngocele. *Retention cysts* ordinarily present no problems in diagnosis because of their typical smooth, yellow-domed appearance. They are most common in the valleculae and on the aryepiglottic folds. The *chronic specific granulomas* may present an identical appearance to cancer and require biopsy for distinction (*syphilis, tuberculosis, actinomycosis,* and *lethal midline granuloma*).

Neoplasms of the nose and paranasal sinuses

Epidermal carcinoma is relatively rare in the nasal chamber but is common in the antrum and the ethmoid sinus. Unfortunately, the cure rate of this lesion is low because it does not produce significant symptoms until it has reached a large size. Ordinarily, an antral carcinoma is not diagnosed or even suspected until it has eroded through one of its bony walls. Any of its walls may be eroded, with the symptoms depending on which wall is involved. When the anterior wall is involved, the symptoms are a fullness in the cheek, a mass, and a numbness of the infraorbital region caused by infiltration of that nerve. Involvement of the inferior wall produces loosening or extrusion of teeth, widening of the alveolar ridge producing a poorly fitting denture, and a mass on the palate. Erosion of the medial wall produces blood-tinged nasal secretions and nasal airway obstruction. Erosion of the superior wall produces infraorbital nerve paresthesias and paralysis, proptosis, and interference with extraocular muscles. Bone destruction is present on appropriate roentgen-ray examination. Treatment is a combination of radiation therapy and maxillectomy, which usually means sacrifice of that side of the hard palate. The patient can be rehabilitated in speech and chewing by the placement of an oral prosthesis that contains teeth.

Adenocystic carcinoma (adenoid cystic carcinoma, pseudoadenomatous basal cell carcinoma, cylindroma) is the most common adenocarcinoma of the region. This may involve any of the paranasal sinuses or the nasal chamber. It is an extremely lethal neoplasm, somewhat sensitive to radiation therapy, but generally treated by surgical means. Other adenocarcinomas may occur here, arising in minor salivary glands, and the types are as listed in the section on neoplasms of the salivary glands (p. 1021).

Solitary myeloma of the respiratory tract (extramedullary myeloma) occurs in the ethmoid sinus or nasal chamber and produces symptoms of epistaxis and airway obstruction. It may exist as a solitary myeloma for many years, but frequently evidence of disseminated myeloma shortly follows. Treatment is by excision or radiation therapy. Fibrosarcoma is another malignant connective tissue neoplasm occasionally arising in this general area.

Olfactory neuroepithelioma (esthesioneuroblastoma) has been described only relatively recently. It is thought to arise from the neural elements of the olfactory epithelium. It is of relatively low-grade malignancy in most patients, although it may metastasize, and it is certainly malignant by position. There appears to be some radiosensitivity to this lesion.

Osteoma is the most common benign tumor of connective tissue origin that arises in the nasal and paranasal cavities. Osteoma usually involves the frontal sinus; it tends to grow slowly but may become very large. Excision must be carried out, especially if it arises adjacent to the nasofrontal duct or threatens to erode the inner wall of the sinus and the dura. *Ossifying fibroma* is one of the bony dysplasias that is not a true neoplasm but tends to act like one. The ethmoid sinus is the most common location, radiographic examination is diagnostic, and treatment is excision by external approach. *Giant cell tumor of bone* may affect any age group, is of generally low-grade malignancy, and may be treated either by surgical excision or by radiation.

Differential diagnosis. *Chronic vestibulitis* of the eczematoid variety is distinguished with difficulty from skin cancer of the nasal vestibule. When seen in a localized area of the nasal vestibule, or particularly when a brief trial of treatment fails, biopsy is mandatory. *Nasal polyposis* of the hyperplastic or allergic types should present no difficulty in distinction from cancer, since a nasal polyp has a striking resemblance to a peeled grape, and the surface epithelium is always intact. Beefy red polyps associated with chronic sinusitis are a different matter, demanding prompt biopsy to rule out neoplasm. The presence of pus with inflammatory polyps does not exclude polypoid nasal malignancy because neoplasms of the nose alter nasal physiology, and infection is the rule. *Nasal glioma,* representing heterotopic glial tissue, may be present anywhere in the nasal chamber and is overlain by normal skin or mucosa. *Meningocele* or *meningoencephalocele* should always be borne in mind when a smooth nonulcerated mass is present in a nasal chamber. Pulsation of the mass is suggestive of meningocele and precludes biopsy. The chronic specific granulomas include *lethal mid-*

line granuloma, sarcoidosis, actinomycosis, and *syphilis. Rhinoscleroma* and *rhinosporidiosis* are rare in this country.

Neoplasms of the salivary glands

Classification

I. Benign
- A. Mixed salivary gland tumor
- B. Benign mucoepidermoid tumor
- C. Adenoma
  1. Papillary cystadenoma lymphomatosum (Warthin's tumor)
  2. Serous cell adenoma
  3. Acidophilic cell adenoma

II. Malignant
- A. Epidermoid carcinoma (well and poorly differentiated, including lymphoepithelioma)
- B. Mucoepidermoid carcinoma
- C. Adenocarcinoma
  1. Adenocystic carcinoma
  2. Acinic (serous) carcinoma
  3. Acidophilic (oxyphilic) cell carcinoma
- D. Unclassified salivary gland carcinoma

Connective tissue tumors also occur in salivary glands, although they are relatively rare. They include neurofibromas, fibromas, and neurofibrosarcomas. Salivary glands may also be the site of infiltration by lymphomas.

About 60% of all salivary gland tumors are the so-called *mixed salivary gland tumor (pleomorphic adenoma),* which is almost always benign (Fig. 42-16). It acquired its name by virtue of an apparent mixture of two germ cell layers in its histological pattern: nests, cords, and sheets of epithelial cells interspersed by a myxomatous stroma that sometimes condenses into pseudocartilage. It is characteristically a slowly growing, firm, freely mobile mass most commonly found in the tail of the parotid gland. When it is less than 2 cm. in size, it may feel so mobile and superficial that the physician is tempted to remove it in the office. *This is always a mistake.* Adequate treatment for a mixed salivary gland tumor is total parotidectomy. In our experience, nothing short of this carries any assurance against recurrence. The mixed salivary gland tumor is notorious for its ability to produce seedling recurrences. This virtually always happens when the tumor capsule is broken at the time of removal, or the tumor is simply shelled out.

Warthin's tumor is characteristically soft and almost cystic and occurs in the tail of the parotid gland, usually in old men. It may be bilateral. Simple excision effects a cure.

The distinction between a benign and a malignant salivary gland

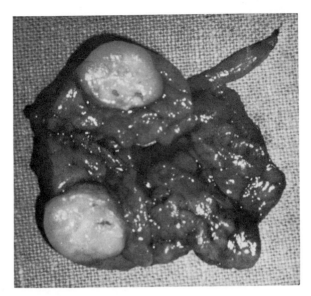

Fig. 42-16. Mixed salivary gland tumor involving the submaxillary salivary gland. This particular neoplasm is much more common in the parotid gland and may also occur in minor salivary glands of the mouth and throat, particularly around the palatine tonsil.

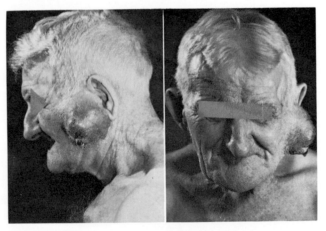

Fig. 42-17. Large, ulcerating adenocarcinoma of the parotid gland.

tumor is frequently a very difficult one. The surgeon is caught between Scylla and Charybdis, where he does not want to biopsy a mass lest it be a mixed tumor, and yet he wants to go to the operating room prepared for whatever radical operation is necessary. Therefore, it is wise to perform total parotidectomy for any parotid tumor. The only characteristic clinical feature of a malignant parotid tumor is a branch paralysis or total paralysis of the facial nerve. Benign tumors reach tremendous size without producing any paralysis of the facial nerve. Other characteristics of malignant tumors are fixation, pain, and tenderness (Fig. 42-17). However, benign tumors may be tender or painful as

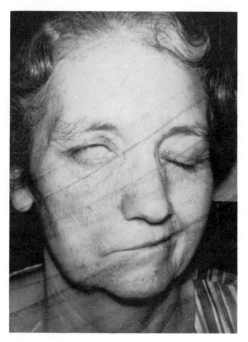

Fig. 42-18. Right complete peripheral facial paralysis with a marked "Bell's phenomenon." This may be due to a lesion anywhere along the course of the facial nerve trunk: internal auditory canal, middle ear, mastoid, or parotid gland. If the cause is not determinable on complete work-up, the diagnosis is Bell's palsy. This patient has just had a parotid malignancy removed and the facial nerve grafted. Facial motion will return in 9 to 12 months.

well, if recent hemorrhage into the tumor produces capsular stretch. If either one of these features is present, the surgeon should assume malignancy and make appropriate preparations. The facial nerve is not sacrificed at operation unless the nerve is stuck to the tumor, in which event it is immediately grafted, using a sensory nerve as donor (Fig. 42-18).

Epidermoid carcinoma is the single most common malignant tumor of salivary glands, but the adenocarcinomas as a group are more common than the epidermoid carcinoma. *Adenocystic carcinoma* is highly lethal, tending to metastasize early in regional lymphatics and to lung. *Mucoepidermoid carcinoma* is rare. Rarer still is *acidophilic cell adenocarcinoma,* which is thought to arise from ductal epithelium, and is a tumor of old men. *Acinic cell adenocarcinoma* is the second most common of the adenocarcinoma group, occurring in females predominantly, and it tends to act more like a sarcoma than a carcinoma in that it metastasizes via the bloodstream.

Benign tumors are more common than malignant tumors in the parotid gland, but in the submaxillary gland approximately 50% of neoplasms are malignant. Well over half of the minor salivary gland tumors are malignant.

Differential diagnosis. Salivary gland calculi may mimic neoplasm by obstruction of salivary flow, but usually a clear history of fluctuation in size of the gland is present. *Mikulicz's disease* and *Sjögren's syndrome* may resemble neoplasms, but they are diffuse diseases of the gland rather than localized; biopsy may be necessary to rule out cancer, and this is permissible in diffuse diseases of the salivary glands. A *high cervical lymph node* may be mistaken for a tumor in the tail of the parotid gland. If the mass can be brought out over the body or ramus of the mandible, it is a parotid gland mass rather than carotid sheath node. A *hypertrophied masseter* or a *wing mandible* may be confused with a diseased parotid gland.

HEARING LOSSES AND MICROSURGERY OF THE EAR
Sensorineural hearing loss

Sensorineural deafness (sensory, or hair cells of the organ of Corti; neural, eighth nerve or above this level in the central nervous system). This is often called "nerve" deafness or perceptive deafness. It is the most common form of deafness. Here are some causes:

1. Congenital
2. Traumatic
3. Toxic
4. Vascular
5. Infection
6. Neoplasm
7. Ménière's disease
8. Degenerative

Congenital sensorineural deafness is usually very severe. As a rule it is bilateral, and so serious that the patient can hear only the loudest of sounds, and of these, only low tones. Such a person will never develop normal speech and needs training in special schools all during his early years. Congenital deafness may be due to Rh incompatibilities, birth trauma, in utero virus infection, malformation of the inner ears, or other causes. Mild forms of congenital deafness also occur. *Traumatic sensorineural deafnesses* are of three kinds: noise-induced deafness, otic concussion, and transverse temporal bone fracture.

The most common is *noise-induced deafness,* commonly called acoustic trauma, which results from an accumulation of the effects of intense sound over months or years. This is becoming more and more prevalent. It is manifest early as a selective 4096 Hz. (Hertz) dip on the audiogram, not impairing speech reception. *Otic concussion* produces a high tone deafness and is the result of either cerebral concussion or the convergence of lines of force through the skull, which center on the temporal bone. *Transverse temporal bone fracture* (see p. 1010) causes a total inner ear deafness. *Toxic deafness* in this country today is generally caused by drugs, the most common of which are aspirin, streptomycin, and kanamycin. This is a direct effect of the drug upon the hair cell. *Vascular deafness* is the result of occlusion of the end artery to the labyrinth and produces total deafness together with loss of vestibular function. It is sometimes called "otic apoplexy." *Viral infection,* the most common of which is the mumps virus, can cause deafness. Fortunately, this almost always spares one ear. It is quite common in children and may not be discovered until adult life or on a routine school audiometric program.

Loss of hearing in one ear produces inability to localize sound and the loss of stereo effect of hearing, preventing the individual from separating out one voice from another when there are multiple conversations in the room; this is sometimes called the "cocktail party effect" of binaural hearing. Bacterial infection from meningitis or from chronic mastoiditis can invade the inner ear and produce immediate total deafness and loss of vestibular function. *Neoplasms* that begin in the middle ear, mastoid, or the auditory nerve produce deafness by growth and infiltration. Of these, the most common are acoustic neuroma, glomus jugulare tumor, and epidermoid carcinoma. *Ménière's disease* is listed separately because we do not know whether it is caused by vascular, toxic, or metabolic factors. It is a pure hair cell deafness, and as such is accompanied by a severe discrimination loss and *recruitment.* Recruitment is the abnormal growth of loudness in a deafened ear. The deafness fluctuates. The disease is characterized by tinnitus and vertigo, the spells lasting 20 minutes to many hours. Treatment is diuretics, vasodilators, and a low-sodium diet. Generally only one ear is affected. If treatment fails, destruction labyrinthotomy may be necessary. *Degenerative sensorineural deafness* is called *presbycusis*. It is the result of gradual loss of hair cells and/or first order neurons, because of the aging process. This strikes virtually all people, and begins in the very high tones. It goes on all through life, but only in the middle-aged or older patient does it produce noticeable deafness by finally involving the upper and then the middle speech frequencies. Even a person 20 years of age does not have as extensive high tone hearing as a younger person. There is no treatment for presbycusis. All the preceding causes of deafness tend to be additive to degenerative deafness, so that presbycusis may occur in such patients at an earlier age than otherwise.

Conductive hearing loss

A *conductive deafness* is any form of deafness that tends to impede sound from reaching the sensorineural apparatus. There are many causes, the more common of which are the following:

    Canal problems, including congenital atresia and stenosis
    Chronic nonsuppurative otitis media
    Chronic suppurative otitis media
    Ossicular destruction or fixation, including otosclerosis
    Trauma

Chronic nonsuppurative otitis media and *chronic suppurative otitis media* have been discussed in the section on *infection. Canal problems* that produce deafness do so by complete blockage of the canal. If even a very small passageway remains for air to reach the tympanic membrane, hearing is unaffected. Wax impactions and acute external otitis are the most common in this category. Other causes are osteomas of the canal, neoplasms of the skin of the canal, neoplasms about the ear such as neurofibromatosis, and congenital atresia, either occurring singly or as a part of a more general anomaly such as Treacher-Collins syndrome. A *perforation* of the tympanic membrane from unresolved middle ear infection or trauma, produces a conductive deafness by virtue of loss of the sound-gathering ability of the tympanic membrane. *Clinical otosclerosis* is a disease of young adults, caused by ankylosis of the stapes by an overgrowth of spongiotic bone from the enchondral layer of otic capsule. It is slowly progressive, and a history of repeated earaches or otorrhea is absent. There is usually a positive family history. It is slightly more common in females than in males. A normal tympanic membrane is compatible with this diagnosis. The deafness is frequently purely conductive, although there may be a mild to moderate sensorineural deafness superimposed. This form of deafness can

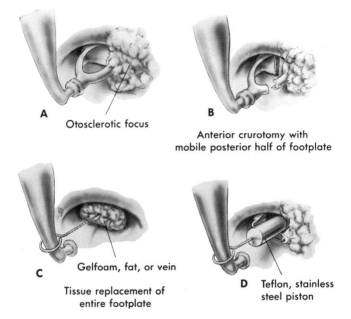

Fig. 42-19. Various methods of handling otosclerotic deafness. **A,** Focus of spongiotic bone is visible at the anterior portion of the footplate binding the stapes in the oval window. **B,** Anterior crurotomy has been done. The footplate is fractured behind the otosclerotic focus, and the posterior assembly is mobile. **C,** Entire stapes has been removed; the footplate is replaced with a tissue graft or Gelfoam and the crura with a stainless steel wire; the knot holding the tissue graft is buried in it. **D,** Teflon piston secured by a wire around the incus replaces the central portion of the footplate.

usually be helped by an operation (see Fig. 42-19). *Traumatic deafness* can be caused by a bursting of the tympanic membrane that has failed to heal, a dislocation of the ossicles in the middle ear, or a temporal bone fracture of longitudinal nature.

Hearing testing

The *decibel* (dB.) is the measure used to describe degrees of hearing loss. It is important to note that the decibel is not a unit of measurement, but a ratio. Hearing loss is expressed logarithmically, because the ear is able to work over a great expanse of energy input.

The decibel is a logarithmic ratio between an observed sound pressure level and a reference level. For every increase in sound of 6 dB., there is a doubling of sound pressure.

The *audiogram* indicates hearing levels at thresholds over a frequency range of 125 to 8000 Hertz. Across the ordinate of the audiogram, the threshold of hearing from 0 to 100 dB. loss is indicated at that frequency. One also measures hearing thresholds at each of the speech frequencies (250, 500, 1000, 2000 Hz.) by bone conduction, placing a transducer over the mastoid bone and stimulating the sensorineural receptor apparatus directly rather than through the ossicular chain and tympanic membrane.

With use of the audiometer, *discrimination testing* can be performed. This is a test of how clearly words are understood by the ear. The volume is raised 40 dB. above the threshold of hearing, and the number of phonetically balanced words the patient can understand is recorded. The normal ear can understand at least 80% of these words. When discrimination ability is definitely impaired, it indicates a sensory or a neural deafness. Conductive deafnesses do not impair word discrimination ability.

Tuning fork tests are important in the identification of hearing loss. The tuning forks most useful are the 512 and 1024 Hz. and frequently the 256 and 2048 Hz. The *Rinne test* is performed by placing the stem of the fork sounded above threshold first over the mastoid bone just behind and above the external canal, and then over the external canal an inch away from the ear. If bone conduction is louder than air conduction, the Rinne test is said to be negative, and if air conduction is louder than bone conduction, it is positive. A negative Rinne test is characteristic of a conductive deafness. A positive Rinne is compatible with normal hearing or a sensorineural deafness. It is important to mask the opposite ear when there is a significant difference of hearing between the two ears, so that during bone conduction testing the sound is not perceived in the opposite or better ear. The *Weber test* is performed by placing the stem of the fork somewhere in the midline: the vertex, the forehead, or the upper incisor teeth. The fork will lateralize to the better ear in a sensorineural deafness, or to the deaf ear in a conductive deafness. It is a rather sensitive test.

Tuning fork tests are supplemented by *whisper and speech tests* to determine the approximate level of the deafness. The normal or very slightly deaf ear can perceive the lightest "residual air" whispered voice. A light-whispered voice audible a few inches from the ear indicates a 20 to 30 dB. deafness, a medium-whispered voice 30 to 40 dB. deafness, a low-spoken voice 50 to 60 dB. deafness, a medium-spoken voice 70 to 80 dB. deafness. If the ear cannot hear a loud-spoken voice or a shout with the other ear properly masked, it is said to be stone deaf.

A number of *special auditory tests* provide a relatively high degree of localization of the lesion, i.e., these special tests may tell us whether the deafness is hair cell in origin, neural, or cortical. Some of them are the short increment sensitivity index (SISI test), tone fatigue testing, Bekesy audiometry, and recruitment. There is also a wide variety of tests available for malingered deafness. There are even special tests available for objective evaluation of auditory acuity, not involving a judgment on the part of the patient. These include psychogalvanic skin response and evoked cortical potential recording using an analog computer.

Tinnitus aurium

Tinnitus aurium means nothing more than ringing in the ears. This is a symptom and not a disease. Tinnitus of varying degree is almost invariably associated with deafness, and it is present to the degree that the ear is deaf. Usually, the tinnitus will be at about the same frequency as the deafness, such that presbycusis or high-tone deafness produces a high-pitched ringing and conductive deafness produces a panfrequency or "white noise" ringing. Tinnitus may be subdivided into *objective* and *subjective*. Subjective tinnitus is that which the patient alone can hear, and the physician is unable to detect any sound using his stethoscope over the external canal or over the temporal region. Objective tinnitus is that which the physician can hear as well. Objective tinnitus always means that there is a physical basis for the tinnitus instead of a sensory or neural lesion. Examples of objective tinnitus are that produced by a cavernous sinus fistula, eddy currents of blood in the carotid system from an arteriosclerotic plaque, eustachian tube clicks, and tympanic muscle clicks from spasm of the tensor tympani muscle or stapedius muscle. The only treatment for tinnitus is detection of the underlying cause, and its correction if possible.

Mastoidectomy

Mastoidectomy is performed for acute or chronic suppurative bone infection of the mastoid portion of the temporal bone (Fig. 42-6). The incidence of mastoidectomy for acute disease has dropped precipitously since antibiotics have become available, but at the same time, mastoidectomy done for chronic bone infection has risen.

A *simple mastoidectomy* is performed for acute osteomyelitis of the mastoid bone. The mastoid cortex is removed and all air cells and diseased bone are removed. This means usually removal of the mastoid tip. The ossicles, tympanic membrane, and the posterior bony canal wall are left intact. If the middle ear becomes well, hearing is unaffected. A simple mastoidectomy is not done for chronic mastoiditis or middle ear disease.

A *modified radical mastoidectomy* is performed for chronic suppurative mastoiditis and otitis media. The mastoid cortex is removed, and a meticulous removal of all mastoid air cells is done as the first step. The posterior canal wall is then removed, with the skin of the posterior and superior canal wall preserved. The epitympanum is then exenterated of disease, and the incus and the head and neck of the malleus is removed. The tympanic membrane is reflected medially until it comes in contact with the head of the stapes, and the skin of the canal is used to line the mastoid cavity, sealing the middle ear from the remaining cavity. This operation joins the external canal and the mastoid cavity, making one large chamber. The cavity then heals by secondary intention, becoming skin-lined in a matter of weeks. Wax and skin debris must be removed from this cavity at twice yearly intervals, because it does not have the normal debris-removing characteristics of the normal ear canal. Excellent hearing may possibly occur after this operation. Theoretically, only the lever ratio of the ossicular chain is sacrificed, and thus it is possible to have as little as a 2 dB. deafness (Fig. 42-20, *B*).

A *radical mastoidectomy* is the same as the modified operation except that portions of the middle ear and tympanic membrane are removed. The contents of the middle ear are exenterated, except for the stapes. Thus one large chamber is created, comprising the external canal, the mastoid cavity, and the middle ear, open for inspection the rest of the patient's life. The consequent hearing loss is, of course, severe: between 45 and 60 dB. (Fig. 42-20, *A*).

Microsurgery of the ear

Deafness is still man's most common physical impairment, despite the myriad ways modern man has found to maim and injure himself. Fortunately, a significant number of deafnesses are surgically correctable, especially those caused by defects in the conducting apparatus (tympanic) membrane, the ossicular chain, and stapedovestibular joint. Since that part of the tympanum containing the hearing mechanism is quite small (Fig. 42-21), these operations are done under magnification and are termed microsurgical operations. Some of the diseases causing deafness that may be helped by microsurgery are (1) tympanic perforation, (2) ossicular chain disruption with or without an intact tympanic membrane, (3) chronic suppurative otitis media (after mastoid disease is controlled), (4) certain varieties of chronic adhesive otitis media, (5) tympanosclerosis, and (6) otosclerosis.

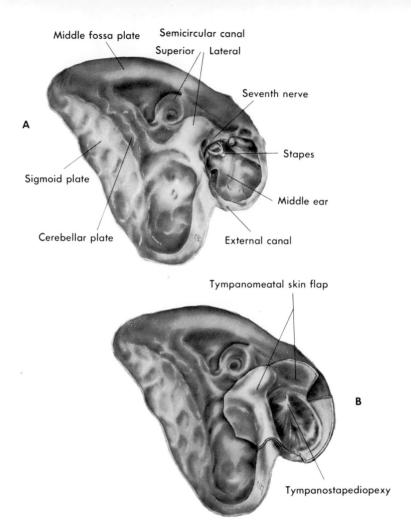

Fig. 42-20. A, The radical mastoidectomy; here, one large common chamber is created, including the mastoid bowl, the middle ear, and the external auditory canal; the ossicles are removed except for the stapes; this is essentially a sculpturing of the bony plates surrounding the temporal bone and is reserved for advanced tympanomastoid disease. **B,** The modified radical mastoidectomy; if the mesotympanum can be preserved, the tympanic membrane is tilted inward to contact the stapes and is held in this new position by reflection of a tympanomeatal canal skin flap onto the facial ridge and roof of the cavity; this preserves hearing.

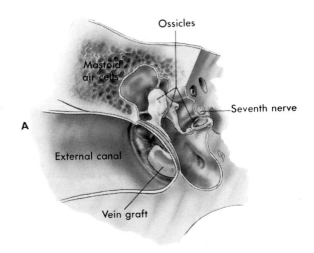

Fig. 42-21. A, Tympanoplasty type I. Note all structures are normal in the middle ear and mastoid, except for the perforation of the tympanic membrane in its lower portion; a vein graft overlies the outer portion of the perforation, after the skin surrounding the perforation has been meticulously removed; it is more common to place the graft material inside the tympanic membrane. **B,** Tympanoplasty type II. The ossicular chain is preserved because it is free of disease; the external auditory canal and the mastoid bowl are one common chamber, from which the middle ear is sealed; normal hearing is obtainable with this operation. **C,** Tympanoplasty type III. Because of disease, the malleus and incus were sacrificed, and the tympanic membrane rests against the head of the stapes; otherwise it is the same as tympanoplasty type II; excellent hearing is attainable, because only the lever ratio of the ossicular chain is sacrificed; the areal ratio (tympanic membrane to footplate) is maintained; this operation is the same as a modified radical mastoidectomy. **D,** Tympanoplasty type IV. The stapedial arch required sacrifice or was absent through disease; the footplate is left exposed to the outside, and the tympanic membrane is sealed against the promontory; the round window (shaded area in center of hypotympanum) is thus joined with the eustachian tube orifice as a closed air-containing chamber; because areal ratio is sacrificed as well as lever ratio, normal hearing is not obtainable; the best level that is theoretically obtainable is 26 dB. below normal.

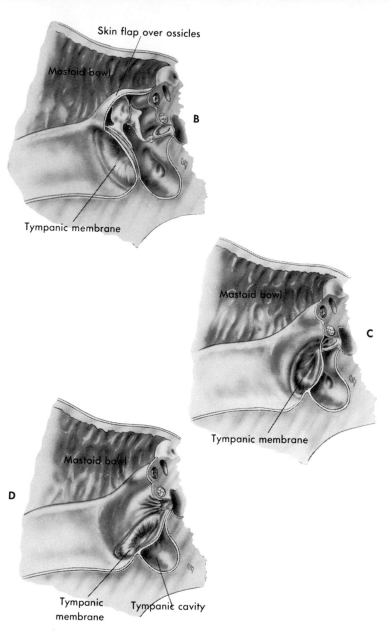

Fig. 42-21, cont'd. For legend see opposite page.

These operations may be performed transmeatally, or across the mastoid after mastoidectomy has been performed. The binocular operating microscope is used, which provides a coaxially lighted image of brilliant intensity, magnified from 6 to 40 times. Operations are done under general or local anesthesia. Where the tympanic membrane is intact, such as in otosclerosis or tympanosclerosis, a skin flap is elevated from the posterior canal wall hinged on the posterior half of the tympanic membrane. Access to the tympanum is gained between the fibrocartilaginous annular ligament and the bony annulus of the tympanum. This renders the posterior half of the tympanum visible, and with it, almost all of the conductive apparatus. A wide variety of special instruments is necessary for these operations. They are electrical and air turbine drills, chisels, needles, picks, hooks, knives, elevators, scissors, saws, suction tips, and various forceps. They are unique primarily in their diminutive size. Since these instruments are all hand-held and not moved by micromanipulators, the surgeon's touch must be developed to an uncommon deftness. This usually takes several years of patient practice.

CHAPTER 43

Gynecology

HERBERT J. BUCHSBAUM
F. K. CHAPLER

Gynecology, a surgical and medical specialty, involves the study, diagnosis, and treatment of disorders of the female reproductive tract. Superficially this discipline appears restricted, but in actuality it includes the total medical, emotional, and physical assessment of the patient. Thoroughness is mandatory, as reproductive tract dysfunction often reflects systemic disease or psychic disturbance. As examples, marital discord can trigger pelvic pain or menstrual dysfunction; a blood dyscrasia may be heralded by menstral hemorrhage; or unsuspected metabolic disease such as diabetes mellitus can perpetuate a vulvovaginitis.

GYNECOLOGICAL HISTORY

The patient should be allowed to present her chief complaint in her own words. Then the physician develops the total history, emphasizing the menstrual, fertility (obstetric), and marital aspects. Particular attention should be given to abnormal vaginal bleeding or discharge, abdominopelvic pain, associated urinary and gastrointestinal tract symptoms, as well as evidence for genital tract relaxation.

GYNECOLOGICAL EXAMINATION

The gynecological examination is performed in the presence of a female attendant after complete physical examination. Proper draping with appropriate regard for the patient's sensitivities is essential. The bladder and rectum should be emptied prior to examination.

An examining table with leg stirrips, a light source, examining gloves, lubricating jelly, bivalve speculums, ring forceps with cotton balls, a single tooth tenaculum, and instruments for obtaining a

Papanicolaou smear and cervical and endometrial biopsies constitute the basic facilities and equipment.

Evaluation of the external genitalia includes visual and palpatory examination of the mons, clitoris, labia, Bartholin glands, urethra, and perineum, in search for anatomic defects (congenital or acquired) or pathological changes. Inflamed vaginal mucosa with a cheesy discharge and a folliculitis is often the only physical evidence of incipient diabetes mellitus. A speculum is next inserted into the introitus and the entire vaginal canal examined (Fig. 43-1, *A*). The cervix is inspected

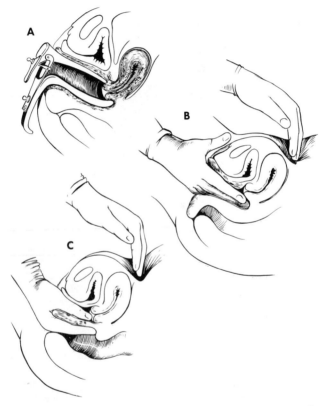

Fig. 43-1. Pelvic examination. **A,** Insertion of the vaginal speculum. **B,** Bimanual abdominovaginal palpation of uterus and adnexa. **C,** Bidigital rectovaginal exam (forefinger in vagina and middle finger in rectum).

and the presence of any lesions noted. A conventional way of recording the site of a lesion is by the face of a clock, with 12 o'clock being anterior on the patient, 6 o'clock posterior. One next carries out bimanual abdominopelvic examination, noting the position of the cervix, consistency, and mobility. Tenderness elicited on lateral motion of the cervix may have great clinical significance. On bimanual examination (Fig. 43-1, *B*), the position (anterior or posterior), size, and contour of the uterine corpus are determined. The adnexal structures, tubes and ovaries, are examined for enlargement, unusual tenderness, or fixation. Positive findings are always reported as right or left of the *patient*.

Bidigital, rectovaginal examination (Fig. 43-1, *C*) completes the routine pelvic examination. In this manner, the uterosacral ligaments, the parametrial and paracervical areas, and the cul-de-sac can be evaluated.

With some experience, the pelvic structures can be palpated and pelvic pathology detected. The size of lesions is always given in centimeters and the shape, consistency, and mobility are described. With greater experience comes increased ability to interpret physical findings.

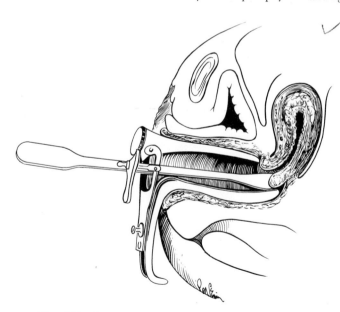

Fig. 43-2. Papanicolaou test—cervical scraping smear.

BENIGN GYNECOLOGICAL CONDITIONS
Useful general gynecological diagnostic procedures and tests

Papanicolaou (Pap) test. The Papanicolaou test, a cytological test, involves glass slide smears of aspirates from the posterior vaginal pool and scrapings from the external cervical os as shown in Fig. 43-2. After appropriate preparation and microscope evaluation, the test is reported as *negative, doubtful* (suspicious or atypical cells), or *positive* (cancer cells). We believe that every sexually active woman should undergo this test annually, regardless of age. The accuracy rate for detecting cervical carcinoma exceeds 90% but is less efficient (60%) for endometrial carcinoma. The management of the patient with an abnormal Pap test will be considered in detail in the oncology section on p. 1059.

Wet vaginal smears. Microscopic evaluation of a wet smear of pathological vaginal discharge (leukorrhea) often elucidates the etiological agent for the following inflammations.

Trichomonas vaginitis. A mixture of 1 drop of discharge and 1 drop of saline solution shows the motile, flagellated, and pear-shaped parasite. Its size is intermediate between that of a while blood cell and a squamous epithelial cell.

Monilial vaginitis. 1 drop of 10% KOH dissolves all but the fungal agent. Long thin septate hyphae and oval yeast buds are seen. Incubation of the vaginal aspirate on Nickerson's medium at room temperature produces dark brown colonies in a few days.

Nonspecific vaginitis (usually cervicitis). A saline wet smear shows an abundance of white blood cells and bacteria.

Atrophic vaginitis. The saline mixture reveals a paucity of superficial (cornified) and many basal epithelial cells, indicative of estrogen deficiency. Many white blood cells, bacteria, trichomonads, or fungal mycelia may be seen.

Schiller's test. The normal squamous epithelium of the vagina and cervix (laden with tissue glycogen) takes on a rich mahogany color when painted with a special iodine solution. Areas that remain light in color (nonstained) are abnormal and the test is considered positive. These areas of epithelial atypicality should be biopsied for microscopic analysis. Cervical biopsies require no anesthesia, and vaginal biopsies only a local anesthetic. This test is particularly useful when the Pap smear is abnormal. Since the columnar epithelium of the endocervical canal does not take up the iodine, exposed canal epithelium in an everted and lacerated cervix will not stain and should not indicate a Schiller positive area.

Pregnancy tests. Pregnancy tests are biological, immunological, and

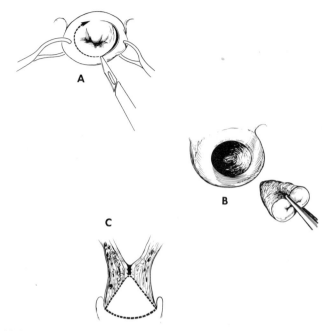

Fig. 43-3. Cone biopsy of the cervix. **A,** Line of incision. **B,** Specimen removed. **C,** Frontal section of cervix and lower corpus demonstrating extent of conization.

radioimmunological assays for detecting human chorionic gonadotropin of placental origin. Quality-controlled tests are reliable about 10 to 14 days after the first missed menstrual period.

Dilatation and curettage (D&C). The diagnostic and therapeutic operative procedure of dilatation and curettage is most adequately performed under general anesthesia. After vaginal antisepsis, the cervix is dilated and the endocervical canal sharply curetted. Then the endometrial cavity is explored for possible polyps with forceps, prior to curettage of the endometrium. The three specimens are submitted separately.

Cone biopsy of the cervix. When more definitive analysis of the cervix is required, a cervical cone is excised by scalpel as shown in Fig. 43-3. This should be done without prior cervical dilatation. Then the endometrium can be curetted and hemostasis of the cone site achieved by heavy figure-of-eight chromic catgut sutures placed laterally at 3 and 9 o'clock.

Laparoscopy. The laparoscope allows the operator to visualize the pelvic organs for diagnostic and therapeutic purposes. The procedure involves general anesthesia, insufflation of the peritoneal cavity with CO_2 through a Verres needle, introduction of the instrument through a small infraumbilical incision, and a fiberoptic light source. Often an accessory probe or instrument is introduced through a second midline suprapubic incision (Fig. 43-4). Table 43-1 lists the indications, uses, complications, and contraindications of this increasingly popular procedure. Constant attention to detail will minimize the complications. Experience in abdominal and/or pelvic surgery is a prerequisite to use of the laparoscope.

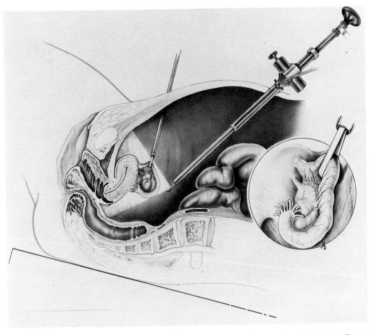

Fig. 43-4. Laparoscopy showing laparoscope and grasping forceps. Inset shows placement for tubal sterilization by coagulation.

Table 43-1. The laparoscope

  I. Indications
    A. Pelvic pain
    B. Infertility
      1. Unexplained
      2. Ovulation disorders
      3. Tubal evaluation
      4. Pre- and post-tuboplasty
    C. Pelvic mass
    D. Pelvic organ abnormalities
    E. Selected amenorrhea cases
    F. Carcinoma follow-up
 II. Operative procedures
    A. Tubal coagulation
    B. Lysis of adhesions
    C. Fulguration of endometriosis
    D. Biopsy of ovary, liver nodule
    E. Peritoneal fluid aspiration
    F. Foreign body recovery
III. Complications
    A. Hemorrhage, hematoma
    B. Bowel perforation
    C. Electrical burns (skin, bowel)
    D. Emphysema
    E. Gas embolism
    F. Cardiorespiratory problems
    G. Infection
    H. Anesthetic incidents
IV. Contraindications
    A. Peritonitis
    B. Ileus
    C. Large abdominal or pelvic mass
    D. Abdominal aneurysm
    E. Failed pneumoperitoneum
    F. Abdominal hernia
    G. Contraindication to general anesthesia
    H. Previous abdominal surgery (relative)
    I. Obesity (relative)

Early pregnancy termination. For whatever reason this procedure is done, it remains very complex and controversial. Revision of existing abortion laws, modified public opinion, and an apparent social need have resulted in an increasing number of hospitals and physicians offering this service. Techniques utilized during the first trimester include menstrual extraction up to 6 weeks' gestation, and vacuum uterine evacuation up to 12 weeks. Midtrimester terminations are more difficult, and the current use of intrauterine instillation of hypertonic saline solution carries a reasonable risk of infection and blood coagulation defects. The use of prostaglandins for midtrimester termination is currently being evaluated. Hysterotomy is rarely done.

Infections and benign disorders of the lower genital tract
Vulva

Chronic vulvar dystrophy. These "white lesions" of the vulva, of unknown etiology, usually appear after the menopause. The term "dystrophy" describes a group of disorders that previously have been designated separately under a variety of terms: leukoplakia, kraurosis, lichen sclerosus et atrophicus, atrophic vulvitis, hyperplastic vulvitis, etc. This classification lumps together the atrophic or hypertrophic changes resulting from a disordered epithelial growth pattern. The surface lesions can be elevated or flat, white (or sometimes red), and are associated with fissuring, weeping, lichenification, and occasionally ulceration. Pruritus is the chief symptom, but soreness and burning can be intense. Multiple biopsies, particularly in suspicious areas, help to evaluate whether the epithelial changes are benign, atypical, or carcinomatous.

Atypia and carcinoma require surgical therapy (see the oncology section on p. 1054); benign changes deserve medical therapy. The latter includes improved local hygiene, treatment of irritating vaginal discharge, and cortisol preparations administered either topically or injected intradermally. More recently, topical 2% testosterone propionate in a petrolatum vehicle has been found to be effective. Treatment results are good in atrophic dystrophy, but less dramatic in the hypertrophic form. Clitoral growth and some increase in facial hair growth have accompanied these hormonal treatments, as a result of systemic absorption of the drugs.

Bartholin's cyst. Bartholin's cyst, a postinflammatory (not necessarily gonococcal) pseudocyst of the Bartholin's gland forms behind a blocked duct. When infected, it is extremely painful and tender, requiring incision and drainage. After subsidence of the inflammation, the cyst should be totally excised. A noninfected cyst, troublesome because of size, should be excised. Some advocate simple marsupialization to form a new duct opening.

Labial agglutination. Agglutination of the labia occurs in infants and young children. It may be asymptomatic or may produce skin irritation from urine collecting behind the agglutination. Since the agglutination usually resolves in later childhood, no treatment of the asymptomatic patient is required. If symptomatic, the physician can usually separate the labia without anesthesia. The mother must maintain separation until healing occurs; judicious application of an estrogen cream to the involved skin areas speeds healing.

Vagina

Trichomonas vaginitis. The trichomonad is transmitted venereally and the diagnosis confirmed by detecting the parasite. The discharge is thin, bubbly, greenish yellow, irritating, and malodorous. The treatment of choice is metronidazole (Flagyl), 250 mg. orally three times daily for 10 days. If it recurs, both the patient and her sexual partner need treatment, since the male is an asymptomatic carrier. Do not use Flagyl in pregnancy, but rather one of the vaginal medications such as furazolidone (Tricofuron) or diiodohydroxyquin (Floraquin).

Monilial vaginitis. Often the discharge from monilial vaginitis resembles cottage cheese and causes severe vulvitis. The male partner may complain of penile glans irritation. One mycostatin vaginal suppository daily for 15 days usually cures most patients. Occasionally a cortisol-like cream is required locally for severe vulvar pruritus. The infection can be resistant or recurrent in patients who are pregnant, diabetic, or taking oral contraceptives. Occasionally diabetic patients require vaginal cleaning with povidone-iodine (Betadine) followed by gentian violet painting of the entire vaginal wall for symptomatic relief.

Atrophic vaginitis. Estrogen deficiency in the post-menopausal or castrated woman may produce atrophic vaginitis. Thinning of the vaginal mucosa leads to infection, synechial formation, and spotting. Associated atrophy of the bladder epithelium evokes symptoms of cystitis. Local treatment by applying dienestrol, an estrogen cream, [Restrol] or conjugated estrogenic substances [Premarin] vaginally every night for 2 to 4 weeks may suffice. The treatment should be repeated every 3 to 4 months to avoid recurrence. Systemic therapy (0.625 or 1.25 mg. Premarin by mouth daily for the first 25 days of each month) alleviates other symptoms of estrogen lack as well.

Nonspecific vaginitis. Nonspecific vaginitis is often associated with cervicitis, and its treatment involves therapy of the cervical infection (see the section on the cervix, p. 1044).

Vulvovaginitis in children. A purulent discharge admixed with blood often suggests a vaginal foreign body. The physician can often palpate the object on rectal examination. Roentgenographic examination helps detect foreign bodies that are radiopaque. A urethroscopic examination of the vagina (occasionally anesthesia is required) detects those objects that are neither palpable nor radiopaque. Manual extraction of the offending foreign object can often be done in the office. Vulvovaginitis may be secondary to a pinworm infestation. Rarely, a gonococcal infection limited to the vagina causes a purulent discharge, resulting from indirect contact with the infected discharge of an adult.

Garter's duct cysts. Garter's duct cysts arise in the anterolateral vaginal wall from Wolffian duct remnants. Total excision is recommended.

Vaginal changes—DES. Changes in the vagina and cervix have been reported in the female offspring of mothers who received diethylstilbestrol (DES) or other nonsteroidal estrogens during pregnancy. These changes include vaginal adenosis, cervical erosion, and vaginal and cervical ridges. The number of cases of clear cell carcinoma of the vagina and cervix in these children suggests a causal relationship with DES. In symptomatic children complete evaluation should be undertaken immediately; in the asymptomatic patient evaluation can be delayed. Evaluation should include cytology, colposcopic examination, differential staining with Lugol's iodine, and biopsy.

Fistulas. Rectovaginal, vesicovaginal, and urethrovaginal fistulas may follow obstetrical and surgical trauma, carcinoma, and heavy pelvic irradiation. Those secondary to operative trauma are surgically repaired after the perifistula inflammation has resolved. Postirradiation fistulas defy correction unless a vascularized pedicle is transposed into the defect from a normal adjacent area.

Cervix

Chronic cervicitis. The majority of parous women, and some sexually active nonparous women, develop some degree of cervical infection. In most it is subclinical, with the only symptom being an increase in mucoid discharge. In the remainder, bacterial infection causes a mucopurulent, malodorous, and irritating discharge. The cervix appears inflamed, edematous, and enlarged. Inflammatory occlusion of glandular ducts produces small yellowish orange nodules called Nabothian cysts. The destruction of squamous epithelium and its replacement by a downgrowth of columnar epithelium from the squamocolumnar junction causes *eversions,* which should be differentiated from true ulcers or *erosions.* Eversions are columnar epithelium in the endocervical canal that becomes visible in the lacerated, parous cervix. Extension of the infection into the endocervical canal can incite endocervical polyp formation. Other repercussions of the cervical infection are parametrial lymphangitis (dyspareunia) and granular urethrotrigonitis (frequency, urgency, and dysuria).

After the physician excludes invasive and intraepithelial cervical neoplasia by Pap smear, colposcopy, and biopsy, he should begin treatment since cervicitis can be the cause of vaginal discharge. Treatment includes nightly douches with povidone-iodine (Betadine) and the application of triple sulfa cream or nitrofurazone (Furacin) suppositories for several weeks. Chronic cervicitis unresponsive to this treatment requires cryosurgery or electrocauterization. These are office procedures and require no anesthesia. Occasionally cases refractory to this treatment respond to cervical conization.

Benign diseases of the uterus
Leiomyomas (fibroids)

Leiomyomas arise from the myometrium. They consist of bundles of smooth muscle cells arranged in a whorl pattern enclosed within a pseudocapsule. Location determines their shape: intramural leiomyomas are spherical, whereas submucosal or subserosal tumors are asymmetrical. The subserosal fibroids may grow into the broad ligament (intraligamentous) or assume a pedunculated shape; uncommonly they derive a blood supply from adjacent tissues with severance of the uterine connection (parasitic). About 5 to 10% of leiomyomas arise in the cervix, and a submucosal pedunculated fibroid may "deliver" through the cervix. They seem to be estrogen dependent, enlarging with pregnancy and receding after the menopause. Benign degenerative changes (hemorrhage, calcification) are common, but sarcomas develop in less than 0.5%. The highest incidence of leiomyomas are found in the black race, nulligravidas, and during the latter portion of reproductive life.

The clinical manifestations of leiomyomas include crampy pain with the menses, heavy menstrual or intermenstrual bleeding, and pressure manifestations because of the enlarged uterine size. During pregnancy, degenerative changes cause pain or the fibroids may impede labor and passage of the baby. Rarely a fibroid uterus is associated with polycythemia (release of an erythropoietin-like material). The diagnosis is usually apparent on pelvic examination, but differentiation between a pedunculated subserosal fibroid and ovarian neoplasm can be difficult.

The treatment is conservative in the small, asymptomatic fibroid uterus. Many gynecologists believe that a fibroid uterus larger than a 3-month gestational size should be removed, even if asymptomatic.

Total abdominal hysterectomy (after a diagnostic D&C) is indicated if symptoms are significant (hemorrhage-induced anemia), regardless of uterine size. Normal ovaries are conserved if the patient is younger than 50 years of age. Fibroids can be "shelled out" (myomectomy) to preserve future childbearing ability.

Adenomyosis

In adenomyosis, endometrial tissue projects into the myometrium. Microscopically this appears as diffuse endometrial islands or localized masses (adenomyomas). Symptoms and pelvic findings consist of increasingly heavy menstrual flow, progressive acquired dysmenorrhea, and an enlarging globular uterus. The uterus occasionally is asymmetrical because of subserosal adenomyomas. The surgeon usually performs total abdominal hysterectomy to relieve symptoms. The diagnosis often depends on the pathologist.

Adenomyosis is also called *endometriosis interna*. The term seems inappropriate, as adenomyosis is dissimilar from endometrial implants, which occur outside of the uterus. Although adenomyosis is most common in multiparous patients in their forties and seems unresponsive to progesterone, "true" endometriosis occurs in younger, infertile women and is hormone responsive.

Endometriosis

Endometriosis is a disorder characterized by hormone-responsive endometrial tissue in extrauterine sites. The most common sites are the ovaries, peritoneal surfaces, uterosacral ligaments and cul-de-sac, posterior lower uterus, and fallopian tubes (Fig. 43-5). Less common sites of endometriosis are the bowel, umbilicus, cervix, external genitalia, abdominal and episiotomy scars, and rarely distant sites like the lungs. Theories of pathogenesis include reflux menstruation through the tubes, lymphatic and hematogenous dissemination, and coelomic epithelial metaplasia. Perhaps several or all mechanisms are operative.

Clinically significant endometriosis is unusual before 20 years of age. It can progress until the menopause, at which time it essentially disappears. The typical patient is in her late twenties or early thirties, nulliparous, and infertile. She complains of severe dysmenorrhea starting just prior to (but terminating with) menstrual flow, dyspareunia, and cyclic bowel and bladder disturbances such as painful defecation and dysuria. Bowel obstruction and cyclic rectal and bladder bleeding are uncommon.

Physical findings include tenderness and nodularity in the cul-de-sac area, retroflexed and fixed uterus, cystic ovarian enlargement (endometrioma), and general pelvic fixation.

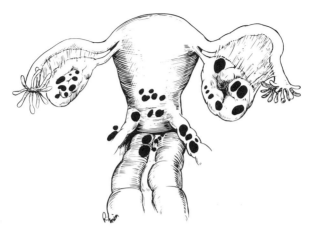

Fig. 43-5. Common sites of pelvic endometriosis.

The diagnosis is suggested by the history and physical findings. Laparoscopy is diagnostic when the typical "powder burn" peritoneal implants permit biopsy. Differential diagnoses include pelvic inflammatory disease, fibroid uterus, and cystic ovarian neoplasm.

Treatment includes observation, analgesics, encouragement of pregnancy if appropriate, and hormones. Palliative hormonal therapy consists of low-dose contraceptive progestins for minimal endometriosis, and large-dose pseudopregnancy progestins for moderate involvement. The pseudopregnancy program consists of gradually increasing doses of combination progestin-estrogen pills to render the patient amenorrheic for 9 months. Intramuscular progestins can also be used. Small doses of estrogen are usually required to prevent spotting. Side effects include weight gain, fluid retention, nausea, and breakthrough bleeding. The rationale for hormonal therapy is the progestin-induced necrobiosis with accompanying atrophy of the endometrial tissue. While successful in many carefully selected patients, it is not generally curative. Temporary symptomatic improvement approaches 75%, while subsequent pregnancies occur in 40%.

Conservative surgery is recommended for moderate and severe endometriosis when reproductive function is to be preserved, or when medical therapy has failed. This involves excision or fulguration of peritoneal implants, resection of endometriomas, lysis of adhesions, suspension of a retroflexed uterus, and occasionally a presacral neurectomy. The extent of the disease markedly influences the postsurgical pregnancy success rate of 50%. When extensive endometriosis exists and/or childbearing is no longer desirable, total abdominal hysterectomy and bilateral salpingo-oophorectomy may be indicated. Residual endometriosis is rarely stimulated by postoperative use of oral estrogen replacement.

Pelvic inflammatory disease (PID) and venereal diseases
Gonorrhea

Gonorrhea now ranks first among communicable diseases, with an estimated three million cases per year. It is epidemic among young men and women, particularly in the 15- to 25-year age group.

The most common sites of infection in the female are the cervix, urethra, Bartholin's and Skene's glands, and rectum. About 1 week after sexual exposure, the female may develop a profuse, thick, irritating vaginal discharge and dysuria, but a significant number of cases are asymptomatic. Ideally, cultures should be obtained from the endocervix, urethra, and rectum. In large screening efforts, the endocervical culture will be the most rewarding. The most effective diagnostic technique is inoculation of Thayer-Martin culture media. The use of Transgrow bottles has facilitated the transport of specimens to the laboratory.

The gonococcus is relatively sensitive to a wide variety of antibiotics. The treatment of choice consists of 4.8 million units of aqueous procaine penicillin given intramuscularly, divided into two doses. One half-hour prior to the injection, 1 Gm. of probenecid should be given orally. This is the most suitable regimen since it will cure incubating syphilis as well as gonorrhea. In the patient allergic to penicillin or penicillin-like drugs alternative regimens utilizing spectinomycin or tetracycline are available.

Upper tract phase. With delayed, inadequate, or no treatment of acute gonorrhea, the organisms ascends along the mucosal surfaces of the uterus and tubes onto the ovaries and pelvic peritoneum. This occurs during the next menses when the cervical mucus barrier is breached, producing acute gonorrheal pelvic inflammatory disease (PID) with the signs, symptoms, and laboratory findings of an acute pelvic peritonitis. The uterus and cervix are exquisitely tender to motion as are both adnexal regions, which may be palpably enlarged. Differential diagnosis includes other acute abdominal infections such as appendicitis, diverticulitis, pyelonephritis, and cystitis.

Treatment is the same as that for peritonitis (see Chapter 20). Wide-spectrum antibiotics are required because of secondary bacterial invaders and should include intramuscular procaine penicillin and streptomycin; initially, aqueous penicillin is given in large doses by the intravenous route. Other antibiotics may be required because of allergy or resistant organisms. The clinical response is usually dramatic in 1 or 2 days, but the antibiotics are continued 5 to 7 days beyond disappearance of the fever. A poor clinical response may herald abscesses in the cul-de-sac or tubo-ovarian area. The former can be drained via the vagina; the latter can be lethal if it ruptures, requiring emergency abdominal surgery. Early and aggressive treatment of acute PID is mandatory to salvage the patient's fertility.

Chronic PID

Repeated attacks of acute PID precipitated by the menses lead to tubal destruction (retort-shaped hydrosalpinx or pyosalpinx), tubo-ovarian abscess, and pelvic viscera fibrosis (Fig. 43-6). The patient is harassed by pain, irregular menstrual bleeding, febrile episodes, and sterility. The causative organisms in this chronic inflammation are nongonococcal. In the early stages, the treatment is medical; in the late stage, it is surgical removal of the uterus, tubes, and ovaries.

Puerperal and postabortal PID

About 20% of the PID cases occur after delivery or abortions. These types of PID are caused chiefly by virulent and invasive gram-

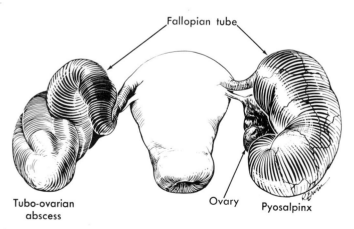

Fig. 43-6. Chronic pelvic inflammatory disease. On biological right, tubo-ovarian abscess. On biological left, pyosalpinx.

negative, endotoxin-producing rods and less often by gram-positive cocci. Uncommonly, a clostridial organism is involved.

The clinical picture is often one of serious sepsis. Once cervical and blood cultures are obtained, vigorous antibiotic and supportive measures are instituted. The infected uterine contents should be evacuated as soon as the patient's condition stabilizes. Urgent treatment can avert septic shock (usually endotoxic with mortality exceeding 50%) and pelvic thrombophlebitis with septic pulmonary embolization. Septic shock demands additional therapy: the use of massive doses of corticosteroids as well as vasomotor drugs. The latter therapy is controversial, but in general try the following therapy:

1. Vasodilator (isoproterenol [Isuprel]) if the central venous pressure is adequate, skin cold and clammy, hypotension increasing.
2. Vasoconstrictor (metaraminol [Aramine]) if CVP is low, skin is warm and dry, and there is hypotension and adequate urine output.

In advanced cases, the infected uterus is removed. When the infection results from *Clostridium,* the medical measures are as outlined in Chapter 6. Early recognition and emergency hysterectomy will avoid an otherwise invariable fatality.

Tuberculous PID

Pelvic tuberculosis is found in 5 to 10% of patients with pulmonary disease. The pelvic structures are secondarily involved by the hematogenous route. Infertility may be its only manifestation, but generally tuberculous PID produces low-grade reproductive tract dysfunction, which includes menstrual irregularities. The best diagnostic approach is to identify the Koch bacillus by culture and animal inoculations of menstrual blood. In minimal cases, antituberculous drugs should be used for at least 6 months. In severe cases, surgery should accompany medical treatment.

Other venereal diseases

Other venereal diseases are syphilis, which is increasing in incidence, and the less common trio chancroid, lymphogranuloma venereum, and granuloma inguinale. Syphilis is caused by the spirochete, *Treponema pallidum,* and is infectious in the primary (hard chancre) and secondary (mucocutaneous patches) stages. History, dark-field microscopy, serological tests, and the clinical manifestations of tertiary lues establish the diagnosis. The antibiotic of choice is penicillin.

Disorders of pelvic support
Retroversion of the uterus

The uterus is anteflexed in 80% of women and retroverted (tilted backward) in the rest. In the past, simple retroversion was blamed for a variety of pelvic complaints including backache, dyspareunia, and heavy menses, as well as infertility, prompting a large number of unnecessary anterior uterine suspensions. Retroversion of the uterus is a normal variation, and surgical correction has been completely abandoned. The uterus may become retroverted by posterior fixation secondary to uterine, adnexal, or cul-de-sac pathological conditions, such as endometriosis.

Pelvic relaxation

Pelvic relaxation results most commonly from obstetrical trauma, with stretching of the pelvic supporting tissues. The bladder and urethra may bulge into the vagina, a result of weakening of the anterior fascia causing a cystourethrocele. Laxity of the perirectal fascia can result in a rectocele. This relaxation of the pelvic outlet is most often accompanied by uterine descensus. The weakened uterine supportive ligaments allow the uterus to descend down the vaginal tube. In its extreme form the uterus may prolapse through the introitus.

The cystocele gives rise to a most distressing symptom: urinary stress incontinence. The involuntary loss of urine occurs with increased intra-abdominal pressure from laughing, coughing, sneezing, or straining. An anatomical defect has been identified which is amenable to surgical correction: obliteration of the normal posterior urethrovesical angle. Stress incontinence must be differentiated from urgency incontinence (severe infection), continuous incontinence (fistula), and overflow incontinence (neurogenic bladder). History and simple laboratory and diagnostic techniques allow the physician to distinguish these entities. Rectoceles are usually asymptomatic, but on occasion may cause problems with bowel movements.

The surgical correction of stress incontinence is by Kelly plication and anterior colporrhaphy. By this technique the posterior urethrovesical angle is restored and the hernia corrected, resulting in relief in 85% of patients. When uterine descensus is present a vaginal hysterectomy should also be performed. Posterior colporrhaphy and perineorrhaphy should be performed when there is a rectocele.

An alternative to this vaginal surgical correction of stress incontinence and uterine descensus is urethropexy (Marshall-Marchetti-Krantz procedure) and abdominal hysterectomy. Colpocleisis, obliteration of the vaginal canal, can be used in the small number of patients in whom medical complications contradict a more definitive operative procedure.

Disorders of early pregnancy
Ectopic pregnancy

Failure of a fertilized ovum to migrate to a normal intrauterine nidation site may result in implantation in an ectopic site—primarily tube, but also ovary, abdominal cavity, or cervix. Most often an ectopic pregnancy occurs because preexisting chronic salpingitis impedes normal passage of the egg.

Classically, the patient relates one or two missed menses followed by the sudden onset of acute lower abdominal pain and signs of hemorrhagic shock. Pelvic examination shows, minimal bleeding from the cervix, and possibly a small, tender adnexal mass. Cul-de-sac needle aspiration returns blood that fails to clot. This confirms intra-abdominal hemorrhage. After blood replacement is begun, the surgeon must excise the ectopic pregnancy, the involved fallopian tube, and sometimes the ovary.

The historical and physical features are often atypical and must be differentiated from other gynecological conditions: early threatened abortion, anovulatory irregular cycles with a painful ovarian follicle cyst, bleeding into or rupture and hemorrhage of a corpus luteum cyst, etc. Particularly difficult to diagnose is the patient with an unruptured ectopic pregnancy. Laparoscopic examination can be helpful in these difficult diagnostic problems.

Abortion (AB)

Abortion is the spontaneous or induced (criminal, therapeutic) termination of pregnancy during the first 20 weeks. Therapeutic abortion is done for medical and, increasingly, for psychosocial reasons.

The spontaneous abortion incidence is about 15%, occurs usually in the first trimester, and is most often caused by blighted ova. The clinical features are a history of one or two missed menses, the onset of spotting or bleeding associated with cramps (threatened AB), beginning cervical dilatation (inevitable AB), and then incomplete or complete passage of the products of conception. Bleeding may be heavy enough to cause hemorrhagic shock. Fever and toxicity should raise the suspicion of criminal intervention. Incomplete abortions require oxytocic infusion and a D&C, whereas complete abortions usually do not. Habitual abortion means three consecutive or nonconsecutive abortions. They usually are first trimester abortions but can be second trimester mishaps because of uterine congenital anomalies (see congenital anomalies, p. 1080) or an incompetent cervix. The patient with cervical incompetence has a history of painless second trimester cervical dilatation, prolapse and rupture of the amniotic sac, and delivery of an immature fetus. Surgical placement of an encircling Mersilene ligature submucosally at the level of the internal os can correct the incompetence. At term the surgeon removes the synthetic ligature.

Molar pregnancy and choriocarcinoma

See the oncology section, p. 1071.

Ovarian tumors

The ovary can be the site of neoplastic and nonneoplastic cysts or tumors. The nonneoplastic or physiological lesions include follicular and corpus luteum cysts. These can cause temporary menstrual aberrations but usually regress and disappear within one or two cycles. The physiological lesions are usually small, less than 5 cm. in size, and can be managed conservatively. Should a corpus luteum cyst rupture with intraperitoneal hemorrhage, surgical intervention is needed. At celiotomy, efforts should be made to preserve the ovary by wedge resection of the involved portion.

A number of classifications of neoplastic ovarian tumors have been proposed. We find the classification based on tissue of origin most useful. Ninety percent of ovarian neoplasms arise from the ovarian epithelium. While the coelomic epithelium is the most common site of origin, benign and malignant tumors can arise from the germ cells, the supporting stromal cells, or ovarian embryonal rests.

Histological classification of ovarian tumors

A. Epithelial tumors
   1. Serous
   2. Mucinous
   3. Endometrioid
   4. Mesonephric
   5. Other
C. Gonadal stromal tumors
   1. Granulosa-theca cell
   2. Arrhenoblastoma
   3. Gynandroblastoma

B. Germ cell tumors
   1. Dysgerminoma
   2. Teratoma
   3. Choriocarcinoma
   4. Endodermal sinus tumor
   5. Other, and mixed forms
D. Congenital rest tumors
   1. Hilus cell
   2. Adrenal rest
   3. Brenner

As a rule, cystic ovarian tumors are far more common than solid tumors, while the latter are more likely to be malignant. Malignant tumors can arise from any of the ovarian tissues. Generally, malignant tumors arise in their benign counterparts, e.g., serous cystadenocarcinoma arises in serous cystadenoma. Some tumors may secrete hormones and have endocrine function: choriocarcinoma (chorionic go-nadotropin); granulosa-theca cell tumors (estrogen); arrhenoblastoma and gynandroblastoma (androgens).

The management of ovarian neoplasms depends on the patient's age and findings on pelvic examination. In the young patients cystic lesions under 5 cm. are ordinarily followed for two cycles. If the lesion persists, laparoscopic examination should be performed. Torsion of the pedicle or rupture of a cyst with bleeding requires laparotomy and surgical excision. The management of malignant ovarian neoplasms is discussed in the following section.

MALIGNANT GYNECOLOGICAL TUMORS AND GYNECOLOGICAL ONCOLOGY
Malignant diseases of the vulva
Intraepithelial lesions

In situ carcinoma, Bowen's disease, and Paget's disease have vary-ing gross and microscopic appearances but share some common fea-tures. They appear about 10 years earlier than invasive vulvar car-cinoma and can properly be called precursors of invasive disease. Bowen's disease and in situ carcinoma occur frequently in dystrophic or leukoplakic areas and produce pain and pruritus.

Microscopically, Paget's disease of the vulva and that of the nipple are similar, with large, oval, or round clear cells in the basal layer. In contrast to breast Paget's, the vulvar counterpart is associated with carcinoma of the underlying apocrine glands in less than one-third of the cases.

The frequent association of in situ carcinoma adjacent to invasive carcinoma requires adequate biopsies to rule out invasive disease. Toluidine blue (1%) solution aids in selecting biopsy sites. After 2 or 3 minutes is allowed for the stain to dry, 1% acetic acid sponging decolorizes normal tissue but leaves a dark blue stain on abnormal epithelium. Since these lesions are likely to be multifocal with a high degree of recurrence after local excision, total vulvectomy is the treat-ment of choice. These lesions represent one phase in the spectrum of malignant disease of the vulva. Thorough histological examination of the surgical specimen should be carried out and the patient closely followed for life.

Invasive carcinoma

The increasing incidence of vulvar carcinoma parallels the increas-ing life expectancy. The average age at the time of diagnosis is slightly over 60 years with approximately 80% of the patients over 50 years of age. Invasive and preinvasive malignancy of the vulva total about 5% of all gynecological malignancies.

Although the disease occurs on the body surface and is accessible to inspection, biopsy, and early diagnosis, 35% of the patients delay over 12 months before seeking medical help. At the University of Iowa, the average stated interval between patient recognition of the lesion and examination by a physician was 10.3 months. False modesty, reluctance to undergo pelvic examination, and self-treatment explain this delay. Even less excusable than patient delay is an average physician delay of over 2 months before a biopsy establishes the diagnosis.

Since vulvar carcinoma is a disease of older women, as many as one-third of the patients have serious medical diseases: diabetes, hypertension, and cardiovascular disease. A thorough pretreatment search

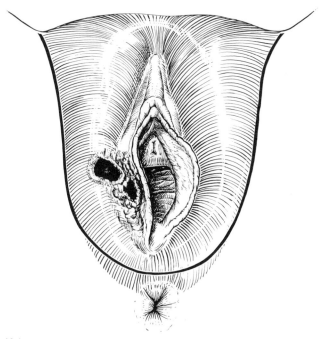

Fig. 43-7. Gross appearance of vulvar carcinoma. Solid line marks perineal resection margin of radical vulvectomy.

should be made for other primary carcinomas. Second primaries have been reported in 16 to 35% of patients. The most common second primaries are other genital carcinomas, particularly cervical carcinoma.

Symptoms and diagnosis. Vulvar carcinoma is heralded by a lump or ulcer on the vulva accompanied by pruritus and pain. The lesion can be ulcerative or papillomatous, white or red, smooth or granular, and appears in a hyperkeratinized or excoriated area present for years. It can arise on any point of the vulva, but the medial aspect of the labia majora is the most common site (Fig. 43-7).

Most lesions are clinically obvious by the time they are seen by the physician, and knife biopsies should immediately be undertaken. One should study the extent of the epithelial changes with toluidine blue as described above to define the margins of disease.

Approximately 90% of the tumors are well-differentiated epidermoid type, with adenocarcinomas, melanomas, and sarcomas being less common.

Treatment. Vulvar carcinoma is a slowly growing malignancy that spreads primarily by direct extension. Lymphatic involvement occurs later, when the lesion enlarges (2 cm. or more). The lymphatic drain-

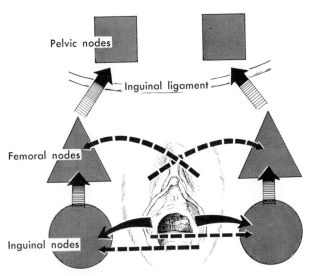

Fig. 43-8. Lymphatic dissemination of vulvar carcinoma. Solid arrows demonstrate most common routes; broken arrows less common routes.

age is via subepithelial, subdermal, and larger subcutaneous plexus to the inguinal and femoral nodes. The channels run anteriorly and laterally always medial to the labiocrural fold and do not extend onto the thigh. There is usually an orderly progression of lymph node involvement: inguinal, femoral, and iliac nodes (Fig. 43-8). When the lesion arises on the anterior portion of the vulva, metastases are more common to the deep pelvic nodes directly and to the contralateral nodes. Involvement of the deep pelvic nodes in the absence of inguinal and femoral node involvement is extremely rare, a factor important in the surgical management of this entity.

The treatment of choice is en-bloc dissection of the vulva including the mons, clitoris, labia and underlying tissues to the periosteum of the symphysis, the efferent lymphatics, and the superficial, deep inguinal, and femoral lymph nodes. This is now the accepted mode of therapy; its superiority over lesser procedures has been adequately demonstrated. We use the Marshall incision (Fig. 43-9) and perform radical vulvectomy and bilateral groin dissection as a single procedure. Should the groin nodes contain tumor, deep pelvic lymph node dissection (obturator, hypogastric, external and internal iliac nodes) is carried out as a second procedure by a transperitoneal approach. Occasionally, extension of the tumor into the vagina and/or anus requires more extensive operative procedures.

Operability is currently limited by size and location of the lesion rather than by the patient's age or condition. The operability rate approaches 90% if concomitant medical diseases can be controlled. Improvements in operative technique have made surgical deaths a rarity and better postoperative care has significantly lowered morbidity. Stainless steel sutures for the skin and suction catheters (under the flaps) have decreased the incidence of seroma or hematoma and wound infection. Prior to the closing of the skin incisions, the sartorius muscles are mobilized at their origin and transposed medially to cover the denuded vessels of the femoral triangle (Fig. 43-10). This maneuver obliterates dead space and protects the major vessels should the skin incisions break down.

Less than half the wounds heal primarily. When the areas of breakdown are small, mechanical and chemical debridement suffice. If there are large areas of separation, split-thickness skin grafts afford adequate coverage.

With extensive disease or when the patient's clinical condition precludes surgical extirpation, radiation therapy is used. External therapy is administered to the vulva and inguinal and deep pelvic lymph node–bearing areas, and the local lesion is treated with radium needles or electron beam irradiation.

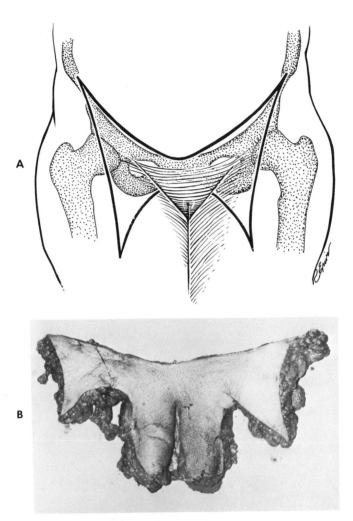

Fig. 43-9. **A,** Marshall incision for radical vulvectomy and bilateral groin dissection. **B,** Radical vulvectomy specimen with en-bloc dissection of vulva, efferent lymphatics, and groin.

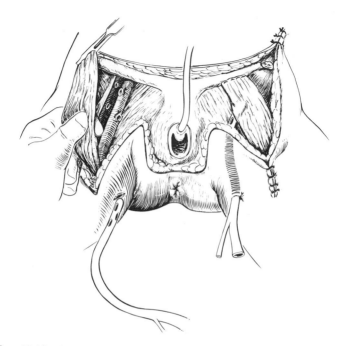

Fig. 43-10. Operative site after removal of specimen. Inguinal and femoral node dissection has been completed, and vessels and nerve are seen´at right. On the left side, sartorius muscle has been transposed, suction catheter is in place, and closure of incision has been started.

Utilizing life-expectancy table methods, we find that early vulvar carcinoma responds well to surgical treatment, with corrected 5-year survivals approaching 90%. The 5-year survival with involvement of the regional lymph nodes is poorer (about 40%). Recurrence occurs within 12 months, generally in patients with positive lymph nodes. A local recurrence suggests inadequate margins of resection.

Malignant diseases of the internal female organs
Cervical carcinoma

Cervical carcinoma is the most common genital malignancy, and the second most common cancer of women, with approximately 30,000 new cases each year. Invasive cervical carcinoma is gradually declining because of the more frequent detection of preinvasive or in situ carcinoma with cytological screening, Pap smear. Earlier detection and improved therapy are reflected in a decreasing number of deaths from cervical carcinoma during the past 20 years.

Epidemiology. Epidemiological studies suggest a correlation between cervical carcinoma and sexual activity. Rare in celibate women, cervical carcinoma is more common in married than in single women, higher in multiparous than nulligravid women, and four to six times more frequent in prostitutes. When all variables are considered, the most significant single factor seems to be the age at first coitus.

Pathology. Much is known about the histogenesis of cervical neoplasm because the cervix is accessible to gross, colposcopic, and colpomicroscopic examination and cytological study. Cervical neoplasm, a spectrum of disease, begins with cellular alterations of dysplasia, progresses to carcinoma in situ and culminates in invasive carcinoma. The common histological alterations include a disorderly array of cells, a lack of maturation, and frequent mitoses. The abnormal cells in the epithelium are characterized by hyperchromasia, nuclear pleomorphism, and increased nucleocytoplasmic ratios.

When these changes involve the entire thickness of the epithelium, but are limited by an intact basement membrane, the condition is referred to as *carcinoma in situ* or *intraepithelial carcinoma* (Fig. 43-11). These changes are less severe with *dysplasia,* and do not necessarily involve the full thickness of epithelium. Delineation between marked dysplasia and carcinoma in situ is a difficult one. Clinically, this distinction is not absolutely necessary since both represent early manifestations of malignancy.

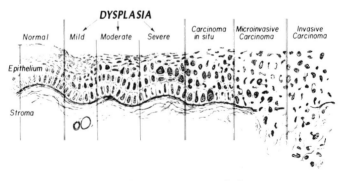

Fig. 43-11. Cervical neoplasia.

Abnormal epithelial elements breaking through the basement membrane into the underlying stroma characterize invasive cervical carcinoma. Though most invasive carcinomas progress through dysplasia and in situ carcinoma, not all dysplastic or in situ carcinomas progress to the invasive stage. The progression rate and the time interval between stages vary; many dysplasias and in situ carcinomas regress. Mild dysplasia regresses most frequently. It occasionally remains static for long periods of time, and in a small percentage of cases progresses. A significant percentage of severe dysplasias and in situ carcinomas will progress to invasive carcinoma if observed long enough undisturbed by biopsy. Although the three lesions often coexist, dysplasia appears approximately 3 to 5 years earlier, on the average, than carcinoma in situ. Carcinoma in situ occurs about 8 years earlier than invasive carcinoma.

Histologically, cervical carcinoma appears to be squamous cell or epidermoid in about 90% of the cases. In 5%, the histology resembles an adenocarcinoma arising from the mucus cells of the endocervix. Adenosquamous carcinoma, a lesion containing malignant components of both squamous and adenomatous epithelium, is increasing in frequency (about 5% of all cases).

Detection. The diagnosis of cervical malignancy depends mainly on the Papanicolaou smear. With this technique, preinvasive forms of this carcinoma can be detected when the patient is asymptomatic. Any ulcerative or cauliflower lesion on the cervix demands a punch biopsy after the Papanicolaou smear. An abnormal smear requires further diagnostic studies (Fig. 43-12).

An abnormal smear in the presence of a normal appearing cervix requires colposcopic examination. The colposcope allows the physician a view of the cervix under 10- to 14-fold magnification. There are colposcopically characteristic cellular and vascular changes of dysplasia, carcinoma in situ, and early microinvasion. The colposcope allows the physician to direct his biopsy to the most abnormal site on the cervix. Colposcopic examination is particularly useful in the pregnant patient with an abnormal cervical smear.

When histological evidence of malignancy has been obtained, the patient must be clinically staged prior to any form of therapy. Staging by the international classification involves physical examination and standard radiographic and endoscopic studies: chest roentgenogram, cystoscopy, intravenous pyelogram, proctoscopy, and barium enema (Table 43-2). This pretreatment survey determines the extent of disease and suggests the appropriate type of therapy. These studies evaluate the structures immediately adjacent to the cervix and the most common sites of metastases.

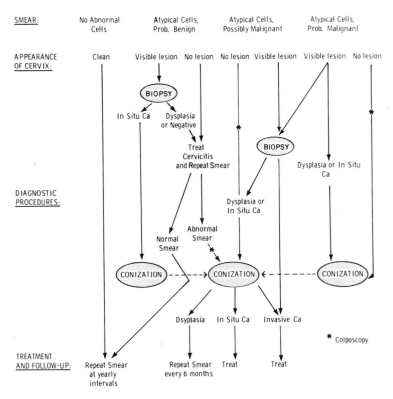

Fig. 43-12. The diagnosis of cervical neoplasm.

Pathophysiology. The intraepithelial asymptomatic stages of this disease are detected only by cytological and colposcopic techniques. Symptoms indicate stromal invasion with disruption of blood vessels. The most frequent complaints are postcoital or contact bleeding and vaginal discharge.

Cervical carcinoma spreads primarily by direct extension to adjacent structures. The most common route of dissemination is via the paracervical tissues laterally along the cardinal ligaments to the lateral pelvic wall. Extension can also take place into the corpus and along the vagina (Fig. 43-13).

Table 43-2. International classification of carcinoma of the cervix uteri (with approximate 5-year survival rates)

Stage 0	Preinvasive carcinoma (carcinoma in situ, intraepithelial carcinoma)	100%
Stage I	Carcinoma strictly confined to the cervix *Stage Ia* The cancer cannot be diagnosed by clinical examination (1) early stromal invasion and (2) occult cancer *Stage Ib* All other cases of Stage I	80-95%
Stage II	The carcinoma extends beyond the cervix but has not extended on to the pelvic wall. The carcinoma involves the vagina, but not lower third. *Stage IIa* No obvious parametrial involvement *Stage IIb* Obvious parametrial involvement	50-75%
Stage III	The carcinoma has extended on to the pelvic wall. On rectal examination, there is no cancer-free space between the tumor and the pelvic wall. The tumor involves the lower third of the vagina.	20-40%
Stage IV	The carcinoma has extended beyond the true pelvis or has involved the mucosa of the bladder or rectum. *Stage IVa* Tumor involves bladder or rectal mucosa *Stage IVb* Distant metastases	Less than 10%

The primary lymph nodes involved in cervical carcinoma are the parametrial nodes. The secondary lymphatics include the obturator, hypogastric, external iliac, and common iliac nodes. From here, dissemination occurs along the para-aortic lymphatics. Involvement of the pelvic lymph nodes occurs in 12 to 15% of stage I cases, 30% of stage II cases and approximately 45 to 60% of stage III cases. The most common sites of distant metastases are lungs, brain, liver, and bone. Involvement of the rectum and/or bladder is rare.

Treatment. Total abdominal hysterectomy is adequate therapy for a stage 0 or carcinoma in situ in any woman over 35 years of age. Ex-

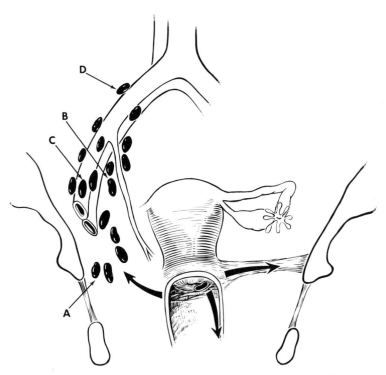

Fig. 43-13. Routes of spread of cervical carcinoma. Left side shows spread by extension along cardinal ligaments to lateral pelvic wall and into vagina. Right side demonstrates commonly involved pelvic lymph nodes. **A,** Obturator. **B,** Hypogastric. **C,** External iliac. **D,** Common iliac.

ceptions to this rule are women who have had conization, are desirous of maintaining their childbearing capacity, and will return for regular cytological examination.

Microinvasive carcinoma appears biologically and histologically to be an intermediary between in situ and frankly invasive carcinoma. Therapy for this stage of disease falls between total abdominal hysterectomy and radical hysterectomy: modified radical hysterectomy. This procedure preserves the adnexal structures in the younger woman; it permits removal of adequate amounts of paracervical tissue and removal of a wide vaginal cuff. In patients unsuited for surgery, radia-

Table 43-3. Radiation therapy—cervical carcinoma

Stage	Radium *Utilizing Fletcher tandem and colpostats*	*External irradiation* ^{60}Co *or linear accelerator, delivered at 200 rad/day; 16 × 16 cm. field*
0, Ia	2 applications, 2 weeks apart, each delivering 4,500 mg. hr.	None
Ib-III	2 applications—at 2,000 rad and at 4,000 rad—of 4,000 mg. hr. each	4,000 rad through anterior and posterior fields; 16 × 16 cm. field

tion therapy is delivered in the form of radium only, as outlined in Table 43-3.

Stages Ib and IIa carcinomas require radical hysterectomy and pelvic lymphadenectomy where no medical contraindications exist. In patients with pelvic inflammatory disease or with pelvic masses, surgery is better than radiation therapy. The procedure as now carried out removes the uterus, tubes and ovaries, suspensory ligaments, and paracervical and parametrial tissues to the lateral pelvic wall, as well as the upper one-third of the vagina. A complete lymphadenectomy is routinely performed to include the obturator, hypogastric, and external and common iliac lymph nodes bilaterally. Radical surgery and radiation therapy have identical results in early cervical carcinoma, i.e., in stages I and II. There is a somewhat higher incidence of ureterovaginal fistulas occurring after surgery, but preservation of ovarian function and maintenance of vaginal patency in the young woman are distinct advantages. Postradiation problems of the bladder and bowel occur as late as $1\frac{1}{2}$ years after therapy. Radiation cystitis, radiation proctitis, rectal strictures, and rectovaginal and vesicovaginal fistulas occur when the dose to the bladder or rectum exceeds 8,000 rad.

Radiation therapy, the most widely used modality of therapy for cervical carcinoma, includes both external radiation and radium (Table 43-3). The field of irradiation encompasses the central cervical lesion as well as the pelvic lymphatics draining the cervix. The radium is applied to both the cervix and vagina.

In stages IIb and III, with extensive paracervical involvement, radiation therapy is the treatment of choice with the technique and doses outlined in Table 43-3. The treatment of stage IV cases is individualized, based on sites of involvement. When disease is limited to the pelvis, one can use radiation therapy, recognizing that there is a great likelihood of fistula formation. In occasional cases, pelvic exenteration may be justified. Metastatic tumor in the brain, lung, or bone can be palliatively treated with radiation.

Chemotherapy is usually ineffective in treating cervical carcinoma. Intra-arterial infusion with cytotoxic agents for the control of nonresectable and radioresistant pelvic carcinoma is, as yet, experimental.

Cervical carcinoma during pregnancy. Rare as it is, when cervical carcinoma arises during pregnancy its treatment should present neither moral nor medical problems. In the first and second trimesters, therapy must be started immediately. When the cancer arises early in the third trimester, a delay of several weeks is justified to allow the fetus to reach viability. With proper treatment, the prognosis in the pregnant patient is no different from that of the nonpregnant patient for a comparable stage of disease. In the first trimester, radical hysterectomy or radiation therapy are performed without prior emptying of the uterus. The slightly enlarged uterus does not compromise the operation. If radiation therapy is used in the second or third trimester, hysterotomy or cesarean section should precede therapy to avoid the considerable cervical dilatation required for delivery. Cervical dilatation favors more rapid dissemination by opening hematogenous and lymphatic channels.

Recurrent carcinoma. About 50% of patients treated for cervical carcinoma return with recurrent disease. When radiation is the primary treatment, repeated courses of radiation are ineffective. Clinical experience suggests that less than 5% of patients survive 5 years. Ultraradical surgery in selected cases is far better, approaching 40% for 5-year survivals.

Rarely, radical hysterectomy might be used, but most surgeons now feel that a more extensive procedure is indicated, especially in patients treated initially with supravoltage radiotherapy. If the abdominal viscera and para-aortic nodes are free of disease and the tumor is not fixed to the bony pelvis, pelvic exenteration can be performed. This procedure removes en bloc the internal genitalia, including uterus, tubes and ovaries, and vagina, rectosigmoid, bladder, and distal ureters. A urinary diversion with ileal or colon conduit and sigmoid colostomy completes the procedure.

This extensive procedure requires experienced surgeons. Although postoperative complications are significant, large series have been reported without an operative death.

Endometrial carcinoma

Endometrial carcinoma, the second most common genital malignancy, is increasing in incidence. The average age at diagnosis is 60 years, so that the higher incidence may merely reflect increased life expectancy. Adenocarcinoma of the endometrium accounts for approximately 95% of uterine corpus malignancies, with the balance being sarcomas.

Epidemiology and etiology. Women who develop endometrial carcinoma have a low fertility index, a higher incidence of menstrual irregularities, and a late menopause. The clinical triad of obesity, diabetes mellitus, and hypertension is frequently associated with endometrial carcinoma, suggesting a pituitary dysfunction. Well-controlled clinical studies have documented its correlation with obesity and large stature only but failed to reveal any higher incidence of hypertension or diabetes. Furthermore, the pituitary gonadotropin levels are identical in cancer patients and in controls.

The search for etiological factors in endometrial carcinoma indirectly implicates estrogen. Endometrial carcinoma occurs rarely in castrated females and more frequently in women with conditions of unopposed estrogen secretion such as polycystic ovary syndrome and granulosa–theca cell tumors. Adenocarcinoma has been experimentally induced in rabbits by prolonged exogenous estrogens.

Diagnosis. Vaginal bleeding, post-menopausal and intermenstrual, occurs in 90% of women with proved endometrial carcinoma. Any episode of bleeding after cessation of normal menses warrants further investigation. Irregular or intermenstrual bleeding in younger women should also be pursued since one-fourth of patients with endometrial carcinoma are premenopausal.

Complete pelvic examination including cervical cytology is the first step in diagnosing endometrial carcinoma. The Papanicolaou smear is ineffective in detecting endometrial carcinoma (60% accuracy). Material can be obtained from the endometrial cavity for histological and cytological examination by two office techniques:

1. Novak endometrial biopsy curette
2. Endometrial lavage utilizing the Gravlee jet washer

Definitive diagnosis and staging of the disease requires sounding of the uterus and dilatation and fractional curettage.

Pathology. Adenocarcinomas of the endometrium demonstrate a varied pattern with change in the epithelial cells as well as in the glands. A well-differentiated tumor retains glandular pattern (grade I), whereas a markedly undifferentiated tumor (grade IV) loses glandular architecture.

Less is known about the natural history of adenocarcinoma of the endometrium than about cervical carcinoma. Women with proved endometrial hyperplasia stand a far better chance of developing carcinoma than control patients. Although cystic hyperplasia appears to be benign and completely reversible, adenomatous hyperplasia can undergo progressive hyperplastic changes under estrogen stimulation. An atypical form of adenomatous hyperplasia is widely accepted as stage 0 endometrial carcinoma.

Prognosis. Endometrial carcinoma spreads locally by extension along the surface of the uterine cavity and by invasion of the myometrium. Later, involvement of the endocervical canal takes place, at which time dissemination can occur by the same routes of spread as cervical carcinoma: paracervical spaces and pelvic lymph nodes. A bulky tumor in the lower segment of the uterus obstructs the internal os to produce symptoms of hematometria or pyometria. The most common sites of spread are the fallopian tube, ovaries, and vagina. Metastatic spread to the lungs, liver, and brain is hematogenous, and lymphatic involvement is uncommon. The most significant prognostic factors in endometrial carcinoma are extent of spread and histological differentiation. The current international classification is as follows:

Stage 0	Carcinoma in situ. Histological findings suspicious of malignancy.
Stage I	The carcinoma is confined to the corpus.
	Stage Ia The length of the uterine cavity is more than 8 cm.
	Stage Ib The length of the uterine cavity is 8 cm. or less.

The Stage I cases should be subgrouped with regard to the histological type of the adenocarcinoma as follows:

	G1 Highly differentiated adenomatous carcinomas
	G2 Differentiated adenomatous carcinomas with partly solid areas
	G3 Predominantly solid or entirely undifferentiated carcinomas
Stage II	The carcinoma has involved the corpus and the cervix.
Stage III	The carcinoma has extended outside the uterus but not outside the true pelvis.
Stage IV	The carcinoma has extended outside the true pelvis or has obviously involved the mucosa of the bladder or rectum.

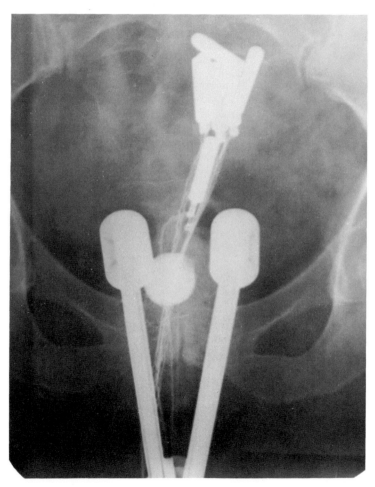

Fig. 43-14. Pelvic roentgenogram showing placement of Heyman capsules and colpostats in endometrial carcinoma. Spherical radiopaque shadow in center is Foley catheter bag filled with contrast media.

A positive correlation exists between lack of differentiation and the extent of myometrial invasion, endocervical involvement, and the occurrence of metastasis.

In summary, the best prognosis (90% for 5-year survival) is seen when the uterus sounds to less than 8 cm., when the tumor is well differentiated, with no involvement of the myometrium or extension into the endocervix. The 5-year survival for all treated cases is approximately 60 to 65%.

Treatment. The preferred treatment for stage I cases is a combination of radium and surgery. The radium capsules are packed into the uterine cavity after dilatation, with one capsule placed into the endocervical canal. Radium is placed in the vaginal fornices and the vagina is packed (Fig. 43-14). By this technique, the radium is delivered more uniformly to the endometrial surface with a reduction of vaginal vault recurrences from approximately 15% to 1 or 2%. Furthermore, the bulk of tumor is reduced and the lymphatic and small vessels draining the tumor are obliterated.

We attempt to deliver 3,000 to 5,000 rad to the serosal surface of the uterus. When the tumor is excessively large, supplemental external radiation is given. For stage I endometrial carcinoma, the radiation therapy is followed in 4 to 6 weeks by total abdominal hysterectomy and bilateral salpingo-oophorectomy.

When endocervical canal and paracervical tissues are involved, additional routes of spread are available via the paracervical tissues and the deep pelvic nodes. These patients receive a full course of radiation therapy: 4,000 rad of ^{60}Co through anterior and posterior ports and two radium applications similar to the dosage in cervical carcinoma.

Treatment of patients with stage IV disease is individualized. A full course of radiation therapy to the pelvis is often combined with systemic hormone therapy or chemotherapy.

Hormone therapy. Cytotoxic agents seldom cure endometrial carcinoma. Potent progestogens are effective in the management of this endocrine-related tumor, inducing a more benign histological appearance to the tumor cells. Well-differentiated tumors respond more promptly, with the histological changes appearing as early as 2 weeks after institution of progestogen therapy. Clinical response may take 3 months to appear. Lung, bone, and lymph node metastases appear to be most responsive, with recurrent pelvic lesions showing the poorest response.

Approximately 35% of patients with metastatic endometrial carcinoma demonstrate objective improvement with progestogens, and one fourth of them have complete remission. The 17-alpha-hydroxylated progesterone esters (hydroxyprogesterone caproate [Delalutin], medroxyprogesterone acetate [Depo-Provera]) have proved very satisfactory in clinical use. They have no estrogen or androgen effect and no evidence of toxicity or side effects. The response to these agents is demonstrated in Fig. 43-15.

Gestational trophoblastic disease

Abnormalities of the placental villi and trophoblast are rare. Gestational trophoblastic disease, as distinguished from primary choriocarcinoma of the ovary and testicle, is a term applied to hydatidiform mole, chorioadenoma destruens, and choriocarcinoma. The normal placenta exhibits some characteristics that are usually ascribed to malignant tumors: local invasiveness and the ability to metastasize. Implantation of the fertilized ovum in the endometrium is an example of local invasiveness, and placenta accreta results from more extensive trophoblastic invasion of the myometrium. Its ability to metastasize is documented by trophoblast and occasionally villi appearing in the lungs in half of normal pregnancies.

Hydatidiform mole. Hydatidiform mole occurs once in approximately 2,000 pregnancies in the United States. Clinical signs appear most commonly between the tenth and thirteenth weeks of pregnancy. Vaginal bleeding occurs in all cases and persists for several weeks, with the passage of molar tissue at 16 to 20 weeks. The tissue has a grapelike appearance composed of translucent vesicles up to 1

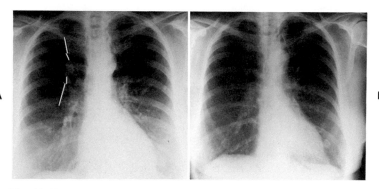

Fig. 43-15. Chest roentgenograms demonstrating regression of pulmonary metatasis in endometrial carcinoma after 3 months of therapy with progestogens.

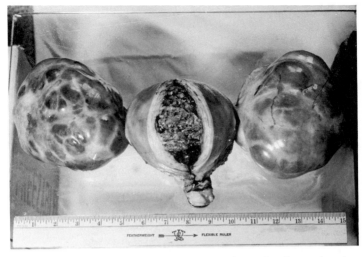

Fig. 43-16. Hydatidiform mole. Surgical specimen showing molar tissue in uterine cavity and bilateral theca-lutein cysts.

cm. in diameter. The incidence of unilateral or bilateral ovarian tumors varies, but can be expected in 20% of cases. The ovarian tumors are theca-lutein cysts resulting from the excessively high level of circulating chorionic gonadotropin (Fig. 43-16).

About one-fourth of the patients complain of hyperemesis and on physical examination half the patients have a larger uterus than anticipated by gestational age. The finding of pregnancy toxemia—hypertension, edema, and albuminuria—early in pregnancy should alert the clinician to the possibility of mole.

The diagnosis is established by a variety of techniques:

1. The absence of fetal parts on roentgenograms and of fetal heart tones on auscultation (limited value in early pregnancy).
2. Pelvic arteriography and amniography are technically difficult to perform and are hazardous if an intrauterine pregnancy is present.
3. Ultrasound scanning is currently the most accurate technique (Fig. 43-17). The accuracy approaches 99% and presents no hazard to mother or fetus.

The most significant study for diagnosis and management is the titer of human chorionic gonadotropin (HCG). In normal pregnancies, the

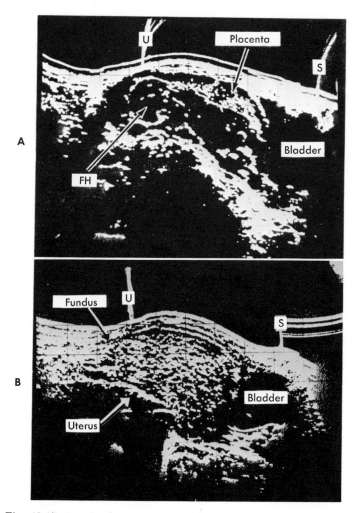

Fig. 43-17. Longitudinal midline ultrasound scans of abdomen. **A,** Normal 22-week gestation showing fetal head, *FH,* and placenta. *U,* Umbilicus. *S,* Symphysis. **B,** Hydatidiform mole showing diffuse homogeneous echo pattern in uterus enlarged to 22-week size with absence of fetal parts.

urinary excretion of HCG peaks between the sixtieth and seventieth days of gestation at 100,000 I.U./24 hr. The level falls to approximately 10,000 I.U./24 hr. by 100 days and plateaus at that level for the remainder of pregnancy. Levels significantly above the normal, in the absence of twin gestation, are highly suggestive of trophoblastic disease. Biological or immunological tests utilizing serial dilution help establish diagnosis and evaluate treatment.

When the diagnosis of mole is established, the uterus should be evacuated by suction curettage, sharp curettage, or hysterotomy depending on the size of the uterus. The lutein cysts require no treatment and regress completely. Prophylactic chemotherapy in hydatidiform mole is presently being evaluated.

Approximately 1 to 2% of moles subsequently develop into choriocarcinoma, but histological appearance does not correlate well with this change. The likelihood increases with the length of time viable trophoblast persists. When viable trophoblast persists for 6 to 8 weeks as measured by HCG titers, the chance of choriocarcinoma developing is about 50%.

Chorioadenoma destruens. Chorioadenoma destruens occupies an intermediary position between hydatidiform mole and choriocarcinoma in histological appearance and biological behavior. It occurs in approximately 1 in 15,000 pregnancies. Chorioadenoma destruens or invasive mole invades the myometrium and produces hemorrhage when tissue destruction is extensive. Histologically, there is maintenance of villous architecture, but now one sees an exuberant trophoblast with marked proliferation. Treatment of this entity is the same as for choriocarcinoma.

Choriocarcinoma. The interest generated by choriocarcinoma among medical scientists is far out of proportion to its incidence. It occurs in about 1 in 50,000 to 100,000 pregnancies, about 500 per year in the United States. Several unique features are responsible for the time and effort expended in studying choriocarcinoma:

1. Prior to the advent of chemotherapy, the outcome was uniformly fatal. Its response to chemotherapy (75% cure) is quite unique among solid tumors.
2. The level of HCG in urine or serum accurately measures response to therapy when clinical criteria are absent.
3. The tumor is properly called an allograft, since half the genetic material is foreign to the host.

The prognosis in choriocarcinoma relates to the time chemotherapy is commenced, the degree of elevation of HCG titer (reflecting extent of disease), and sites of metastasis. There are no suitable histological criteria for prognosis. Nearly half the cases follow a molar pregnancy,

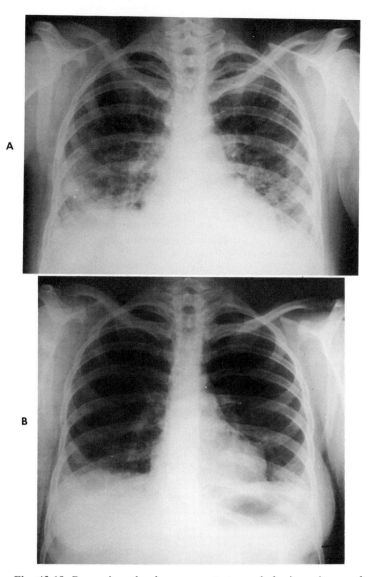

Fig. 43-18. Regression of pulmonary metastases of choriocarcinoma after treatment with methotrexate. **A,** Chest roentgenogram prior to chemotherapy. **B,** Appearance after three courses of methotrexate.

with the balance occurring after abortion or term pregnancy. The most common sites of metastases are lungs, vagina, brain, and liver, with the last two having the poorest prognosis. The histological appearance is that of a markedly malignant tumor with sheets of trophoblastic tissue. Finding villi by no means rules out the diagnosis, but the total absence of villi is more characteristic.

Chemotherapy is the treatment of choice in patients with localized or metastatic disease. With methotrexate alone, one can anticipate complete and sustained remission in 70% of patients (Fig. 43-18). This increases to 85 to 90% when actinomycin D is used sequentially. Prior to the start of therapy, a complete blood count and tests of liver and renal function must be obtained. Bone marrow depression, stomatitis, nausea and vomiting, and alopecia are the most common side effects. Toxic effects can occur as late as 5 to 10 days after completion of therapy. The patient is treated by repeated courses of methotrexate until the HCG titer reaches normal levels. One additional course of therapy is administered after a negative titer is obtained.

Should the disease prove refractory to methotrexate, the drug of next choice is actinomycin D.

With chemotherapy, surgery is avoided and women maintain their childbearing capacity. Pregnancy should be avoided for the first posttherapy year. During this period, HCG titers are obtained monthly for the first 6 months and every 2 months for the balance of the year. There is no change in the fertility index after treatment, nor has there been an increase in congenital anomalies in their offspring.

Ovarian carcinoma

Ovarian carcinoma is the third most common gynecological cancer, with approximately 14,000 new cases annually. This figure represents half the number of new cases of cervical carcinoma, yet deaths from ovarian malignancy exceed those of cervical carcinoma. A comparison of the adjusted death rates from ovarian carcinoma between 1952 and 1967 reveals a 12% increase. This increased death rate has occurred despite improved surgical, chemotherapeutic, and radiation therapy techniques.

The risk of a female developing ovarian carcinoma approaches 1%, with the peak incidence in the fifth and sixth decades. Although the number of patients under 25 is small, they are prone to develop the more malignant germ cell tumors and therefore have a disproportionally high death rate.

Approximately 90% of ovarian carcinomas are of epithelial origin (Table 43-4) and can be grossly classified as solid or cystic. The cystic form is twice as common as solid carcinomas and develops in preexist-

Table 43-4. Common ovarian carcinomas

Histological type	Incidence	5-year survival
Serous cystadenocarcinoma	50%	30%
Solid adenocarcinoma	30%	10%
Mucinous cystadenocarcinoma	10%	50%
Endometrioid carcinoma	Less than 5%	70%
Others	Less than 10%	10%
Malignant teratoma		
Dysgerminoma		
Granulosa–theca cell		
Mesonephroma		

ing cystic tumors, i.e., mucinous cystadenocarcinoma develops in a previously existing mucinous cystadenoma.

The poor prognosis of ovarian carcinoma is related to the late stage of diagnosis. During the early stages, growth is insidious. Although a cystic tumor is most likely benign, solid ovarian tumors exceeding 5 cm. in diameter are highly suspicious. Even the most careful pelvic examination often fails to detect early neoplasms. Cul-de-sac aspiration has been used to obtain material from the peritoneal cavity for cytological examination in the early detection of ovarian carcinoma. As a large scale screening technique, this is unsatisfactory. The most promising area of investigation in the early diagnosis of ovarian carcinoma lies in immunological techniques related to tumor specific antigens.

Diagnosis and therapy. The most common complaints are related to ascites, pleural effusion, or intestinal tract involvement:

1. Increasing abdominal girth
2. Abdominal pain
3. Shortness of breath
4. Vaginal bleeding
5. Nausea and vomiting

The patient with ascites should have the fluid examined cytologically. More adequate pelvic and abdominal examination can then be performed. On examination, one finds the physical signs of intraperitoneal fluid, pelvic masses, and often a solid, slightly mobile epigastric mass that represents an omentum completely replaced by tumor. The preoperative evaluation should include a small bowel series and barium enema as evidence of bowel involvement.

Laparotomy establishes the histological diagnosis and determines the extent of disease. Eighty-five percent of patients have spread of tumor beyond the genital structures, and nearly 70% have extensive intraperitoneal disease. Total abdominal hysterectomy and bilateral salpingooophorectomy is the treatment of choice in all but a few cases of ovarian carcinoma. When the disease is extensive, every attempt should be made to excise the bulk of tumor including involved omentum and peritoneal implants. Bowel resection is dictated by metastases that are producing actual or impending intestinal obstruction. Since ovarian carcinoma spreads by surface implantation, any serosal surface may be involved.

Radiation therapy and chemotherapy have produced small but significant improvement in 5-year survivals and are indicated in all but stage Ia carcinomas. Radiosensitivity of ovarian tumors is unpredictable and its location often precludes adequate radiation therapy, but dysgerminoma is one histological type that is uniquely sensitive.

The radiation therapy can be delivered by one of several methods:

1. Large-field total abdominal irradiation, delivering 3,000 rad to the total abdomen (shielding the kidney and liver) and an additional 2,000 rad to the pelvis.
2. Radioactive isotopes sometimes help to control ascites and to treat small serosal implants. Radioactive gold and chromic phosphate have limited penetration of the radiation and may produce bowel obstruction, bowel necrosis, and fistula formation.

Chemotherapy often satisfactorily palliates patients with distant metastases. The chemotherapeutic agents most suitable and effective are the alkylating agents (chlorambucil, cyclophosphamide, nitrogen mustard and thio-tepa). These agents are administered systemically by the oral and intravenous routes, and some can be instilled into the peritoneal or pleural cavities. Nitrogen mustard has most effectively controlled pleural effusion because of its local vesicant action. When there is no response to a single chemotherapeutic agent, a combination of the agents is administered.

Prognosis. Ovarian carcinoma is perhaps the most frustrating malignancy the gynecologist deals with. Despite the three currently available modalities of therapy, the death rate continues to climb. The prognosis appears to be related to three factors:

1. *Stage of disease.* The international classification of ovarian carcinoma is shown in Table 43-5.
2. *Histological type.* Table 43-4 demonstrates that the 5-year survival varies significantly with the histological appearance of the tumor. Mucinous cystadenocarcinomas and endometrioid carcinoma have a significantly better prognosis at each stage of disease than solid undifferentiated adenocarcinomas.
3. *Histological grade.* In each histological type of tumor and within each stage of disease, the prognosis is significantly affected by the

histological grade of tumor. The 5-year survival in a well-differentiated stage IIa mucinous cystadenocarcinoma is more than double that for a similar stage and histological type of tumor that is poorly differentiated.

Carcinoma metastatic to the ovary

The ovary can be the site of metastasis from other genital carcinomas, particularly the endometrium. The most common extragenital

Table 43-5. Classification of carcinoma of the ovary

Stage I	Growth limited to the ovaries
Stage Ia	Growth limited to *one* ovary; no ascites
	(i) No tumor on the external surface; capsule intact
	(ii) Tumor present on the external surface or/and capsule ruptured
Stage Ib	Growth limited to *both* ovaries; no ascites
	(i) No tumor on the external surface; capsule intact
	(ii) Tumor present on the external surface or/and capsule(s) ruptured
Stage Ic	Tumor either stage Ia or stage Ib, but with ascites* present or positive peritoneal washings
Stage II	Growth involving one or both ovaries with pelvic extension
Stage IIa	Extension and/or metastases to the uterus and/or tubes
Stage IIb	Extension to other pelvic tissues
Stage IIc	Tumor either stage IIa or stage IIb, but with ascites* present or positive peritoneal washings
Stage III	Growth involving one or both ovaries with intra-peritoneal metastases outside the pelvis and/or positive retroperitoneal nodes
	Tumor limited to the true pelvis with histologically proven malignant extension to small bowel or omentum
Stage IV	Growth involving one or both ovaries with distant metastases
	If pleural effusion is present there must be positive cytology to allot a case to stage IV
	Parenchymal liver metastases equals stage IV
Special category	Unexplored cases which are thought to be ovarian carcinoma

*Ascites is peritoneal effusion which in the opinion of the surgeon is pathological and/or clearly exceeds normal amounts.

carcinomas that metastasize to the ovary arise in the gastrointestinal tract and the breast. About 10% of ovaries removed for the treatment of breast carcinoma are found to contain metastatic carcinoma.

CONGENITAL ANOMALIES, ENDOCRINOLOGY, AND INFERTILITY
Congenital anomalies
Vaginal anomalies

1. Failure of fusion of the urogenital sinus and Müllerian duct systems can result in imperforate hymen or transverse vaginal septum. It is usually detected after menarche when the accumulation of menstrual flow collects above the obstruction causing pain and a cystic mass. These patients with cryptomenorrhea must be distinguished from primary amenorrhea. Surgical removal of the barrier is curative.
2. Congenital absence of the upper two-thirds of the vagina usually coexists with an absent or rudimentary uterus and normal ovaries. Correction is achieved by pressure with Silastic dilators progressively increased in length (Frank method) or surgical opening of the space and placement of a split-thickness skin graft. Infrequently a normal uterus and small segment of upper vagina are present. If neglected, the ensuing collection of blood can cause irreparable uterotubal damage and endometriosis.
3. Total absence of the ovaries, tubes, uterus, and vagina is rare.

Uterine anomalies—duplications

Failure of fusion or incomplete fusion of the two Müllerian ducts can result in a spectrum of anomalies ranging from a uterus with a small intrauterine vertical septum in the upper fundus to two separate uteri, cervices, and vaginas. These anomalies may cause no problem or result in repeated midtrimester abortions or infertility. The uterus may be reunified surgically by excision of the septum. If a vaginal septum exists, it should be removed. Obstetrical delivery is by cesarean section.

In all anomalies of the female reproductive tract, except for an imperforate hymen, preoperative intravenous pyelograms must rule out associated urinary tract malformations.

Endocrinology
Useful endocrine tests and procedures

1. Saturation analysis, including radioimmunoassay and competitive protein binding, has gradually replaced the older, less precise

methods of bioassay in determining blood levels of hormones. Although more specific and sensitive, the newer methods measure immunological not biological activity, and require great precision and care to minimize the frequent laboratory problems.

   a. *Gonadotropins.* Serum determinations of FSH and LH are helpful if extremely low or high. Normal range values and the FSH:LH ratio are hard to interpret, especially in view of the apparent pulsatile release of the gonadotropins into the bloodstream.

   b. *Steroid hormones.* Plasma progesterone rises during the postovulatory phase and correlates well with the urinary measurement of its metabolite, pregnanediol. Plasma estrogen levels have limited value at present, but are useful in conjunction with other assessments of estrogen activity. Measurement of the plasma androgens is useful in severe cases of hirsutism, ruling out tumors, determining the source, and guiding therapy. 17-OH progesterone in the blood and its urinary metabolite pregnanetriol are markedly elevated in congenital adrenal hyperplasia. Elevated levels of cortisol are found in Cushing's disease. (Other tests of adrenal function are found in Chapter 15.)

2. Urinary 17-ketosteroids test is a 24-hour urine assay that indirectly evaluates the androgen status of the female. Normal values range from 5 to 10 mg.; 85% come from the adrenal gland and 15% come from the ovary. With elevated levels and differential adrenal and ovarian suppression, one can ascertain the source of abnormal androgen production.

3. Vaginal maturation index—a smear from the upper lateral vaginal wall can estimate estrogen status.

   a. Estrogen deficiency is indicated by less than 20% superficial cells (cornified) and the presence of parabasal cells.

   b. A good estrogen effect shows 50 to 70% superficial cells, with the rest being intermediate cells (precornified).

   c. A shift to a predominance of intermediate cells is seen after ovulation (progesterone) or in an androgenic disorder (testosterone) and indicates a relative estrogen deficiency.

4. Progesterone challenge test—oral Provera 10 mg. per day for 5 days, or 50 to 100 mg. I.M. progesterone in oil, will cause withdrawal bleeding in an amenorrheic patient if she has adequate estrogen production.

5. Endometrial biopsy—an office procedure in which an endometrial sample is obtained in the postovulatory part of the cycle. It reflects progesterone effect and ovulation by the secretory endometrial changes.

6. Buccal smear—when appropriately prepared, a dark-staining chromatin mass (Barr body) adjacent to the nuclear membrane in over 20% of the cells indicates a chromatin-positive individual or genetic female. Two X chromosomes are required for presence of the Barr body. Fluorescent staining techniques now allow demonstration of the Y chromosome in sex chromatin–negative smears.

7. Karyotype—with a cell "squash" preparation the forty-four autosomal chromosomes and two sex chromosomes can be lined up in pairs. This technique is valuable in assessing mosaicism.

8. Bone age—roentgenographic films of the hand, wrist, and knee can be used to evaluate bone maturation by noting appearance of ossification centers and epiphyseal changes. Osseous development is accelerated by estrogen and androgens.

Primary amenorrhea

If menarche has not occurred by age 16 the patient should be considered to have primary amenorrhea. Since this is a symptom of an underlying disorder involving the hypothalamic-hypophyseal-gonadal-genital axis, appropriate investigation should be done to identify the area involved. Most often it will result from a gonadal or ovarian problem, congenital anomalies of the Müllerian ductal system, hypogonadotropic states, or an intersex (hermaphroditic) problem (Fig. 43-19). In addition to a history, physical, and pelvic examination, the following tests are helpful: sex chromatin count, gonadotropins, estrogen assessment, skull film, bone age, and an androgen evaluation if indicated.

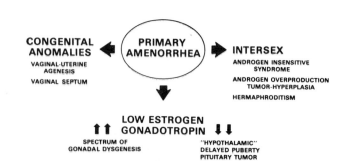

Fig. 43-19. Principal causes of primary amenorrhea.

1. Congenital anomalies. These patients have a normal sex chromatin count, physical findings, and endocrine evaluation. Pelvic or rectal examination will detect the problem, which can be corrected by surgery.

2. Gonadal dysgenesis. Abnormal gonadal differentiation results from sex chromatin errors. Disorders range from the classic "Turner's" monosomic (XO) condition with short stature and other somatic abnormalities, to mosaic variants that can appear normal. Patients with hypoestrogenism and hypergonadotropinism should have a chromosome karyotype. If an XY line of cells is identified, gonadectomy is indicated because of potential neoplasm formation. Additional treatment consists of estrogen replacement. Except in rare cases, patients with gonadal dysgenesis are infertile.

3. Intersex. These patients have phenotypes that do not completely correlate with their gonads. The testicular feminizing patient, or male intersex, presents as a normal female lacking pubic and axillary hair. Actually, he is an XY male whose cells are insensitive to androgens. The explanation lies in deficient intracellular androgen binding problems. There may also be an enzyme deficiency preventing the conversion of testosterone to its active form, dihydrotestosterone. These patients have no uterus and upper vagina because they do respond to the Müllerian inhibiting substance secreted by the testes. The gonads are either intra-abdominal or located in the inguinal canal. They should be removed because of potential tumor formation. Estrogen replacement therapy is indicated and formation of a vagina is usually necessary.

An overproduction of androgens from either an adrenal or ovarian tumor can present with masculinizing or defeminizing signs as hirsutism, acne, deep voice, and clitoral hypertrophy, in conjunction with primary amenorrhea. Benign ovarian androgenic hyperfunction, or the polycystic ovarian syndrome patient, can occasionally present with a similar but less severe picture. Rarely the adrenogenital syndrome, caused by congenital adrenal hyperplasia, may present undiagnosed and complain only of signs of hyperandrogenism and lack of menses. Appropriate androgen evaluation is necessary to determine the cause in these cases.

4. Hypothalamic amenorrhea. Patients with normal sex chromatin, low gonadotropins, and low estrogen levels, usually have a suppression of hypothalamic releasing hormone levels. Psychogenic stress and certain drugs can alter the synthesis and metabolism of the monoamine neurotransmitters—dopamine, norepinephrine, and serotonin—thus producing the functional abnormality which alters the hypothalamic gonadotropin regulating centers. Pituitary or parapituitary lesions, al-

though rare, can also produce this state. Skull films and indicated neurological evaluation should be obtained. Delayed onset of menarche should be included in the differential diagnosis. It is often difficult to rule out. Treatment varies from observation to estrogen replacement for developmental purposes. Low doses should be used so bone growth is not jeopardized.

Secondary amenorrhea

Once established, menses may cease on a prolonged or intermittent basis. Anovulation is often the cause and is related to a variety of endocrine disorders. Fig. 43-20 is a diagnostic flow sheet for the secondary amenorrheas. The three most common causes are discussed here briefly.

1. Hypothalamic amenorrhea. Hypothalamic amenorrhea encompasses the largest group of patients. Because of either overt or insidious emotional tensions, the pituitary secretion of gonadotropins is suppressed, with resultant ovarian underactivity. Therapy includes low doses of estrogen to stimulate gonadotropin secretion, psychotherapy,

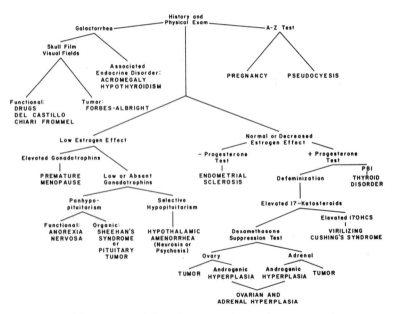

Fig. 43-20. Determining the cause of secondary amenorrhea.

and watchful waiting. Cyclic uterine bleeding should not be induced by the oral contraceptives since these hormone combinations contain dosages high enough to further decrease gonadotropin production. If a pregnancy is desired, ovulation induction can be attempted with clomiphene citrate (Clomid) or menotropins (Pergonal) plus human chorionic gonadotropin (HCG) as discussed in the infertility section of this chapter.

2. Galactorrhea and amenorrhea. This symptom combination is associated with utero-ovarian atrophy. It can be secondary to drugs (phenothiazines), an associated endocrine disease (hypothyroidism), a pituitary tumor, or idiopathic. The treatment for the first three is obvious. Suppression of idiopathic galactorrhea is currently unsatisfactory. Dopaminergic drugs may prove to be useful. Hyperprolactinemia and abnormal sella tomograms help diagnose pituitary microadenomas.

3. Androgenic disorders. The overwhelming majority of androgenic disorders are not caused by virilizing ovarian or adrenal neoplasms, congenital adrenal hyperplasia, or Cushing's syndrome. Rather, they are the result of hypothalamopituitary-induced androgen hypersecretion by either the ovaries, adrenals, or both. The differential diagnosis can be made from the urinary 17-ketosteroid values as shown in Table 43-6. Plasma androgen determination is helpful.

The signs and symptoms of these androgenic hyperfunction problems include hirsutism, amenorrhea or dysfunctional uterine bleeding, and infertility, but no virilization. Therapy is as follows:

    a. Ovarian androgenic hyperfunction. Control hirsutism with a nonandrogenic contraceptive pill. For desired pregnancy, stop the "pill" and induce ovulation with Clomid.

    b. Adrenal androgenic hyperfunction. Control hirsutism; regularize menses with maintenance corticosteroid.

    c. Combination of both entities. Combine the above two modes of treatment.

The ovarian androgenic neoplasms include arrhenoblastoma, adrenal-like tumors, etc. They cause virilization by secreting male levels of testosterone; treatment is excision of the involved ovary.

Miscellaneous gynecological endocrine disorders

1. *Dysfunctional uterine bleeding (DUB)* is irregular and occasionally heavy uterine bleeding that can complicate any anovulatory endocrine disorder. The uninterrupted estrogen effect can cause endometrial hyperplasia. Two special forms are the anovulation of the adolescent before she develops full ovarian maturation and of the premenopausal women as ovarian function begins to decline. Both age

Table 43-6. Interpretation of the differential suppression studies 17-ketosteroid values in mg./24 hours

Baseline	Dexamethasone	Dexamethasone and Enovid E	Diagnosis
<10 (normal range 5-10)	<3	—	Androgenic disorder unlikely
15-25	<3	—	Adrenal androgenic hyperfunction
10-20	5-10 (decrease 10 or less)	Further suppression <3	Ovarian androgenic hyperfunction
15-35	5-10 (decrease is >10)	Further suppression <3	Both adrenal and ovarian androgenic hyperfunction
15-30 (>30 = adrenal rest tumors)	10-20	Essentially no change	Ovarian virilizing neoplasm
>40	<3	—	Congenital adrenal hyperplasia
>80	Essentially no change	—	Adrenal virilizing neoplasm

The above values are presented as "general rules of thumb" and should not be construed as being absolute for every patient.

groups' excessive bleeding can be managed by the temporary use of hormones cyclically, but the older woman needs a D&C to rule out endometrial carcinoma.

2. In *menopause,* ovarian function has declined to the point that uterine bleeding ceases. As the estrogen levels fall, the patient may be bothered with "hot flushes." Ultimately her estrogen deficiency manifests a variety of other problems such as atrophic vaginitis, regression of breast size, some facial hirsutism, and dysuria. Therapy is cyclic estrogen replacement systemically or topically as indicated. Postmenopausal bleeding requires a D&C to rule out endometrial carcinoma.

3. *Precocious puberty* is defined as the appearance of secondary sexual development and menstrual flow prior to 9 years of age. It can result from an estrogen-secreting tumor (granulosa cell tumor or thecoma) or an irritative peripituitary lesion such as craniopharyngioma. The treatment is obvious. More frequently it is attributable to premature activation of the hypothalamic-pituitary-ovarian axis culminating in ovarian estrogen production. This causes the signs and symptoms of isosexual precocity. Normal serum levels of FSH and LH support this diagnosis, while low levels suggest a tumor. I.M. medroxyprogesterone acetate (Devo-Provera) administration inhibits the hypothalamus and gonadotropin secretion. Menstruation ceases, breast development regresses, and the accelerated bone growth is often slowed. Pubic hair growth is not affected. Treatment is continued until the bone age approximates 12 years.

Contraception

The most effective method of contraception is the oral combination progestin-estrogen pill. Its primary action is hypothalamic suppression of releasing factors with subsequent decreased gonadotropin secretion, resulting in ovulation inhibition. In addition to the effects on the female genital tract, the pill alters many physiological and metabolic processes. Common benign side effects include nausea, spotting, and weight gain. Potentially more serious problems include thromboembolism, increased serum lipids, hypertension, and altered liver function. Since these are associated with the estrogen component, it has been recommended that pills containing 50 μg. of estrogen be initially prescribed. In an effort to eliminate estrogen, the minipill has been introduced. It contains a small amount of progestin and is taken daily. A slightly higher failure rate and breakthrough bleeding problems constitute drawbacks to its use.

The inert plastic intrauterine device (IUD) is the next most effective method. Its effects are limited to the female genital tract, including an inflammatory endometrial reaction and cervical mucus alteration. These are the causative factors for its effectiveness. Problems associated with the IUD include uterine perforation, cramping, bleeding, and activation of pelvic inflammatory disease. Changes in design and composition are being made, such as the addition of copper wire and impregnating the plastic with progesterone.

Less effective methods include the diaphragm with spermicidal jelly, vaginal foam, and the condom.

Permanent conception control can be achieved by surgical sterilization. Tubal ligation can be done by either an abdominal or vaginal route with low rates of morbidity or mortality. The availability of fiberoptic instruments has made tubal coagulation with the laparoscope a very widespread procedure. While it offers the patient a shortened hospital stay, it is still to be considered a major surgical procedure.

Table 43-7. Factor analysis

Factor	Test	Normal findings
I. Male	Seminogram	20 million sperm with 75% motility and normal forms/cc.
II. Cervical	Sims-Huhner Obtain endocervical mucus at ovulation time, 2-6 hrs. post-coitus	Clear elastic mucus containing 2-20 motile sperm/hpf; minimal cells; few nonmotile sperm
III. Tubal	Rubin's CO_2 uterotubal insufflation	Shoulder pain; normal tracing on machine
	Hysterosalpingogram Water soluble radiopaque medium instilled under fluoroscopy	Normal uterine cavity, tubes, and intra-peritoneal spill
IV. Ovulatory	Basal body temperature Endometrial biopsy Plasma progesterone Urinary pregnanediol	Biphasic pattern with 14-day rise; dated secretory changes; 2-20 ng./ml on day 22; over 3 mg./24 hr.
V. Miscellaneous	Laparoscopy	No evidence of endometriosis, adhesions, or ovarian pathology

Infertility

One year of unprotected intercourse without pregnancy defines infertility, which affects 10% of couples. More than a third of these involve a male factor problem, which has been discussed in the chapter on urology. The primary causes of female infertility are anovulation and tubal pathology, while a cervical problem is occasionally found. Fifteen percent of infertile couples will have no demonstrable cause.

Evaluation of the infertile female

Following a complete medical, sexual, and psychological history, physical and pelvic examination, a "Factor Analysis" should be done (Table 43-7).

Therapy

1. Male—Urologist.
2. Cervical—Cervicitis should be treated with proper antibiotics. Thick mucus can be improved with estrogen. If an immunological problem is suggested, by the observation of all sperm being nonmotile in the cervical mucus, condoms can be used for 6 months. Sperm antibody titers will decrease in many of these patients.
3. Tubal—Tuboplasty procedures including salpingolysis, fimbrioplasty, salpingostomy, anastomosis, and cornual implantation, are available. Antiadhesive programs utilizing corticosteroids, antihistamines, and antibiotics are often used. Postoperative tubal hydrotubation seems helpful. Patency rates average 40%, while pregnancy rates are nearer 20%. The most important factors influencing these rates are the extent of the disease and experience of the surgeon.
4. Ovulation—The most commonly used agent to correct anovulation is clomiphene citrate. Its antiestrogenic effect in the hypothalamus results in an increase in gonadotropin releasing factors and gonadotropins. An intact hypothalamic-pituitary-ovarian axis is necessary. Adequate endogenous estrogen production is preferable. Success rate is 80% for ovulation, but only 40% for pregnancy. The incidence of spontaneous abortion and twin gestation is increased. Ovarian cysts occasionally form and can be treated conservatively. Other agents used to induce ovulation include gonadotropin releasing factors (not yet available for general use), Pergonal (a combination of FSH and LH), and human chorionic gonadotropin (HCG) (LH substitute). Pergonal requires daily injections and monitoring and is associated with hyperstimulation of the ovaries and multiple pregnancies. It can be used in pituitary failure patients.

Patients with polycystic ovarian disease (ovarian androgenic hyperfunction) are candidates for bilateral wedge resection of the ovaries.

Most often a trial of clomiphene is given before the surgical approach is undertaken. Both have similar success rates.

5. Miscellaneous—If no causative factor is found or a tubal or peritoneal factor is suspected, laparoscopy should be performed. Positive findings approach 20%. (See section on laparoscopy.)

References

Chapter 1: Origin of surgical disease

Ackerman, L. V., in collaboration with Rosai, J.: Surgical pathology, ed. 5, St. Louis, 1974, The C. V. Mosby Co.

Anson, B. J., and McVay, C. P.: Surgical anatomy, Philadelphia, 1971, W. B. Saunders Co.

Artz, C. P., and Hardy, J. D.: Complications in surgery and their management, ed. 3, Philadelphia, 1975, W. B. Saunders Co.

Dunphy, J. E., and Botsford, T. W.: Physical examination of the surgical patient, Philadelphia, 1975, W. B. Saunders Co.

Egdahl, R. H., and Mannick, J. A.: Modern surgery, New York, 1970, Grune & Stratton, Inc.

Egdahl, R. H., and Mannick, J. A.: Readings in modern surgery, New York, 1973, Grune & Stratton, Inc.

Maingot, R.: Abdominal operations, ed. 6, New York, 1974, Appleton-Century-Crofts.

Sabiston, D. C.: Christopher's textbook of surgery, ed. 10, Philadelphia, 1972, W. B. Saunders Co.

Schwartz, S. I., Lillehei, R. C., et al., editors: Principles of surgery, ed. 2, New York, 1974, McGraw-Hill Book Co.

Shackelford, R. T.: Bickham-Callander's surgery of the alimentary tract, Philadelphia, 1955, W. B. Saunders Co.

Thorek, P.: Anatomy in surgery, ed. 2, Philadelphia, 1962, J. B. Lippincott Co.

Zimmerman, L., and Levine, R.: Physiologic principles of surgery, ed. 3, Philadelphia, 1974, W. B. Saunders Co.

Zollinger, R. M, and Cutler, E. C.: Atlas of surgical operations, ed. 3, New York, 1967, The Macmillan Co.

Chapter 2: Wounds, wound healing, and drains

Chen, R. W., and Postlethwait, R. W.: The biochemistry of wound healing, Monogr. Surg. Sci. 1(3):215-276, September 1964.

DeVito, R. V.: Healing of wounds, Surg. Clin. N. Amer. **45:**441, 1965.

Dunphy, J. E: The fibroblast—a ubiquitous ally for the surgeon, N. Engl. J. Med. **268:**1367, 1963.

Peacock, E. E.: Wound healing and wound care. In Schwartz, S. I., Lillehei, R. C., et al., editors: Principles of surgery, ed. 2, New York, 1974, McGraw-Hill Book Co.

Chapter 3: Fluids and electrolytes

Bland, J. H.: Clinical metabolism of body water and electrolytes, Philadelphia, 1963, W. B. Saunders Co.

Eichenholz, A.: Why a symposium on acid-base balance? Arch. Intern. Med. **116:**647, 1965.

Goldsmith, R. S., and Ingbar, S. H.: Inorganic phosphate treatment of hypercalcemia of diverse etiologies, N. Engl. J. Med. **274:**1, 1966; **274:**284, 1966.

Hackney, J. D., Sears, C. H., and Collier, C. R.: Estimation of arterial CO_2 tension by rebreathing technique, J. Appl. Physiol. **12:**425, 1958.

Kinney, J. M., Lister, J., and Moore, F. D.: Relationship of energy expenditure to total exchangeable potassium, Ann. N. Y. Acad. Sci. **110:**711, 1963.

Leaf, A.: The clinical and physiological significance of the serum sodium concentration N. Engl. J. Med. **267:**24, 77, 1962.

Mason, E. E., and Dryer, R. L.: The implications of abnormal sodium concentration, Surg. Gynec. Obstet. **105:**273, 1957.

Mason, E. E.: Fluid, electrolyte and nutrient therapy in surgery, Philadelphia, 1974, Lea & Febiger.

Moyer, C. A., Margraf, H. W., and Monafo, W. W., Jr.: Burn shock and extravascular sodium deficiency—treatment with Ringer's solution with lactate, Arch. Surg. **90:**799, 1965.

Shires, T.: The role of sodium-containing solutions in the treatment of oligenic shock, Surg. Clin. N. Amer. **45:**365, 1965; in same volume see also: Butcher, H. R.: The pathophysiology of sodium depletion in man, p. 345; Zimmerman, B.: Pituitary and adrenal function in relation to surgery, p. 299.

Siggaard-Andersen, O.: The acid-base status of the blood, Baltimore, 1964, The Williams & Wilkins Co.

Chapter 4: Hemostatic defects and bleeding: diagnosis and treatment

Deykin, D.: Current concepts in the use of heparin, N. Engl. J. Med. **280:**937, 1969.

Laufman, H., and Erichson, R. B.: Hematologic problems in surgery, Philadelphia, 1970, W. B. Saunders Co.

Mollison, P. L.: Blood transfusion in clinical medicine, Oxford, Eng., 1967, Blackwell Scientific Publications.

Thompson, J. S., Severson, C. D., Parmely, M. J., Marmorstein, B. L., and Simmons, A.: Pulmonary "hypersensitivity" reactions induced by transfusion of non–HL-A leukoagglutinins, N. Engl. J. Med. **284:** 1120, 1971.

Verstraete, M., Vermylen, C., Vermylen, J., and Vandenbroucke, J.: Excessive consumption of blood coagulation components as cause of hemorrhagic diathesis, Amer. J. Med. 38:899, 1965.

Wasserman, L. R., and Gilbert, H. S.: Surgical bleeding in polycythemia vera, Ann. N. Y. Acad. Sci. 115:122, 1964.

Wintrobe, M. M.: Clinical hematology, Philadelphia, 1974, Lea & Febiger.

Chapter 5: Shock

Altemeier, W. A., Todd, J. C., and Wellford, W. I.: Gram-negative septicemia; a growing threat, Ann. Surg. 116:530, 1967.

Blalock, A.: Experimental shock, the cause of the low blood pressure produced by muscle injury, Arch. Surg. 20:959, 1930.

Cannon, W. B.: Traumatic shock, New York, 1932, D. Appleton and Co.

Dillon, J., et al.: A bioassay of treatment of hemorrhagic shock, Arch. Surg. 93:537, 1966.

Fine, J.: Septic shock, J.A.M.A. 188:427, 1964.

Hardaway, R. M., et al.: Intensive study and treatment of shock in man, J.A.M.A. 199:779, 1967.

Lillehei, R. C., et al.: The nature of irreversible shock; experimental and clinical observations, Ann. Surg. 160:682, 1964.

MacLean, L. D., et al.: Patterns of septic shock in man; a detailed study of 56 patients, Ann. Surg. 166:543, 1967.

Palmerio, C., and Fine, J.: The nature of resistance to shock, Arch. Surg. 98:679, 1969.

Shoemaker, W. C.: Shock, Springfield, Ill., 1967, Charles C Thomas, Publisher.

Siegel, J. H., et al.: A bedside computer and physiologic nomogram; guides to the management of the patient in shock, Arch. Surg. 97:480, 1968.

Swan, H. J. C., et al.: Catheterization of the heart in man with use of a flow-directed balloon-tipped catheter, N. Engl. J. Med. 283:447, 1970.

Wilson, J. N., et al.: Central venous pressure in optimal blood volume maintenance, Arch. Surg. 85:563, 1962.

Chapter 6: Surgical infections

Alexander, J. W.: Nosocomial infections, In current problems in surgery, New York, 1973, Year Book Medical Publishers, Inc.

Ben-Shoshan, M., Gius, J. A., and Smith, I. M.: Exploratory laparotomy for fever of unknown origin. Surg. Gynec. Obstet. 132:994-996, June 1971.

Burke, J. F.: Use of preventive antibiotics in clinical surgery, Am. Surg. 39(1):6-11, January 1973.

MacLennan, J. D.: The histotoxic clostridial infections of man, Bacteriol. Rev. **26**(2), June 1962.

Neu, H. C.: Antimicrobial agents—mechanism of action and clinical usage. In Current problems in surgery, New York, 1973, Year Book Medical Publishers, Inc.

Robson, M. C., Krizek, T. J., and Heggers, J. P.: Biology of surgical infection. In Current problems of surgery, New York, 1973, Year Book Medical Publishers, Inc.

Roding, B., Graenveld, P. H. A., and Borema, I.: Ten years of experience in the treatment of gas gangrene with hyperbaric oxygen, Surg. Gynec. Obstet. **134**:579-585, April 1972.

Wangensteen, O. H., Wangensteen, S. D., and Klinger, C. F.: Surgical cleanliness, hospital solubrity, and surgical statistics historically considered, Surgery **71**:477, 1972.

World Health Organization Committee and Rabies Fourth Report, Technical Series, No. 201, 1960.

Chapter 7: Total parenteral feeding

Boeckman, C. R., and Krill, C. E., Jr.: Bacterial and fungal infections complicating parenteral alimentation in infants and children, J. Pediat. Surg. **5**:117, 1970.

Dudrick, S. J., and Rhoads, J. E.: New horizons for intravenous feeding, J.A.M.A. **215**:939, 1971.

Filler, R. M., and Eraklis, A. J.: Care of the critically ill child: Intravenous alimentation, Pediatrics **46**:456, 1970.

Freeman, J. B., and MacLean, L. D.: Intravenous hyperalimentation: a review, Canadian J. Surg. **14**:180, 1971.

Freeman, J. B., LeMire, A., and MacLean, L. D.: Intravenous alimentation and septicemia, Surg. Gynec. Obstet. **135**:708, 1972.

Freeman, J. B., and Litton, A. A.: The preponderance of gram-positive infection associated with intravenous alimentation, Surg. Gynec. Obstet. **139**:905, 1974.

Freeman, J. B., Wienke, J., and Soper, R. T.: *Candida* osteomyelitis associated with intravenous alimentation, J. Pediat. Surg. **9**:783, 1974.

Johnson, D. G.: Total intravenous nutrition in newborn surgical patients: A three-year perspective, J. Pediatr. Surg. **5**:601, 1970.

Wilmore, D. W., Groff, D. B., Bishop, H. C., and Dudrick, S. J.: Total parenteral nutrition in infants with catastrophic gastrointestinal anomalies, J. Pediatr. Surg. **4**:181, 1969.

Chapter 8: Preoperative care

American College of Surgeons Committee on Pre- and Postoperative care, Kinney, J. M., et al. Manual of preoperative and postoperative care, ed. 2, Philadelphia, 1971, W. B. Saunders Co.

Gibbel, M. I.: Pitfalls in preoperative and postoperative care, Surg. Clin. N. Amer. **38**:41, 1958.

Hurd, J. B.: The diabetic patient and surgery, Postgrad. Med. **32:**370, 1962.

Miller, R. D.: Effect of pulmonary impairment on the surgical candidate, Med. Clin. N. Amer. **46:**885, 1960.

Ralston, L. S.: Medical evaluation of patients before operation, Postgrad. Med. **26:**484, 1959.

Schumer, W.: Metabolic considerations in the preoperative evaluation of the surgical patient, Surg. Gynec. Obstet. **121:**611, 1965.

Stein, M., et al.: Preoperative pulmonary function tests, J.A.M.A. **181:** 765, 1962.

Veidenheimer, M. C., editor: Evaluation of the surgical patient, Surg. Clin. N. Amer. **50:**539-748, June 1970.

Chapter 9: Anesthesia

Bendixen, H. H., Egbert, L. D., Hedley-Whyte, J., Laver, M. B., and Pontoppidan, H.: Respiratory care, St. Louis, 1965, The C. V. Mosby Co.

Cullen, S. C., and Larson, C. P.: Essentials of anesthetic practice, Chicago, 1974, Year Book Medical Publishers, Inc.

Dripps, R. D., Eckenhoff, J. E., and Vandam, L. D.: Introduction to anesthesia. The principles of safe practice, ed. 4, Philadelphia, 1973, W. B. Saunders Co.

Moore, D. C.: Regional block. A handbook for use in the clinical practice of medicine and surgery, ed. 5, Springfield, Ill., 1973, Charles C Thomas, Publisher.

Chapter 10: Postoperative care

Arkins, R., Smessaert, A. A., and Hicks, R. G.: Mortality and morbidity in surgical patients with coronary artery disease, J.A.M.A. **190:**485, 1964.

Artz, C. P., and Hardy, J. D.: Management of surgical complications, ed. 3, Philadelphia, 1975, W. B. Saunders Co.

Bryant, L. R., Griffith, R., Harris, R., and Eiseman, B.: Effect of major surgical stress on chronic psychosis, Amer. Surg. **31:**359, 1965.

Coon, W. W., and Willis, P. W.: Deep venous thrombosis and pulmonary embolism, Amer. J. Cardiol. **4:**611, 1959.

Engler, H. C., Kennedy, T. E., Ellison, L. T., Purvis, J. G., and Moretz, W. H.: Hemodynamics of experimental acute gastric dilatation, Amer. J. Surg. **113:**194, 1967.

Hamilton, W. K., McDonald, J. S., Fischer, H. W., and Bethards, R.: Postoperative respiratory complications. A comparison of arterial gas tensions, radiographs and physical examination, Anesthesiology **25:**607, 1964.

Strode, J. E.: Acute cholecystitis as a complication following surgery unrelated to the biliary tract, Surgery **59:**195, 1966.

Thomas, P. A., and Merrigan, E. H.: Prevention of postoperative pulmonary atelectasis, Amer. Surg. **32:**301, 1966.

Chapter 11: Malignant neoplasms

Ansfield, F. J.: Chemotherapy of disseminated solid tumors, ed. 2, Springfield, Ill., 1973, Charles C Thomas, Publisher.

Boyd, W.: The spontaneous regression of cancer, Springfield, Ill., 1966, Charles C Thomas, Publisher.

Brodsky, I. and Kahn, S. B., editors: Cancer chemotherapy, II, New York, 1972, Grune & Stratton, Inc.

Clark, R. L., Jr.: Cancer chemotherapy, Springfield, Ill., 1961, Charles C Thomas, Publisher.

Cole, W. H., McDonald, G. O., Roberts, S. S., and Southwick, H. W.: Dissemination of cancer: prevention and therapy, New York, 1961, Appleton-Century-Crofts.

Daicoff, G. R., Harmon, R., and Van Prohaska, J.: Effect of adrenalectomy on mammary carcinoma, Arch. Surg. 85:800, 1962.

Everson, T. C., and Cole, W. H.: Spontaneous regression of cancer, Philadelphia, 1966, W. B. Saunders Co.

Gilman, A.: The initial clinical trial of nitrogen mustard, Amer. J. Surg. 105:574, 1963.

Goodall, G. M.: A review on para-endocrine cancer syndromes, Int. J. Cancer 4:1-13, 1969.

Holland, J. F., and Frei, E.: Cancer medicine, Philadelphia, 1973, Lea & Febiger.

Humphrey, L. J., Murray, D. R., and Boehm, O. R.: Effect of tumor vaccines in immunizing patients with cancer, Surg. Gynec. Obstet. 132:437-442, March 1971.

Karnofsky, D. A.: Problems and pitfalls in the evaluation of anticancer drugs, Cancer 18:1517, 1965.

Lawton, R. L., Latourette, H. B., and Collier, R. G.: Simultaneous high-energy irradiation and chemotherapy, Arch. Surg. 91:155, 1965.

Moore, T. L., Kupchik, H. Z., Marcon, N., and Zamcheck, N.: Carcinoembryonic antigen assay in cancer of the colon and pancreas and other digestive tract disorders, Amer. J. Dig. Dis. 16(1):1-7, January 1971.

Raven, R. W., editor: Modern trends in oncology, 1. Part II: Clinical progress, Scarborough, Ont., 1973, Butterworth & Co.

Rubin, P., editor: Current concepts in cancer, Chicago, 1974, American Medical Association.

Stehlin, J. S., Jr., Smith, J. L., Jr., Jing, B.-S., and Sherrin, D.: Melanomas of the extremities complicated by in-transit metastases, Surg. Gynec. Obstet. 122:2, 1966.

Stillman, A., and Zamcheck, N.: Recent advances in immunologic diagnosis of digestive tract cancer, Amer. J. Dig. Dis. 15(11):1003-1018, November 1970.

Chapter 12: The skin

Allen, A.: The skin, New York, 1966, Grune & Stratton, Inc.

Conway, H. E., Hugo, N. E., and Tulenko, J. F.: Surgery of tumors of the skin, ed. 2, Springfield, Ill., 1966, Charles C Thomas, Publisher.

Lever, W. F.: Histopathology of the skin, ed. 4, Philadelphia, 1967, J. B. Lippincott Co.

Lund, H. B.: Tumors of the skin. In Atlas of tumor pathology, Washington, D.C., 1957, Armed Forces Institute of Pathology, sect. 1, fasc. 2.

Lund, H. B., and Kraus, J. M.: Melanotic tumors of the skin. In Atlas of tumor pathology, Washington, D. C., 1962, Armed Forces Institute of Pathology, sect. 1, fasc. 3.

McGovern, V. J., Mihm, M. C., et al.: The classification of malignant melanoma and its histologic reporting, Cancer **32**:1446, December 1973.

Chapter 13: The thyroid gland

Astwood, E. B., Cassidy, C. E., and Aurbach, G. D.: Treatment of goiter and thyroid nodules with thyroid, J.A.M.A. **174**:459, 1960.

Beahrs, O. H., Woolner, L. B., Engel, S., and McConahey, W. M.: Needle biopsy of the thyroid gland and management of lymphocytic thyroiditis, Surg. Gynec. Obstet. **144**:636, 1962.

Graverman, L. F.: Consequences of thyroid radiation in children, N. Engl. J. Med. **292**:204, 1975.

Carneiro, L., Dorrington, K. J., and Munro, D. S.: Relation between long-acting thyroid stimulator and thyroid function in thyrotoxicosis, Lancet **2**:878, 1966.

Crile, G.: Endocrine dependency of papillary carcinomas of the thyroid, J.A.M.A. **195**:721, 1966.

Editorial: Hypothyroidism after treatment of thyrotoxicosis, Lancet **1**: 637, 1965.

Glassford, G. H., Fowler, E. F., and Cole, W. H.: The treatment of nontoxic nodular goiter with desiccated thyroid: results and evaluation, Surgery **58**:621, 1965.

Harness, J. K., Thompson, N. W., and Nishiyama, R. H.: Childhood thyroid carcinoma, Arch. Surg. **102**:278, 1971.

Hayles, A. B., Johnson, L. M., Beahrs, O. H., and Woolner, L. B.: Carcinoma of the thyroid in children, Amer. J. Surg. **106**:735, 1963.

Kogut, M. D., Kaplan, S. A., Collipp, P. J., et al.: Treatment of hyperthyroidism in children, N. Engl. J. Med. **272**:217, 1965.

Lee, T. C., et al.: The use of propranolol in the surgical treatment of thyrotoxic patients, Ann. Surg. **177**:643, June 1973.

Liechty, R. D.: Myxedema causing adynamic ileus, serous effusions, and inappropriate secretion of antidiuretic hormone, Surg. Clin. N. Amer. **50**:1087, 1970.

Liechty, R. D., Graham, M., and Freemeyer, P.: Benign solitary thyroid nodules, Surg. Gynec. Obstet. **121**:571, 1965.

Machin, J. F., Canary, J. J., and Pittman, C. S.: Thyroid storm and its manageemnt, N. Engl. J. Med. **291**:1396, 1974.

Nofal, M. M., Bierwaltes, W. H., and Patno, M. E.: Treatment of hyperthyroidism with sodium iodide I^{131} (16-year experience), J.A.M.A. **197**:605, 1966.

Welch, C.: Therapy for multinodular goiter, J.A.M.A. **195**:339, 1966.

Werner, S. C., and Ingbar, S. H.: The thyroid, ed. 3, New York, 1971, Harper & Row, Publishers.

Winship, T., and Rosvoll, R. V.: Childhood thyroid carcinoma, Cancer **14:**734, 1961.

Chapter 14: The parathyroid gland

Aurbach, G. D., et al.: Polypeptide hormones and calcium metabolism, Ann. Intern. Med. **70:**1243-1265, 1969.

Block, M. A., et al.: The extent of operation for primary hyperparathyroidism, Arch. Surg. **109:**798, December 1974.

Cope, O.: Hyperparathyroidism: Diagnosis and management, Am. J. Surg. **99:**394-398, 1960.

Foster, G. V.: Calcitonin, N. Engl. J. Med. **279:**349-360, 1968.

Goldsmith, R. S.: Evaluation and treatment of hypercalcemia, Mod. Med., pp. 104-109, September 22, 1969.

Goldsmith, R. S.: Hyperparathyroidism (a discussion of diagnostic tests), N. Engl. J. Med. **281:**367-374, 1969.

Haff, R. C., and Ballinger, W. F.: Causes of recurrent hypercalcemia after parathyroidectomy for primary hyperthyroidism, Ann. Surg. **173:**884, 1971.

Paloyan, E., Lawrence, A. M., and Straus, F. H.: Hyperparathyroidism, New York, 1973, Grune & Stratton, Inc.

Potts, J. T., and Deftos, L. J.: Parathyroid hormone, thyrocalcitonin, vitamin D, bone and bone mineral metabolism. In Duncan, G. G.: Diseases of metabolism, ed. 7, Philadelphia, 1974, W. B. Saunders Co.

Pyrah, L. N., Hodgkinson, A., and Anderson, C. K.: Primary hyperparathyroidism, Brit. J. Surg. **53:**245, 1966.

Chapter 15: The adrenal glands

Biglieri, E. G.: Aldosterone, Ciba Clin. Sympos. **15:**23, 1963.

Beierwaltes, W. H., et al.: Visualization of human adrenal glands in vivo by scintillation scanning, J.A.M.A. **216:**275, 1971.

Conn, J. W., Rovner, D. R., Cohen, E. L., and Nesbit, R. M.: Normokalemic primary aldosteronism, J.A.M.A. **195:**21, 1966.

Egdahl, R. H.: Surgery of the adrenal gland, N. Engl. J. Med. **278:**939, 1969.

Eisenstein, A. B.: The adrenal cortex, Boston, 1967, Little, Brown & Co.

Forsham, P. H.: The adrenal gland, Ciba Clin. Symp. **15:**3, 1963.

Hume, D. M.: Pheochromocytoma in the adult and in the child, Am. J. Surg. **99:**458, 1960.

Kirkendall, W. M., Liechty, R. D., and Culp, D. A.: Diagnosis and treatment of patients with pheochromocytoma, Arch. Intern. Med. **115:**529, 1965.

Marks, L. J., King, D. W., Kingsbury, P. F., Boyett, J. E., and Dell, E. S.: Physiological role of the adrenal cortex in the maintenance of plasma volume following hemorrhage or surgical operation, Surgery **58:**510, 1965.

O'Neal, L. W.: Pathological anatomy in Cushing's syndrome, Ann. Surg. **168:**860, 1964.

Treadwell, B. L. J., Savage, O., Sever, E. D., and Copeman, W. S. C.: Pituitary-adrenal function during corticosteroid therapy, Lancet **1:**355, 1963.

Van Way, C. W., et al.: Pheochromocytoma—current problems in surgery, Chicago, 1974, Year Book Medical Publishers, Inc.

Webb, W. R., Degerli, I. U., Hardy, J. D., and Umal, M.: Cardiovascular responses in adrenal insufficiency, Surgery **58:**273, 1965.

Chapter 16: The breast

Atkins, H., and Wolff, B.: Discharges from the nipple, Brit. J. Surg. **51:**602, 1964.

Brinkley, D., and Haybittle, J. L.: Treatment of stage II carcinoma of the female breast, Lancet **2:**291, 1966.

Copeland, M. M.: American Joint Committee on Cancer Staging and End Results Reporting: Objectives and progress, Cancer **18:**1637, 1965.

Crile, G.: A biological consideration of treatment of breast cancer, Springfield, Ill., 1967, Charles C Thomas, Publisher.

Haagensen, C. D.: Cancer of the breast in pregnancy and lactation, Am. J. Obstet. Gynec. **98:**141, 1967.

Haagensen, C. D.: Diseases of the breast, Philadelphia, 1971, W. B. Saunders Co.

Leis, H. P.: Diagnosis and treatment of breast lesions, Flushing, N. Y., 1970, Medical Examination Publishing Co., Inc.

Liechty, R. D., Davis, J., and Gleysteen, J.: Cancer of the male breast, Cancer **20:**1617, 1967.

Macdonald, I.: The natural history of breast cancer, Am. J. Surg. **3:**435, 1966.

McDivitt, R. W., Urban, J. A., and Farrow, J. H.: Cystosarcoma phyllodes, Johns Hopkins Med. J. **120:**33, 1967.

McWhirter, R.: Simple mastectomy and radiotherapy in the treatment of breast cancer, Brit. J. Radiol. **28:**128, 1955.

Moore, F. D., et al.: Carcinoma of the breast, N. Engl. J. Med. **277:** 293, 343, 411, 460, 1967.

Rosemond, G. P., Maier, W. P., and Brobyn, T. J.: Needle aspiration of breast cysts, Surg. Gynec. Obstet. **128:**351, February 1969.

Shapiro, S., Strax, P., and Venet, L.:Periodic breast cancer screening in reducing mortality for breast cancer, J.A.M.A. **215:**1777, March 15, 1971.

Shimkin, M. B.: Cancer of the breast: some old facts and new perspectives, J.A.M.A. **183:**358, 1963.

Urban, J. A.: Clinical experience and results of excision of internal mammary lymph node chain in primary operable breast cancer, Cancer **12:**14, 1959.

Wolfe, J. N.: Analysis of 462 breast carcinomas, Am. J. Roentgenol. **121:**846, August 1974.

Chapter 17: Liver and biliary tract

Child, C. C., III: The liver and portal hypertension, Philadelphia, 1964, W. B. Saunders Co.

Conn, H. O., and Lindenmuth, W. W.: Prophylactic portacaval anastomosis in cirrhotic patients with esophageal varices, N. Engl. J. Med. **279:**725, 1968.

DenBesten, L., and Liechty, R. D.: Cancer of the biliary tree, Am. J. Surg. **109:**587, 1965.

Fonkalsrud, E. W., and Boles, E. T.: Choledochal cysts in infancy and childhood, Surg. Gynec. Obstet. **121:**733, 1965.

Foster, F., Lawles, M. R., Wellborn, M. B., Holcomb, G. W., and Sawyers, J. L.: Recent experience with major hepatic resection, Arch. Surg. **167:**651, 1968.

Glenn, F., McSherry, C. K., and Dineen, P.: Morbidity of surgical treatment for nonmalignant biliary tract disease, Surg. Gynec. Obstet. **126:**15, 1968.

Hermann, R. E., Rodriguez, A. E., and McCormack, L. J.: Selection of patients for portal-systemic shunts, J.A.M.A. **196:**1039, 1966.

Linton, R. R., Ellis, D. S., and Geary, J. E.: Surgical treatment of portal cirrhosis, Ann. Surg. **154:**446, 1961.

Mason, E. E.: Splenectomy and side-to-side splenorenal shunt for portal hypertension, Surgery **60:**536, 1966.

McDermott, W. V., Palazzi, H., Nardi, G. H., and Mondet, A.: Elective portal systemic shunt: an analysis of 237 cases, N. Engl. J. Med. **264:**419, 1961.

Menken, M., Barrett, P. V. D., and Berlin, N. I.: Bilirubin production and excretion: clinical considerations, J.A.M.A. **198:**1273, 1966.

Morfin, E., Ponka, J. L., and Brush, B. E.: Gangrenous cholecystitis, Arch. Surg. **96:**567, 1968.

Orloff, M. J.: Emergency portacaval shunt, Ann. Surg. **166:**456, 1967.

Popper, H., and Schaffner, F.: Progress in liver disease, New York, 1970, Grune & Stratton, Inc.

Ravdin, I. S.: Surgical jaundice; factors influencing injury and repair of liver (collective review), Surg. Gynec. Obstet. (Int. Abst.) **89:**209, 1949.

Sherlock, S.: Diseases of the liver and biliary system, Oxford, 1968, Blackwell Scientific Publications.

Small, D. M.: Gallstones, N. Engl. J. Med. **279:**588, 1968.

Snell, A. M.: Liver function tests and their interpretation, Gastroenterology **34:**675, 1958.

Thorbjarnarson, B.: The anatomical diagnosis of jaundice by percutaneous cholangiography and its influence on treatment, Surgery **61:**347, 1967.

Chapter 18: The pancreas

Anderson, M. D.: Review of pancreatic disease, Surgery, **66:**434, 1969.

Baker, R. J.: Newer considerations in the diagnosis and management of fasting hypoglycemia, Surg. Clin. N. Amer. **49:**191, 1969.

Carey, L. C.: The pancreas, St. Louis, 1973, The C. V. Mosby Co.

Creutzfeldt, W., and Schmidt, H.: Aetiology and pathogenesis of pancreatitis (current concepts), Scand. J. Gastroent. 6(suppl.):47, 1970.

dePeyster, F. A.: Planning the appropriate operation for islet cell tumors of the pancreas, Surg. Clin. N. Amer. 50:133, 1970.

Drash, A., and Wolff, F.: Drug therapy in leucine-sensitive hypoglycemia, Metabolism 13:487, 1964.

Editorial: Streptozotocin for metastatic insulinoma, J.A.M.A. 214:907, 1970.

Ellison, E. H., and Wilson, S. D.: The Zollinger-Ellison syndrome updated, Surg. Clin. N. Amer. 47:1115, 1967.

Fry, W. J., and Child, C. G.: Ninety-five percent distal pancreatectomy for chronic pancreatitis, Ann. Surg. 162:543, 1965.

Jordan, G. L.: The current status of pancreatoduodenectomy for malignant lesions of the pancreas, Surg. Gynec. Obstet. 127:598, 1968.

Liechty, R. D., Alsever, R. N., and Burrington, J.: Islet cell hyperinsulinism in adults and children, J.A.M.A. 230:1538, December 16, 1974.

McCutcheon, A. D.: A fresh approach to the pathogenesis of pancreatitis, Gut 9:296, 1968.

McGuigon, J. E., and Trudeau, W. L.: Elevated serum levels of gastrin in Zollinger-Ellison syndrome, N. Engl. J. Med. 278:1308, 1968.

Mongé, J. J., Dockerty, M. B., Wollaeger, E. E., et al.: Clinicopathologic observations on radical pancreatoduodenal resection for peripapillary carcinoma, Surg. Gynec. Obstet. 118:275, 1964.

Paloyan, E.: The forms of pancreatitis, Curr. Probl. Surg., pp. 3-66, June 1967.

Puestow, C. R., and Gillesby, W. J.: Retrograde surgical drainage of the pancreas for chronic relapsing pancreatitis, Arch. Surg. 76:898, 1958.

ReMine, W. H., Priestly, J. T., Judd, E. S., and King, J. N.: Total pancreatectomy, Ann. Surg. 172:595, 1970.

Warren, K. W.: Surgical management of chronic relapsing pancreatitis, Amer. J. Surg. 117:24, 1969.

Warren, K. W., Braasch, J. W., and Thum, C. W.: Diagnosis and surgical treatment of carcinoma of the pancreas, Curr. Probl. Surg., pp. 3-70, June 1968.

Wermer, P.: Genetic aspects of adenomatosis of endocrine glands, Amer. J. Med. 16:363, 1954.

Zollinger, R. M., and Ellison, E. H.: Primary peptic ulcerations of the jejunum associated with islet cell tumors of the pancreas, Ann. Surg. 142:709, 1955.

Chapter 19: The spleen

Ashby, W. B., and Ballinger, W. F.: Indications for splenectomy, Arch. Surg. 85:913, 1962.

Block, G. E., Evans, R., and Zajtchuk, R.: Splenectomy for idiopathic thrombocytopenic purpura, Arch. Surg. 92:484, 1965.

Erkalis, A. J., and Filler, R. M.: Splenectomy in childhood: a review of 1413 cases, J. Pediat. Surg. 7:382, 1972.

Keisewetter, W. B., and Patrick, D. B.: Childhood splenectomy: indications for and results from, Ann. Surg. **37**:135, 1971.

McClure, P. D.: Idiopathic thrombocytopenic purpura in children: diagnosis and management, Pediatrics **54**:68, 1975.

Sandusky, W. R., Leavell, B. W., and Benjamin, B. I.: Splenectomy: Indications and results in hematologic disorders, Ann. Surg. **159**:695, 1964.

Sizer, J. S., Wayne, E. R., and Frederick, E. R.: Delayed rupture of the spleen, Arch. Surg. **92**:362, 1966.

Smith, C. H.: Indications for splenectomy in the pediatric patient, Amer. J. Surg. **107**:523, 1964.

Willox, G. L.: Nonpenetrating injuries of abdomen causing rupture of spleen, Arch. Surg. **90**:498, 1965.

Wilson, H.: Splenectomy for traumatic injury of the spleen, Surg. Clin. N. Amer. **46**:1311, 1966.

Chapter 20: The peritoneum and acute abdominal conditions

Botsford, T. W., and Wilson, R. E.: The acute abdomen, Vol. X, Major problems in clinical surgery, Philadelphia, 1969, W. B. Saunders Co.

Campbell, J. A., and McPhail, D. C.: Acute appendicitis, Brit. Med. J. **1**:852, 1958.

Cope, Z.: The early diagnoses of the acute abdomen, ed. 14, New York, 1972, Oxford University Press.

Fry, W. J., and Kraft, R. O.: Visceral angina, Surg. Gynec. Obstet. **117**:417, 1963.

Jones, P. F., and Dudley, H. A.: Emergency abdominal surgery in infancy, childhood and adult life, Philadelphia, 1974, J. B. Lippincott Co.

Lichtenstein, M. E.: Abdominal emergencies requiring immediate operation, Surg. Clin. N. Amer. **34**:27, 1954.

Requarth, W.: Indications for operation for abdominal trauma, Surgery **46**:461, 1959.

Warren, K. W.: Acute surgical conditions of the abdomen in the aged and the poor risk patient, Surg. Clin. N. Amer. **34**:745, 1954.

Chapter 21: Intestinal obstruction

Berry, R. E. L.: Obstruction of the small and large intestine. Physiopathology and treatment, Surg. Clin. N. Amer. **39**:1267, 1959.

Crowley, R. T., and Johnston, C. G.: Physiological principles in intestinal obstruction, Surg. Clin. N. Amer. **26**:1427, 1946.

Quan, S. H. Q., and Stearns, M. W., Jr.: Early postoperative intestinal obstruction and postoperative intestinal ileus, Dis. Colon Rectum **4**:307, 1961.

Wangensteen, O. H.: Intestinal obstruction, ed. 3, Springfield, Ill., 1955, Charles C Thomas, Publisher.

Welch, C. E.: Intestinal obstruction, Chicago, 1958, Year Book Medical Publishers, Inc.

Chapter 22: Gastrointestinal hemorrhage

Albo, R. J., Grimes, O. F., and Dunphy, J. E.: Management of massive lower gastrointestinal hemorrhage. Am. J. Surg. 112:264, 1966.

Baum, S.: Angiography of localized gastric lesions, Semin. Roentgenol. 6:207, April 1971.

Baum, S., and Nusbaum, M.: The control of gastrointestinal hemorrhage by selective mesenteric arterial infusion of vasopressin, Radiology 98:497, 1971.

Baum, S., et al.: Selective mesenteric arterial infusions in the management of massive diverticular hemorrhage, N. Engl. J. Med. 288:1269, June 1973.

Berkowitz, D.: Fatal gastrointestinal hemorrhage: diagnostic implications from a study of 200 cases, Am. J. Gastroent. 40:372, 1963.

Calem, W. S., and Jiminez, F. A.: Vascular malformations of the intestine, Arch. Surg. 86:571, 1963.

Corry, R. J., Bartlett, M. K., and Cohen, R. B.: Erosions of the cecum: a cause of massive hemorrhage, Am. J. Surg. 119:106, January 1970.

Corry, R. J., Mundth, E. D., and Bartlett, M. K.: Massive upper gastrointestinal tract hemorrhage, Arch. Surg. 97:531, October 1968.

Drapanas, T., et al.: Experiences with surgical management of acute gastric mucosal hemorrhage: a unified concept in the pathophysiology, Ann. Surg. 173:628, 1971.

Freeark, R. J., Norcross, W. J., Baker, R. J., and Strohl, E. L.: The Mallory-Weiss syndrome, Arch. Surg. 88:882, 1964.

Hedberg, S. E.: Early endoscopic diagnosis in upper gastrointestinal hemorrhage: an analysis of 323 cases, Surg. Clin. N. Amer. 46:499, 1966.

Hoar, C. S., and Bernard, W. F.: Colonic bleeding and diverticular disease of the colon, Surg. Gynec. Obstet. 99:101, 1954.

Jackson, F. C., et al.: A clinical investigation of the portacaval shunt, V. Survival analysis of the therapeutic operation. Ann. Surg. 174:672, 1971.

Linton, R. R.: The treatment of esophageal varices, Surg. Clin. N. Amer. 46:485, 1966.

Malt, R. A.: Medical intelligence—current concepts: control of massive upper gastrointestinal hemorrhage, N. Engl. J. Med. 286:1043, 1972.

Mendeloff, A. I.: Gastrointestinal bleeding: a symposium, Curr. Med. Dig., p. 1527, October 1966.

Noer, J. J., Hamilton, J. E., Williams, D. J., and Broughton, D. S.: Rectal hemorrhage: moderate and severe, Ann. Surg. 155:794, 1962.

Orloff, M. J.: Emergency portacaval shunt: a comparative study of shunt, varix ligation and nonsurgical treatment of bleeding esophageal varices in unselected patients with cirrhosis, Ann. Surg. 166:456, 1967.

Raffensperger, J. G.: Gastrointestinal bleeding in children, N. Carolina Med. J. 30:44, February 1969.

Spencer, R.: Gastrointestinal hemorrhage in childhood, Surgery 55:718, 1964.

Wolff, W. I., and Shinya, H.: Polypectomy via the fiberoptic colonoscope, N. Engl. J. Med. **288**:299, 1973.
Zollinger, R. M., and Nick, W. V.: Upper gastrointestinal tract hemorrhage, J.A.M.A. **212**:2251, 1970.

Chapter 23: The stomach and duodenum

Amdrup, E., et al.: Clinical results of parietal cell vagotomy (HSV)
two to four years after operation, Ann. Surg. **180**:279, September
1974.
Buchwald, H.: The dumping syndrome and its treatment, Amer. J. Surg.
116:81, 1968.
De La Rosa, C., et al.: Experimental gastric ulcers produced by pyloric
stenosis, Arch. Surg. **88**:927, 1964.
Dragstedt, L. R.: Section of the vagus nerves to the stomach in the
treatment of peptic ulcer, Surg. Gynec. Obstet. **83**:547, 1946.
Dragstedt, L. R.: Gastrin and peptic ulcer, Arch. Surg. **91**:1005, 1965.
Eiseman, B., and Heyman, R. L.: Stress ulcer—a continuing challenge,
N. Engl. J. Med. **282**:372, February 12, 1970.
Farmer, D. A.: Surgical treatment of duodenal ulcer, Postgrad. Med. J.
38:233, 1965.
Farris, J. M., and Smith, G. K.: Treatment of gastric ulcer (in situ) by
vagotomy and pyloroplasty, Ann. Surg. **158**:461, 1963.
Frankel, A., Finkelstein, J., and Kark, A.: Selection of operations for
peptic ulcer, Amer. J. Gastroent. **46**:206, 1966.
Fry, W. J., and Thompson, N. W.: Vagotomy and pyloroplasty for
duodenal ulcer, Surg. Clin. N. Amer. **46**:359, 1966.
Goligher, J. C.: A technique for highly selective (paraietal cell or proximal gastric) vagotomy for duodenal ulcer, Brit. J. Surg. **61**:337, May
1974.
Herrington, J. L.: Vagotomy-pyloroplasty for duodenal ulcer: a critical
appraisal of early results, Surgery **61**:698, 1967.
Kelly, K. A., Nyhus, L. M., and Harkins, H. N.: Reappraisal of in-
testinal phase of gastric secretion, Amer. J. Surg. **109**:1, 1965.
Moore, F. D.: Surgery in search of a rationale. Eighty years of ulcero-
genic surgery, Amer. J. Surg. **105**:304, 1963.
Rosato, F. E., and Noto, J. A.: Gastric polyps, Amer. J. Surg. **111**:647,
1966.
Schofield, B.: Vagal release of gastrin, Gastroenterology **39**:511, 1960.
Skillman, J. J.: Pathogenesis of peptic ulcer: a selective review, Surgery
76:515, September 1974.
Weinberg, J. A.: Pyloroplasty and vagotomy for duodenal ulcer, Curr.
Probl. Surg., pp. 3-36, April 1964.
Welch, C. E.: Surgery of the stomach and duodenum, ed. 5, Chicago,
1973, Year Book Medical Publishers, Inc.
Woodward, E. R.: The postgastrectomy syndromes, Springfield, Ill.,
1963, Charles C Thomas, Publisher.
Zollinger, R. M., and Ellison, E. H.: Primary peptic ulcerations of the

jejunum associated with islet cell tumors of the pancreas, Ann. Surg. **142:**709, 1955.

Chapter 24: The small intestine

Colcock, B. P., and Braasch, J. W.: Surgery of the small intestine in the adult, Philadelphia, 1968, W. B. Saunders Co.

Colcock, B. P., and Fortin, C.: Surgical treatment of regional enteritis: review of 85 cases, Ann. Surg. **161:**812, 1965.

Kutscher, A. H., Zegardli, E. V., Rankow, R. M., and Mercandante, J. L.: Peutz-Jeghers syndrome: follow-ups on patients reported on in the literature, Amer. J. Med. Sci. **238:**180, 1959.

Rankin, G. B., and Turnbull, R. B., Jr.: Transmural colitis: medical and surgical management, Hosp. Practice, p. 65, January, 1971.

McPeak, C. J.: Malignant tumors of the small intestine, Amer. J. Surg. **114:**402, 1967.

Ottinger, L. W., and Austin, W. G.: A study of 136 patients with mesenteric infarction, Surg. Gynec. Obstet. **124:**251, 1967.

Read, J. D.: Intestinal carcinoma in the Peutz-Jeghers syndrome, J.A.M.A. **229:**833, 1974.

Sherman, N. J., et al.: Regional enteritis in childhood, J. Pediat. Surg. **7:**585, 1972.

Skinner, D. B., et al.: Mesenteric vascular disease, Am. J. Surg. **128:**835, December 1974.

Chapter 25: The large intestine

Bacon, H. E., and Pezzutti, J. E.: Granulomatous ileocolitis, J.A.M.A. **198:**1330, 1966.

Burkitt, D. P.: Epidemiology of cancer of the colon and rectum, Cancer **28:**3, 1971.

Coller, F. A., Ransom, H. K., and Regan, W. J.: Cancer of the colon and rectum, Monograph, American Cancer Society, 1956.

Goltzer, et al.: Comparative features and course of ulcerative and granulomatous colitis, N. Engl. J. Med. **282:**582, 1970.

Hawk, W. A., Turnbull, R. B., and Farmer, R. G.: Regional enteritis of the colon, J.A.M.A. **201:**738, September 4, 1967.

Liechty, R. D., and Raterman, L.: Villous adenoma, a surgical dilemma, Arch. Surg. **87:**107, 1963.

Miller, F. E., and Liechty, R. D.: Adenocarcinoma of the colon and rectum in persons under thirty years of age, Amer. J. Surg. **113:**507, 1967.

Ransom, H. K.: Treatment of diverticulitis of the colon; choice of operation, Amer. J. Surg. **92:**672, 1956.

Spratt, J. S., Ackerman, L. V., and Moyer, C. A.: Relationship of polyps of the colon to colonic cancer, Ann. Surg. **148:**682, 1958.

Sugarbaker, P. H., et al.: Colonoscopy in the management of diseases of the colon and rectum, Surg. Gynec. Obstet. **139:**341, 1974.

Turnbull, R. B., Jr., et al.: Cancer of the colon: the influence of the no-touch isolation technique on survival rates, Ann. Surg. **166:**420, 1967.

Turrell, R.: Diseases of the colon and anorectum, ed. 2, Philadelphia, 1969, W. B. Saunders Co.

Welch, C. E.: Polypoid lesions of the gastrointestinal tract, Philadelphia, 1968, W. B. Saunders Co.

Wolff, W. I., and Shinya, H.: A new approach to colonic polyps, Ann. Surg. **178:**3, 1973.

Wolff, W. I., and Shinya, H.: Modern endoscopy of the alimentary tract—current problems in surgery, Chicago, 1974, Year Book Medical Publishers, Inc.

Zetzel, L.: Granulomatous (ileo) colitis, N. Engl. J. Med. **282:**600, 1970.

Chapter 26: The anorectum

Beahrs, O. H.: Complete rectal prolapse: an evaluation of surgical treatment, Ann. Surg. **161:**221, 1965.

Buckwalter, J. A., and Jurayj, M. D.: Relationship of chronic rectal disease to carcinoma, Arch. Surg. **75:**352, 1957.

Dunphy, J. E.: Surgical anatomy of the anal canal, Arch. Surg. **57:**791, 1948.

Dunphy, J. E., and Pikula, J.: Fact and fancy about fistula-in-ano, Surg. Clin. N. Amer. **35:**1469, 1955.

Goligher, J. C.: Surgery of the anus, rectum and colon, ed. 3, Springfield, Ill., 1972, Charles C Thomas, Publisher.

Goligher, J. C., Leacock, A. G., and Brossy, J. J.: The surgical anatomy of the anal canal, Brit. J. Surg. **43:**51, 1955.

Harkins, H. N.: Correlation of the newer knowledge of surgical anatomy of the anorectum, Dis. Colon Rectum **8:**154, 1965.

Milligan, E. T., and Morgan, C. M.: Surgical anatomy of the anal canal, Lancet **2:**1150, 1213, 1934.

Nesselrod, J. P.: Clinical proctology, ed. 3, Philadelphia, 1964, W. B. Saunders Co.

Page, B. H.: The entry of hair into a pilonidal sinus, Brit. J. Surg. **56:**32, 1969.

Parks, A. G.: Haemorrhoidectomy, Surg. Clin. N. Amer. **45:**1305, 1965.

Patey, D. H.: A reappraisal of the acquired theory of sacrococcygeal pilonidal sinus, Brit. J. Surg. **56:**462, 1969.

Philips, S. F.: Some aspects of anal continence and defecation, Gut **6:**396, 1965.

Sawyers, J. L.: Epidermoid cancer of the perianus and the anal canal, Surg. Clin. N. Amer. **45:**1173, 1965.

Shropshear, G.: Anatomic basis for anorectal disease, Dis. Colon Rectum **7:**399, 1964.

Turrell, R.: Diseases of the colon and anorectum, ed. 2, Philadelphia, 1969, W. B. Saunders Co.

Turrell, R.: Epidermoid Ca of anus and perianus, Postgrad. Med. **40:**210, 1966.

Walker, G. L., and Nigro, N. D.: The choice of operation for massive rectal prolapse, Surg. Clin. N. Amer. **45**:1293, 1965.

Chapter 27: Abdominal hernia

Anson, B. J., Morgan, E. H., and McVay, C. B.: Surgical anatomy of the inguinal region based upon a study of 500 body halves, Surg. Gynec. Obstet. **111**:707, 1960.

Herrington, J. L.: Treatment of esophageal hiatal hernia, Arch. Surg. **84**:379, 1962.

Iason, A. H.: Inguinal and femoral hernias, Ciba Clin. Sympos. **18**:35, 1966.

Johnston, J. H.: Hiatus hernia in childhood, Arch. Dis. Child. **35**:61, 1960.

McVay, C. B.: Inguinal and femoral hernioplasty, Surgery **57**:615, 1965.

Nyhus, L. M., and Harkins, H. N.: Hernia, Philadelphia, 1964, J. B. Lippincott Co.

Ryan, E. A.: An analysis of 313 consecutive cases of indirect sliding inguinal hernias, Surg. Gynec. Obstet. **102**:45, 1956.

Snyder, W. H., and Greaney, E. M.: Congenital diaphragmatic hernia, Surgery **57**:576, 1965.

Soper, R. T.: Hernia in infants and children, Postgrad. Med. **40**:523, 1966.

Zimmerman, L. M., and Aanson, B. J.: The anatomy and surgery of hernia, ed. 2, Baltimore, 1967, The Williams & Wilkins Co.

Chapter 28: Pediatric surgery

Babson, S. G., Osterud, H. T., and Thompson, H.: The congenitally malformed. IX. Congenital malformation and the low birth weight infant, Northwest Med. **65**:729, 1966.

Bain, K.: The physically abused child, Pediatrics **31**:895, 1963.

Benson, C. D., Mustard, W. T., Ravitch, M. M., Snyder, W. H., and Welch, K. J.: Pediatric surgery, ed. 2, Chicago, 1970, Year Book Medical Publishers, Inc.

Cox, J. A., and Soper, R. T.: Malrotation of the midgut, J. Iowa Med. Soc. **60**:317, 1970.

Ederer, F., Miller, R. W., and Scotto, J.: U. S. childhood cancer mortality patterns, 1950-1959, J.A.M.A. **192**:593, 1965.

Froehlich, L. A., and Fujikura, T.: Significance of a single umbilical artery, Amer. J. Obstet. Gynec. **92**:274, 1966.

Gross, R. E.: The surgery of infancy and childhood, Philadelphia, 1953, W. B. Saunders Co.

Izant, R. J., and Hubey, C. A.: Annual injury of 15,000,000 children, J. Trauma **6**:65, 1966.

Louw, J. H., and Barnard, C. N.: Congenital intestinal atresia: Observations on its origin, Lancet **2**:1065, 1955.

Raffensperger, J. G., and Jones, J. Z.: Gastroschisis, Surg. Gynecol. Obstet. **138**:230, 1974.

Rickham, P. P., Soper, R. T., and Stauffer, U.: Synopsis of pediatric surgery, Stuttgart, 1975, Georg Thieme Verlag.

Rubin, P.: Cancer of the urogenital tract: Wilms' tumor and neuroblastoma, J.A.M.A. **205:**103, 1968.

Stephens, F. D., and Smith, E. D.: Ano-rectal malformations in children, Chicago, 1971, Year Book Medical Publishers, Inc.

Swenson, O.: Pediatric surgery, ed. 3, New York, 1973, Appleton-Century-Crofts.

Young, D. G.: Fluid balance in pediatric surgery, Brit. J. Anaesth. **45:**953, 1973.

Chapter 29: Geriatric surgery

Arkins, R., Smessaert, A. A., and Hicks, R. G.: Mortality and morbidity in surgical patients with coronary artery disease, J.A.M.A. **190:**485, 1964.

Comfort, A.: The biology of senescence, New York, 1956, Rinehart & Co., Inc.

Metropolitan Life Insurance Co., Statistical Bulletin, New York.

Powers, J. H., editor: Surgery of the aged and debilitated patient, Philadelphia, 1968, W. B. Saunders Co.

Worcester, A.: The care of the aged, the dying and the dead, ed. 2, Springfield, Ill., 1961, Charles C Thomas, Publisher.

Ziffren, S. E.: Management of the aged surgical patient, Chicago, 1960, Year Book Medical Publishers, Inc.

Chapter 30: Thoracic and pulmonary surgery

Bates, D. V., Macklem, P. T., and Christie, R. V.: Respiratory function in disease, ed. 2, Philadelphia, 1971, W. B. Saunders Company.

Blades, B., editor: Surgical diseases of the chest, ed. 2, St. Louis, 1966, The C. V. Mosby Co.

Comroe, J. L., Jr., Foster, R. E., II, DuBois, A. B., Brisco, W. A., and Carlson, E.: The lung, ed. 3, Chicago, 1965, Year Book Medical Publishers, Inc.

Doty, D. B., Anderson, A. E., Rose, E. F., Go, R. T., Chiu, C. L., and Ehrenhaft, J. L.: Cardiac trauma: Clinical and experimental correlations of myocardial contusion, Ann. Surg. **180:**452, 1974.

Edwards, F. R.: Foundations of thoracic surgery, Baltimore, 1966, The Williams & Wilkins Company.

Flavell, G.: An introduction to chest surgery, New York, 1957, Oxford University Press.

Gibbon, J. H.: Surgery of the chest, Philadelphia, 1962, W. B. Saunders Co.

Johnson, J., and Kirby, C. K.: Surgery of the chest, ed. 4, Chicago, 1970, Year Book Medical Publishers, Inc.

Lindskog, G., Liebow, A., and Glenn, W.: Thoracic and cardiovascular surgery with related pathology, New York, 1962, Appleton-Century-Crofts.

References 1109

Slonim, N. B., and Hamilton, L. H.: Respiratory physiology, ed. 3, St. Louis, 1976, The C. V. Mosby Company.
West, J. B.: Ventilation/blood flow and gas exchange, ed. 2, Philadelphia, 1970, F. A. Davis Company.
Zavala, D. C., and Rossi, N. P.: Nonthoracotomy diagnostic techniques for pulmonary disease, Arch. Surg. 107:152, 1973.

Chapter 31: Cardiac surgery

Ad Hoc Committee, National Academy of Sciences, National Research Council: Cardiopulmonary resuscitation, J.A.M.A. 198:372, 1966.
Berne, R. M., and Levy, M. N.: Cardiovascular physiology, ed. 2, St. Louis, 1972, The C. V. Mosby Co.
Blalock, A., and Taussig, H. B.: Surgical treatment of malformation of the heart in which there is pulmonic stenosis or pulmonic atresia, J.A.M.A. 128:189, 1945.
DeWall, R. A., Grage, T. V., McFee, A. S., and Chiechi, M. A.: Theme and variations on blood oxygenators. I, Bubble oxygenators, Surgery 50:931, 1961.
Doty, D. B., Rossi, N. P., and Ehrenhaft, J. L.: Which patients need coronary artery surgery? J. Iowa Med. Soc. 63:477, 1973.
Gentsch, T. O., Bopp, R. K., Siegel, J. H., Cev, M., and Glenn, W. W. L.: Experimental and clinical use of a membrane oxygenator, Surgery 45:301, 1960.
Heart transplantation, Med. World News 15:25, 1974.
Hung, J., Willis, J., and Tague, R. B.: The heart, arteries and veins, New York, 1966, McGraw-Hill Book Co.
Hurst, J. W., and Logue, R. B., editors: The heart, ed. 2, New York, 1970, McGraw-Hill Book Co.
Kirklin, J. W., editor: Advances in cardio-vascular surgery, New York, 1973, Grune & Stratton, Inc.
Kirklin, J. W., and Archie, J. P., Jr.: The cardiovascular subsystem in surgical patients, Surg. Gynec. Obstet. 139:17, 1974.
Kirklin, J. W., and Pacifico, A. D.: Surgery for acquired valvular heart disease, N. Engl. J. Med. 288:133, 1973.
Kirklin, J. W., and Karp, R. B.: The tetralogy of Fallot—from a surgical viewpoint, Philadelphia, 1970, W. B. Saunders Co.
Lindskog, G. E.: Thoracic and cardio-vascular surgery with related pathology, ed. 3, New York, 1975, Appleton-Century-Crofts.
Neville, W. E.: Extracorporeal circulation (Current problems in surgery—monograph), Chicago, 1967, Year Book Medical Publishers, Inc.
Potts, W. J., Smith, S., and Gibson, S.: Anastomosis of aorta to pulmonary artery, J.A.M.A. 132:627, 1946.
Sloan, H., Morris, J. D., Vander Woude, R., Hewitt, H., and Long, G. L.: Clinical experience with a rotating disc oxygenator, Surgery 45:138, 1959.
Watson, H., editor: Paediatric cardiology, St. Louis, 1968, The C. V. Mosby Co.

Weber, K. T., and Janicki, M. S.: Intra-aortic balloon counter pulsation: a collective review, Ann. Thorac. Surg. **17:**602, 1974.

Wright, K. E., Jr., and McIntosh, H. D.: Artificial pacemakers—indications and management, Circulation **47:**1108, 1973.

Chapter 32: Peripheral arteries

Barker, W. F.: Peripheral arterial disease, ed. 2, Philadelphia, 1975, W. B. Saunders Co.

Blaisdell, F. W., and Hall, A. D.: Axillary-femoral artery bypass for lower extremity ischemia, Surgery **54:**563-568, 1963.

Burgess, E. M., Romano, R. L., and Zettl, J. H.: The management of lower extremity amputations, TR 10-6, Washington, D.C., 1969, U. S. Government Printing Office.

Dale, W. A., and Lewis, M. R.: Management of ischemia of the hand and fingers, Surgery **67:**63-79, 1970.

Eastcott, H. H. G.: Arterial surgery, Philadelphia, 1969, J. B. Lippincott Co.

Eastcott, H. H. G., Pickering, G. W., and Rob, C. G.: Reconstruction of internal carotid artery in a patient with intermittent attacks of hemiplegia, Lancet **2:**994-996, 1954.

Fairbairn, J. F., et al., editors: Allen-Barker-Hines peripheral vascular disease, ed. 4, Philadelphia, 1972, W. B. Saunders Co.

Fogarty, T. J., Cranley, J. J., Krause, R. J., Strasser, E. S., and Hafner, C. D.: A method for extraction of arterial emboli and thrombi, Surg. Gynec. Obstet. **116:**241-244, 1963.

Linton, R. R., and Wilde, W. L.: Modifications in the technique for femoral popliteal saphenous vein bypass autografts, Surgery **67:**234-248, 1970.

Linton, R. R.: Atlas of vascular surgery, Philadelphia, 1973, W. B. Saunders Co.

Pilcher, D. B., Barker, W. F., and Cannon, J. A.: An aorto-iliac endarterectomy case series followed 10 years or more, Surgery **67:**5-17, 1970.

Stoney, R. J., and Wylie, E. J.: Surgical treatment of ruptured abdominal aneurysms, Calif. Med. **111:**1-4, 1969.

Strandness, D. E.: Peripheral arterial disease, London, 1969, J. & A. Churchill Ltd.

Szilagyi, D. E., Smith, R. F., DeRusso, F. J., Elliott, J. P., and Sherrin, F. W.: Contribution of abdominal aortic aneurysmectomy to prolongation of life, Ann. Surg. **164:**678-699, 1966.

Weale, F. E.: An introduction to surgical haemodynamics, Chicago, 1967, Year Book Medical Publishers, Inc.

Wylie, E. J., and Ehrenfeld, W. K.: Extracranial occlusive cerebrovascular disease, diagnosis and management, Philadelphia, 1970, W. B. Saunders Co.

Chapter 33: Peripheral veins

Dodd, H., and Cockett, F. B.: Pathology and surgery of veins of the lower limb, ed. 2, Edinburgh, 1970, The Williams & Wilkins Co.

Donaldson, G. A., Linton, R. R., and Rodkey, G. V.: A twenty-year survey of thrombcembolism at the Massachusetts General Hospital. 1932-1959, N. Engl. J. Med. **265:**208, 1961.

Fairbairn, J. F., et al., editors: Allen-Barker-Hines peripheral vascular disease, ed. 4, Philadelphia, 1972, W. B. Saunders Co.

Goldsmith, H. S., de los Santos, R., and Beattie, E. J., Jr.: Relief of chronic lymphedema by omental transposition, Ann. Surg. **166:**573, 1967.

Gurewich, V., Thomas, D. P., and Stuart, R. K.: Some guidelines for heparin therapy of venous thromboembolic disease, J.A.M.A. **199:**116, 1967.

Lansing, A. M., and Davis, W. M.: Five-year follow-up study of ileo-femoral venous thrombectomy, Ann. Surg. **168:**620, 1968.

Lofgren, K. A.: Pitfalls in vein surgery, J.A.M.A. **188:**17, 1964.

Stallworth, J. M., Bradham, G. B., Kletke, R. R., and Price, R. G.: Phlegmasia cerulea dolens: a ten year review, Ann. Surg. **161:**802, 1965.

Chapter 34: Plastic and reconstructive surgery

Converse, J. M., editor: Reconstructive plastic surgery, Philadelphia, 1964, W. B. Saunders Co., 5 vols.

Longmire, W. P., Jr.: A current survey of clinical experiences in tissue and organ transplantation, Surg. Clin. N. Amer. **45:**407, 1966.

McGregor, I. A.: Fundamental techniques of plastic surgery and their surgical applications, ed. 3, Baltimore, 1965, The Williams & Wilkins Co.

Russell, P. S., and Monaco, A. P.: The biology of tissue transplantation, Boston, 1964, Little, Brown and Co.

Woodruff, M. F. A.: The transplantation of tissues and organs, Spring-field, Ill., 1960, Charles C Thomas, Publisher.

Chapter 35: Care of the acutely injured patient

American College of Surgeons, Committee on Trauma: Emergency care of the sick and injured, ed. 2, Philadelphia, 1972, W. B. Saunders Co.

Ballinger, W. F., et al.: The management of trauma, Philadelphia, 1973, W. B. Saunders Co.

Shires, G. T.: Care of the trauma patient, New York, 1966, Blakiston Division, McGraw-Hill Book Co.

Walt, A. J., and Wilson, R.: Management of trauma, Philadelphia, 1974, Lea & Febiger.

Chapter 36: Transplantation

Billingham, R. E., and Silvers, W. K.: The immunobiology of tissue transplantation. In Samter, M., editor: Immunological diseases, ed. 2, Boston, 1971, Little, Brown and Co.

Najarian, J. S., and Simmons, R. L.: Transplantation, Philadelphia, 1972, Lea & Febiger.

Penn, I.: Malignant tumors in organ transplant recipients, New York, 1970, Springer-Verlag.

1112 *Synopsis of surgery*

Penn, I.: Transplantation. In Hill, G. J., editor: Outpatient surgery, Philadelphia, 1973, W. B. Saunders Co.

Starzl, T. E.: Experience in renal transplantation, Philadelphia, 1964, W. B. Saunders Co.

Starzl, T. E.: Experience in hepatic transplantation, Philadelphia, 1969, W. B. Saunders Co.

Chapter 37: Thermal injuries

Achauer, B. M., Allyn, P. A., Furnas, D. W., and Bartlett, R. H.: Pulmonary complications of burns: The major threat to the burn patient, Ann. Surg. 177:311, 1973.

Andreasen, N. J. C., Norris, A S., and Hartford, C. E.: Incidence of long-term psychiatric complications in severely burned adults, Ann. Surg. 174:785, 1971.

Andreasen, N. J. C., Noyes, R., Jr., Hartford, C. E., Brodland, G., and Proctor, S.: Management of emotional reactions in seriously burned adults, N. Engl. J. Med. 286:65, 1972.

Artz, C. P., and Moncrief, J. A.: The treatment of burns, Philadelphia, 1969, W. B. Saunders Co.

Bromberg, B. E., and Song, I. C.: Homografts and heterografts as skin substitutes, Am. J. Surg. 112:28, 1966.

Burke, J. F., Bondoc, C. C., and Quinby, W. C.: Primary burn excision and immediate grafting: A method shortening illness, J. Trauma 14:389, 1974.

Burke, J. F., May, J. W., Jr., Albright, N., Quinby, W. C., and Russell, P. S.: Temporary skin transplantation and immunosuppression for extensive burns, N. Engl. J. Med. 290:269, 1974.

Collentine, G. E., Waisbren, B. A., and Mellender, J. W.: Treatment of burns with intensive antibiotic therapy and exposure, J.A.M.A. 200:939, 1967.

Colocho, G., Graham, W. P., III, Greene, A. E., Matheson, D. W., and Lynch, D.: Human amniotic membrane as a physiologic wound dressing, Arch. Surg. 109:370, 1974.

Curreri, P. W., Asch, M. J., and Pruitt, B. A.: The treatment of chemical burns: Specialized diagnostic, therapeutic, and prognostic considerations, J. Trauma 10:634, 1970.

Evans, E. B., Larson, D. L., Abston, S., and Willis, B.: Prevention and correction of deformity after severe burns, Surg. Clin. N. Amer. 50:1361, 1970.

Evans, E. I., Purnell, O. J., Robinett, P. W., Batchelor, A., and Martin, M.: Fluid and electrolyte requirements in severe burns, Ann. Surg. 135:804, 1952.

Foley, F. D.: Pathology of cutaneous burns, Surg. Clin. N. Amer. 50:1201, 1970.

Hartford, C. E.: Fluid resuscitation of the burned patient. In Mason, E. E., editor: Fluid, electrolyte and nutrient therapy in surgery, Philadelphia, 1974, Lea & Febiger, p. 286.

Hartford, C. E., and Ziffren, S. E.: Electrical injury, J. Trauma 11:331, 1971.

Jelenko, C., III: Chemicals that "burn," J. Trauma **14:**65, 1974.

Law, E. J., Kim, O. J., Stieritz, D. D., and MacMillan, B. G.: Experience with systemic candidiasis in the burned patient, J. Trauma **12:**543, 1972.

Lund, C. C., and Browder, N. C.: The estimation of areas of burns, Surg. Gynec. Obstet. **79:**352, 1944.

Mason, A. D., Jr., Pruitt, B. A., Jr., Lindberg, R. B., Moncrief, J. A., and Foley, F. D.: Topical sulfamylon chemotherapy in the treatment of patients with extensive thermal burns. In Matter, P., Barclay, T. L., and Konickova, Z., editors: Research in burns, Berne, 1971, Hans Huber Publishers, p. 120.

Moyer, C. A., and Butcher, H. R.: Burns, shock, and plasma volume regulation, St. Louis, 1967, The C. V. Mosby Co.

Polk, H. C., Jr., and Stone, H. H., editors: Contemporary burn management, Boston, 1971, Little, Brown and Co.

Pruitt, B. A., Jr., Foley, F. D., and Moncrief, J. A.: Curling's ulcer: A clinical-pathological study of 323 cases, Ann. Surg. **172:**523, 1970.

Reiss, E., Stirman, J. A., Artz, C. P., Davis, J. H., and Amspacher, W. H.: Fluid and electrolyte balance in burns, J.A.M.A. **152:**1309, 1953.

Sevitt, S.: Burn pathology and therapeutic applications, London, 1957, Butterworth and Co., Ltd.

Stone, H. H., and Humphrey, C. P.: Burn septicemia—a clinical and bacteriological study. In Matter, P., Barclay, T. L., and Konickova, Z., editors: Research in burns, Berne, 1971, Hans Huber Publishers, p. 201.

Sturim, H. S.: The treatment of electrical burns, Surg. Gynec. Obstet. **128:**129, 1969.

Teplitz, C.: Pathogenesis of pseudomonas vasculitis and septic lesions, Arch. Path. **80:**297, 1965.

Wilmore, D. W.: Nutrition and metabolism following thermal injury, Clin. Plast. Surg. **1:**603, 1974.

Zaroff, L. E., Mills, W., Jr., Duckett, J. W., Jr., Switzer, W. E., and Moncrief, J. A.: Multiple uses of viable cutaneous homografts in the burned patient, Surgery **59:**368, 1966.

Chapter 38: Orthopedics

American Orthopaedic Association: Manual of orthopaedic surgery, 1966.

Blount, W. P.: Fractures in children, Baltimore, 1955, The Williams & Wilkins Co.

Cooper, R.: Fractures in children: Fundamentals of management, J. Iowa Med. Soc. **54:**472, 1964.

Cooper, R.: Management of common forearm fractures in children, J. Iowa Med. Soc. **54:**689, 1964.

Crenshaw, A. H., editor: Campbell's operative orthopaedics, ed. 5, St. Louis, 1971, The C. V. Mosby Co., 2 vols.

Flatt, A. E.: The care of minor hand injuries, ed. 3, St. Louis, 1972, The C. V. Mosby Co.

Hart, V. L.: Acute osteomyelitis in children, J.A.M.A. **108:**524, 1937.

Jaffe, H. L.: Metabolic, degenerative and inflammatory diseases of bones and joints, Philadelphia, 1972, Lea & Febiger.

Larson, C. B.: Low back pain, disease a month, Chicago, 1957, Year Book Medical Publishers, Inc.

Mercer, W., and Duthie, R. B.: Orthopedic surgery, Baltimore, 1964, The Williams & Wilkins Co.

Ponseti, I. V.: Congenital dislocation of the hip in the infant, American Academy of Orthopaedic Surgeons Instructional Course Lectures, vol. 10, Ann Arbor, March, 1953, J. W. Edwards.

Ponseti, I. V.: Legg Perthes disease. Observations on the pathological changes in two cases, J. Bone Joint Surg. **38A:**739, 1956.

Ponseti, I. V., and Friedman, B.: Prognosis in idiopathic scoliosis, J. Bone Joint Surg. **32A:**381, 1950.

Ponseti, I. V., and Smoley, E. N.: Congenital club foot. The results of treatment, J. Bone Joint Surg. **45A:**261, 1963.

Raney, R. B., Brashear, H. R., and Shands, A. R.: Shands' handbook of orthopaedic surgery, ed. 8, St. Louis, 1971, The C. V. Mosby Co.

Stone, D. B., and Bonfiglio, M.: Pyogenic vertebral osteomyelitis. A diagnostic pitfall for the internist, Arch. Intern. Med. **112:**491, 1963.

Turek, S. L.: Orthopaedics: Principles and their application, ed. 2, Philadelphia, 1967, J. B. Lippincott Co.

Chapter 39: The hand

Bunnell, S.: In Boyes, J. H., editor: Surgery of the hand, ed. 5, Philadelphia, 1970, J. B. Lippincott Co.

Chase, R. A.: Atlas of hand surgery, Philadelphia, 1973, W. B. Saunders Co.

Flatt, A. E.: The care of minor hand injuries, ed. 3, St. Louis, 1972, The C. V. Mosby Co.

Littler, J. W.: The hand and upper extremity. In Converse, J. M., editor: Reconstructive plastic surgery, Philadelphia, 1964, W. B. Saunders Co., vol. 4.

Chapter 40: Neurosurgery

Davis, L., and Davis, R. A.: Principles of neurological surgery, Philadelphia, 1963, W. B. Saunders Co.

Ingraham, F. D., and Matson, D. D.: Neurosurgery of infancy and childhood, Springfield, Ill., 1954, Charles C Thomas, Publisher.

Jackson, F. E.: The pathophysiology of head injuries, Clin. Sympos. **18:**67, 1966.

Jackson, F. E.: The treatment of head injuries, Clin. Sympos. **19:**4, 1967.

Kernohan, J. W., and Sayre, G. P.: Tumors of the central nervous system, Washington, 1952, Armed Forces Institute of Pathology.

Mullan, S.: Essentials of neurosurgery for students and practitioners, New York, 1961, Springer Publishing Co., Inc.

Nulsen, F. E.: Pitfalls in peripheral nerve surgery. In Artz, C. B., and

Hardy, J. D.: Complications in surgery and their management, Philadelphia, 1961, W. B. Saunders Co., chap. 56.

White, J. C., and Sweet, W. H.: Pain and the neuro-surgeon, Springfield, Ill., 1969, Charles C Thomas, Publisher.

Youmans, J. T., editor: Neurological surgery, Philadelphia, 1973, W. B. Saunders Co.

Chapter 41: Urology

Abeshouse, B. S., and Abeshouse, G. A.: Sponge kidney, J. Urol. **84:**252, 1960.

Ansell, J. S., Geist, R. W., and Creevy, C. D.: Estimation of total body potassium in patients with ureterosigmoidostomies, Surg. Gynec. Obstet. **112:**322, 1961.

Campbell, M. F., and Harrison, J. H.: Urology, ed. 3, Philadelphia, 1970, W. B. Saunders Co.

Creevy, C. D.: Hypospadias, Urol. Survey **8:**2, 1958.

Culp, D. A.: The histology of the exstrophied bladder, J. Urol. **91:**538, 1964.

Culp, D. A., and Flocks, R. H.: The diversion of urine by the Heitz-Boyer procedure, Trans. Amer. Ass. Genitourin. Surg. **57:**25, 1965.

Culp, D. A., Graf, R. A., and Haschek, H.: Testicular tumor, J. Urol. **89:**843, 1963.

Emmett, J. L.: Clinical urography, Philadelphia, 1971, W. B. Saunders Co.

Emmett, J. L., and McDonald, J. R.: Urethral caruncle, Surg. Gynec. Obstet. **87:**611, 1948.

Flocks, R. H.: The treatment of urethral tumors, Trans. Amer. Ass. Genitourin. Surg. **47:**166, 1955.

Flocks, R. H.: Carcinoma of the prostate, J.A.M.A. **163:**709, 1957.

Flocks, R. H.: Clinical cancer of the prostate, a study of 4,000 cases, J.A.M.A. **193:**559, 1965.

Flocks, R. H., and Culp, D. A.: Surgical urology, ed. 4, Chicago, 1975, Year Book Medical Publishers.

Flocks, R. H., and Kadesky, M. C.: Malignant neoplasms of the kidney: an analysis of 353 patients followed five years or more, Trans. Amer. Ass. Genitourin. Surg. **49:**105, 1957.

Glenn, J. F., editor: Diagnostic urology, New York, 1964, Harper & Row, Publishers.

Hamm, F. C., and Lavalle, L. I.: Tumors of the ureter, J. Urol. **61:**493, 1949.

Hamm, F. C., and Waterhouse, K.: Changing concepts in lower urinary tract obstruction in children, J.A.M.A. **175:**854, 1961.

Hinman, F., Jr.: Surgical disorders of the bladder of urachal origin, Surg. Gynec. Obstet. **113:**605, 1961.

Huggins, C., and Hodges, C. V.: Studies on prostatic cancer. I. The effect of castration, of estrogens, etc., Cancer Res. **1:**293, 1941.

Jewett, H. J.: Perineal prostatectomy for cancer, J. Urol. **61:**277, 1949.

Kimbrough, J. C., and Reed, J. F., Jr.: Treatment of undescended testes, J.A.M.A. **163**:621, 1957.

Marshall, V. F.: Textbook of urology, ed. 2, New York, 1964, Harper & Row, Publishers.

Marshall, V. F.: Symposium on bladder tumors, Cancer **9**:543, 1956.

Spence, H. M., Baird, S. D., and Ware, E. W.: Cystic disorders of the kidneys, J.A.M.A. **163**:1466, 1957.

Straffon, R. A.: Cancer chemotherapy in the urologic patient, J. Urol. **86**:259, 1961.

Swenson, O., Fisher, J. H., and Cendron, J.: Megaloureter: results of newer forms of treatment, Surgery **40**:223, 1956.

Whitmore, W. F.: Hormone treatment in prostatic cancer, Amer. J. Med. **21**:697, 1956.

Winter, W. C.: Advances in the radioisotope renogram, J. Urol. **85**:683, 1961.

Chapter 42: Head and neck surgery

Anson, B. J., and Donaldson, J. A.: Surgical anatomy of the temporal bone and ear, Philadelphia, 1973, W. B. Saunders Co.

Bradley, W. H.: Practical office audiometry, New York, J. Med. **56**:2975, 1956.

DeWeese, D. D., and Saunders, W. H.: Textbook of otolaryngology, ed. 4, St. Louis, 1973, The C. V. Mosby Co.

Harrison, M. S., and Naftalin, L.: Meniere's disease, Springfield, Ill., 1968, Charles C Thomas, Publisher.

Ogura, J. H., Saltzstein, S. L., and Spjut, H. J.: Experiences with conservation surgery in laryngeal and pharyngeal carcinoma, Laryngoscope **71**:258, 1961.

Paparella, M. M., and Shumrick, D. A., editors: Otolaryngology, Philadelphia, 1973, W. B. Saunders Co.

Second Workshop on Reconstructive Middle Ear Surgery, Arch. Otolaryng. **78**:4, 1963.

Chapter 43: Gynecology

Danforth, D. N., editor: Textbook of obstetrics and gynecology, ed. 2, New York, 1971, Harper & Row, Publishers.

Goplesud, D. R., and Keettel, W. C.: Carcinoma of the vulva, Amer. J. Obstet. Gynec. **100**:550, 1968.

Green, T. H.: Gynecology, essentials of clinical practice, ed. 2, Boston, 1971, Little, Brown & Co.

Gusberg, S. B., and Frick, H. C., II: Corscaden's gynecologic cancer, ed. 3, Baltimore, 1970, The Williams & Wilkins Co.

Julian, C. G., and Woodruff, J. D.: The role of chemotherapy in the treatment of primary ovarian malignancy, Obstet. Gynec. Survey **24**:1307, 1969.

Ketcham, A. S., Deckers, P. J., Sugarbaker, E. V., Hoye, R. C., Thomas, L. B., and Smith, R. R.: Pelvic exenteration for carcinoma of the uterine cervix. A 15-year experience, Cancer **26**:513, 1970.

Nelson, J. H., Jr.: Atlas of radical pelvic surgery, New York, 1969, Appleton-Century-Crofts.

Novak, E. R., et al., editors: Textbook of gynecology, ed. 9, Baltimore, 1975, The Williams & Wilkins Co.

Varga, A., and Henriksen, E.: Histologic observations on the effect of 17-alpha-hydroxyprogesterone-17-n-caproate on endometrial carcinoma, Obstet. Gynec. **26:**656, 1965.

Index

Ileocolic intussusception, 469
Ileum obstruction, 453
Ileus
  adynamic ; *see* paralytic *below*
  gallstone, and intestinal obstruc-
      tion, 302, 305
  meconium, congenital, 429
  neurogenic ; *see* paralytic *below*
  paralytic, 307-308
    differentiated from mechanical
        intestinal obstruction, 308-
        309
    etiology of, 308
    postoperative, 128
Iliac artery occlusion, 579, 586
Immobilization
  atrophy after, 771
  fracture, 754
Immune response
  cancer and, 153
  transplantation and ; *see* Trans-
      plantation, immune response
      and
Immunoglobulin A-deficient trans-
      fusion recipient, anti-IgA in,
      63-64
Immunological enhancement of
      transplants, 650-651
Immunological tolerance of trans-
      plants, 650
Immunology and cancer, 152-155
Immunosuppression ; *see* Transplan-
      tation, immunosuppression
Immunotherapy, cancer, 153-155
Implantation defects and congenital
      anomalies, 423
Incisions
  camouflaged, 14
  Marshall, for vulvectomy and
      groin dissection, 1058
  placement of, 13-14
Infant
  branchial fistula in, 459
  branchial remnants in, 458-459
  hernia in
    inguinal, repair of, 404-405
    umbilical, 410-411
  hygroma of neck in, cystic, 459-
      462
  lymph nodes in, 457-458
  lymphadenitis in ; *see* Lymph-
      adenitis, cervical
  neck masses in, 457-462
  rhabdomyosarcoma in, 436
  thyroglossal duct remnants in,
      461, 462
Infections
  abdomen, causing lung abscess,
      497
  anomalies due to, congenital, 423
  anus, 395
  bone, 739-745

Infections—cont'd
  breast, 226
  breast cancer and, 218
  burn ; *see* Burn, infection
  differentiated from gastrointes-
      tinal obstruction, 438
  ear, 998-1003
  epidermis, 156
  fractures and, 771
  genital tract, lower, 1042-1045
  hand, 826-827
  head ; *see* Head, infections
  head injury and, 860
  intestine
    large, 371-372
    small, 348-354
  intracranial, 888-889
  liver, surgical, 243-245
  lung, due to atypical mycobac-
      teria, 506
  medical, vs. surgical, 78-79
  neck ; *see* Neck, infections
  palmar space, 826, 827
  rectum, 359
  surgical, 78-95
    antibiotics in, 91-95
    classification of, 80-81
    fungal, 86-90
    liver, 243-245
    pathophysiology of, 79-80
    treatment of, 91-95
    vs. medical infections, 78-79
  urethra, 967-968
  urinary
    postoperative, 125
    tract ; *see* Urinary tract, infec-
        tions
  wound ; *see* Wound, infections
Infectious diseases after transfu-
      sion, 64
Infectious mononucleosis, 995-996
Infertility, 1088, 1089-1090
Inguinal
  hernia ; *see* Hernia, inguinal
  lymphadenitis differentiated from
      inguinofemoral mass, 409
Inguinofemoral hernia, 400, 409
Inhalation injury and burns, 678-
      679
Injury ; *see* Trauma
Insemination, artificial, 985
Inspiratory flow, mean maximal,
      490
Insulinoma, pancreas, 277, 279, 280
Interatrial septal defect, 424
Intercostal drainage in pneumotho-
      rax, 517
Interphalangeal joints, 797
Intertrochanteric fracture, 762-764
Intervertebral disc
  degeneration, 696-697, 709-710
  herniation ; *see* Herniation

Neurological examination in orthopedics, 693
Neuroma, 172, 872
  digital, 738-739
  hand, 835
  -in-continuity, 875
  Morton's, 738-739
Neuromuscular
  disorders, 782-788
  system, peripheral, and anesthe-
    sia, 112
Neuropathies, 788
Neuroses, postoperative, 131
Neurosurgery, 837-899
  diagnostic studies, 838-845
Neutropenia, idiopathic splenic,
  288
Nevi
  "bathing trunk," 165, 169
  blue, 165
  compound, 165, 167
  description of, 168
  flammeus, 173
  hairy, giant, 165, 169
  intradermal, 165, 166-167
  junctional, 165, 166-167
  pigmented, 165-169
  strawberry, 172, 173
Newborn
  atresia in
    anal, 453-454
    rectal; *see* Atresia, rectal, in
      newborn
  colon obstruction in, 453-457
  duodenal obstruction in, 451-452
  fluid therapy, 418-419
  gastrointestinal obstruction; *see*
    Gastrointestinal, obstruction,
    in newborn
  gastroschisis in, 443
  ileal obstruction in, 453
  jaundice in, 241, 254
  jejunal obstruction in, 453
  meconium plug syndrome in, 453-
    454
  operating room and, 421-422
  postoperative care, 421-422
  respiration in, 420
  surgical disease, rapid progres-
    sion of, 420-421
  surgical patient, 417-421
  surgery in, 420-421
Nipple discharge, 216
Nitrogen test, single-breath, 491
Nocardia asteroides, 89
Nocardiosis of lung, 503
Noise-induced deafness, 1025
Nonunion of fractures, 769
North American blastomycosis of
  lung, 505
Nose
  carcinoma; *see* Carcinoma, nose
  cold, viral, 994-995

Nose—cont'd
  fracture; *see* Fracture, nose
  glioma, 1020
  granulomas, 1020-1021
  hump, plastic surgery, 612
  meningocele, 1020
  meningoencephalocele, 1020
  oronasopharyngeal bleeding, 315
  osteoma, 1020
  polyposis, 1020
  "saddle" deformity, 1005
  septum, 1006
  trauma, 1004-1006
  tumors, 1019-1021
  vestibulitis, chronic, 1020
Nosebleed; *see* Epistaxis
Nursemaid's elbow, 701-702
Nutrition
  burns and, 689-690
  deficiencies and congenital anom-
    alies, 423
  malnutrition and sodium, 28
  preoperative, in aged, 477-478
  status and preoperative care, 108

O

Obstetric palsy, 699
Obstipation in intestinal obstruction, 305
Obstruction and surgical diseases,
  1-2
Obturation and intestinal obstruction, 305
Obturator hernia, 413
Occlusion, arterial, 578-587
  amputation in, 587
  chronic, 582-583
  of extremities, lower, 578-580
  iliac artery, 579, 586
  sympathectomy in, 587
  treatment of, 584-587
Occlusion, vascular, superior mesenteric, 354-356
Occult carcinoma, 601
17-OHCS in diagnosing Cushing's
  syndrome, 201
Olfactory neuroepithelioma, 1020
Oliguria, 906
Omphalocele, 410, 431, 441, 442-
  443
Oncology, gynecological, 1054-1080
Open heart surgery, consequences
  of, 546-547
Operating room
  management of anesthesia, 119-
    121
  newborn and, 421-422
Operative problems in aged, 478-
  479
Oral; *see also* Mouth
  contraceptives and breast cancer,
    218

Pour en Y 278